Anesthesia complications in the dental office

Anesthesia complications in the dental office

Editors:

Robert C. Bosack, DDS

Clinical Assistant Professor
College of Dentistry
University of Illinois
Chicago, Illinois, USA

Private Practice
Oral and Maxillofacial Surgery
Chicago, Illinois, USA

Stuart Lieblich, DMD

Clinical Professor
Department of Oral and Maxillofacial Surgery
University of Connecticut
Avon, Connecticut, USA

Private Practice
Oral and Maxillofacial Surgery
Avon, Connecticut, USA

WILEY Blackwell

This edition first published 2014 ©2014 by John Wiley & Sons, Inc.

Editorial offices: 1606 Golden Aspen Drive, Suites 103 and 104, Ames, Iowa 50010, USA
The Atrium, Southern Gate, Chichester, West Sussex, PO19 8SQ, UK
9600 Garsington Road, Oxford, OX4 2DQ, UK

For details of our global editorial offices, for customer services and for information about how to apply for permission to reuse the copyright material in this book please see our website at www.wiley.com/wiley-blackwell.

Library of Congress Cataloging-in-Publication Data

Anesthesia complications in the dental office / editors, Robert C. Bosack, Stuart Lieblich.
p. ; cm.
Includes bibliographical references and index.
ISBN 978-0-470-96029-5 (cloth)
I. Bosack, Robert C., editor. II. Lieblich, Stuart E., editor.
[DNLM: 1. Anesthesia, Dental–adverse effects. 2. Anesthesia, Dental–contraindications. 3. Intraoperative Complications–prevention & control. 4. Postoperative Complications–prevention & control. 5. Risk Factors. WO 460]
RK510
617.9'676–dc23

2015000738

A catalogue record for this book is available from the British Library.

Wiley also publishes its books in a variety of electronic formats. Some content that appears in print may not be available in electronic books.

Set in 9/11pt MinionPro-Regular by Laserwords Private Limited, Chennai, India
Printed and bound in Malaysia by Vivar Printing Sdn Bhd

3 2016

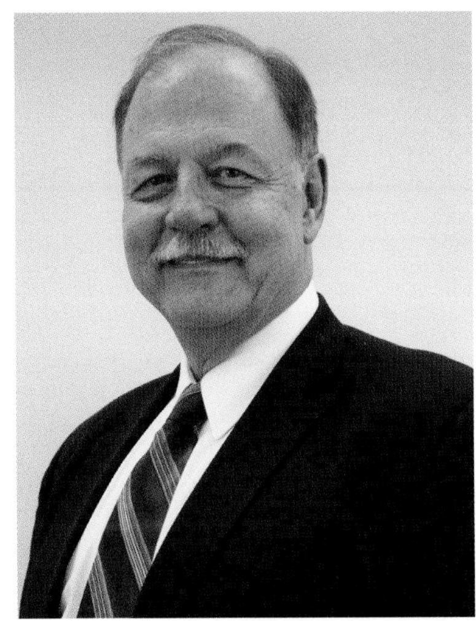

To my family, with special remembrance for my Dad, S. Richard Bosack, DDS (1921–2011), to whom I promised this dedication.

Robert C. Bosack

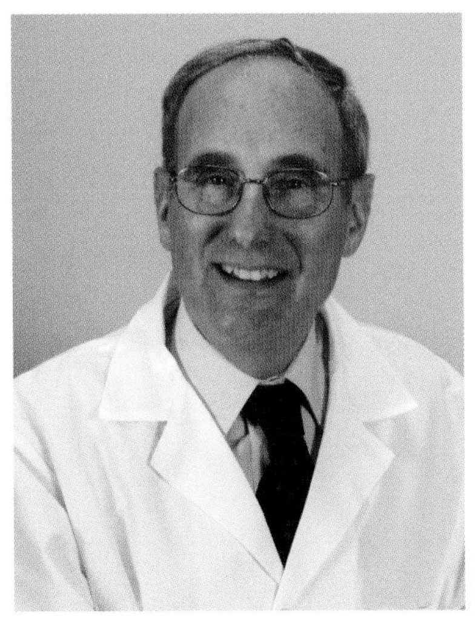

To my family, teachers, and students; but most importantly to the patients who have trusted me with their care.

Stuart Lieblich

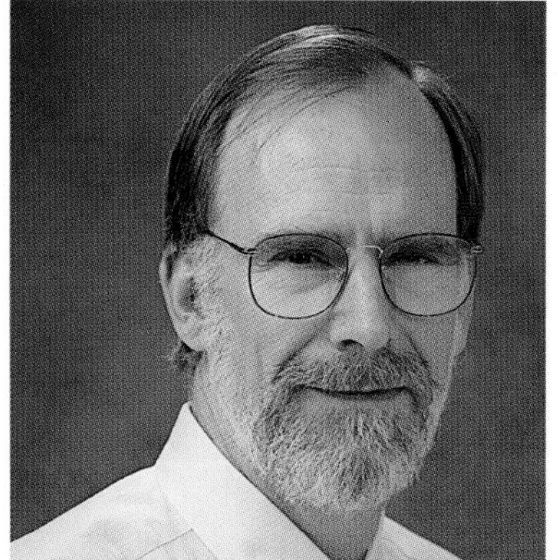

In memory of John Yagiela, DDS (1947–2010).

Contents

Contributors, ix

Foreword, xiii

Preface, xv

Acknowledgment, xvii

Section 1: Introduction

1 Anesthetic complications—how bad things happen, 3
Robert C. Bosack

Section 2: Patient risk assessment

2 History and physical evaluation, 9
Kyle Kramer, Trevor Treasure, Charles Kates, Carrie Klene, and Jeffrey Bennett

3 Laboratory evaluation, 15
Kyle Kramer and Jeffrey Bennett

4 NPO guidelines, 19
Kyle Kramer and Jeffrey Bennett

Section 3: Anesthetic considerations for special patients

5 Anesthetic considerations for patients with cardiovascular disease, 25
Erik Anderson and Robert Bosack

6 Anesthetic considerations for patients with respiratory disease, 49
Robert C. Bosack and Zak Messieha

7 Anesthetic considerations for patients with endocrinopathies, 61
Daniel Sarasin, Kevin McCann, and Robert Bosack

8 Anesthetic considerations for patients with psychiatric illness, 71
Daniel L. Orr, Robert C. Bosack, and John Meiszner

9 Anesthetic considerations for patients with neurologic disease, 79
Joseph A. Giovannitti

10 Anesthetic considerations for patients with hepatic disease, 85
Jeffrey Miller and Stuart Lieblich

11 Anesthetic considerations for patients with renal disease, 89
Marci H. Levine and Andrea Schreiber

12 Anesthetic considerations for pediatric patients, 93
Michael Rollert and Morton Rosenberg

13 Anesthetic considerations for geriatric patients, 97
Andrea Schreiber and Peter M. Tan

14 Anesthetic considerations for patients with bleeding disorders, 103
O. Ross Beirne

15 Anesthetic considerations for patients with cancer, 113
Andrea M. Fonner and Robert C. Bosack

16 Anesthetic considerations for pregnant and early postpartum patients, 117
Robert C. Bosack

Section 4: Review of anesthetic agents

17 Clinical principles of anesthetic pharmacology, 123
Richard C. Robert

18 Local anesthetic pharmacology, 129
Roy L. Stevens and Robert C. Bosack

19 Enteral sedation agents, 133
Richard C. Robert

20 Parenteral anesthetic agents, 135
Richard C. Robert

21 Inhalational anesthetic agents, 143
Charles Kates, Douglas Anderson, Richard Shamo, and Robert Bosack

22 Antimuscarinics and antihistamines, 151
Richard C. Robert

23 Drug interactions, 155
Kyle Kramer and Richard C. Robert

Section 5: Monitoring

24 Limitations of patient monitoring during office-based anesthesia, 163
Robert C. Bosack and Ken Lee

Section 6: Preparation for adversity

25 Crisis resource management, 173
Joseph Kras

26 Simulation in dental anesthesia, 177
Joseph Kras

27 Airway adjuncts, 181
H. William Gottschalk

28 Intravenous fluids, 185
Cara Riley, Kyle Kramer, and Jeffrey Bennett

29 Emergency drugs, 189
Daniel A. Haas

Section 7: Anesthetic adversity

30 Failed sedation, 201
Roy L. Stevens and Kenneth L. Reed

31 Complications with the use of local anesthetics, 207
M. Anthony Pogrel, Roy L. Stevens, Robert C. Bosack, and Timothy Orr

32 Anesthetic adversity – cardiovascular problems, 219
Robert C. Bosack and Edward C. Adlesic

33 Anesthetic adversity—respiratory problems, 231
Charles F. Cangemi, Edward C. Adlesic, and Robert C. Bosack

34 Allergy and anaphylaxis, 251
H. William Gottschalk and Robert C. Bosack

35 Anesthetic adversity – neurologic problems, 257
Michael Trofa and Robert C. Bosack

36 Acute, adverse cognitive, behavioral, and neuromuscular changes, 261
Edward Adlesic, Douglas Anderson, Robert Bosack, Daniel L. Orr, and Steven Ganzberg

37 Anesthetic problems involving vasculature, 271
Stuart Lieblich

Section 8: Post-anesthetic adversity

38 Nausea and vomiting, 277
Edward Adlesic

39 Post-anesthetic recall of intraoperative awareness, 283
Robert C. Bosack

40 Delayed awakening from anesthesia, 287
Stuart E. Lieblich

41 Safe discharge after office-based anesthesia, 291
Stuart Lieblich and Peter M. Tan

Section 9: When bad things happen

42 Morbidity and mortality, 295
Lewis Estabrooks

43 Death in the chair: a dentist's nightmare, 299
Glen Crick

44 Legal issues of anesthesia complications: risks or malpractice, 307
Arthur W. Curley

Section 10: When should you say no

45 When should you say no? 315
Andrew Herlich and Robert C. Bosack

Section 11: Appendices

Appendix A A pilot's perspective on crisis resource management, 323
David Yock

Appendix B Medical emergency manual for the general practitioner, 325
Robert C. Bosack

Appendix C Malignant hyperthermia Q & A, 337
Edward C. Adlesic and Steven I. Ganzberg

Index, 339

Contributors

Edward C. Adlesic, DMD
Assistant Clinical Professor
Department of Oral and Maxillofacial Surgery
University of Pittsburgh School of Dental Medicine
Pittsburgh, PA
USA

Douglas W. Anderson, DMD
Clinical Assistant Professor (Ret)
Department of Anesthesiology and Peri Operative Medicine
Oregon Health Sciences University
Portland, OR
USA

Erik P. Anderson, MD
Assistant Professor
Department of Anesthesiology
University of Vermont College of Medicine
Burlington, VT
USA

O. Ross Beirne, D.M.D., Ph.D.
Professor
Department of Oral and Maxillofacial Surgery
University of Washington
Seattle, WA
USA

Jeffrey D. Bennett, DMD
Professor
Department of Oral Surgery and Hospital Dentistry
Indiana University
Indianapolis, IN
USA

Robert C. Bosack, DDS
Clinical Assistant Professor
University of Illinois
College of Dentistry
Chicago, IL,
USA
Private Practice
Oral and Maxillofacial Surgery
Orland Park, IL,
USA

Charles F. Cangemi Jr., DDS, MS
Dentist-Anesthesiologist
Private Practice, Dental Anesthesiology
Charlotte, NC
USA

Glen Crick, esq. (dec.)
Chicago, IL
USA

Arthur W. Curley, JD
President and Managing Partner
Bradley, Curley, Asiano, Barrabee, Abel & Kowalski, PC
Larkspur, CA
USA

Lewis N. Estabrooks DMD, MS
Board of Directors
OMSNIC
Rosemont, IL
USA

Andrea M. Fonner, DDS
Dentist Anesthesiologist
Private Practice
Seattle, WA
USA

Steven Ganzberg, DMD, MS
Director of Anesthesiology
Century City Outpatient Surgery Center
Clinical Professor of Anesthesiology
UCLA School of Dentistry
Los Angeles, CA
USA

Joseph A. Giovannitti, Jr., DMD
Professor
Department of Dental Anesthesiology
University of Pittsburgh School of Dental Medicine
Pittsburgh, PA
USA

H. William Gottschalk, DDS
Assistant Clinical Professor
University of Southern California School of Dentistry
Los Angeles, CA
USA

Daniel A. Haas, DDS, PhD, FRCD(C)
Professor and Dean
Faculty of Dentistry
University of Toronto
Toronto, ON
Canada

Andrew Herlich, DMD, MD, FAAP
Professor and Vice-Chair for Faculty Development
Department of Anesthesiology
University of Pittsburgh School of Medicine
Staff Anesthesiologist, UPMC Mercy
Pittsburgh, PA
USA

Charles H. Kates, DDS
Associate Professor, Anesthesiology and Surgery
Departments of Anesthesiology and Surgery
University of Miami Miller School of Medicine
Chief of Anesthesiology and Pain Management, Section of Oral/Maxillofacial Surgery, Department of Surgery
Jackson Memorial Hospital
Miami, FL
USA

Carrie Klene, DDS
Program Director
Clinical Assistant Professor
Oral and Maxillofacial Surgery
Indiana University
Indianapolis, IN
USA

Kyle J. Kramer, DDS, MS
Assistant Clinical Professor
Department of Oral Surgery and Hospital Dentistry
Indiana University
Indianapolis, IN
USA

Joseph F. Kras, MD, DDS, MA
Associate Professor
Department of Anesthesiology
Washington University in St. Louis
St. Louis, MO
USA

Kenneth K. Lee, DDS
Attending in Dental Anesthesia, NYU-Lutheran Medical Center
Associate Clinical Professor
Ostrow School of Dentistry at USC
Los Angeles, CA
USA

Marci H. Levine, DMD, MD
Clinical Assistant Professor
Department of Oral and Maxillofacial Surgery
New York University College of Dentistry
New York, NY
USA

Stuart Lieblich, DMD
Clinical Professor
Oral and Maxillofacial Surgery
University of Connecticut
Farmington, CT
Private Practice
Avon Oral and Maxillofacial Surgery
Avon, CT,
USA

Kevin J. McCann, DDS, FRCD(C)
Private Practice
Waterloo, ON
Canada

John W. Meiszner, MD
Private Practice in General and Addiction Psychiatry
Forensic Psychiatrist for State of Illinois, retired
Orland Park, IL
USA

Zakaria Messieha, DDS
Clinical Professor of Anesthesiology
Colleges of Dentistry & Medicine
University of Illinois at Chicago
Private Practice, Dental Anesthesiology
Chicago, IL
USA

Jeffrey Miller, DMD, MD, MPH
Chief Resident
Department of Oral and Maxillofacial Surgery
University of Connecticut Health Center
Farmington, CT
USA

Daniel Orr II, DDS, PhD, JD, MD
Professor and Director
Oral and Maxillofacial Surgery and Advanced Pain Control
UNLV School of Dental Medicine
Clinical Professor
Oral and Maxillofacial Surgery and Anesthesiology for Dentistry
University of Nevada School of Medicine
Las Vegas, NV
USA

Timothy M. Orr, DMD
Dentist Anesthesiologist
Austin, TX
USA

M. Anthony (Tony) Pogrel, DDS, MD
Professor
Department of Oral and Maxillofacial Surgery
University of California
San Francisco, CA
USA

Kenneth Reed, DMD
Associate Program Director
Dental Anesthesiology
Lutheran Medical Center
Brooklyn, NY
USA

Cara J. Riley, DMD, MS
Assistant Professor
Children's Hospital Colorado
Department of Anesthesiology
Aurora, CO
USA

Richard C. Robert, DDS, MS
Clinical Professor
Department of Oral and Maxillofacial Surgery
University of California at San Francisco
San Francisco, CA
USA

Michael K. Rollert, DDS
Private Practice
Denver, CO
USA

Morton Rosenberg, DMD
Professor of Oral and Maxillofacial Surgery
Head, Division of Anesthesia and Pain Control
Tufts University School of Dental Medicine
Associate Professor of Anesthesiology
Tufts University School of Medicine
Boston, MA
USA

Daniel S Sarasin, DDS
Private Practice OMFS
Cedar Rapids, IA
USA

Andrea Schreiber DMD
Associate Dean for Post-Graduate and Graduate Programs
Clinical Professor of Oral and Maxillofacial Surgery
New York University College of Dentistry
New York, NY
USA

Rick Shamo DDS, MD
Director of Oral & Maxillofacial Surgery
Memorial Hospital of Sweetwater County
Rock Springs, WY
USA

Roy L. Stevens, DDS
Private Practice
General Dentistry for Patients with Special Health Care Needs
Oklahoma City, OK
USA

Peter M. Tan DDS, MSHS
Mid-Maryland Oral and Maxillofacial Surgery, P.A.
Frederick, MD
USA

Trevor E. Treasure, DDS, MD
Assistant Professor
Department of Oral and Maxillofacial Surgery
University of Texas – School of Dentistry
Houston, TX
USA

Michael Trofa, DMD, MD
Department of Oral and Maxillofacial Surgery
University of Connecticut
Farmington, CT
USA

Captain David Yock, ATP
Southwest Airlines
Dallas, TX
USA

Foreword

The publication *Anesthesia Complications in the Dental Office* covers a wide range of topics beneficial to all levels of anesthesia care providers, be they students, residents, academics, or clinical practitioners. The book begins with the preoperative issues that play a role in evaluating the difficulties in safeguarding the patients, many of whom present with medical problems that were far less common a couple of years ago. Modern medicine has extended our longevity but now the patients present to our offices with an extended list of medications for diseases that were less recognized in the past decades and they are often diagnosed with behavioral and obesity issues.

Pharmacology of anesthesia practice has frequently met the challenges of modern societal problems with newer, more efficient shorter acting agents than what was available in the 1960s and 1970s. These are discussed in the middle chapters of the book. While basic physiology has not changed much, our understanding of the new drugs available and the way they affect the safety of patients under anesthesia has. Since the 1980s, monitoring the effects of all anesthesia drugs with pulse oximetry, capnography, and even bispectral analysis for special situations has set the scene for improved safety.

Despite the improvement in airway management techniques and skills learned, complications, both common and far less common, are still of great concern. The final chapters in the book deal with the need for prompt recognition and treatment of anesthesia-related urgencies and emergencies. While death "is not an option" so to speak, it is discussed and put in proper perspective when comparing the risks of air travel, driving, and even exercising to those of undergoing anesthesia in the office.

This first edition of *Anesthesia Complication in the Dental Office* offers a wide variety of subject material and should be on the library shelf of every anesthesia care provider working in the dental office. The names of the contributors are well known in academia and in clinical practice and have great credibility in the field of office-based anesthesia practice to make this book worthy of acquiring.

Robert Campbell DDS
Emeritus Professor of Anesthesiology and Oral and Maxillofacial Surgery
Departments of Anesthesiology and Oral and Maxillofacial Surgery
Virginia Commonwealth University/Medical College of Virginia
Richmond, Virginia, USA

Preface

Anesthesia is a unique discipline in dentistry. We all take it for granted, yet little can be done without it. The only time we ever really pay attention to it is when it does not work as planned. Anesthetic complications, which range from simple annoyances to patient mortality, are inevitable, given the many and complex interactions of doctor, patient, personnel, and facility. Our intent is to minimize the frequency and severity of adverse events, by providing concise and clinically relevant information that can be put to everyday use.

This book is intended for all dental professionals, who already have a working knowledge of anesthesia at their level of practice. Most of the 10 sections are relevant to all levels of anesthesia practice – including patient risk assessment (Section II) and a review of common pathophysiologic problems (Section III). The review of anesthetic agents includes chapters on local anesthesia, nitrous oxide analgesia, and both enteral and parenteral agents. Emphasis in Section IV is placed on pharmacology, with the hope that appropriate and successful use of these agents will limit adverse and sometimes unexpected side effects. Sections V–X are more relevant to parenteral techniques, with the notable exception of the robust Chapter (31) on problems associated with the use of local anesthesia. We were pleased to have the opportunity to review the Standing Medical Orders of the Emergency Medical System from a major metropolitan region. Knowing what paramedics would do when called validated our recommendations for the initial management of anesthesia-related emergencies.

The appendices contain an interesting submission on crisis resource management by an airline pilot. We have learned much from the groundbreaking safety protocols that have transformed the airline industry. A brief emergency manual, suitable for general practitioners, has also been provided.

We have taken several liberties with this publication. Focus has been directed to the office setting, with its obvious and inherent limits on diagnosis and treatment. We have used the words anesthesia and sedation interchangeably, with the understanding that drug use may be limited by training or license. Wherever possible, we have attempted to include references to key or seminal articles, to provide direction to those practitioners seeking further information.

Over the years, we have been given the wonderful opportunity to present to and interact with a great number of dentists of all specialties on the topic of anesthesia. Interest always piqued with the word "complication," so that fueled the content of this project. Over the past 32 years, we have accumulated a fair amount of practice experience, either first hand or by listening to your sometimes painful stories, which many have unabashedly shared. We have learned more than we taught and it is our hope to share all of this information with you. We are grateful and humbled to be among our 43 contributors, who so graciously accepted the invitation to also share their knowledge, experience, and expertise with us.

If but one life can be saved, or one patient managed better, then this book is well worth the effort. We both assiduously embrace the statement: "Patient Safety through Education." Thank you for your interest and dedication to improving the delivery of anesthesia in the dental office. Our best wishes to your continued successful professional practice.

Robert C. Bosack
University of Illinois
College of Dentistry
Chicago, Illinois, USA

Stuart Lieblich
University of Connecticut
Department of Oral and Maxillofacial Surgery
Farmington, Connecticut, USA

Acknowledgment

Mr. Brian Stafford, who so patiently created many of the illustrations in this book making "comprehension at a glance" an art form.

Unless otherwise indicated, all pictures are courtesy of Dr. Robert C. Bosack.

SECTION 1

Introduction

1 Anesthetic complications—how bad things happen

Robert C. Bosack
University of Illinois, College of Dentistry, Chicago, IL, USA

The delivery of anesthesia in any setting is not without risk. The environment is complex, uncertain, and ever-changing. Human performance of this potentially hazardous task can be unpredictable and imperfect, especially in times of urgency, intensity, and time pressure. Risk and human error cannot be eliminated, but can be reduced and managed by eliminating a culture of blame and punishment and replacing it with a culture of vigilance and cooperation to expose and remediate system weaknesses, which, in combination, often lead to error and injury.

The concept is straightforward. Most patients do not enjoy going to the dentist. Although patients understand that pain can be eliminated with local anesthesia, fear and anxiety still fuel avoidance of necessary care. Dentistry has responded to these issues by providing options for various levels of sedation, analgesia, or general anesthesia in the dental office. Usually, all goes well. Patients are satisfied; necessary dental work gets done. Sometimes, however, things do not go well.

Complications (adverse events, sentinel events) are defined as unplanned, unexpected, unintended, and undesirable patient outcomes: death, physical/psychological injury, or any unexpected variation in a process or outcome that demands notice. *Errors* are deviations from accuracy or correctness, usually, caused by a fault (mistake) for example, carelessness, misjudgment, or forgetfulness. Most errors have no obvious effect on patients, yet most (82%) preventable complications in the past involved human error (Cooper et al., 1978).

Errors are categorized according to persons or systems (Reason, 2000). Person approach refers to individual human error: forgetfulness, inattention, lapses (temporary failure of memory), preoccupation, violation (conscious deviation from a rule), loss of situational awareness, and fixation errors. Human errors lead to specific technical, judgmental, or monitoring mistakes, examples of which are given in Table 1.1. System approach refers to practice conditions: staff training, equipment, schedule density, health history gathering, policies, procedures, checklists, and so on. Latent errors can lay dormant in practices for years, only to be exposed during a triggering event, which then leads to an adverse outcome in a susceptible patient.

Although it is tempting to blame a complication on a single human error (e.g., the practitioner gave the wrong drug and the patient died), seldom is this the case. Most complications are now known to be due to an unfortunate temporal alignment of a *series of errors*, which results in injury. These errors can arise from multiple sources, which include *latent errors* (overbooking, failure to update medical histories, failure to check equipment, lack of training, poor communication), *psychological precursors* (fear of lawsuit, embarrassment), *system defects* (staff not trained in emergency protocols, failure to use checklists, failure to update medical emergency drugs), *triggering factors* (loss of airway, unintended drug overdose, hypotension, etc.), *atypical conditions* (key staff member absent), and *outright unsafe acts* (lack of knowledge, errors of the moment, ignoring a monitor, failure to address a problem, wrong drug given, etc.)

Scope of errors

Unfortunately, errors are a normal part of human behavior, and their causes are not obscure. Habit intrusion, stress, anger, fatigue, boredom, fear, time urgency, illness, and haste increase the odds of faulty performance.

The extent of errors documented to have contributed to anesthetic complications is great. All six major areas of anesthetic practice are implicated: inadequate pre-anesthetic evaluation, faulty patient selection, poor anesthetic management, inadequate monitoring, hurried recovery, and faulty recognition and inappropriate management of complications. Specific examples of errors are noted in Table 1.2.

The human condition

Homo sapiens is the only species that understands the concept of risk; however, habituation blunts this worry. The sense of having control over risk feeds the illusion of preparedness and prompts feelings of denial – "it won't happen (to me)"; or "if it happens to me, it won't be that bad".

Once the error cascade begins, numerous opportunities arise to stop its progression. Many times, however, these opportunities are ignored. Impending doom, coupled with the high stakes environment and time urgency, overwhelms and short circuits the human mind, which makes the most conservative (not necessarily correct) decision more attractive, ultimately leading to situational paralysis. Individuals with increased "cognitive horsepower" tend to be more susceptible to this shortfall, as worry about legal recourse, shame, and personal doom overpower rational thoughts and interfere with concentration on the task at hand (Bielock, 2010; Figure 1.1). Management of these "necessary fallibilities" is possible with repeated

Anesthesia Complications in the Dental Office, First Edition. Edited by Robert C. Bosack and Stuart Lieblich.

Table 1.1 Triggering events.

- Technical
  - Drug overdose
  - Failed airway management technique
  - Oxygen source disconnection
  - Equipment failure
- Judgmental
  - Inadequate patient history
  - Wrong drug/technique
  - Wrong airway management technique
  - Delay or failure to adequately treat abnormality
- Monitoring/vigilance
  - Failure to detect abnormality
  - Failure to accept abnormality
  - Alarm "saturation"

Table 1.2 Examples of anesthetic errors (Cooper et al., 1984).

- Loss of oxygen supply (tanks empty, not turned on, tubes disconnected)
- Drug error – wrong drug, wrong dose, syringe swap (unlabeled)
- Wrong choice of airway maintenance
- Careless, lack of vigilance haste
- Faulty information gathering and assimilation
- Lack of preparation, scenario rehearsal
- Poor communication among team members
- Unreliable intravenous access
- Unfamiliarity with drugs

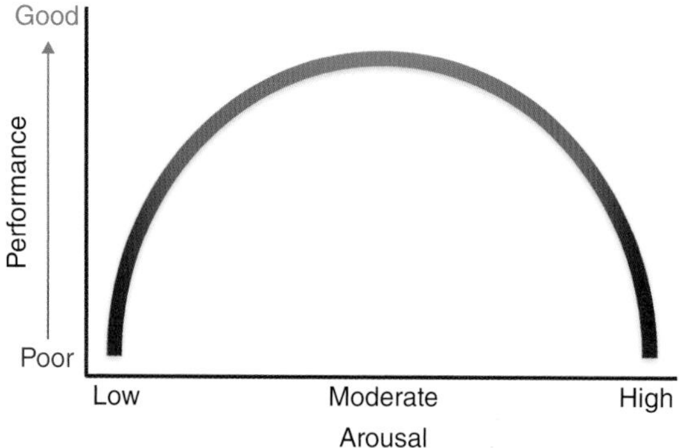

Figure 1.1 Performance decrement at extremes of arousal. Adapted from (Bielock, 2010).

practice under stress, periodic "pauses" to collect thoughts, a focus on outcome rather than mechanics, continual self-assurance of one's ability, and the use of memory guides.

Currently, there is a national focus on checklists (Gawande, 2009) as part of a cognitive safety net to provide protection against necessary fallibility by outlining the minimum necessary steps, especially important during times of adversity and complexity, when worry short-circuits the brain.

Scope of complications

The dental community provides a wide range of anesthesia: local anesthesia only, local anesthesia with nitrous oxide, enteral sedation, parenteral sedation, and anesthesia. It naturally follows that the complications associated with these techniques are also highly variable. These complications range from inability to anesthetize, failed sedation, syncope, and pressure or rhythm disorders to hypoxia and death.

It remains impossible to accumulate complete data on the nature and frequency of anesthetic errors/complications in the dental office. Errors are often managed without patient injury. Most dental anesthetics are administered in private practices (often by solo practitioners) which have sparse reporting requirements. Voluntary reporting is stifled due to fear of further inquiry and punishment. Learning from errors including changing of systems does not occur. Insurance companies also have no obligation to report closed claims, and many malpractice cases are settled and sequestered.

Perianesthetic complications are rare in the dental office, with most reports showing similar data. Perrott et al. (2003) reported on a prospective study of 34,391 ASA I and II patients and showed a complication rate of 1.3 per 100 cases. These included, in approximate order of decreasing frequency, vomiting, laryngospasm/bronchospasm, prolonged recovery, vascular injury, syncope, arrhythmia, seizure, and neurologic impairment. D'Eramo et al. (2008) reported similar complication rates from a survey of 169 oral and maxillofacial surgeons. Other examples of complications are noted in Table 1.3. However, a true mortality rate is not readily obtainable. The most current data from OMSNIC (the malpractice insurance company that covers approximately 80% of US oral and maxillofacial surgeons) estimates the likelihood of an office-anesthetic-related death to be 1/365,554 anesthetic cases (Estabrooks, 2011).

The prevention, diagnosis, and management of anesthetic complications are the focus of this book, and are addressed from multiple perspectives. Patient evaluation and selection, with emphasis on common comorbidities, knowledge of drug action, limitations of office-based anesthesia, monitoring, and preparation and management of adversity are addressed. Crisis resource management during error/complication evolution is not taught in dental school or residency programs. It is included here as the most important asset for complication management.

Table 1.3 Examples of anesthetic complications.

- Syncope
- Laryngospasm
- Bronchospasm
- Upper airway obstruction
- Allergy
- Seizure
- Tachycardia/bradycardia
- Cardiac arrhythmia
- Hypertension/hypotension
- Myocardial infarction/cardiac death
- Malignant hyperthermia
- Aspiration
- Post-anesthetic recall of intraoperative awareness

References

Bielock, S. *Choke: What the Secrets of the Brain Reveal about Getting it Right When You Have to*. New York: Free Press, 2010.

Cooper, J. B., et al. Preventable anesthesia mishaps: a study of human factors. *Anesthesiol* **49**: 399–406, 1978.

Cooper, J. B., et al. An analysis of major errors and equipment failures in anesthesia management : considerations for prevention and detection. *Anesthesiol* **60**: 34–42, 1984

Reason, J. *Human Error*. New York: Cambridge University Press, 1990.

Reason, J. *Human Error*: models and management. *Br Med J* **320**: 768–770, 2000.

D'Eramo, E. M., et al. Anesthesia morbidity and mortality experience among massachusetts oral and maxillofacial surgeons. *J Oral Maxillofac Surg.* **66**: 2421–2433, 2008.

Estabrooks, L. Redefining the standards of office anesthesia: supporting data to adapt higher standards. Presented at the 93rd AAOMS annual meeting, Philadelphia, PA, 2011.

Gawande A. *The Checklist Manifesto: How to Get Things Right*. New York: Metropolitan Books, 2009.

Perrott, D. H., et al. Office-based ambulatory anesthesia : outcomes of clinical practice of oral and maxillofacial surgeons. *J Oral Maxillofac Surg* **61**: 983–995, 2003.

SECTION 2

Patient risk assessment

2 History and physical evaluation

Kyle Kramer[1], Trevor Treasure[2], Charles Kates[3], Carrie Klene[4], and Jeffrey Bennett[1]

[1]Indiana University, Department of Oral Surgery and Hospital Dentistry, Indianapolis, IN, USA
[2]University of Texas – School of Dentistry, Department of Oral and Maxillofacial Surgery, TX, USA
[3]University of Miami Miller School of Medicine, Departments of Anesthesiology and Surgery, FL, USA
[4]Indiana University, Indianapolis, IN, USA

Introduction

The risks associated with office-based anesthesia are greater than the risk of dental surgery. Preanesthetic patient evaluation and appropriate case selection maximize safety, efficacy, and efficiency of office-based anesthesia and surgery. It provides a basis for case refusal or limit setting on the depth of anesthesia.

Accurate patient evaluation requires effective communication with patients by ensuring complete patient comprehension by "repeat back" questions, enhanced listening skills of the doctor, and effective team communication. Unfortunately, some patients will be less than forthright in disclosing their diseases or medication adherence. In other cases, patients may be unaware of their disease or will have yet-to-be-diagnosed disease. Suspicion of any disease in the dental patient should help diagnosis and trigger appropriate referral as necessary.

Cardiovascular, pulmonary, and upper airway complications are three major causes of morbidity and mortality in the dental office. Together with NPO status, these comprise the core elements of pre-anesthesia patient evaluation.

The American Society of Anesthesiologists recommends the following sequence for preoperative evaluation:

- Patient interview and review of the medical/surgical/anesthetic history
- Physical examination
- Assigning of an ASA physical status score
- Formulation and discussion of the anesthetic plan

Consideration of the anticipated physiologic and anatomic disruptions of both surgery and anesthesia is the first aspect of patient evaluation. Preoperative patient evaluation is an opportunity to identify previously diagnosed diseases; to assess patients for signs and symptoms of occult diseases; to determine the need for focused preoperative laboratory or diagnostic studies; and to review patient medications. This is done in order to preoperatively optimize the patient and prevent exacerbation of existing disorders. Ultimately, this will guide decisions regarding refusal of anesthesia, limit setting on the depth of anesthesia, and location of care. This process is called *risk assessment*.

The ASA physical status is assigned to a patient in order to stratify the risk of the anesthesia and planned surgery. In the operating room setting, where the majority or anesthetics are given, the ASA score (Table 2.1) is known to correlate with morbidity and mortality, unplanned ICU admissions, longer hospital stays, and adverse cardiopulmonary outcomes (Sweitzer et al., 2008). Though the majority of outpatient dental procedures may be minor in comparison to an inpatient surgical procedure, the anesthetics given (and thus the risk profile) in either setting may be similar.

Cardiovascular risk assessment

History

Direct office-based anesthetic cardiovascular risks include adverse heart rate and blood pressure changes, with tachycardia and hypotension being more worrisome in the adult patient. Patients with coronary artery disease (diagnosed or undiagnosed) are less able to tolerate increased oxygen demand associated with tachycardia. Any decrease in oxygen delivery to vital organs, due to a decrease in cardiac output or blood pressure, is also worrisome.

Cardiovascular evaluation for dental patients undergoing office-based anesthesia is used to screen those patients with major issues who will benefit from further testing and disease optimization management prior to surgery and anesthesia. The presence of "minor" symptoms also may prompt a delay in office-based anesthesia, pending further evaluation.

Direct questions should screen for the presence of preexisting diseases, including hypertension, coronary artery disease, prior myocardial infarction, heart failure, arrhythmias, valvulopathy, hyperlipidemia, and prior cardiac intervention (stents, bypass grafts, cardiac implantable electronic device). Physical symptoms of angina, shortness of breath, level of exercise tolerance, palpitations, irregular heartbeat, cough, dizziness, orthostatic hypotension, syncope, smoking, sedentary life style, and family history of sudden cardiac death are significant findings (Table 2.2). The patient's medication list can also provide insight into the presence of disease state.

Case selection and management are guided by estimates of patient resilience and patient reserve. *Resilience* refers to the patient's ability to tolerate hypoxia and heart rate and/or blood pressure changes without decompensation. The ability to tolerate adversity depends on both the duration and the severity of the challenge. As an example, a patient with obesity and coronary artery

Anesthesia Complications in the Dental Office, First Edition. Edited by Robert C. Bosack and Stuart Lieblich.

Table 2.1 ASA physical status score (American Society of Anesthesiologists, available at www.asahq.org).

ASA I	Healthy patient without organic, biochemical, or psychiatric disease
ASA II	Mild systemic disease, without significant impact on daily activity, e.g., mild asthma or well-controlled hypertension. Unlikely impact on anesthesia and surgery
ASA III	Significant or severe systemic disease that limits normal activity. Likely impact on anesthesia and surgery
ASA IV	Significant and severe systemic disease that is a constant threat to life.
ASA V	A moribund patient that is not expected to survive without the operation
ASA VI	A patient declared brain-dead whose organs are being harvested for donation

disease is challenged by decreased functional residual capacity (due to cephalad displacement of the diaphragm, especially during anesthesia) leading to quick onset hypoxemia with apnea and an inability to tolerate the subsequent sustained tachycardia. *Reserve* refers to the ability to physiologically compensate hypoxemia and/or adverse cardiovascular changes via arousal and ventilatory and/or cardiovascular changes. As examples, the elderly may be unable to compensate for hypoxemia with tachycardia, while the infants have an invariate stroke volume and will be unable to tolerate a bradycardia.

Cardiovascular disease (hypertension, atherosclerosis (coronary artery disease, CAD, and ischemic heart disease), valvulopathy, heart failure, and rhythm disorders) affects up to one-third of patients presenting for dental care, which puts them at increased risk for cardiovascular complications (Pasternak, 2002). As "Baby Boomers" age and thresholds for performing procedures on the elderly ease, increased numbers of patients with cardiovascular disease will be presenting for dental care under anesthesia.

Goldman et al. (1977) was the first to prospectively evaluate 1001 patients over age 40 who underwent non-cardiac surgery. They documented nine preoperative variables that were associated with a higher risk of cardiac events in the perioperative period. These findings, revised in 1999 by Lee (known as the Revised Cardiac Risk Index), led to the 2007 American College of Cardiology/American Heart Association guidelines on perioperative cardiovascular evaluation for non-cardiac surgery (Fleisher et al., 2007). These guidelines help estimate the risk of a cardiac event during non-cardiac surgery, help define risk with selective testing, suggest intervention to lower risk as necessary, and assess long-term risk and modify risk factors. Three elements are assessed to determine the extent of risk – the presence of active cardiac conditions, exercise capacity, and surgery-specific risk (Table 2.3). This algorithm suggests immediate referral and refusal of all elective surgery for patients with active cardiac conditions and referral and refusal for intermediate risk surgery for patients who cannot function at least at a 4 MET level. Further action or referral for patients without active cardiac conditions and low risk surgery (office-based dental surgery) is seldom required.

There are, however, other factors that can introduce unnecessary risk during office-based anesthesia (Kheterpal et al., 2009). These factors include age >68 years, BMI > 30 kg/m^2, previous cardiac intervention, cerebrovascular disease, hypertension, and operative duration >3.8 hours. Obesity, obstructive sleep apnea, and diabetes mellitus are also strongly associated with cardiovascular disease.

Cardiovascular examination

Core elements of cardiovascular examination include inspection, palpation, and auscultation. Vital signs, including blood pressure,

Table 2.2 Significance of screening questions.

Disease	Select cardiovascular concerns
Atherosclerosis, coronary artery disease (CAD)	Inability to tolerate increased cardiac work (increased rate or force of contraction)
Hypertension	Increased cardiac workload, known risk factor for CAD, MI, HF; perianesthetic hypotension
Prior myocardial infarction (MI)	Post infarct irritability, arrhythmia, re-infarction with recent MI (<30 days)
Heart failure (HF)	Level of compensation, exercise tolerance
Arrhythmias	Level of control, side effects of anti-arrhythmic medication, symptoms, possibility of recurrence during anesthesia
Valvulopathy	Increased cardiac workload, aortic stenosis limits cardiac output
Hyperlipidemia	Atherosclerosis, CAD
Prior cardiac intervention – stents, bypass, CIED	Stent re-thrombosis, compliance with anti-platelet therapy, device efficacy, battery life
Angina	Never normal, could indicate coronary artery disease
Shortness of breath	Never normal, non-specific symptom, cardiac and/or pulmonary origin
Level of exercise tolerance	Should be able to take care of self, ascend one flight of stairs (4 METS)
Palpitations; unprovoked episodic tachycardia	Atrial fibrillation, PVCs, supraventricular tachycardia
Irregular heart beat	Atrial fibrillation, PVCs
Cough	Non-specific symptom, decompensated heart failure, COPD
Dizziness	Arrhythmia, pre-syncope, hypotension
Orthostatic hypotension	Side effect of anti-hypertensive medications
Syncope	Vasovagal syncope, carotid sinus hypersensitivity
Smoking	Atherosclerosis, COPD, increased airway irritability, sympathomimetic, falsely elevated SpO_2
Sedentary life style	Atherosclerosis, obesity
Family history of sudden cardiac death	Hereditary long QT syndrome

Table 2.3 Three elements of risks for surgery and anesthesia (Fleisher, 2007).

1	Active cardiac conditions that require evaluation and treatment prior to non-cardiac surgery		Unstable coronary syndromes—severe angina, MI within 1 month
			Decompensated, worsening or new-onset heart failure
			Significant arrhythmias—high grade AV block, symptomatic ventricular arrhythmias, SVT with rates >100 bpm, symptomatic bradycardia
			Severe valvular disease—aortic stenosis and symptomatic mitral stenosis
2	Exercise capacity (Hlatky et al., 1989) (1 MET = 3.5 ml O_2 uptake/kg/min	1 MET	Eat, dress, use the toilet
		4 MET	Light housework, climb a flight of stairs, walk up a hill
		10 MET	Dancing, doubles tennis
3	Surgery-specific risk	High risk	Major vascular surgery
		Intermediate risk	Head and neck surgery, abdominal or thoracic or orthopedic surgery
		Low risk	Ambulatory surgery, endoscopic procedures, superficial procedures

pulse, and respiratory rate are obtained on all patients, ideally at a preoperative visit (Bickley and Szilagyi, 2009). Inspection of the patient includes identification of any signs of distress, shortness of breath, inappropriate sweating (a fight or flight response), pallor, cyanosis, ankle edema, or obesity. Palpation of the radial pulse is done to determine rate (normal is 60 to 100 bpm) and regularity. Most irregular pulses are due to atrial fibrillation (irregularly irregular) or occasional premature atrial or ventricular beats. Blood pressure is obtained manually or with a machine from the right arm with the patient seated and arm at heart level. Cuffs that are too small falsely elevate the value; cuffs that are too big falsely reduce the value. Normal pressures are <120 mmHg systolic AND <80 mmHg diastolic (Chobanian et al., 2003).

Table 2.4 Risk factors for perioperative pulmonary complications in patients undergoing general anesthesia in a hospital setting (Arozullah et al., 2000; Khan and Hussain, 2005).

- Chronic obstructive pulmonary disease (COPD)
- Age >70 years
- Cigarette use, current or >20 pack years
- ASA 2 or 3
- Upper respiratory tract infection
- Heart Failure
- Obstructive sleep apnea
- Smoking
- <4 METS exercise capacity
- Poorly controlled asthma
- BMI >30
- Site of surgery—head and neck
- Depth of anesthesia
- Procedure duration >2 hours

Pulmonary risk assessment

History

Risks to the pulmonary system during office anesthesia are primarily due to ventilatory depression by blunting of the ventilatory response to hypercarbia and hypoxemia by the medications administered. Less common issues are a decrease in functional residual capacity due to the relaxation of the diaphragm causing caudal movement of the abdominal contents, which can lead to atelectasis and exacerbation of underlying chronic disease.

Pulmonary history seeks to identify disease states below the vocal cords that could interfere with airflow and therefore oxygenation. Several authors (Arozullah et al., 2000; Khan and Hussain, 2005) have identified risk factors for perioperative pulmonary complications in patients undergoing general anesthesia in a hospital setting (Table 2.4). Most patients anesthetized in dental offices are maintained breathing spontaneously without intubation, which mitigates some of these risks.

The most common pulmonary symptoms include dyspnea (breathing discomfort), cough, wheezing, chest tightness, and exercise intolerance. Specific diseases include obstructive diseases (asthma, chronic bronchitis, and emphysema), restrictive diseases (obesity, advanced pregnancy, skeletal malformation, fluid accumulation in the lungs, interstitial disease), and upper respiratory tract infections (URTIs). Diseases of the respiratory system frequently have an insidious onset; severe disease can be present without obvious symptoms or signs, as patients equilibrate to their limitations and feel normal. This is especially true with advanced chronic bronchitis and chronic cough. When challenged with upper airway obstruction or respiratory depression, these patients may rapidly desaturate.

Most anesthetic drugs used in the dental office depress the ventilatory drive, reduce functional residual capacity, and relax the muscles that maintain upper airway patency, leading to hypoventilation and hypoxemia. As such, it is ideal to confirm that concurrent medical conditions are optimized prior to elective or semi-elective surgery/anesthesia. Poorly controlled asthma (recent exacerbation <4 weeks), especially with concomitant URTI, can increase the likelihood of an attack with even mild triggers.

Smoking (active or passive) (within hours of anesthesia) can increase the likelihood of laryngospasm and bronchospasm in susceptible patients and falsely elevate the SpO_2.

Patients with URTIs can be at increased risk of laryngospasm, bronchospasm, and diminished oxygen diffusibility across respiratory membranes. Both severity and rate of onset of hypoxemia will increase when these patients are challenged by hypoventilation or apnea.

Pulmonary examination

Physical pulmonary examination includes inspecting the patient with clothes on. Examination can reveal the barrel chest of emphysema, thoracic spine distortion, supraclavicular retraction of airway obstruction, the worried look of air hunger, cyanosis, and abnormal respiratory rate (adult normal is 12–20 breaths per minute). Ankle edema, if visible, can be a sign of fluid retention, which affects the entire body, including the lungs. Auscultation of the lungs should be performed with any suspicion of disease. Obstruction or airway fluid can cause adventitious (abnormal) breath sounds, including wheezing or crackles. Oxygen saturation on room air is an important baseline vital sign, and is needed as a baseline reference for patients who experience respiratory trouble during or after anesthesia/sedation.

Upper airway risk assessment

The most important preanesthetic/sedation evaluation is that of the upper airway. The second most important is a detailed medical history. Whether the plan is a simple, one-drug, conscious sedation or a full general anesthetic, preparation and airway evaluation remain the same.

Past medical history as it relates to the airway includes a screening for obstructive sleep apnea, including the presence of snoring, excessive daytime sleepiness, and hypertension. Any adverse outcome with prior anesthetics, including airway compromise, is worrisome.

Any cervical spine pathology may signal the inability to perform a chin-lift, head tilt maneuver.

Assessment of the upper airway is divided into four specific elements (Strauss, 2010):

1. The ability to perform mask ventilation
2. The ability to utilize an extraglottic device
3. The ability to perform laryngeal exposure and intubation
4. The ability to perform an emergency surgical airway

In order to accomplish the above, rapid and reproducible upper airway evaluation is essential, so that anticipated airway problems can be quickly assessed prior to sedation or general anesthesia.

Mask ventilation requires an adequate mask seal to allow for positive pressure ventilation, and a simultaneous ability to perform a jaw thrust, head tilt, and chin lift maneuver. The following parameters must be assessed:

- The presence of abnormal facial form or jaw deformities.
- The presence of facial hair.
- The presence of foreign bodies in the pharynx with potential for upper airway obstruction.
- The presence of obesity, which can limit airway diameter and increase resistance to air flow.
- The presence of edentulism, which allows the lips to prolapse into the oral cavity. Stable full dentures should be retained during induction to expand the lips and allow for a better mask seal.
- Loss of tissue elasticity (increased resistance to airflow) and flexibility of the neck and temporomandibular joint (inability to open the airway) in patients older than 60 years of age.
- Cervical range of motion.

Problems with placement of extraglottic devices are similar to those encountered with mask ventilation, and additionally, are complicated by restricted mouth opening, abnormal oral and pharyngeal anatomy, and obstruction of the upper airway by foreign bodies, swelling, and/or oropharyngeal deviation.

Prediction of successful laryngoscopy and intubation is divided into five key elements:

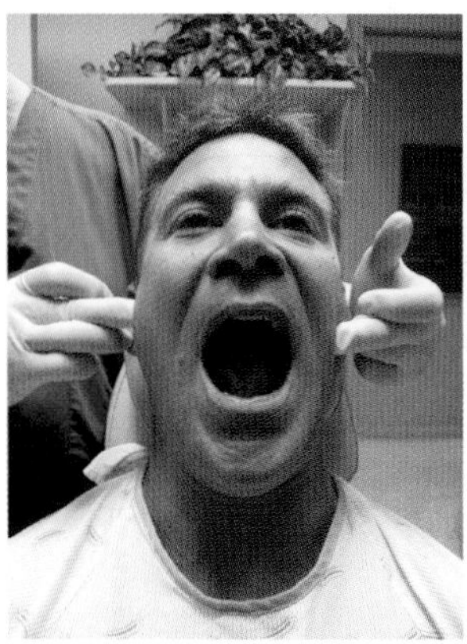
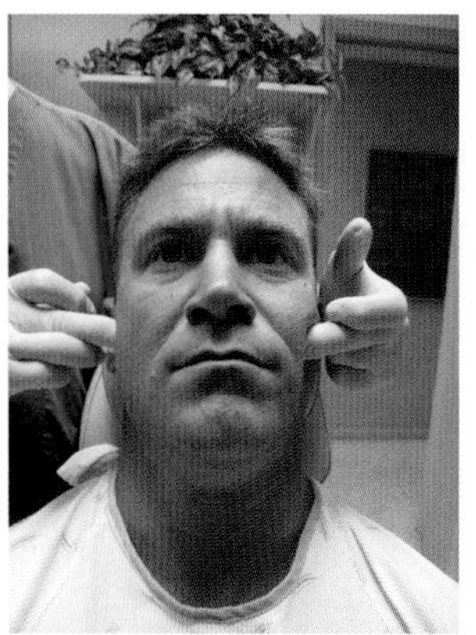
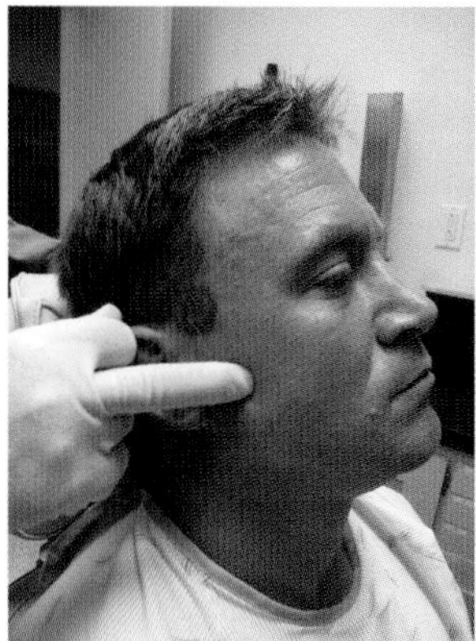
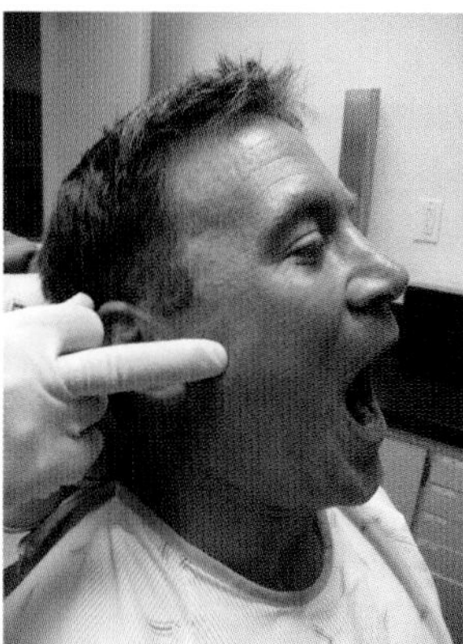

Figure 2.1 Predicting successful visualization of the vocal cords with a traditional laryngoscope utilizing condylar translation in the glenoid fossa of the TMJ.

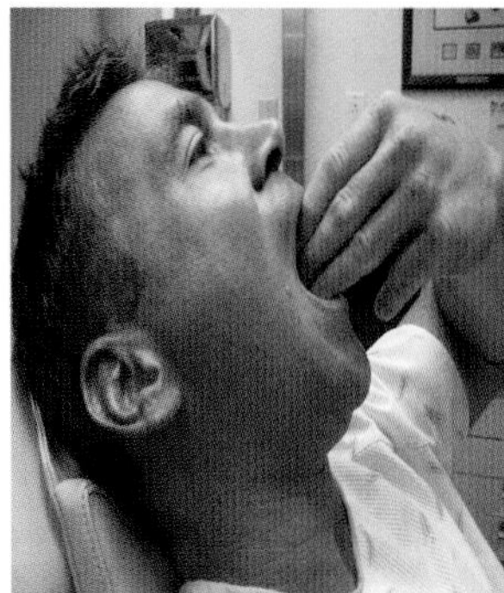
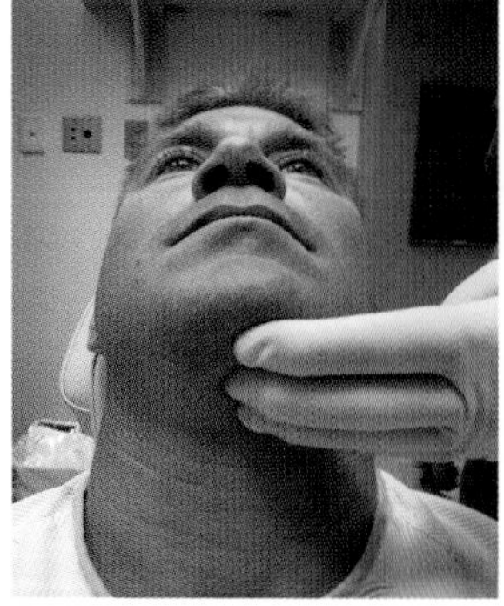
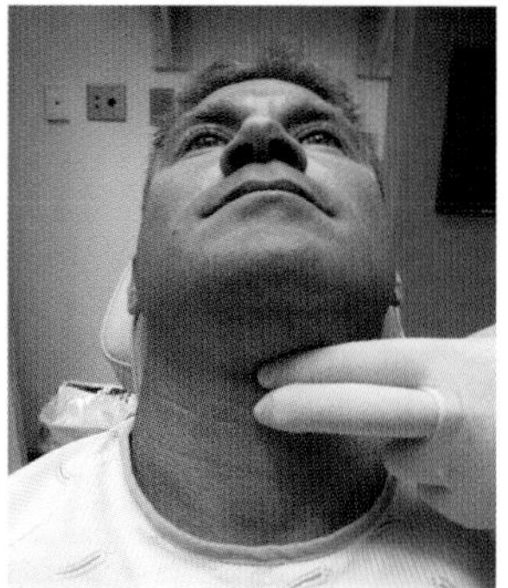

Figure 2.2 Rapid assesment of airway. (A) interincisive distance (3 fingers), (B) chin to neck (3 fingers), (C) neck to thyroid (2 fingers).

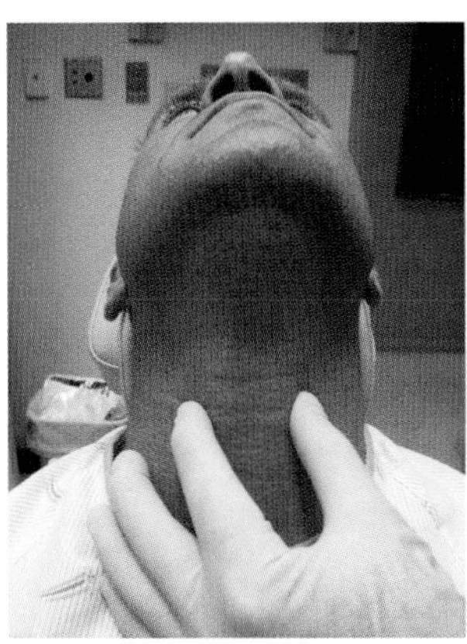
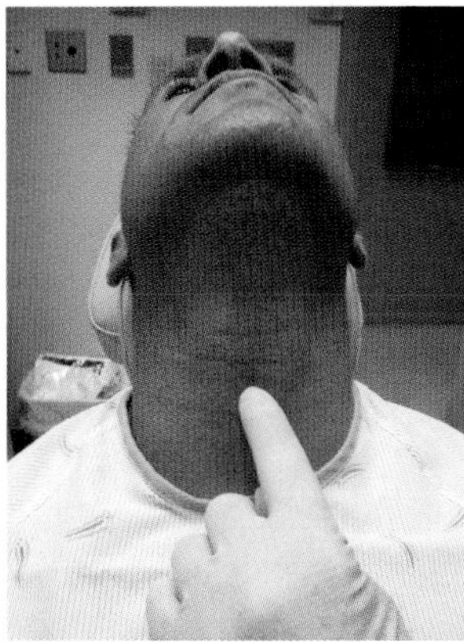

Figure 2.3 Cricothyroid location. Finding the cricothyroid depression for emergency surgical airway.

1 Patient appearance: a maxillary protrusion or a mandibular retrognathia, loose teeth, high palatal vault, and maxillary/mandibular tori will interfere with proper insertion and manipulation of a traditional laryngoscope.
2 Evaluation of the relationship between the uvula, soft palate, hard palate, and tongue is referred to as the *Mallampatti classification*. While this classification has become very popular and, in fact, is always recorded on anesthesia records in the hospital, it only has value if it is POSITIVE and EXTREME. In other words, a "Mallampatti III or IV," where only the soft and/or hard palate is visible, is the only reliable predictor. The reason for this is that patient positioning and evaluation varies so much from examiner to examiner that a reliable, reproducible prediction is usually not possible (Kates and Gayer, 2010).
3 The most important predictor of laryngoscopy with a traditional laryngoscope is translation of the mandibular condyles in the temporomandibular joint. The patient is asked to open the mouth while the examiner palpates the mandibular condyles. There should be a normal anterior/inferior movement of the condyle, which predicts the ability of the operator to visualize the larynx. If the patient has a hinge axis rotation, it will not be possible to visualize the larynx with a traditional laryngoscope (Figure 2.1).
- Measure the interincisive distance. Anything less than 20 mm is problematic. The patient should open his/her mouth as widely as possible and place his/her three fingers vertically between the upper and lower incisors. Two fingers measure approximately 20 mm, and three fingers measure approximately 30 mm.
- Evaluate the mandible to larynx relationships. The distance between the chin and where the neck begins should measure another three finger breadths. This is approximately 30–35 mm.

The third parameter is the distance from where the neck begins to the thyroid cartilage; that should be about two fingers breadths, or about 20 mm. The operator can use his own three fingers for these measurements. This method is superior to the popular "thyromental distance" measurement. It gives added information: the length of the mandible in relation to the cricothyroid apparatus and the approximate angle of the neck (about 90 degrees is normal) (Figure 2.2).

The last issue to evaluate is whether it would be possible to do a rapid emergency surgical airway, should it become necessary. The simplest way to do this is to have the patient hyperextend his/her head and neck. Palpate the cricothyroid depression that occurs between the cricoid and thyroid cartilages. This is a well-defined entrance through the cricothyroid membrane, and in an emergency, is quickly and efficiently located (Figure 2.3).

The above predictors for a difficult airway should be accomplished in less than a minute, recorded in the patient's record, and always performed on every patient who will be sedated, or who will have a general anesthetic.

Reference

Arozullah, A. M., et al. Multifacyorial risk index for predicting postoperative respiratory failure in men after major non-cardiac surgery. *Ann Surg* **232**: 242–253, 2000.

Bickley, L. S. and Szilagyi, P. G. *Bates' Guide to Physical Examination and History Taking*. 10th edn Philadelphia: Lippincott Williams and Wilkens, 2009.

Chobanian, A. V., et al. The seventh report of the Joint National Committee on prevention, detection, evaluation and treatment of high blood pressure: the JNC 7 report. *J Am Med Assoc* **289**: 2560, 2003.

Fleisher, L. A., et al. ACC/AHA 2007 guidelines on perioperative cardiovascular evaluation and care for noncardiac surgery: executive summary: a report on the American College of Cardiology/American Heart Association Task Force on practice guidelines (Writing Committee to revise the 2002 guidelines on perioperative cardiovascular evaluation for noncardiac surgery) *Circ* **116**: 1971–1996, 2007.

Goldman, L., et al. Multifactorial index of cardiac risk in noncardiac surgical procedures. *New Engl J Med* **297**: 845, 1977.

Hlatky, M. A., et al. A brief self-administered questionnaire to determine functional capacity. *Am J Cardiol* **64**: 651–654, 1989.

Kates, C. H. and Gayer, S. Recognition and management of the difficult airsay. In: Shaw, I., ed. *Oxford Textbox of Anaesthesia for Oral and Maxillofacial Surgery* Vol. 1. Oxford: Oxford University press, 2010.

Khan, M. A. and Hussain, S. F. Pre-operative pulmonary evaluation. *J Ayub Med Coll Abbottabad* **17**: 82–86, 2005.

Kheterpal, S., et al. Preoperative and intraoperative predictors of cardiac adverse events after general, vascular and urological surgery. *Anesthesiol* **110**: 58–66, 2009.

Pasternak, L.R. ASA Practice Guidelines for Preanesthetic Assessment. *Int Anesthesiol Clin* **40**: 31–46, 2002.

Strauss RA Noordhoek R: Management of the difficult airway. *Atlas Oral Maxillo Surg Clin NA*. **18**: 11–28, 2010.

Sweitzer, B.J., et al. *Anesthesiology*. New York: McGraw-Hill, 2008.

3 Laboratory evaluation

Kyle Kramer[1] and Jeffrey Bennett[2]
[1]Indiana University, Indianapolis, IN, USA
[2]Indiana University, Department of Oral Surgery and Hospital Dentistry, Indianapolis, IN, USA

Introduction

Preoperative laboratory evaluation is seldom indicated prior to dental procedures. Occasionally, certain medical conditions may indicate a need for further, more specific evaluations to determine the severity or control of concomitant disease, for example, INR in patients taking coumadin or white blood cell count (WBC) in a patient undergoing chemotherapy (Table 3.1). Most studies (Kumar and Srivastava, 2011) agree that routine laboratory testing is unnecessary and often times harmful to patients as 5% of normal patients will have abnormal findings, and that these abnormal findings often trigger further testing, which is both costly and may lead to unnecessary additional intervention (Munro et al., 1997). Preoperative tests are ordered only when indicated by the history and physical examination, which will likely identify factors impacting perioperative management (Fattahi, 2006). The need for or interpretation of laboratory tests can be done in consultation with the patient's physician as per the knowledge and scope of practice of the dental practitioner. Patients may present with copies of recent, but unrequested laboratory information. This chapter reviews the commonly used preoperative laboratory tests to aid in their interpretation.

Table 3.1 Pre-anesthetic testing rationale (Pasternak, 2003).

Rationale supporting the need for preanesthetic testing
• Previous or existing medical comorbidities • High risk, extensive, prolonged or invasive surgical plan • Anesthetic plan with inherently higher risk • High risk stratification based on patient demographics • Need to establish a baseline prior to surgery due to risk of postoperative complications

Basic metabolic panel

These studies (Table 3.2) are useful in helping to identify or quantify common metabolic and electrolyte imbalances along with providing a crude indication of renal function (Giannakopoulos et al., 2006).

Sodium

Sodium is the main extracellular cation that is chiefly responsible for maintaining osmotic hemostasis and neuronal impulse transmission. Sodium serum concentration is regulated by dietary intake and renal excretion. Extracellular sodium concentrations are closely regulated, with normal values ranging between 135 and 145 mEq/L. *Hyponatremia*, defined as serum sodium levels below 135 mEq/L, may reflect a variety of conditions including renal disease, excess intake of free water, or as a side effect from various medications, including some diuretics and anticonvulsants (carbamazepine, valproate). Elective procedures in patients presenting with a serum sodium level below 130 mEq/L are postponed until further consultation and optimization/sodium normalization occurs. Acute and chronic hyponatremia usually remain asymptomatic until sodium levels drop below 130 mEq/L and 120 mEq/L respectively (Giannakopoulos et al., 2006) Clinical manifestations of acute hyponatremia can clinically manifest as lethargy, cramps, seizures, and altered mental status, especially if serum sodium levels decrease quickly. Chronic hyponatremia may be symptomless. *Hypernatremia*, defined as serum sodium level above 145 mEq/L, typically reflects a hypovolemic state (inadequate intake of free water or excessive free water loss followed by renal reabsorption of sodium to compensate), a euvolemic state (diabetes insipidus), or a hypervolemic state (ingestion of saltwater, Cushing's disease). Hypernatremia may present as agitation, altered mental status, or seizures.

Potassium

Potassium, the main intracellular cation, is intimately involved with maintaining polarization of the cell membrane and subsequent transmission of neuronal impulses, especially the cardiac conduction system. The normal value of extracellular potassium is 3.5–5.0 mEq/L. As a positive intracellular cation, potassium has the capacity to shift concentrations depending on the presence of positive hydrogen ions. An increase in serum H^+ ions (decrease pH) will lead to a shift (increase) in extracellular K^+. Alkalosis produces the opposite ion-swapping scenario and can lead to hypokalemia. Hypokalemia is associated with patients taking potassium-wasting diuretics (hydrochlorothiazide) and loop diuretics (furosemide). Patients with a serum potassium level below 3.5 mEq/L may require correction preoperatively with either oral supplements or intravenous potassium, which must be done slowly to prevent cardiac complications. Hypokalemia below 3.0 mEq/L leads to prolongation of the PR interval, ST depression, T wave flattening and/or inversion, and the appearance of prominent U waves (Dubin, 2000). Hyperkalemia may be noted in a multitude

Anesthesia Complications in the Dental Office, First Edition. Edited by Robert C. Bosack and Stuart Lieblich.

Table 3.2 Basic Metabolic Panel

Components	Reference range	Possible indications
Sodium	135–145 mEq	Fluid imbalance
Potassium	3.5–5.2 mEq/L	Electrolyte abnormality
Chloride	100–108 mEq/L	Diabetes
Bicarbonate	22–28 mEq/L	Acute or chronic renal impairment
Blood urea nitrogen (BUN)	8–23 mg/dL	
Creatinine	0.6–1.2 mg/dL	
Glucose	70–110 mg/dL	

of clinical situations, most commonly in patients who have chronic kidney disease requiring dialysis. A serum potassium level above 5.5 mEq/L will require correction preoperatively, which, for this select group of patients, means postponement of the surgery and undergoing dialysis. Hyperkalemia will initially trigger a reduction in the amplitude of the P waves, followed by the development of peaked T waves. As hyperkalemia worsens, the QRS complex begins to widen, ultimately progressing into a sinusoidal pattern (Dubin, 2000).

BUN and creatinine

Serum creatinine and blood urea nitrogen (BUN) provide insights into renal function. Creatinine is a byproduct of skeletal muscle breakdown (and is directly related to the quantity of skeletal muscle) and is excreted by the kidneys. Normal serum creatinine values range from 0.7–1.2 mg/dL (Faust and Cucchiara, 2002). Serum creatinine can be interpreted as an index of glomerular filtration rate. BUN is a byproduct of protein metabolism. Normal serum BUN values range from 8–20 mg/dL. BUN measurements are not as reliable an index of GFR as serum creatinine. Elevated BUN may reflect dehydration, a diet high in protein, situations resulting in massive quantities of protein breakdown (burns, muscle injury), or possibly decreased renal function. Both BUN and creatinine are rather poor indicators of *acutely* changing renal function, and typically, increases in serum concentrations are not noted until glomerular filtration rates drop by approximately 75%. As such, abnormally high BUN and creatinine values tend to suggest chronically decreased renal function.

Serum glucose

Normal fasting (8–12 hours) blood glucose (FBG) level is 70–100 mg/dL, pre-diabetes occurs when FBG is between 101 and 125 mg/dL and diabetes with an FBS > 125 mg/dL. Patients with diabetes are usually aware of their blood glucose levels and are knowledgeable in the use of glucometers to manage their blood levels. Knowledge of pre- and postanesthetic blood glucose is highly desirable to avoid complications associated with excessively high or low levels. Patients who undergo invasive oral procedures may have significant postoperative oral discomfort and are at risk for hypoglycemia due to decreased oral intake secondary to pain. Pain can trigger postoperative hyperglycemia due to release of counter-regulatory hormones (glucagon, cortisol, epinephrine, and growth hormone) that elevate blood sugar and cause insulin resistance. Patients should closely monitor their blood glucose at home in the postanesthetic period in order to prevent complications.

Glycosylated hemoglobin (HbA1c)

Glycosylated hemoglobin (HbA1c) has become the gold standard for evaluating a diabetic patient's long-term glucose control and is

Table 3.3 Gylcosylated Hemoglobin and Average Serum Glucose

HbA1c (%)	Mean blood glucose (mg/dL)	Interpretation
4*	60	*Non-diabetic range
5*	95	
6*	130	
7+	160	+Target range for diabetics
8**	195	**Therapy needed
9**	225	
10**	260	

typically measured every 3–6 months depending upon the level of control (Table 3.3). Glucose irreversibly binds to hemoglobin. As the average life span of a red blood cell is 120 days, the HbA1c value reflects a "report card" of the average plasma glucose concentration over the past 3 months. Elevated values will heighten suspicion of the presence of cardiovascular and other comorbidities.

Complete blood count

The complete blood count measures many hematologic parameters. In the dental office, focus is usually directed to WBC, hematocrit, hemoglobin (Hgb), and platelet count. Evaluation of the WBC count can help identify a patient with an active bacterial infection (elevation), side effects of chemotherapy (depression), or malignancy (elevation or depression) (Table 3.4). Hematocrit and hemoglobin establish a baseline for procedures where blood loss is anticipated and will also help identify any underlying hematologic disorders such as anemia (Hgb <10 g/dL) or polycythemia (Stoelting and Miller, 2007). Platelet counts less than 50,000/mm^3 can result in prolonged postoperative bleeding.

Coagulation studies

Coagulation studies, typically an INR and/or PTT, are used to screen patients with a history of bleeding tendencies, hepatic disease, coagulopathy, or comorbidities requiring treatment with anticoagulants. Patients taking coumadin are often at supratherapeutic or subtherapeutic levels because of the delay of drug onset and magnitude of drug interactions affecting coumadin levels. More information can be found in Chapter 14.

Liver function tests (Table 3.5)

Patients with a history of hepatic diseases (hepatitis, cirrhosis, etc.) can have disruptions of normal hepatic function, notably plasma

Table 3.4 Complete blood count.

Components	Reference range	Possible indications
White blood cells (WBC)	4,500–11,000/mm^3	Infection Anemia Immunodeficiency hemorrhage
Hemoglobin	Male: 13.5–17.5 g/dL Female: 12–16 g/dL	
Hematocrit	Male: 41–53% Female: 36–46%	
Platelets	150,000–400,000/mm^3	

Table 3.5 Additional Tests.

Additional tests Components	Reference range	Possible indications
Liver function tests Albumin	3.5–5.0 g/dL	Acquired or congenital hepatic disease Malnutrition
Serum hCG	Negative: <5 IU/L Indeterminate: 5–25 IU/L Positive: >25 IU/L	Pregnancy (unexpected or expected)

protein synthesis and drug metabolism. Liver function tests, or a hepatic panel, typically evaluate transaminase levels, albumin, total protein, and bilirubin along with several other factors.

Transaminases

Transaminase (alanine transaminase, aspartate transaminase) enzymes are relatively selective for hepatocytes. ALT and AST are sensitive tests and elevated values indicate that the hepatocytes have been damaged, resulting in spillage of the intracellular enzymes into the systemic circulation. Causes of elevated transaminases may include hepatitis, cirrhosis, chronic heavy alcohol consumption, obesity, and diabetes.

Albumin

Albumin, the main protein component in blood plasma, is produced by the liver. Low albumin concentrations, as seen in prolonged fasting, eating disorders, malignancy, and old age, increase the availability of protein-bound drugs, leading to an unexpectedly increased clinical effect and decreased duration.

Pregnancy tests

Many dental anesthesia providers will commonly treat female patients that are of child-bearing age. Since several medications (benzodiazepines, NSAIDs) commonly used during sedations/anesthesia are contraindicated in pregnant patients, it is imperative that clinicians have a plan in place to identify pregnant females preoperatively. Most commonly, this is done with direct questioning, such as "are you or could you be pregnant?" Take-home pregnancy tests that evaluate β-hCG levels in the urine are usually reliable and accurate relatively early, often within 10–14 days of conception (Tintinalli and Stapczynski, 2011). Patients may actually be pregnant but not have a positive β-hCG very early during pregnancy because the hormone concentrations have not increased enough at the time of the test to trigger a "positive" result.

Cardiac and cardiovascular studies

Electrocardiogram: preoperative studies

Preoperative ECG is unlikely to uncover significant findings that would result in case of cancellation or altered anesthetic management and is therefore not indicated in ASA I or II patients without risk factors (Practice Guidelines, 2002). The same practice advisory published by the ASA recognized that age alone is not an indication for obtaining a preoperative ECG. However, increasing age, along with existing comorbidities or risk factors, does increase the likelihood of underlying cardiovascular disease (Richman, 2010). A normal ECG does not guarantee the absence of cardiovascular disease. Once the clinician has determined the indication for preoperative ECG evaluation, several options exist. Patients who have received a 12-lead ECG within the last 12–18 months may not require a new study, depending on the severity and stability of the patient's health and risk factors. Significant findings on a preoperative ECG may include evidence of ischemia, left ventricular hypertrophy, arrhythmias, conductions blocks, previous myocardial infarction, or the presence of a pacemaker. It is advisable for patients who present with novel, significant ECG findings immediately prior to the start of a dental procedure/anesthetic to seek reevaluation prior to continuing treatment. This is especially true for patients with existing comorbidities, with significant risk factors, or whose new ECG findings vary greatly from previous ECG results. Should a new study be indicated, the patient should be sent to his primary care provider or possibly referred to a cardiologist for evaluation, depending on the situation.

Additional studies

There currently exist several methodologies used to identify the presence and severity of cardiovascular diseases that could potentially affect the perioperative management of dental patients. Some common examples of available studies include transthoracic or transesophageal echocardiogram (TTE or TEE), stress tests, and cardiac catheterization.

An echocardiogram provides a structural image of the heart and surrounding structures using an ultrasound probe, placed in the esophagus or outside the chest wall. Echocardiograms also provide information relating to ejection fraction (EF), valve function, wall motions, flow disturbances during contraction and relaxation, along with several other clinical abnormalities (pulmonary hypertension, flow disturbances, etc.). Normal EFs range from 55–70%. An EF below 40% may require modifications in the surgical and/or anesthetic plan (Stoelting et al., 2008). Reductions in EF indicate damage and/or impairment of the myocardium to effectively pump blood, possible due to previous infarction or cardiomyopathy.

Stress tests are commonly utilized preoperatively to identify patients in whom a previously identified comorbidity (e.g. coronary artery disease) may predispose the patient for perioperative complications. Stress tests commonly include either an exercise (treadmill) or pharmacologic (dobutamine or adenosine) component, depending on the presence of other health concerns (severe osteoarthritis, claudications, lower extremity amputations, etc.). The classic finding with stress testing is ST segment changes. ST depression indicates subendocardial ischemia, and testing enhances our ability to diagnose coronary artery disease. Information obtained from the stress test includes peak heart rate and blood pressure, depth, morphology, and persistence of ST segment depression. This added information gives anesthesia providers insight pertaining to the patient's ability to respond to and handle stress related to the planned procedure. When combined with an echocardiogram or other studies used to visualize cardiac function and/or coronary arterial flow, stress tests can provide detailed information about myocardial differences both at rest and during exertion.

Radionucleotide tests and cardiac catheterizations are more invasive studies performed by cardiologists to further evaluate cardiac abnormalities. Radionucleotide angiography involves intravenous administration of radioactive materials (e.g., Thallium 201) during cardiovascular imaging in order to visualize areas of ischemia, infarction, or other abnormalities. Imaging will increase sensitivity and specificity when combined with stress test results. Commonly performed in conjunction with cardiac catheterization, these imaging studies can provide extremely accurate information about cardiac function. Dental anesthesia providers who are treating medically compromised patients, usually with a history of cardiovascular or pulmonary disease, can request the results of any previous studies. A consultation with the patient's cardiologist is also recommended in order to further evaluate the patient's underlying medical conditions and augment the planned procedures accordingly.

References

American Society of Anesthesiologists Task Force on Preanesthesia Evaluation. Practice Advisory for preanesthesia evaluation: a report. *Anesthesiol* **96**: 485–496, 2002.

Dubin, D. *Rapid Interpretation of EKG's: An Interactive Course*. Tampa: Cover Publishing Co., 2000.

Fattahi, T. Perioperative laboratory and diagnostic testing – what is needed and when? *Oral Maxillofac Surg Clin Am* **18**: 1–6, 2006.

Faust, R. J. and Cucchiara, R. F. *Anesthesiology Review*. New York: Churchill Livingstone, 2002.

Giannakopoulos, H., et al. Fluid and electrolyte management and blood product usage. *Oral Maxillofac Clin N Am* **18**: 7–17, 2006.

Kumar, A. and Srivastava, U. Role of routine laboratroy investigations in preoperative evaluation. *J Anaesthesiol Clin Pharmacol* **27**: 174–179, 2011.

Munro, J., et al. Routine preoperative testing: a systematic review of the evidence. *Health Technol Assess* **12**: 1–2, 1997.

Pasternak, L. R. Preoperative screening for ambulatory patients. *Anesthesiol Clin North America* **21**: 229–42, vii., 2003.

Richman, D. C. Ambulatory surgery: how much testing do we need? *Anesthesiol Clin* **28**: 185–97, 2010.

Stoelting, R. K., et al. *Stoelting's Anesthesia and Co-exisiting disease*. Philadelphia: Churchill Livingstone/Elsevier, 2008.

Stoelting, R. K. and Miller, R. D. *Basics of Anesthesia*. Philadelphia: Churchill Livingstone, 2007.

Tintinalli, J. E. and Stapczynski, J. S. *Tintinalli's Emergency Medicine: a Comprehensive Study Guide*, 7th edn. New York: McGraw-Hill, 2011.

4 NPO guidelines

Kyle Kramer[1] and Jeffrey Bennett[2]
[1]Indiana University, Indianapolis, IN, USA
[2]Indiana University, Department of Oral Surgery and Hospital Dentistry, Indianapolis, IN, USA

The concept of preoperative fasting prior to a patient receiving sedation or anesthesia for elective procedures, including dentistry, has been around since the 1850s (Maltby, 2006). NPO orders were initially given to reduce the likelihood of postoperative nausea and vomiting, which was considered rather unpleasant. Progression into the modern medical age brought forth the belief that a prolonged fasting period would favorably alter the pH and volume of gastric contents, thus reducing the risk of pulmonary complications should aspiration occur. Roberts and Shirley (1974) addressed critical pH and gastric volume as risk factors for complications stemming from pulmonary aspiration. They extrapolated data from animal studies utilizing rhesus monkeys and stated that adult female patients with residual gastric volumes consisting of 0.4 mL/kg or 25 mL of gastric juice with a pH below 2.5 were likely to have respiratory complications should aspiration of gastric contents occur. They disclosed several years later that they instilled the entire volume directly into the monkey's right mainstem bronchus rather than stimulating regurgitation. The initial study from 1974 therefore failed to establish a direct relationship between residual gastric volume and the volume of aspirated material. Nonetheless, these "critical values" quickly became anesthesia dogma. This paved the way for the common "NPO after midnight" guidelines. This dogmatic approach has been successfully challenged and refuted in recent years.

A multitude of clinical research articles have demonstrated the fallacy that prolonged fasting would lead to decreased residual gastric volumes and increased gastric pH. In 2003, 2005, and 2009 (Brady), the Cochrane database compiled a review of randomized and quasi-randomized clinical trials specifically evaluating the preoperative fasting guidelines for adults and children. Regarding gastric volume or pH, there was no evidence that pediatric patients with a prolonged preoperative fasting period of 6 hours or more had any benefit when compared to those receiving unlimited clear liquids up to 2 hours preoperatively (Brady, 2005, 2009). In adults, not only was there no benefit, patients who were permitted clear liquids up to 2 hours preoperatively actually had significantly *lower* gastric volumes (Brady et al., 2003). Of note, however, is the lack of research on patient populations deemed at high risk for aspiration.

The current ASA guidelines (Table 4.1) discuss preoperative fasting for clear liquids, breast milk, infant formula, nonhuman milk, and solids (Practice Guidelines, 2011). These guidelines are not intended for patients with any increased risk factors for regurgitation and/or pulmonary aspiration (Table 4.2). Patients with comorbidities impacting normal gastric physiologic function may require NPO guideline adjustments in addition to the utilization of appropriate adjunctive treatment modalities to lessen aspiration risk.

Clear liquids

Clear liquids empty at a rapid rate dependent primarily on the pressure gradient between the duodenum and the stomach. The emptying halftime is approximately 10–20 minutes, which results in 90% of the volume being passed within 1 hour and complete passage after 2 hours (Maltby, 2006; Hellstrom et al., 2006). Clear liquids include water, carbonated beverages, fruit juice without pulp, and black coffee or tea. Alcohol, while a clear liquid, is not permitted (Practice guidelines, 2011). The ASA guidelines do not discuss the allowable volume of clear liquids, only that they must be held at least 2 hours preoperatively for patients scheduled to undergo sedation or anesthesia. Preoperative oral medications taken with a small amount of water within the 2-hour window are not considered violations of NPO status and are permissible.

Breast milk and infant formula

Guidelines state that breast milk is allowed up to 4 hours preoperatively while infant formula must be held at least 6 hours preoperatively (Practice guidelines, 2011). Clearly, these recommendations are typically pertinent for a select patient population (infants, neonates, etc.) and may not be applicable for the typical dental patient receiving sedation/anesthesia.

Solid foods and nonhuman milk

While solid foods are permitted up to 6 hours prior to surgery, the ASA guidelines discuss limiting the solids to a light meal, consisting of dry toast and clear liquids. Nonhuman milk, when consumed and mixed with gastric fluid, congeals into a semisolid mass and should be considered a solid rather than a liquid (Maltby, 2006). The rate at which solid foods and nonhuman milk pass from the stomach into the small intestine differs drastically from that of clear liquids. Additional factors of importance to the rate of gastric emptying include the volume of food ingested, type of food, and the size of the ingested particles. Liquids, semisolids, and solids smaller than 2 mm in diameter pass from the stomach initially in a linear manner. The pyloric sphincter prevents particles smaller than 2 mm from easily passing from the stomach, first requiring further digestion

Anesthesia Complications in the Dental Office, First Edition. Edited by Robert C. Bosack and Stuart Lieblich.

Table 4.1 Current ASA NPO guidelines (Practice Guidelines, 2011).

Substance	NPO recommendation (hours)	Examples
Clear liquids	2	Water, black coffee, tea, juice without pulp
Breast milk	4	
Non-human milk	6	Baby formula
Light breakfast	6	Dry toast with black coffee
Fatty foods	8+	Bacon, eggs, milk, cream, butter

and breakdown into a smaller passable size. This process can take as long as 4 hours to complete (Maltby, 2006; Hellstrom et al., 2006). Indigestible solids, such as fat and cellulose-containing vegetables, may not be broken down further and require additional time to pass from the stomach. Only after the stomach is empty of all other passable (<2 mm) substances does the process of actively passing the indigestible material begin. This may take well beyond 8 hours to complete (Maltby, 2006).

Preoperative therapeutics

Historically, a variety of approaches have been implemented to reduce complications stemming from perioperative pulmonary aspiration. Measures have included pharmacotherapeutics such as antacids, gastric prokinetics, proton pump inhibitors (PPIs), and histamine blockers. In addition, protective anesthetic techniques include cricoid pressure (Sellick's maneuver, Sellick, 1961), rapid sequence induction, and awake fiberoptic intubations. Several of these treatment modalities are summarized in Table 4.3.

Antacids

The rationale behind the use of antacids is to neutralize the acidic environment of the gastric contents. By ingesting the basic salt compounds contained within the various antacid formulations, the gastric pH is raised. This reduces the risk of possible damage, should aspiration of gastric contents occur. Available antacids include both insoluble, particulate (aluminum or magnesium hydroxide) and soluble, nonparticulate (sodium citrate or sodium bicarbonate) formulations. Particulate matter, if aspirated, is capable of producing localized inflammation and tissue damage, potentially equal to that produced by aspiration of acidic gastric fluid (Apfel and Roewer, 2005; Morgan et al., 2006). As such, the use of particulate antacids is no longer encouraged, and is replaced instead with nonparticulate antacid solutions (Apfel and Roewer, 2005). Moreover, nonparticulate solutions are more effective than particulate antacids, primarily due to increased ease of mixing with gastric fluid (Morgan et al., 2006). Preoperative administration of antacid solutions, such as sodium citrate (BiCitra), is recommended only for patients with an increased risk of aspiration (Apfel and Roewer, 2005).

Gastric prokinetics

The prototypical gastric prokinetic (gastrointestinal stimulant) used today is metoclopramide (Reglan®), a dopamine antagonist (Faust and Cucchiara, 2002). Preoperative administration of metoclopramide is thought to promote gastric motility and emptying, thus reducing the volume of residual gastric contents (Page, 2002). As a dopamine antagonist, metoclopramide administration may be associated with several notable complications including akathisia, oculogyric crisis, muscle spasms, and other extrapyramidal effects. Gastrointestinal stimulants are contraindicated in patients with bowel obstruction and are associated with an increased risk of cramping (Faust and Cucchiara, 2002). Use of metoclopramide is typically reserved only for patients deemed at increased risk of

Table 4.2 Patients at high risk for pulmonary aspiration.

Disease process	Pathophysiology	Possible adjunctive therapy
Diabetes	Gastroparesis, delayed gastric emptying	Prolonged NPO duration, gastric prokinetic
Bowel obstruction	Impaired peristalsis	Prolonged NPO duration, preoperative gastric suction
Pregnancy	↑Intra-abdominal pressure	Prolonged NPO duration
Obesity	Impairment of lower esophageal sphincter ↓pH and ↑volume of gastric fluid	Avoid supine position Nonparticulate antacid PPI, H2 blocker
GERD, acid reflux	Incompetent lower esophageal sphincter	Prolonged NPO duration PPI, H_2 blocker Avoid supine position
Peptic ulcer disease	↓pH and ↑volume of gastric fluid	Nonparticulate antacid PPI, H_2 blocker
Pain Severe anxiety Narcotic use/abuse	Delayed gastric emptying	Prolonged NPO duration Gastric prokinetic
Trauma or emergency patients	Possible full stomach, delayed gastric emptying (pain)	Gastric prokinetic Nonparticulate antacid PPI, H_2 blocker Postpone procedure?
Cerebral palsy Multiple sclerosis Paralysis	Musculoskeletal impairment Dysphagia Impairment of airway reflexes	Prolonged NPO duration Nonparticulate antacid PPI, H2 blocker

Note: Patients at high risk for pulmonary aspiration may not be appropriate for office-based sedation and may require advanced anesthesia management (i.e. rapid sequence induction and intubation, awake fiberoptic intubation)

Table 4.3 Treatment options for patients at risk for aspiration.

Modality	Comment
Antacids	Not recommended for low risk patients
PPIs	Clinical effects may require sufficient
H2 blockers	time after administration
Gastric prokinetics	
Gastric suction	NG/OG tube placement requires advanced training and equipment
Cricoid pressure (Sellick's maneuver)	Reserved for rapid sequence induction and intubation
	Does not halt active regurgitation
Rapid sequence induction and intubation	Requires advanced anesthesia training
Awake fiberoptic intubation	

regurgitation and pulmonary aspiration. Current evidence and guidelines do not promote the routine use of metoclopramide preoperatively for low risk patients (Practice Guidelines, 2011). However, if deemed appropriate, these medications do require sufficient time to work. As such, they should be given early in the preoperative period, ideally 15–30 minutes prior to induction, depending on the route administered (Faust and Cucchiara, 2002; Morgan et al., 2006).

PPIs and H_2 blockers

While these medications are typically used to manage symptomatic gastroesophageal reflux disease (GERD), they can also be useful for reducing the risk of complications from pulmonary aspiration. PPIs function by irreversibly inhibiting the H^+/K^+-dependent ATPase proton pumps located within the gastric parietal cells (Page, 2002; Neidle et al., 2004). H_2 blockers are reversible, competitive antagonists that work selectively on gastric parietal cell histamine-2 (H_2) receptors (Page, 2002; Neidle et al., 2004). Both PPIs and H_2 antagonists produce a decrease in acid secretion by the parietal cells, which increases the gastric pH. Patients currently on PPI or H_2 therapy should be advised to continue use throughout the perioperative period. Elective use in the preoperative periods for patients deemed at higher risk for pulmonary aspiration is appropriate, but requires sufficient time for maximum effectiveness. The routine administration of PPIs and H_2 antagonists in patients at low risk of pulmonary aspiration undergoing sedation or anesthesia is not recommended (Practice Guidelines, 2011).

Cricoid pressure

In 1961, Sellick originally described success in preventing the reflux of gastric contents by applying posterior pressure to the cricoid, effectively "sealing off" the esophagus (Sellick, 1961). Ideally, cricoid pressure should be applied immediately prior to induction and maintained until successful intubation has been confirmed and the risk of aspiration negated (Morgan et al., 2006; Stoelting and Miller, 2007). The recommended amount of pressure to utilize has been described as 30–40 N (10 N = 1 kg of force). Ideally, pressure should be applied lightly (~10 N) while the patient is conscious, and then increased (30–40 N) once the patient is unconscious (Ovassapian and Salem, 2009). Despite the current widespread use of cricoid pressure during rapid sequence inductions for patients deemed to be at high risk for aspiration, this remains a controversial technique mainly due to the lack of conclusive data stemming from the difficulty designing ethical clinical research evaluating the prevention of aspiration while applying cricoid pressure (Lerman, 2009; El-Orbany and Connolly, 2010).

Summary

Current NPO guidelines are presented to help reduce the risk of perioperative complications, specifically regurgitation and pulmonary aspiration. These guidelines have recently undergone review and significant revision when compared with the traditional "nothing by mouth after midnight." However, strict adherence does not relieve the anesthesia provider of all responsibility. Prudent anesthesia providers must evaluate each patient and *tailor* the guidelines accordingly to achieve maximal results regarding perioperative safety and patient comfort. Determining appropriate NPO guidelines for each patient and relaying the particular information to the patient preoperatively is a crucial step in the development of an anesthetic plan for all dental anesthesia providers. Failure to adhere to the recommended guidelines may put the patient at risk for intraoperative complications. Therefore, it is also imperative that the clinician be able to relay the importance of following the preoperative NPO instructions. Although strategies such as the use of antacids and prokinetics for patients at a higher risk of aspiration have been reviewed, consideration of these interventions may caution the provider that a secured airway may be indicated, that is, endotracheal intubation with a cuffed tube.

References

Apfel, C. C. and Roewer, N. Ways to prevent and great pulmonary aspiration of gastric contents. *Curr Opin Anaesthesiol* **18**: 157–162, 2005.

Brady, M., et al. Preoperative fasting for preventing perioperative complications in children. *Cochrane Database Syst Rev*, CD005285, 2009.

Brady, M., et al. Preoperative fasting for preventing perioperative complications in children. *Cochrane Database Syst Rev*, CD005285, 2005.

Brady, M., et al. Preoperative fasting for adults to prevent perioperative complications. *Cochrane Database Syst Rev*, CD004423, 2003.

El-Orbany, M. and Connolly, L. A. Rapid sequence induction and intubation: current controversy. *Anesth Analg* **110**: 1318–1325, 2010.

Faust, R. J. and Cucchiara, R. F. *Anesthesiology Review*. New York: Churchill Livingstone, 2002.

Hellstrom, P. M., et al. The physiology of gastric emptying. *Best Pract Res Clin Anaesthesiol* **20**: 397–407, 2006.

Lerman, J. On cricoid pressure: "May the force be with you." *Anesth Analg* **109**: 1363–1366, 2009.

Maltby, J. R. Fasting from midnight - the story behind the dogma. *Best Pracxt REs Clin Anaesthesiol* **20**: 363–378, 2006.

Morgan, G. E., et al. *Clinical Anesthesiology*. New York: Lange Medical Books/McGraw Hill, 2006.

Neidle, E. A., et al. *Pharmacology and therapeutics for dentistry*. St. Louis: Mosby, 2004.

Ovassapian, A. and Salem, M. R. Sellick's maneuver: to do or not do. *Anesth Analg* **109**: 1360–1362, 2009.

Page, C. P. *Integrated Pharmacology*. Edinburgh: Mosby, 2002.

American Society of Anesthesiologists Committee on Standards and Practice Parameters Practice guidelines for preoperative fasting and the use of pharmacologic agents to reduce the risk of pulmonary aspiration: application to healthy patients undergoing elective procedures. An updated report. *Anesthesiol* **114**: 495–511, 2011.

Roberts, R. B. and Shirley, M. A. Reducing the risk of acid aspriation during cesarean section. *Anesth Analg* **53**: 859–868, 1974.

Sellick, B. A. Cricoid pressure to control regurgitation of stomach contents during induction of anaesthesia. *Lancet* **2**: 404–406, 1961.

Stoelting, R. K. and Miller, R. D. *Basics of Anesthesia*. Philidelphia: Churchill Livingstone, 2007.

SECTION 3

Anesthetic considerations for special patients

5 Anesthetic considerations for patients with cardiovascular disease

Erik Anderson[1] and Robert Bosack[2]
[1]Oregon Health Sciences University, Department of Anesthesiology and Peri Operative Medicine, Portland, OR, USA
[2]University of Illinois, College of Dentistry, Chicago, IL, USA

Introduction

Advances in modern medicine have allowed many patients with cardiovascular disease to lead normal and productive lives. What remains in stark contrast, unfortunately, is the changing canvas of the American way: sedentary lifestyle, poor dietary choices, smoking, and alcohol consumption, which contribute to increased incidence of obesity, diabetes, and cardiovascular disease. A clinical understanding of the pathophysiology and treatment options for common cardiovascular diseases (hypertension, coronary artery disease (CAD), valvulopathy, cardiac rhythm disorders, and heart failure) facilitates risk stratification. Although pathologic processes will be considered separately, such delineations are impossible in clinical practice.

The cardiovascular system serves as a transport system to deliver nutrients (oxygen and glucose) to cells and remove waste products (carbon dioxide and metabolic by-products.) The system consists of the heart (cardiac muscle, coronary blood supply, valves, and electrical conduction system) and the peripheral vasculature (with musculoelastic walls to maintain pressure and direct blood flow). Dysfunction in any component can eventually result in decreased forward flow and reduced oxygen delivery: chest pain, dizziness, dyspnea, exercise intolerance, or fatigue; and/or volume backup in the lungs and peripheral circulation: shortness of breath and peripheral edema.

Systemic blood pressure (see Figure 5.1) is regulated by cardiac output (heart rate × stroke volume) and systemic vascular resistance. Stroke volume (SV) is assessed by echocardiographically measuring the ejection fraction. At the end of diastole, the left ventricle contains a volume of blood. At the end of systole, a certain fraction of that blood volume is ejected into the systemic circulation. This fraction, calculated by dividing the SV by the end diastolic volume (EDV), is called the *ejection fraction*. A normal EF is approximately 55–75%.

$$EF = \frac{SV}{EDV}$$

Heart rate, SV, and vascular resistance are modulated by the autonomic nervous system (rapid). Blood volume and vascular resistance are modulated by the kidney (delayed and rapid). The sympathetic nervous system increases the heart rate (direct action at the sinoatrial and atrioventricular node), increases the strength of cardiac contraction (β_1-cardiac receptors), dilates skeletal muscle blood vessels (β_2-vascular receptors), and constricts peripheral blood vessels (α_1-vascular receptors), as would be expected in a "fight or flight" situation (Table 5.1). The parasympathetic nervous system slows down the heart rate by direct action at the sinoatrial node and atrioventricular node, but does not innervate the vasculature. The kidney regulates blood pressure by sensing hypotension, which triggers the release of renin, stimulating the production of angiotensin II, a powerful vasoconstrictor (immediate effect). Angiotensin II also stimulates the release of aldosterone, which promotes retention of salt and water (delayed effect).

Coronary perfusion occurs during diastole and is driven by diastolic aortic pressure. Ventricular wall tension, filling pressures, and atherosclerotic hardening and narrowing of the coronary arteries also affect coronary blood flow. Faster heart rates tend to limit the time spent in diastole, and hence coronary perfusion. Hypertension and tachycardia, resulting from the neuroendocrine stress response from inadequate anesthesia during surgery thus becomes a double insult.

Hypertension and/or narrowing of valves or blood vessels increases afterload (resistance to blood flow), which increases the pressure work done by the heart. Sustained increases in afterload eventually lead to *cardiac muscle hypertrophy* accompanied by a resultant decrease in chamber size, inability to relax fully (diastolic dysfunction), and a thick muscle that can outgrow its blood supply, making it more susceptible to ischemia. This is in comparison to *cardiac dilatation*, secondary to fluid overload (increased volume work) due to valvular regurgitation or extrinsic insult, where the chamber tends to get lax and limited in its ability to contract and expel its blood volume (systolic dysfunction). It is important to note that pressure work (increased afterload, stenotic valves) is metabolically more costly and therefore more worrisome than volume work (increased preload, valvular regurgitation).

Anesthesia Complications in the Dental Office, First Edition. Edited by Robert C. Bosack and Stuart Lieblich.

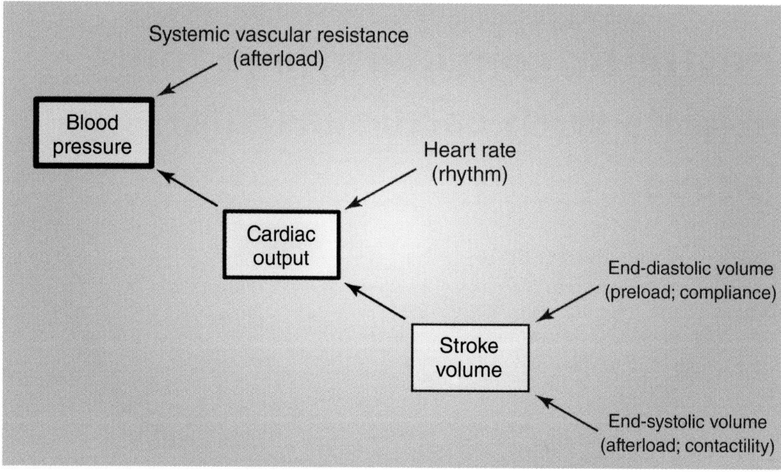

Figure 5.1 Determinants of blood pressure.

Table 5.1 The sympathetic nervous system—"fight or flight".

- α_1 - peripheral vasoconstriction
- β_1 - increased heart rate and force of contraction
- β_2 - skeletal muscle vasodilation, bronchiolar dilation

Table 5.2 Blood pressure classification (Chobanian et al., 2003).

Classification	Systolic (mmHg)		Diastolic (mmHg)
Normal	< 120	and	< 80
Prehypertension	120–139	or	80–89
Stage I hypertension	140–159	or	90–99
Stage II hypertension	≥ 160	or	≥ 100

Hypertension

Definition

Hypertension is arbitrarily defined as a sustained increase in arterial blood pressure greater than 140 mmHg systolic or 90 mmHg diastolic (Chobanian et al., 2003; Table 5.2). Approximately one-third of adults in the United States are considered hypertensive, with this number likely to grow as the population ages and the prevalence of obesity increases. Unfortunately, only a limited percentage of hypertensive patients are adequately controlled because of factors such as poor access to care (undiagnosed disease) and suboptimal medication adherence for a symptomless disease, secondary to cost or adverse side effects of drugs. Risk factors for the development of hypertension include genetic predisposition, excess salt and/or alcohol consumption, obesity, aging, inactivity, dyslipidemia, and African-American heritage. Hypertension (especially systolic) is a primary and powerful risk factor for atherosclerosis and cardiovascular disease, including acute myocardial infarction, heart failure, renal failure, aortic aneurysm, and stroke. The degree of risk appears to be directly related to the severity of hypertension. The goal of antihypertensive therapy is to reduce the incidence or severity of these diseases.

Primary essential hypertension (95%) often starts insidiously and is idiopathic, although there are attempts to implicate factors such as increased sympathetic tone, increased angiotensin II activity, overproduction of Na^+-retaining hormones, high Na^+ intake, or deficiency of endogenous vasodilators, among others. Secondary hypertension (5%) has an identifiable cause, oftentimes presenting more abruptly, as seen in cases of renal artery stenosis, pheochromocytoma, Cushing's syndrome, sleep apnea, drugs, and coarctation (narrowing) of the aorta, among others. Correction of the causative disease resolves secondary hypertension.

Hypertensive crises refer to pressure elevations greater than 180 mmHg systolic and/or 110 mmHg diastolic. Urgencies (no evidence of target organ damage) can be asymptomatic or associated with vague symptoms such as headache, nosebleed, or shortness of breath. Hypertensive emergencies can present with chest pain, neurologic deficit, retinal hemorrhage, or papilledema. Peripheral or pulmonary edema can present with concomitant heart failure.

Pathophysiology

Although causality is difficult to prove, it is thought that hypertension exposes conduit vessels to repeated pulsatile stress. This can lead to dilation, stiffening, endothelial dysfunction, atherosclerosis, plaque fatigue, and fracture with subsequent thrombosis (MI, stroke, cerebrovascular event). Sustained hypertension increases afterload, which, over time, can provoke ominous left ventricular hypertrophy and resultant ischemia, dysrhythmia, and heart failure.

Diagnosis of this usually asymptomatic disease is made with serial blood pressure measurements over two or more visits. Accurate pressures are measured with patients sitting, back supported, arm held passively at heart level with a properly sized cuff that covers 80% of the upper arm. Cuffs that are too small can falsely elevate systolic pressures by up to 50 mmHg. Blood pressures measured at the wrist can falsely elevate systolic and reduce diastolic measurements. Blood pressures measured in the immediate preanesthetic period are often elevated due to stress levels associated with the dental visit. Not knowing a "true" baseline pressure blurs treatment goals during the acute management of pressure disorders during anesthesia.

Cardiovascular risk assessment proceeds with a search for a history of smoking, and presence of obesity, inactivity, diabetes mellitus, kidney disease, family history, and dyslipidemia. Medical work-up involves a search for secondary causes as well as a determination of the existence or extent of target organ damage – eyes, kidney, heart (heart failure, CAD, left ventricular hypertrophy), brain (stroke, TIA), and peripheral blood vessels (claudication—exercise-induced pain, cramping, or tired feeling in the legs).

Treatment

Satisfactory treatment of hypertension is associated with a 25% reduction in the incidence of major cardiovascular events (stroke, heart failure, myocardial infarction) (Turnbull et al., 2008). Primary hypertension is managed initially with lifestyle modification, followed by antihypertensive medication if needed. Lifestyle changes include salt restriction, weight loss, diet modification (fruits, vegetables, whole grains, beans, fish, poultry, saturated fat restriction), exercise, limited alcohol consumption, and smoking cessation.

If necessary, the goal of further medical management is to consistently achieve blood pressure readings less than 150/90 mmHg in patients over the age of 60 and less than 140/90 mmHg for all other patients (James et al. 2014) with one or more antihypertensive agents. These agents are also useful in the treatment of myocardial dysfunction, left ventricular hypertrophy, heart failure, and some types of renal disease. Beta-adrenergic blockers have a wider range of indications, but have fallen out of favor for the treatment of isolated hypertension because of adverse side effects. There are five major classes (Table 5.3) of frequently used antihypertensive agents. The list of combination drugs is continually growing.

Diuretics

Diuretics are often the first line therapy for the treatment of hypertension. Drugs in this class include thiazides (hydrochlorothiazide and chlorthalidone), loop diuretics (furosemide), potassium-sparing diuretics (amiloride, triamterene), and aldosterone antagonists (spironolactone.) Diuretics are the mainstay in the treatment of both hypertension and heart failure. Diuretics enhance the renal tubular elimination of sodium and water. Initially, diuretics lower blood pressure by reducing intravascular volume, but this action is not sustained. They work well in combination with other antihypertensive agents and are thought to activate vascular endothelial channels to reduce systemic vascular resistance. Side effects of diuretics include hypotension, potassium and magnesium depletion, hyperkalemia (with potassium-sparing drugs), and impaired glucose tolerance with insulin resistance. Both orthostatic hypotension (dizziness upon standing upright) and hypovolemia remain clinical concerns. Excess plasma potassium (also associated with ACE inhibitors, ARBS and β-blockers) is usually excreted in the urine. Diuretics are one of only a few drug classes that can be withheld prior to anesthesia in NPO patients who are already volume depleted.

Angiotensin-Converting Enzyme (ACE) Inhibitors

ACE inhibitors block the formation of angiotensin II, which is both a potent vasoconstrictor and a trigger for aldosterone-mediated sodium and water retention. These drugs prolong survival in patients with heart failure with left ventricular dysfunction, reduce overall mortality in high risk patients, and are considered "renoprotective" in patients with diabetes mellitus and nephropathy. These drugs end in "-pril." Examples include captopril, enalapril, lisinopril, ramipril, fosinopril, quinapril, benazepril, and trandolapril. Side effects include hypotension, hyperkalemia (especially with K^+ sparing diuretics), dry cough, loss of taste, and angioedema (Stojiljkovic, 2012), especially of the face and mouth (Chiu et al., 2001) (Figure 5.2). Interestingly, ACE inhibitors, ARBS, and β-blockers are frequently less effective in African-American patients.

Table 5.3 Commonly prescribed drugs for the treatment of hypertension

Drug class	Category	Generic name	Trade name™
Diuretics	Thiazides	Hydrochlorothiazide	Hydrodiuril
		Chlorthalidone	Hygrotin
	Loop	Furosemide	Lasix
	K^+ sparing	Amiloride	Midamor
		Triamterene	Dyrenium
	Aldosterone antagonist	Spironolactone	Aldactone
ACE inhibitors		Captopril	Capoten
		Enalopril	Vasotec
		Lisinopril	Zestril, Prinivil
		Ramipril	Altace
		Fosinopril	Monopril
		Quinapril	Accupril
		Benazepril	Lotensin
		Trandolapril	Mavik
Angiotensin receptors blockers		Losartan	Cozaar
		Candesartan	Atacand
		Irbesartan	Avapro
		Valsartan	Diovan
		Olmesartan	Benicar
		Telmisartan	Micardis
		Eprosartan	Teveten
β-blockers	Non-cardioselective	Labetolol	Normodyne
		Carvedilol	Coreg
		Propranolol	Inderal
		Nadolol	Corgard
		Timolol	Blockadren
		Pindolol	Visken
	β1 cardioselective	Bisoprolol	Zebeta
		Atenolol	Tenormin
		Metoprolol	Lopressor
		Acebutolol	Sectral
		Betazolol	Kerlone
		Esmolol	Breviblock
Calcium channel blockers	Dihydopyridines	Nifedipine	Procardia
		Amlodipine	Norvasc
		Felodipine	Plendil
		Isradipine	Dynacirc
		Nicardipine	Cardene
		Clevidipine	Cleviprex
	non-Dihydopyridines	Verapamil	Isoptin, Calan
		Diltiazem	Cardizem

Angiotensin Receptor Blockers (ARBs)

ARBs block the AT1 receptor, which mediates the vasoconstrictive effects of angiotensin II. ARBS are considered as effective as ACE inhibitors with fewer and milder side effects; however, hypotension and hyperkalemia still remain possibilities. These drugs end in "-sartan." Examples include losartan, candesartan, irbesartan, valsartan, olmesartan, telmisartan, and eprosartan.

Beta-adrenergic blockers

β-blockers can be useful in the management of hypertension in patients who have other indications for β-blockade, such as angina or migraine, but their isolated use for the initial treatment of hypertension has fallen out of favor, due in part to adverse side effects. They are indicated for treatment of CAD, tachydysrhythmias, tremor, thyrotoxicosis, and neurocardiogenic syncope. β-blockade can be nonspecific or β_1-selective. β_1-receptor blockade decreases

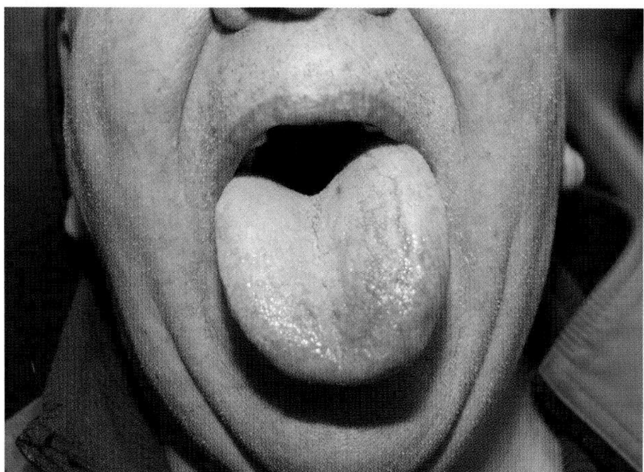

Figure 5.2 Angioedema of the left tongue in a patient taking an ACE inhibitor, 24 hours after routine dental extraction with local anesthesia. This patient was urgently admitted to an intensive care unit for airway monitoring.

heart rate and contractility, thereby reducing oxygen demand and consumption. The decrease in rate also prolongs diastolic coronary perfusion time, which improves cardiac oxygen delivery. Blood pressure is decreased, in part due to a reduction in cardiac output, and by other mechanisms, which have yet to be fully elucidated. β_1-blockade also reduces renin secretion, which inhibits the formation of the vasoconstrictive angiotensin II. β_2-receptor blockade interferes with skeletal muscle vasodilation and can cause bronchiolar constriction, especially in susceptible patients. This leaves α_1 vasoconstriction unopposed and can lead to coronary spasm and aggravation of Raynaud's peripheral vasoconstriction and other forms of peripheral vascular disease.

Labetolol and carvedilol are non-selective β-blockers with some α-adrenergic blocking activity. Labetolol is useful for hypertensive emergencies in patients without bronchospastic disease.

Non-cardioselective β-blockers include propranolol, nadolol, timolol, and pindolol. Pindolol possesses some "intrinsic" sympathomimetic activity, which attenuates the β-blockade to minimize peripheral vasoconstriction while causing less of a decline in heart rate.

Cardioselective (β_1) blockers include bisoprolol, atenolol, metoprolol, acebutolol, betaxolol, and esmolol. These drugs have a diminished β_2-blocking action when used in lower doses; selectivity diminishes with increasing dose.

In addition to the side effects discussed previously, β-blockade can trigger or exacerbate heart failure, bradycardia, heart block, hyperkalemia, and peripheral vascular disease. B-blockade can also facilitate hypoglycemia and attenuate the associated norepinephrine-induced signs including sweating and anxiety. Depression, weight gain, fatigue, and sexual dysfunction can also occur with the use of β-blockers.

Calcium channel blockers (CCBs)

As their name implies, CCBs block the inward movement of Ca^{++} ions across cell membranes. This confers several advantages to the use of this heterogeneous group of medications. These drugs inhibit the action potentials (contractility) of vascular smooth muscle cells, cardiac muscle cells, and nodal pacemakers, which results in vasodilation, decreased cardiac contractility, and decreased heart rate, respectively. Vasodilation improves coronary blood flow and decreases both preload and afterload by lowering blood pressure. The decrease in both inotropy (contractility) and chronotropy (heart rate) decreases myocardial oxygen demand. There are two classes of CCBs: the dihyropyridines, which are used primarily as vasodilators, and the non-dihydropyridines, which are used primarily to lower heart rates. Dihyropyridines (end in "-pine") include nifedipine, amlodipine, felodipine, isradipine, nicardipine, and clevidipine. Non-dihydropyridines include verapamil and diltiazem.

Risk assessment

Risk assessment explores the likelihood of undesirable consequences of a planned action (severity, duration and tolerability). It begins with a thorough history, based on interview, and is supplemented with a written questionnaire. Patients who are already diagnosed and aware of their hypertension should be questioned about their adequacy of control, adherence to medication, side effects of the medication, and recent changes in dose or drug. Blood pressure should be measured preoperatively with an appropriately sized cuff, seating the patient with back supported and arm at heart level. Often times, pre-procedural readings are higher due to anxiety and attendant increased sympathetic outflow. In this instance, a concomitant elevation in heart rate is often noted.

Optimization of the patient's health, including treatment of hypertension, is a priority before any surgical or anesthetic intervention. Although mild to moderate hypertension is not considered a risk factor for office-based anesthesia (Royster et al., 2011), intraoperative blood pressure swings are commonly seen in these patients, regardless of the level of pressure control (Goldman and Caldera, 1979). Prys-Roberts et al. (1971), Roizen and Fleisher (2010), and many others have noted that in the absence of comorbidities, patients with preanesthetic pressures as high as 180/110 mmHg with a normal sinus rhythm should be able to tolerate these levels during a well-conducted anesthetic that minimizes further increases in blood pressure or increases in heart rate. Measurements above this level often invite significant intraoperative pressure swings.

There are three distinct risks of treating patients with hypertension: the risk of further increasing the blood pressure with either anesthesia or surgery, the risk of decreasing the blood pressure leading to hypoperfusion of critical organs and the risk of increasing heart rate in the presence of hypertension, drastically increasing oxygen demand. In addition to surgical bleeding, increases in blood pressure augment both preload and afterload, increasing myocardial oxygen demand and inviting ischemia in patients with preexisting CAD. In rare instances, severe, rapid, and/or sustained increases in blood pressure can cause rupture of compromised vasculature, leading to end-organ ischemia (stroke). Pressure decreases in hypertensive patients, which can occur during the administration of many anesthetic agents, exposes critical organs to the risk of hypoperfusion, as blood flow becomes dependent on higher pressures. This is graphically depicted in the flow–pressure autoregulation curve, which shifts to the right in patients with preexisting hypertension (Figure 5.3). Tachycardia decreases the time for diastolic coronary perfusion, which decreases myocardial oxygen supply. The presence of these risks gives clear reason to optimize blood pressures prior to anesthetic or surgical intervention.

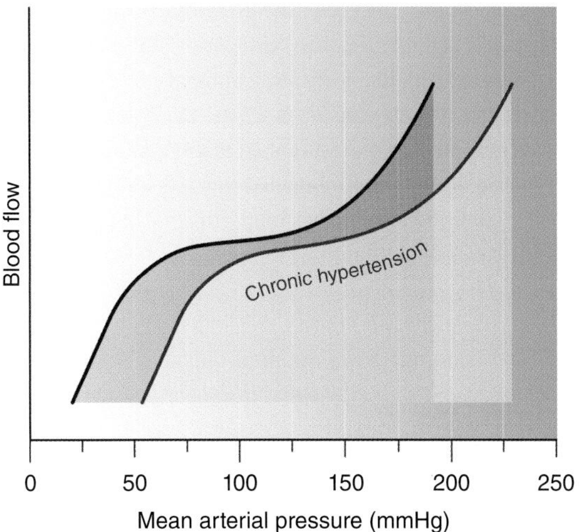

Figure 5.3 Autoregulation. The body is capable of normalizing blood flow and oxygen delivery at mean arterial pressures between 50 and 150 mmHg. In patients with longstanding hypertension, cerebral blood flow can be compromised at higher pressures in hypertensive patients as compared to normotensives, as the flow–pressure curve shifts to the right (Strandgaard, 1976, Paulson et al., 1990, Immink et al., 2004, Cheung, 2006).

Anesthetic concerns

All patients with hypertension should be rendered normotensive if possible, prior to either local or intravenous anesthesia. All blood pressure medications, with the possible exception of diuretics, should be taken per usual schedule, with two caveats. Rapid induction to full general anesthesia, although rarely performed in the dental office, can lead to hypotension in patients taking ACE inhibitors or ARBs (Coriat et al., 1994). Abrupt discontinuation of β-blockers or clonidine (Catapres™, an alpha 2 agonist) can result in an exaggerated rebound sympathetic surge (Krukemyer et al., 1990). Perianesthetic exposure to diuretics can exaggerate hypovolemia and may trigger a disruptive need to void in the midst of sedation or early recovery.

Adequate local anesthesia minimizes the possibility of pain, attendant sympathetic discharge, and resultant increases in blood pressure and heart rate for all patients, irrespective of whether the procedures are performed with local anesthesia only, local and nitrous oxide, or local and intravenous anesthesia (Wolfsthal, 1993). Epinephrine should be used cautiously in patients taking non-selective β-blockers. In this circumstance, unopposed α_1 stimulation can lead to hypertension and reflex bradycardia, exacerbating the β-blocker-induced bradycardia.

Additional concerns arise when patients with hypertension undergo intravenous anesthesia. Most sedative and analgesic drugs, with ketamine being a notable exception, lower blood pressure by direct action and by obtunding anxiety-induced sympathetic discharge. In addition, many hypertensive patients are volume depleted. These three factors make the hypertensive patient particularly vulnerable to hypotension during IV anesthesia. Slow titration of anesthetic drugs, avoidance of deeper levels of anesthesia if possible, and adequate hydration can mitigate these risks. Finally, hypotension is less tolerated in patients taking β-blockers, which can inhibit a compensatory tachycardia.

Hypertension during IV anesthesia can be caused by sympathetic discharge secondary to pain, agitation, hypoxia, hypercarbia, hypervolemia, or bladder distension. Adequate ventilation and oxygenation, together with careful control of hemodynamic responses to noxious stimuli with local anesthetics and narcotics will eliminate many of these factors.

Coronary artery disease

Definition

Coronary artery disease (CAD) refers to hardening, narrowing, and/or dysfunction of the blood vessels that supply oxygen to cardiac muscle. The presence and severity of symptoms depend on the degree of interruption of the balance between cardiac oxygen supply and oxygen demand, and can range from none to sudden cardiac death. The American Heart Association estimates that as of 2008 approximately 7% of the US population over age 20 has some form of cardiovascular disease and that every 25 seconds an American will experience a coronary event. The AHA further estimates that every minute one American will die from a coronary event (Roger et al., 2012). Given the prevalence of cardiovascular disease, especially in older patients, it is important to understand this pathophysiology to improve management decisions in patients undergoing elective dental procedures with sedation or general anesthesia. Risk factors that lead to blood vessel injury and inflammation, often resulting in atherosclerotic plaques, are listed in Table 5.4.

Pathophysiology

In all instances, CAD reduces blood flow (hence oxygen supply) to the myocardium and is most commonly due to atherosclerosis – hardening of the internal lining of the coronary arteries (which limits vasodilation) and narrowing of the lumens by focal atheromatous plaques. Further reduction in coronary blood flow occurs with increased heart rates and/or decreased diastolic pressure. Metabolic oxygen demand (consumption) is proportional to the cardiac workload, which increases with heart rate, contractility, and blood pressure (afterload), often resulting from pain-induced increased sympathetic tone. Myocardial ischemia is a dynamic process that occurs when the oxygen supply cannot meet the metabolic oxygen demand of the heart muscle (see Table 5.5).

During ischemia, cardiac muscle releases mediators, which stimulate nociceptors and cause typical chest pain. These mediators typically slow down conduction and decrease contractility, which decreases oxygen demand. Although variability is the rule, the usual presenting complaint ("classic angina") is crescendo–decrescendo dull, retrosternal discomfort, pain, or heaviness that can radiate (angina equivalents) to the neck (choking sensation), jaw (toothache, Kreiner et al., 2007), left shoulder or arm (tingling,

Table 5.4 Risk factors for coronary artery disease.

- Male gender
- Advanced age
- Hypercholesterolemia
- Hypertension
- Diabetes mellitus
- Genetics
- Obesity
- Poor lifestyle choices
  - Sedentary lifestyle
  - Cigarette smoking
  - Alcohol consumption
  - High fat, high carbohydrate diet

Table 5.5 Myocardial oxygen balance.

↓ O_2 supply	↑ O_2 demand
↓ Coronary blood flow (vessel radius)	↑ Afterload (systolic blood pressure) (valvular stenosis)
↑ Heart rate	↑ Preload (ventricular volume, filling pressure)
↓ Diastolic pressure	↑ Heart Rate
↓ Oxygen delivery (O_2 saturation, [Hgb])	↑ Contractility

numbness), or epigastrum (heartburn). Onset occurs over minutes, and if relief occurs, it happens over the next hour. "Soft" angina equivalents may also be a presenting complaint, which include shortness of breath (the need to take a deep breath), diaphoresis, pallor, and/or anxiety. Table 5.6 illustrates the spectrum of this disease. Stable angina is thought to occur from a fixed, flow-limiting plaque, which predictably causes symptoms during increased oxygen demand and is relieved by rest or vasodilators. Mixed angina presents similarly, but with overlying coronary vasoconstriction, which decreases predictability of symptoms, triggers, or relief. Unstable angina includes new onset of symptoms, angina at rest, or angina that becomes more severe, more often or lasts longer. Unstable angina is thought to be triggered by intermittent coronary occlusion. Myocardial infarction (cell death) occurs when there is total or near total intermittent or permanent occlusion of a coronary artery due to rapid plaque growth or plaque rupture/clot occlusion offsetting the balance of oxygen supply and demand in the distal myocardium.

The diagnosis of CAD is often challenging, depending on the severity of a patient's symptoms as discovered in the medical history. Unfortunately, many dental patients needing medical care do not access it (Greenberg et al., 2007) and may present with "undiagnosed disease" that insidiously decreases their exercise tolerance. This underscores the importance of a meticulous medical history, which questions previous heart attacks, palpitations, dizziness, shortness of breath, prior episodes of chest pain, and activity level. Activity (exercise tolerance) at the 4 MET level (one metabolic equivalent of task consumes 3.5 ml O_2/kg/min) is generally accepted to imply that the patient probably has an adequate cardiac reserve to tolerate a well-managed low risk surgery, where oxygenation is continuously maintained and tachycardia and hypotension are avoided (see Table 5.7).

A preoperative resting electrocardiogram (ECG) is not likely to help in the diagnosis of chronic stable CAD, as ST segment changes (elevation or depression) generally manifest only during periods of high oxygen demand and/or inadequate supply. New onset Q waves, T wave inversion, new AV nodal blocks, and a new left bundle branch block may indicate a recent cardiac event and warrant further evaluation by the patient's cardiologist. Correll, et al. (2009) determined that age greater than 65 years was an independent predictor for significant preoperative ECG abnormalities. Suspicion of new, poorly managed, unstable, or progressively worsening symptoms related to CAD warrants postponement of elective procedures and referral to the patient's primary care physician or cardiologist for further evaluation.

Treatment

Similar to the initial treatment of hypertension, management of CAD begins with lifestyle modification (achieve an ideal body weight, low fat diet, regular aerobic exercise), optimal management of comorbid diseases (e.g., hypertension, diabetes), and subsequent pharmacological and/or invasive interventions such as the placement of a coronary stent or open heart surgery with a coronary artery bypass graft. A wide variety of medications are prescribed to improve overall long-term survival for patients with CAD. Therapeutic interventions include reducing myocardial oxygen demand, increasing oxygen supply (coronary perfusion), inhibiting platelet activity, and limiting thrombus formation, among others.

Table 5.6 Spectrum of coronary artery disease.

Severity →					
Fixed atherosclerotic plaque			Plaque rupture and thrombosis (acute coronary syndrome)		
Asymptomatic Coronary artery disease	Stable angina "ischemia of demand"	Mixed angina "ischemia of demand and supply"	Unstable angina	Acute myocardial infarction	Sudden cardiac death
	↑ oxygen demand Fixed threshold **Triggers** • Exertion • Exercise • Exposure to temperature extremes • Eating a heavy meal • Emotional stress **Relief** • Rest • vasodilators	↑ oxygen demand with ↓ oxygen supply from variable coronary vasoconstriction Variable threshhold	New onset angina Angina at rest Crescendo angina • Severity • Frequency • Duration	Cardiac muscle injury	Lethal ventricular tachydysrhythmias

Table 5.7 Estimated functional capacity in METs (Data from Fleisher, 2007).

1 MET	Eating, getting dressed, using the bathroom
2-3 METS	Walking slowly on level ground, up to 1–2 blocks
4 METS	*Doing light housework*
	Climbing 1–2 flights of stairs without stopping
4–10 METS	Walking > 2 blocks at normal pace
	Doing heavy housework
	Running short distances
	Golf, bowling, social dancing
	Competitive sports

Beta-blockers

The primary purpose of β-blockade in a patient with CAD is to slow down the heart rate, thereby decreasing oxygen consumption and prolonging coronary diastolic perfusion. The target heart rate is between 60 and 80 bpm with blood pressure parameters discussed in the section on hypertension. β-blockers should always be continued throughout the perioperative period, as abrupt discontinuation can precipitate acute hypertensive episodes because of receptor upregulation.

Angiotensin-Converting Enzyme (ACE) Inhibitors

In addition to the management of hypertension, ACE inhibitors have been shown to reduce ventricular remodeling after acute myocardial infarction and to improve long-term survival (Beckwith and Munger, 1993). Left ventricular remodeling results in hypertrophy or scarring of the myocardium and can lead to functional or electrical abnormalities. ACE inhibitors are often withheld on the day of surgery, when hypotension can occur after rapid bolus induction prior to endotracheal intubation. This practice may not be necessary for most dental cases involving open airway anesthesia or sedation where rapid bolus inductions are not commonplace. Oftentimes, patients will take their ACE inhibitors at night, thus negating the concern.

Antiplatelet therapy

Patients with a history of myocardial infarction, coronary angiography, coronary artery stent placement, coronary artery bypass graft surgery, stroke, or peripheral vascular disease may be taking antiplatelet medication. Antiplatelet therapy consisting of thienopyridines (clopidogrel, [Plavix™] or ticlopidine [Ticlid™]), in combination with aspirin following coronary stent placement or coronary artery bypass graft surgery, has been shown to dramatically reduce adverse cardiac events compared with aspirin alone or with warfarin (Ten Berg et al., 2001). As a general rule, antiplatelet medications should be continued during routine oral surgery, as the risk of stent thrombosis, reinfarction, and death greatly outweigh the benefit of reducing minor, easily controllable post-operative bleeding (Grines et al., 2007; Valerin et al., 2006; Lockhart et al., 2003). Elective procedures for which there is a significant risk of surgical bleeding should be delayed until the patient has completed his/her course of antiplatelet therapy recommended by the cardiologist (12 months following placement of a drug eluting stent or 1–6 months following placement of a bare metal stent). For those procedures that mandate cessation of thienopyridine therapy within the recommended post-stent time period, aspirin should be continued if at all possible and thienopyridine therapy should be restarted as soon as possible post procedure. This should be done in consultation with the patient's cardiologist (Grines et al., 2007).

Nitrates

This class of medication is used almost exclusively in patients with coronary disease. Common medications in this class include sublingual nitroglycerin for acute relief of angina (Nitrostat™, Nitroquick™, Nitrobid™, Nitrodur™, Minitran™, Deponit™, Nitrol™, Nitrolingual™), and daily isosorbide mononitrite (Imdur™) or isosorbide dinitrate (Isordil™) to decrease episodes of angina and improve exercise tolerance.

Nitroglycerin works at several different sites to reduce symptoms of angina. It is a known venodilator, thus increasing venous compliance and reducing preload. This reduction in preload decreases myocardial oxygen demand by reducing left ventricular filling pressure. Nitroglycerin also works by coronary vasodilatation, improving coronary perfusion. It is not known if nitroglycerin can dilate an obstructed coronary artery due to atherosclerotic narrowing or if it improves normal perfusion to ischemic territories by collateral perfusion. However, it is known to improve anginal symptoms in the acute phase and is often carried by patients with stable angina as a rescue medication. It can cause a decrease in blood pressure and has a duration of action of approximately 20 minutes when taken via the sublingual route. Its onset is rapid (within minutes) when taken sublingually (Katzung, 2001).

Isosorbide mononitrate and isosorbide dinitrate work by a similar mechanism as nitroglycerin but are prescribed in patients in whom a longer duration of action is needed. They are often prescribed as adjuvant therapy in patients with refractory, advanced, or medically managed CAD. Usually, these medications are continued in the perioperative period. Any concern for hypotension related to these medications should be referred to the patient's cardiologist.

Risk assessment

The importance of medical history cannot be overstated, which, in many cases will guide the clinician to an accurate diagnosis in most instances. Physical examination can boost this rate by 20–25%. In contrast, studies such as a chest X-ray and an ECG may only help with 3% of diagnoses and an exercise tolerance test may help only 6% of the time (Sandler, 1980).

The American College of Cardiology and the American Heart Association (Fleisher, 2007) published guidelines to help determine cardiac risk (the combined incidence of cardiac death and non-fatal cardiac infarction) in patients undergoing non-cardiac surgery. The guidelines provide a basis regarding decisions to proceed with or cancel surgery. They are based on three parameters: the patient's cardiac status, functional capacity, and the level of surgery planned. In the absence of a true surgical emergency, attention should be given to establishing the presence of active cardiac conditions, which, if present should provoke cancellation of elective procedures and referral for further evaluation and treatment. These conditions are listed in Table 5.8.

The type of surgery is also integral to establishing risk. The ACC/AHA guidelines divide surgical risk into three categories: low, intermediate, and vascular (formerly "high"). Low risk surgery carries a cardiac risk of less than 1%, intermediate 1–5%, and vascular surgery 5% or greater. In the absence of active cardiac conditions, office dental procedures (low risk) can be performed without any further preoperative cardiac testing, assuming a well-executed anesthetic plan. Non-cardiac symptom or disease-prompted laboratory assessments such as INR, fasting blood glucose, platelet number, or WBC levels are still determined as necessary.

Extensive and invasive oral maxillofacial surgeries of the head and neck, which occasionally are performed in an office setting, fall into

Table 5.8 Active cardiac conditions. Presence of these conditions warrants further evaluation prior to surgery.

Unstable coronary syndromes
- Unstable or severe angina
- Recent MI (7–30 days)

Decompensated heart failure (NYHA class IV, worsening or new onset HF)
Significant dysrhythmias
- Mobitz II AV block
- Third degree AV block
- Symptomatic bradycardia
- Symptomatic ventricular dysrhythmias
- Supraventricular dysrhythmias
  - Atrial fibrillation with ventricular rates > 100 bpm at rest

Severe valvular disease
- Severe aortic stenosis
- Symptomatic mitral stenosis

the intermediate cardiac risk category. In this case, a minimum functional capacity of 4 METs (climbing 1–2 flights of stairs without interruption, chest pain or shortness of breath) indicates a patient should be able proceed with surgery without further testing or intervention. It is important to determine whether limitations in functional capacity are due to true cardiopulmonary symptoms or from other medical problems, such as osteoarthritis of the knees and hips. In the case of poor functional capacity, a search for other clinical risk factors will help guide the decision process. These clinical risk factors include ischemic heart disease, compensated or prior heart failure, diabetes mellitus, renal insufficiency, and cerebrovascular disease. In the absence of any of these clinical risk factors, surgery may be performed as planned without further testing. In any case of doubt, consultation with medical care providers can be most helpful.

Anesthetic concerns

There is no single perfect anesthetic for a patient with ischemic heart disease. Adequate ventilation, oxygenation, analgesia, amnesia (if appropriate), and maintenance of a stable hemodynamic profile are all tenets of a well-delivered anesthetic in any patient, not just one with cardiac disease. This can be achieved in many different ways and must be tailored to the individual patient's surgical needs and disease processes. The key concept in delivering anesthesia to patients with CAD is the maintenance of balance between myocardial oxygen supply and demand, by providing tight control of vital signs, especially heart rate and blood pressure. Anxiety or inadequate anesthesia (pain) will trigger the neuroendocrine stress response of surgery, leading to sympathetic-mediated tachycardia and hypertension, which increases myocardial oxygen demand. Hypoxia is a double insult, which triggers a sympathetic response while decreasing oxygen supply. Prolonged hypoxia eventually gives way to bradycardia, cerebral ischemia, cardiac dysrhythmia, and death.

Tight control of vital signs is achieved by minimizing hemodynamic variation. Relative or absolute diastolic hypotension reduces coronary perfusion. Hypertension decreases coronary perfusion and increases oxygen demand by an increase in ventricular wall tension and work in overcoming higher aortic pressures. Uncompensated bradycardia not only reduces cardiac output but also decreases coronary perfusion by extending ventricular filling time, which increases ventricular wall tension. Tachycardia increases myocardial work and oxygen demand, while reducing ventricular filling time and SV, which can lead to hypotension.

A commonly accepted range of hemodynamic variation is 20% from normal preanesthetic values. It is understood that in the immediate pre-surgical period heart rate and blood pressure may be artificially elevated due to anxiety, commonly referred to as *white coat syndrome*. Currently, the guidelines for cancellation of an elective procedure on the day of surgery are a systolic blood pressure of 180 mmHg or diastolic pressure of 110 mmHg (Sear, 2008). Clinical judgment should be used, however, and poorly managed blood pressure or blood pressure far outside the patient's normal range should raise suspicion for potential challenges with hemodynamic management and may necessitate further workup prior to proceeding with the procedure.

Oral anxiolytics taken with adequate time to reach peak effect prior to the start of the procedure, coupled with local anesthesia, may be sufficient for the majority of dental procedures. Regardless of the anesthetic plan, patients with limited or reduced cardiac reserve (ischemic heart disease, cardiomyopathy, valvular disease, etc.) may not tolerate the same anesthetic plan that a "normal" healthy patient would. This should be a significant consideration when providing care for these patients.

Volatile anesthetic agents (isoflurane, sevoflurane, and desflurane) are peripheral and coronary vasodilators, which also reduce or eliminate the neuroendocrine stress response. The mechanism of the general cardioprotective effects of volatile anesthetics is not clear but may be due to activation of ATP-sensitive potassium channels and stimulation of specific adenosine receptors (Yost, 1999). Although volatile anesthetics are known to be direct myocardial depressants, they have a greater effect on reducing systemic vascular resistance (Stoelting and Miller, 2007). Propofol and intravenously administered narcotics (with the exception of meperidine) can be expected to cause a dose- and rate-of-administration-dependent drop in blood pressure and heart rate. Benzodiazepines can lead to a more attenuated cardiovascular depressant effect, again, based on dose, rate of administration, and fluid status of the patient.

Nitrous oxide has very little effect on systemic vascular resistance and myocardial contractility. When used in combination with intravenous opioids and benzodiazepines is often a well-tolerated anesthetic, particularly in the dental population where surgical stimulus is often easily mitigated with the use of local anesthetics. With any anesthetic, intravenous or inhalational, SVR and myocardial contractility may be reduced secondary to the effects of a depressed consciousness and reduced sympathetic tone. Nitrous oxide should be used with caution in patients with known pulmonary hypertension as it can cause a slight increase in pulmonary vascular resistance.

The use of local anesthetics can be a tremendous aid in the dental setting when treating a patient with cardiovascular disease. Adequate blockade of painful stimuli can reduce or eliminate the need for adjuvant anesthetic agents in many dental procedures. There is no convincing evidence to avoid the use of vasoconstrictors with local anesthetics in patients with cardiovascular disease (Brown and Rhodus, 2005; Bader et al., 2002), as they have not been shown to reduce coronary blood flow or worsen cardiac ischemia. Alpha 1-blockade often minimizes surgical bleeding in patients on anticoagulants or antiplatelet medication.

Monitoring is essential when administering any medication that can alter the cardiovascular or pulmonary systems. Lead II can be helpful in detecting inferior ischemia related to cardiac muscle perfused by the right coronary artery, but is of limited value to detect ischemia in other areas of the heart. Frequent measurement of the patient's blood pressure is useful in assuring adequate perfusion pressure to the myocardium and can be useful in alerting the clinician to hemodynamic swings.

Valvular heart disease

Properly functioning cardiac valves should facilitate orthograde (forward) blood flow. They should not impede forward blood flow nor should they allow retrograde (backward) leakage. As such, common end points of all valvular pathology are either stenosis (narrowing) and/or incompetence (leaking.) Stenosis impedes forward flow, which increases the work (oxygen demand) done by the antecedent chamber and typically leads to chamber dilation if atrial or chamber hypertrophy if ventricular. Regurgitation also decreases orthograde blood flow and often dilates the antecedent chamber. In many cases, valvular pathology develops insidiously over a number of years, initially without symptoms, and is then treated with medical management, and ultimately managed with surgical valve replacement when the patient can no longer function in daily life.

A heart murmur is a "swoosh" sound originating from turbulent (vs. laminar) blood flow as would occur with a decrease in valve diameter (stenosis), a leaky (incompetent, regurgitant) valve, or an increase in blood flow rate (Lessard et al., 2005). Murmurs can also arise from abnormal openings between the heart chambers. A systolic murmur can be found in nearly all children and in up to 44% of adults. Because many murmurs are benign, it has been suggested that only those people with a systolic murmur associated with symptoms of dyspnea, chest pain, or lower extremity edema be considered to have a pathological murmur and warrant referral to a cardiologist (Attenhofer Jost et al., 2000). All diastolic murmurs are considered pathological and warrant further evaluation prior to elective surgery.

This section addresses the more common and more hemodynamically significant valvular lesions, typically occurring on the left side of the heart because of higher pressures. Diagnosis of valvular lesions or auscultatory detection of cardiac murmurs is beyond the scope of the dental practitioner. Questions regarding angina, shortness of breath, and exercise tolerance are indicated in all patients, regardless of the presence of diagnosed or undiagnosed valvulopathy. In all cases, anesthetic goals target a normal sinus rhythm (60 – 80 bpm) and maintenance of blood pressure within 10–15% of the preanesthetic values (Bonow et al., 2006; see Figure 5.4). This is most readily accomplished by intravenous fluid replacement of fasting losses, slow titration of benzodiazepines, narcotics and hypnotics (as per training, licensure, and individual comfort level), supplemented with profound local anesthesia. Rarely will vital signs be controlled with non-anesthetic agents during office-based procedures, and if this is deemed necessary or likely, consideration should be given to conducting the procedure in other locations together with other health care providers.

Aortic stenosis

Aortic stenosis is a serious and progressive condition hallmarked by compensatory changes in the heart muscle and function, ultimately leading to symptoms of heart failure. Without surgical treatment, most patients with symptomatic aortic stenosis will die within 2–5 years after diagnosis. Cardinal symptoms of aortic stenosis include dyspnea with exertion, angina, and orthostatic syncope. Aortic stenosis causes an increase in the pressure gradient between the left ventricle and aorta, which results in pressure overload, ventricular hypertrophy, wall stiffness, and increased diastolic filling pressure. Compensation by left ventricular hypertrophy eventually fails, leading to ventricular dilation, increased left atrial pressures, and increased pulmonary arterial pressures. The left atrium compensates for this increase in filling pressure by contracting more forcefully. In aortic stenosis, this atrial contraction (commonly referred to as the "atrial kick") may contribute up to 40% of the left ventricular SV. Atrial fibrillation is common in this setting, resulting in the loss of the atrial kick and a severe reduction in the ejection fraction and cardiac output. Because blood flow through the stenotic aortic valve is limited, cardiac output is essentially fixed and the heart is unable to meet any increase in the body's metabolic demands.

Patients with aortic stenosis often have concomitant CAD. This is a serious comorbidity because of the pressure gradient between the left ventricle and the aorta. Aortic diastolic pressures are much lower in aortic stenosis and thus the driving force for coronary artery perfusion is reduced. Moreover, because of the thickened left ventricle, the patient is at much greater risk for subendocardial ischemia (Kodama-Takahashi et al., 2003).

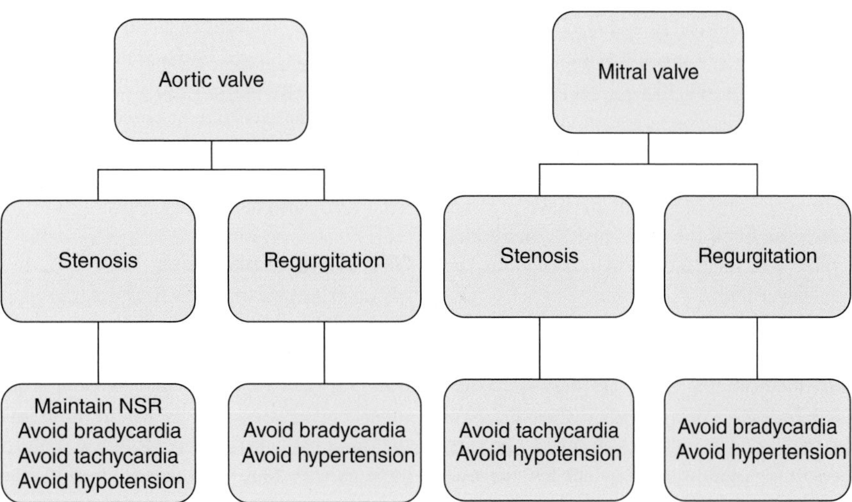

Figure 5.4 Anesthetic goals in patients with valvulopathy.

As aortic stenosis is the most important valvular lesion, which often leads to significant cardiac complications, appropriate consultation with the patient's cardiologist will help estimate the patient's ability to tolerate unintended cardiovascular changes occasionally associated with office-based anesthesia. Targeted concerns during intravenous anesthesia include the maintenance of a normal sinus rhythm and the avoidance of hypotension beyond 10–15% of preanesthetic values.

Properly timed atrial contractions are needed to provide adequate fill of the stiff left ventricle. Loss of atrial contraction in cases of atrial fibrillation or the appearance of nodal rhythms will result in hypotension, further embarrassing coronary perfusion. Fast heart rates limit the time for adequate diastolic fill and will similarly result in hypotension, often with attendant decrease in coronary perfusion and dysrhythmia. Bradycardia also results in hypotension.

Profound local anesthesia can reduce or eliminate the neuroendocrine stress response. A careful technique will minimize inadvertent intravascular injection of vasoconstrictors. With the exception of ketamine and meperidine, most intravenous anesthesia drugs used in the dental office are cardiovascular depressants. The resultant decrease in sympathetic tone in patients with autonomic compensation can also lead to hypotension. For this reason, preanesthetic fluid replacement to compensate for hypovolemia is desirable. Positive pressure ventilation, should it be necessary, increases intrathoracic pressure and can reduce venous return (preload), also causing hypotension. Finally, chest compressions, should they be necessary, can be ineffective in overcoming the pressure needed to eject blood through the stenotic aortic valve.

Aortic regurgitation

Aortic regurgitation occurs when the aortic valve allows blood from the aorta to flow back into the left ventricle during diastole. This process decreases cardiac output and diastolic blood pressure [and increases pulse pressure, (systolic–diastolic)], and eventually results in left ventricular hypertrophy followed by dilation, due to both pressure and volume overload. As expected, the volume regurgitated back into the left ventricle increases with slower heart rates and increased systemic vascular resistance. The combination of increased oxygen demand from a hypertrophied ventricle and decreased oxygen supply from decreased diastolic coronary perfusion can result in ischemia and angina, even in the absence of CAD. As the left ventricle increases in size, both from hypertrophy and dilation, it is prone to dysrhythmias. In addition, the increase in left ventricular filling pressures is transmitted back to the left atrium and to the pulmonary circulation, placing the patient at risk for pulmonary edema.

Medical therapy for chronic aortic regurgitation is often based on lowering the systemic arterial pressure to facilitate forward flow of blood through the aortic valve and reduce the diastolic pressure gradient between the aortic root and the left ventricle. Increasing left ventricular contractility with medication such as digitalis can also help with improving forward flow.

As with all valvulopathies, patients with chronic aortic regurgitation should be medically optimized at the time of elective procedures, often with medications such as digitalis, ACE inhibitors, and diuretics. Anesthetic goals include the avoidance of bradycardia and avoidance of sudden increases in blood pressure, as both facilitate increases in regurgitant flow into the left ventricle placing the patient at risk for heart failure, pulmonary edema, and hemodynamic compromise. Hypotension can further aggravate diastolic coronary perfusion, while tachycardia can precipitate ischemia.

Mitral stenosis

Mitral stenosis results from thickening of the valve leaflets (typically a result of rheumatic fever), which obstructs blood flow to the left ventricle. This obstruction decreases left ventricular filling (preload) and results in pressure buildup in the left atrium, pulmonary vasculature, and eventually the right side of the heart. This loss of dynamic variation in left ventricular filling results in a fixed cardiac output, limiting exercise tolerance. In severe or longstanding cases, shortness of breath results from pulmonary hypertension and transudation of fluid into the interstitial spaces. The left atrium usually dilates to accommodate the increase in pressure due to the stenotic mitral valve. This left atrial stretch puts the patient at risk for atrial dysrhythmias (supraventricular tachycardia, atrial fibrillation) and embolic events. An important component of the atrial contraction, known as the *atrial kick*, can contribute up to 40% of the left ventricular EDV. The atrial kick does not occur in atrial fibrillation, severely compromising left ventricular filling pressures and cardiac output when mitral stenosis is present.

As with all anesthetics, tight control over vital signs is desirable. In the setting of mitral stenosis, tachycardia (stress response, ketamine, intravascular epinephrine, hypoxia) should be avoided to allow adequate time for ventricular fill. Ideal heart rates are between 60 and 80 bpm. Hypotension is worrisome as it may trigger reflex tachycardia. Hypertension should also be avoided, as this increases afterload, which increases cardiac oxygen demand and decreases peripheral perfusion. Fluid overload secondary to over-administration of IV fluids or Trendelenburg positioning is not tolerated well in patients with mitral stenosis.

Mitral regurgitation

Chronic MR permits a portion of the left ventricular SV to return to the left atrium during systole, reducing the SV to systemic circulation. The end result is a reduced forward flow of blood (cardiac output) into the systemic circulation and an increase in pressure in the left atrium, pulmonary circulation, and the right side of the heart. The regurgitant flow of blood causes the left atrium to dilate, predisposing the patient to atrial dysrhythmias, including atrial fibrillation.

Anesthetic concerns relate to the maintenance of cardiac output. This is best achieved by avoidance of bradycardia (increased filling time) and hypertension (resistance to ejection), both of which tend to increase left ventricular blood volume. As the left ventricle faces higher pressures in forcing open the aortic valve, more of the SV ends up in the left atrium through the lower pressure mitral valve, left atrium, and pulmonary veins.

Mitral valve prolapse

Mitral valve prolapse (MVP) is the most common valvular cause of chronic MR. As the left ventricle contracts, a portion of the mitral valve billows back into the left atrium and may lead to regurgitation. Patients with MVP and no other comorbidities will tolerate most anesthetic plans; however, in some cases a similar approach as that for a patient with chronic MR is appropriate. Not infrequently, patients with MVP will complain of anxiety, dizziness, and occasional palpitations. Benign cardiac dysrhythmias are also possible (Schaal, 1992).

Prosthetic heart valves

Prosthetic heart valves are either mechanical or bioprosthetic. Mechanical valves include metal structures, such as a caged ball or tilting discs. These valves are more durable, but also more thrombogenic. These valves are expected to last 20–30 years, and are preferred for younger patients who can tolerate long-term anticoagulation. Bioprosthetic valves include bovine or porcine heterografts mounted on metal rings or non-pathologic sections of native valves. They are less thrombogenic when compared to mechanical valves. A typical life span of only 10–15 years renders bioprosthetic valves preferable for elderly patients or those who cannot tolerate anticoagulation. Regardless of the type, valves at the mitral position are more thrombogenic than those at the aortic position. All patients with prosthetic valves require prophylactic antibiotics prior to invasive procedures. As the cross-sectional area of all prosthetic valves is smaller than that of the native valve, screening questions of angina, dyspnea, dizziness, and exercise tolerance are still appropriate.

Cardiac rhythm disorders

An understanding of normal and abnormal cardiac rhythms is necessary to assess patient suitability for office-based sedation/anesthesia. This insight further informs management decisions when confronted with perianesthetic rhythm disturbances; decisions that might include cancellation and referral, close observation without treatment, cessation of surgery/anesthesia, medical treatment, or emergency medical triage.

Rhythm disorders [anything other than a normal sinus rhythm (Figure 5.5)] are common during anesthesia. Fortunately, most are short lived and hemodynamically insignificant. Avoidance or remediation of hypoxia and sympathetic stimulation, both common dysrhythmia triggers, often averts or resolves the problem. Unfortunately, those patients who tend to be more susceptible to rhythm disorders (e.g., disease affecting the conduction system) are often the ones least able to tolerate them.

The heart consists of three non-discrete groups of excitable cells that orchestrate a coordinated, rhythmic tempo of contractions that optimizes chamber filling and ejection of blood: pacemaker cells, fast conducting cells, and contractile myocytes (see Figure 5.6). The pacemaker cells include the SA node and the AV node, both capable of spontaneous depolarization because of leaky calcium influx channels. The fast conducting cells that populate conduction pathways (atrial intermodal tracts, Bachmann's bundle, HIS bundle, right and left bundle branches and Purkinje fibers) depolarize by means of Na^+ influx, when stimulated by adjacent cellular, ionic, or electrical activity. The wave of stimulation continues, albeit at a slower rate, to the cardiac myocytes, which subsequently depolarize, contract, and further conduct impulses to adjacent myocytes.

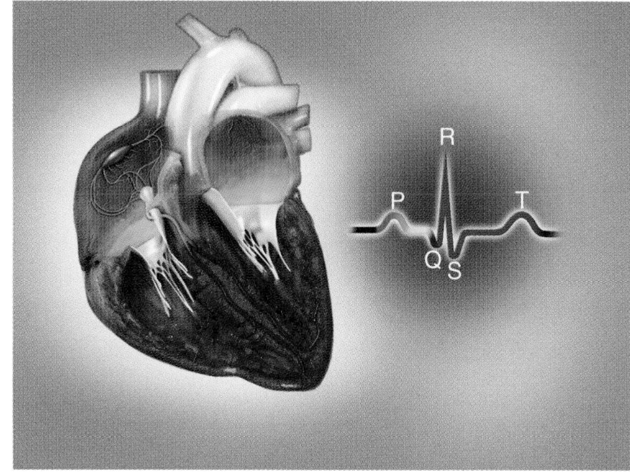

Figure 5.6 Electrical system of the heart.

The SA node is the primary site for impulse initiation, which spontaneously depolarizes at an intrinsic normal sinus rate of 60–100 bpm, and sends an electrical impulse down specialized neuronal pathways to stimulate the AV node. Here, a short delay occurs (to allow atrial contraction to augment ventricular fill and to prevent conduction of rapid supraventricular rhythms) prior to progression to the HIS bundle, right and left bundle branches, and Purkinje fibers. This wave disperses to adjacent myocytes, albeit at a slower rate, resulting in their progressive contraction, and literal squeezing of blood from the respective chamber. As the fastest intrinsic pacemaker, the SA node leads to overdrive suppression of (prevents) spontaneous activity from other slower potential pacemaker cells, as they remain refractory to further stimulation until repolarization is complete. Should the SA node fail, other foci (from the atria, AV node or ventricles) become capable of initiating "ectopic" impulses, which are allowed to "escape" when higher foci do not depolarize, also at a slower rate.

These electrical events can be measured at the skin and amplified to yield the standard ECG tracing (See Figure 5.7). The events occurring in the SA node and AV node are electrocardiographically silent. The P wave represents electrical depolarization of the atria (right followed by left atria) that occurs just prior to contraction. The PR interval (0.12–0.2 seconds) includes the normal impulse

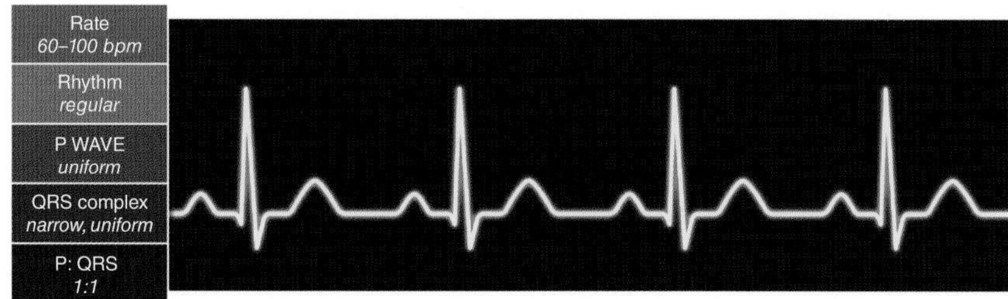

Figure 5.5 Normal sinus rhythm
- 60 – 100 bpm.
- Identical P waves, upright in lead II, at regular intervals.
- Each P is followed by a narrow QRS (<0.12sec).
- Each QRS is preceded by a P wave.
- QRS waves occur at regular intervals.

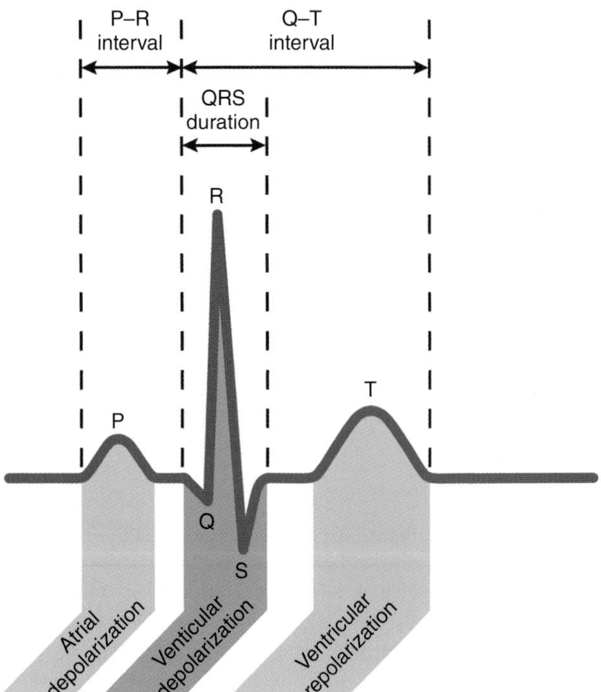

Figure 5.7 ECG tracing.

delay that occurs at the AV node as well as the subsequent spread of depolarization up to and including the terminal Purkinje fibers. Conduction blocks prolong the PR interval. The QRS complex (<0.12 seconds) represents depolarization of the ventricular myocytes. It is much larger than the P wave, as the ventricular muscle mass is much larger than the mass of the atria. The T wave represents ventricular repolarization. The electrical events associated with atrial repolarization are overshadowed and hidden in the QRS complex. The ST segment represents the time between the end of the S wave (end of ventricular depolarization) and the beginning of the T wave (beginning of ventricular repolarization). It is important to note that the ECG reflects the electrical depolarization of the cardiac muscle, and NOT the muscular contraction, which fortunately, usually follows.

After electrical depolarization, cells become refractory to further stimulation until repolarization is complete or nearly complete when resting concentrations of ions are restored. Hypoxia and sympathetic stimulation can both lead to irritable foci producing ectopic beats out of sequence, usually earlier than anticipated. Stimulus strength is directly related to both severity and duration of insult.

Interpretation of a dynamic ECG (see Table 5.9) tracing as displayed on a monitor during office-based sedation includes determination of rate, rhythm and presence, morphology, consistency, and relationship of P waves and QRS complexes. Lead II (see Figure 5.8) (right arm negative, left leg positive) most closely follows the usual path of cardiac depolarization. This lead facilitates dysrhythmia detection during anesthesia as it easily tracks heart rate, clearly demonstrates an upright P wave, and exposes the R wave for synchronized cardioversion in most patients. It is difficult to accurately measure the P–R interval and T wave morphology on a lead II oscilloscopic tracing without gridlines, although monitor printouts will place the ECG deflections on paper with gridlines.

Table 5.9 Dynamic ECG Interpretation.

- Rate—is it too fast (>100bpm) or too slow (<60bpm)?
- Rhythm—is it regular or irregular? (visual inspection of R-R′ intervals)
- Morphology and consistency—are P waves present and uniform? Are QRS complexes present, uniform and narrow?
- Sequence—is each P wave followed by a QRS at a consistent interval? Is each QRS complex preceded by a P wave?
- Intervals—PR < 0.2 sec, QRS < 0.12sec

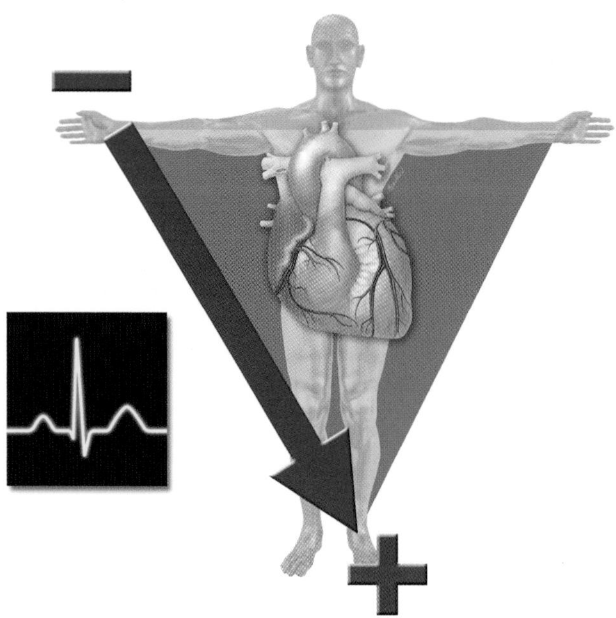

Figure 5.8 Lead II configuration parallels the net vector of depolarization.

P–R intervals are used to measure the presence of cardiac conduction blocks. ST segment alterations (elevation or depression) are monitored with chest lead V together with lead II; therefore, accurate and complete assessment of cardiac ischemia is not possible with an isolated lead II. The ST segment (early ventricular repolarization) is normally isoelectric in lead II, and depression of this segment is never normal; however, slight elevation can occur without abnormality. Ischemia, hypokalemia, or myocardial injury can displace the ST segment. It is important to be mindful of the fact that the ECG can lack sensitivity, which can overlook significant cardiac disease.

The heart enjoys robust autonomic innervation, allowing it to pump faster and stronger to meet increasing oxygen demands of the body in times of stress or increased physical activity. Sympathetic nerves innervate the SA and AV nodes to increase the spontaneous firing rate of the SA node and decrease the conduction lag in the AV node. Sympathetic nerves also directly innervate cardiac muscle, leading to an increase in the strength of contraction. High sympathetic tone, either from exogenous epinephrine or from the endogenous neuroendocrine surgical stress response, can promote ectopy (abnormal, usually premature impulse generation.) Parasympathetic nerves innervate only the SA node (slowing down the rate) and AV node (further increasing the conduction lag).

Cardiac dysrhythmias

Any rhythm other than normal sinus rhythm is termed a dysrhythmia (arrhythmia) (see Table 5.10). These include variances in rate, interval length, or conduction path. They are further categorized by duration (fleeting or prolonged) and location (supraventricular or ventricular). Atrial dysrhythmias usually have less hemodynamic significance than ventricular dysrhythmias and cause only mild increases in oxygen demand. In general, dysrhythmias that are fast, prolonged, and originating in the ventricles tend to be more worrisome. Stated differently, in most instances, the more obvious the rhythm disturbance, the more harmful. From a clinical standpoint, rhythm disorders interfere with the normal fill-eject cycle and become significant when they lead to a decrease in cardiac output, and hence a decrease in blood pressure and organ perfusion. Dysrhythmias can also interfere with coronary perfusion, lead to increased myocardial oxygen demand, and deteriorate to a more hemodynamically significant (worse) dysrhythmia, due to interference with the orderly, sequenced movement of ions (see Table 5.11).

Preanesthetic screening not only identifies preexisting rhythm disorders, for example, heart block, atrial fibrillation, or PVCs, but also helps identify those patients who might be at increased risk of dysrhythmias, as well as those who might be less able to tolerate them during the course of the office-based anesthetic. A partial list of risk factors for perianesthetic dysrhythmias are listed in Table 5.12–5.14. Palpitations are an awareness of one's own heartbeat, and can be due to a variety of dysrhythmias, often times provoked by caffeine, tobacco, or alcohol ("Holiday Heart"). Similarly to many rhythm disturbances, palpitations are sporadic and are rarely "caught" on an ECG. In the same context, abnormal beats during anesthesia can also be fleeting, allowing the anesthetist only seconds to identify, in the absence of a physical paper tracing or a 12-second ECG display. Physical examination for preexisting dysrhythmias is accomplished with a radial artery pulse check or preanesthetic rhythm strip, screening for the irregularly irregular atrial fibrillation or occasional extra or skipped beats, whose origin can only be identified with an ECG.

Table 5.10 Common perianesthetic dysrhythmias.

Tachydysrhythmias
- Supraventricular
  - Sinus tachycardia
  - Ectopic beats
    - Premature atrial complex
    - Premature junctional complex
  - Atrial fibrillation
  - PSVT—paroxysmal supraventricular tachycardia
  - Pre-excitation syndromes
- Ventricular
  - Ectopic beats
    - PVC—premature ventricular complex
- Bradydysrhythmias
- Sinus bradycardia
- Escape beats
- Conduction disturbances
  - Sinus pause
  - Heart block
    - First degree
    - Second degree, Mobitz 1

Table 5.11 Significance of cardiac dysrhythmias

1 Decrease cardiac output (stroke volume), blood pressure and organ perfusion
2 Increase cardiac oxygen demand
3 Interfere with coronary perfusion
4 Can deteriorate to worse dysrhythmias

Table 5.12 Risk factors for perianesthetic dysrhythmias.

- Advancing age (fibrosis of conduction system)
- Male gender
- Smoking
- Sympathomimetic drugs
- Sedentary life style
- Ttype A personality
- Obstructive sleep apnea
- Structural heart disease (see Table 5.13)
- Electrolyte disturbances (hypokalemia, see Table 5.14)
- Absolute hypovolemia
- Relative hypovolemia (venous pooling during "beach chair" positioning)
- Diuretic usage
- Illicit drug use
- History of palpitations
- Postural dizziness
- Unexplained syncope
- Ischemia or infarct

Table 5.13 Stuctural heart disease that can predispose to cardiac rhythm disorders.

- Prior myocardial infarction
- Left venticular hypertrophy
- Coronary artery disease
- Prior cardiac surgery
- Recent stent
- Cardiomyopathy
- Congenital heart disease
- Valvulopathy
- Heart failure

Rhythm disturbances are common during anesthesia or sedation. Transient mild increases in rate often accompany inspiration (Bainbridge reflex), as negative intrathoracic pressure augments venous return (preload), which stimulates an increase in heart rate. Two of the most potent triggers of perianesthetic dysrhythmias are hypoxia and the neuroendocrine sympathetic stress response to surgery, typically worse with inadequate local anesthesia and/or during lighter planes of anesthesia. Hypoxia is avoided through maintenance of adequate ventilation with supplemental oxygen via a fully patent upper airway.

Most anesthetic agents have cardiovascular depressant effects, which alter homeostasis of the myocardium and reduce vascular tone. Volatile anesthetics are often associated with nodal rhythms. Ketamine, meperidine, and methohexital can increase heart rates, while opioids tend to slow down the heart rate, via a central vagotonic action. Fortunately, a vast majority of these perianesthetic

Table 5.14 Possible causes of transient or persistent hypokalemia.

- β_2-adrenergic stimulation
- Non K^+-sparing diuretics
- Hyperventilation
- Dumping s/p bariatric surgery
- Eating disorders

dysrhythmias are short lived and have little effect on perfusion. Dysrhythmias that can be encountered in the dental office during the administration of anesthetic agents are listed in Table 5.10.

Tachydysrhythmias

Supraventricular tachydysrhythmias

Sinus tachycardia is regular heart rate greater than 100 bpm, originating at the sinoatrial node, thereby displaying identical P waves (Figure 5.9). At faster heart rates (~150bpm), the P wave may not be obvious as it becomes hidden in the prior T wave. In these cases, the rhythm is referred to as *supraventricular tachycardia*, as one is not sure if the origin is from the SA node. As expected, the QRS complex is narrow as the impulse originates above the bifurcation of the HIS bundle. Tachycardias increase myocardial oxygen consumption and reduce the time spent in diastole, decreasing venous fill (hence cardiac output) and diastolic coronary perfusion. Normal "physiologic" causes arise from excess sympathetic stimulation triggered by pain, hypoxia, hypoglycemia, hypotension, hypovolemia, exercise, or sympathomimetic or anti-muscarinic drug effect. Typically, the heart rate will increase gradually in response to the intensity and duration of the trigger. Remediation occurs with stimulus removal, by oxygen administration with adequate ventilation and/or by deepening anesthesia, IV fluid challenge or administration of a dextrose solution as clinically indicated. Administration of β-blockers to slow down the heart rate is contraindicated in these instances, as that will only mask the etiology. "Pathologic" tachycardias, as seen in cases of hyperthyroidism, atrial fibrillation, or paroxysmal supraventricular tachycardias (PSVT), may require additional treatment (drugs, vagal maneuvers) as the trigger is either not necessary to sustain the problem or it cannot be readily managed.

Ectopic beats

All cardiac cells are capable of spontaneous depolarization, albeit at slower rates than the SA node, which leads to overdrive suppression of all other potential pacemakers. When irritated by hypoxia, hypoglycemia, hypokalemia, light anesthesia, or excessive sympathetic stimulation due to pain, exogenous epinephrine, or stimulant medication (ketamine, caffeine or illicit drugs), potential pacemaker cells become irritable and can fire and trigger a QRS complex earlier than expected. As the name implies, supraventricular beats arise above the bundle of HIS.

A premature (earlier than anticipated) atrial complex (PAC) (see Figure 5.10) displays a different P wave morphology (unlike sinus dysrhythmia, which has identical P waves), but usually conducts to a normal QRS complex unless the AV node is refractory from the prior beat, in which case the beat will not conduct. Unlike a premature ventricular complex, there is no compensatory pause, and the next sinus beat (if it occurs) begins one normal cycle length after the premature beat. The PR interval is variable, depending on the distance between the ectopic foci and the AV node. In general, supraventricular ectopic beats only modestly compromise ventricular fill at rates less than 100 bpm, and blood pressure should not be affected as long as narrow QRS complexes are present in sufficient number to maintain that pressure. PACs are not considered a risk factor for progression to more hemodynamically significant dysrhythmias; however, they can be associated with acute infarction. PACs should be monitored with an effort to remediate possible triggers as clinically indicated.

A premature nodal (junctional) beat (see Figure 5.11.11) originates from an irritable AV node and can conduct a normal or slightly widened QRS complex, with the latter occurring when one of the bundle branches is still refractory from the prior beat. P waves are absent or may conduct in a retrograde manner.

Premature beats usually increase the rate of ventricular contraction; however, an atrial escape *rhythm* or junctional (nodal) *rhythms* (see Figure 5.12) typically (but not always) are slower than sinus rhythms, all other things being equal. Junctional rhythms are common under anesthesia, presenting normal QRS complexes in the absence of P waves. At faster rates, loss of atrial kick can compromise ventricular fill, cardiac output, and blood pressure. Atropine or ephedrine can be considered with significant decrease in blood pressure, and often times will trigger return of a sinus beat. Junctional rates can vary between 40 and 180 bpm.

Atrial fibrillation

Atrial fibrillation is the uncoordinated atrial activation from many different foci, which prevents atrial contraction and normal pumping of blood (Nathanson and Gajraj, 1998) Distinct P waves are absent, and the QRS complex usually remains narrow, but conducts with haphazard frequency; hence the term "irregularly irregular." (Figure 5.13) Since atrial contraction is not possible, ventricular fill depends only on passive blood flow, which becomes compromised at faster heart rates. Therefore, tachycardias in patients with atrial fibrillation become a triple threat: decreased cardiac output, decreased diastolic coronary perfusion, and increased myocardial oxygen consumption, all of which can lead to ischemia. Clots tend to develop in fibrillating atria, increasing the risk of pulmonary or cerebral emboli. Therapy consists of elimination of possible triggers, prevention of embolization, rate control, and then rhythm control, as driven by patient history and symptoms. Anesthetic concerns for patients presenting with rate-controlled atrial fibrillation include maintaining adequate preload to maximize cardiac output and keeping the heart rate less than 90 bpm, by judicious use of vasoconstrictors and anti-muscarinics, and by providing adequate anesthesia and analgesia. New onset of atrial fibrillation during office-based sedation warrants immediate transfer to a hospital setting, which facilitates early rate/rhythm control and prevention of clot formation or embolization, as these usually do not develop acutely.

Paroxysmal supraventricular tachycardia (PSVT)

As the name implies, this dysrhythmia presents as a sudden, unexpected onset of tachycardia originating somewhere above the ventricles (at or above the HIS bundle), as evidenced by a narrow QRS complex. Unlike sinus tachycardia, sympathetic triggers are absent, onset is rapid, and rates are typically faster than 150 bpm in younger patients. Hypotension is more likely because of decreased diastolic fill. The substrate for this disorder is the presence of two electrophysiologically dissimilar (conduction rates and refractory periods are not the same) bidirectional pathways, most often within the AV

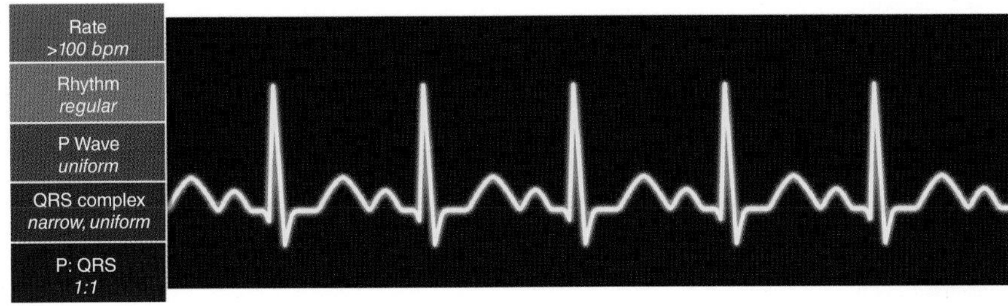

Figure 5.9 Sinus tachycardia.

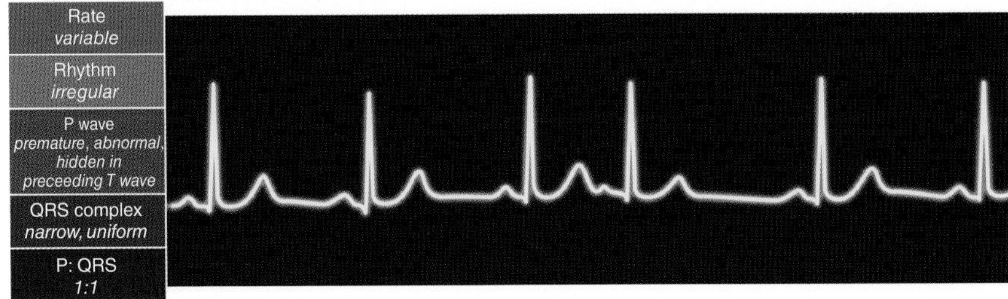

Figure 5.10 PAC - premature atrial complex.

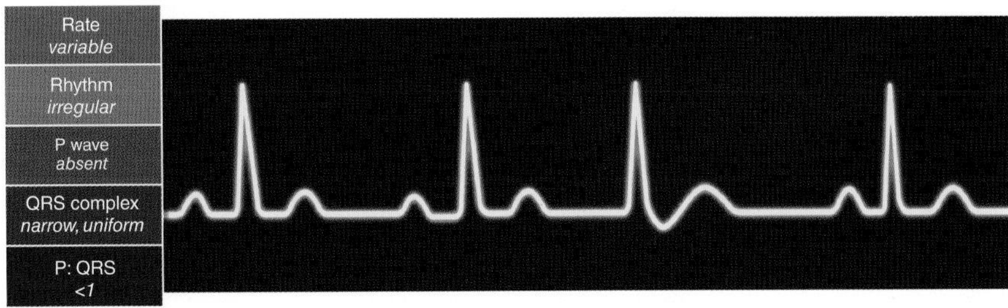

Figure 5.11 PJC - premature junctional complex.

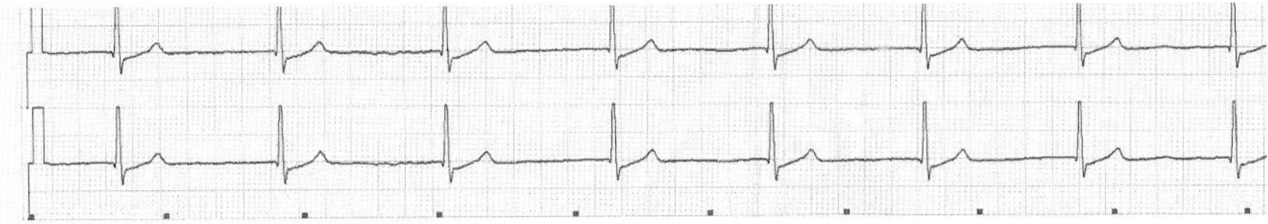

Figure 5.12 Junctional rhythm.

node. When an impulse conducts earlier than expected (e.g., a crucially timed PAC or an abrupt change in heart rate), it meets the refractory limb and conducts down the alternate limb to the ventricle and simultaneously up the previously refractory limb to set up a self-propagating circular pattern of stimulation. This phenomenon is called re-entry (see Figure 5.15).

Patients presenting with a history of PSVT (sudden, unprovoked onset of tachycardia) will typically report spontaneous palpitations, shortness of breath, light-headedness, and chest discomfort. Fleeting episodes may go unnoticed, while prolonged bouts prompt emergency medical care. Recurrent cases often undergo radiofrequency ablation, which destroys one of the pathways, thereby eliminating the substrate. Ablations are successful in most but not all cases. Sudden onset of persistent tachycardia during anesthesia, in the absence of triggers, requires immediate attention. Therapy is aimed at slowing down conduction through the AV node or electrical interruption of the re-entry circuit during severe hemodynamic compromise. (see Figure 5.14)

Pre-excitation syndromes

Normally, the atria and ventricles are electrically isolated from each other by dense fibrous tissue supporting the AV valves. As such, the only way an electrical signal can reach the ventricle is via the AV node and HIS bundle, which perforate this fibrous tissue. In approximately 1% of patients, an abnormal muscular bridge exists outside of the AV node, which can become a potential path for electrical conduction between the atria and the ventricles. The presence of this abnormal bridge gives rise to the Wolff–Parkinson–White syndrome. At normal heart rates, the accessory pathway is either concealed (non-conducting) or manifest (conducting). In the latter instance, the PR interval will be shortened and a delta wave will slur the upstroke of the QRS

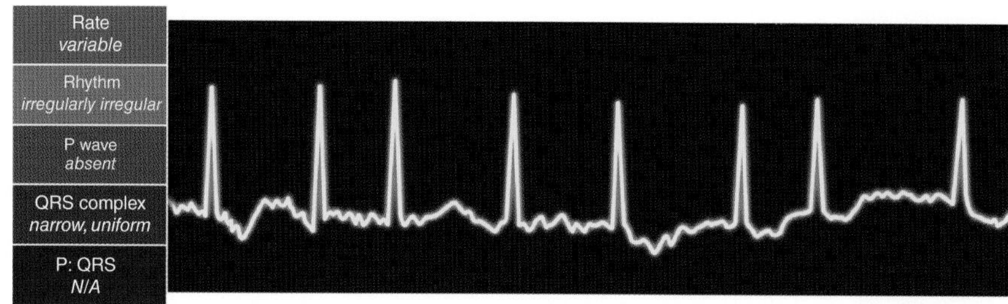

Figure 5.13 Atrial fibrillation.

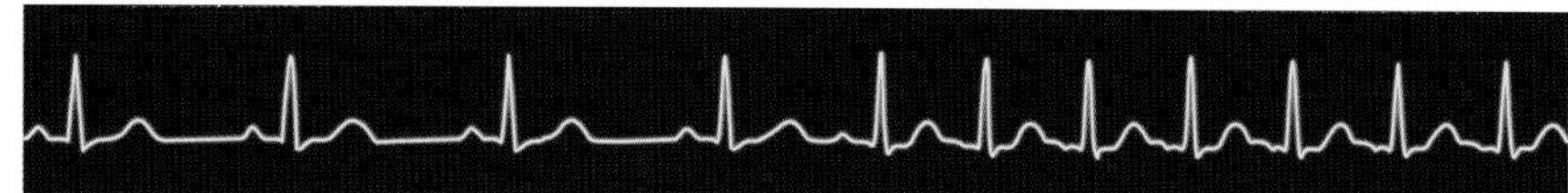

Figure 5.14 Paroxysymal supraventricular tachycardia.

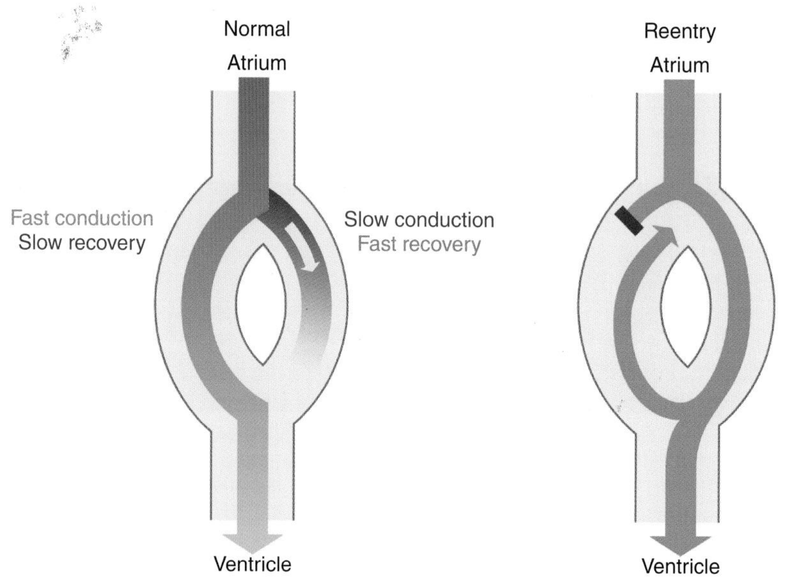

Figure 5.15 Reentry circuit.

as the ventricle becomes "pre-excited"(Figure 5.16) At faster heart rates (reciprocating tachycardias), the nomenclature changes to orthodromic (conduction down the AV node and return up the accessory pathway) or antidromic, where the impulse travels down the accessory pathway and up the AV node. Orthodromic tachycardias are treated similarly to PSVT, while antidromic tachycardias, which occur much less frequently, can be aggravated by that therapy (Stahmer and Cowan, 2006).

Ventricular tachydysrhythmias

Ectopic beats

Premature ventricular complex(Figure 5.17)

The term *premature ventricular complex* (PVC) unambiguously characterizes the cardiac electrical event that occurs earlier than expected, which arises from irritable ectopic foci or diseased conduction systems *below* the bifurcation of the bundle branches (Watson, 2012). Since conduction does not follow the bundle branch – Purkinje system, the QRS complex is bizarre and significantly widened as the spread of electrical activity is slower (see Table 5.15). A compensatory pause follows as the atrial cycle is not disturbed, but the following beat fails to conduct. It is thought that the ejection fraction of a PVC is less than the normal QRS beat; however, PVC-associated hemodynamic compromise appears to occur infrequently, unless the PVC burden is high or where the ejection fraction is low. If a palpitation (awareness of one's own heartbeat) occurs, it results from the normal contraction following the PVC, where end-diastolic volume is increased following the inefficient PVC. PVCs can be classified according to severity as simple or complex (see Table 5.16).

Simple PVCs are common and usually asymptomatic in most patients, regardless of the presence of cardiac disease. Prevalence increases with age, electrolyte disturbances, sympathetic stimulation secondary to pain, stimulants, exercise, and/or the presence of cardiac disease, such as hypertension and resultant LVH, ischemia, conduction abnormalities, healed infarction, or valvulopathy, among others (Simpson et al., 2002). Concern

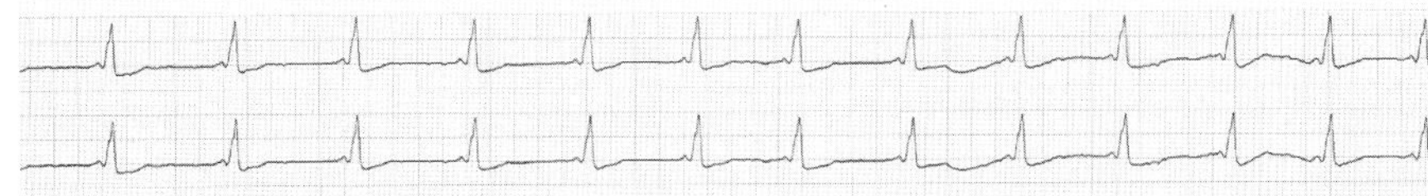

Figure 5.16 *WPW* – This rhythm strip depicts a shortened PR interval with a delta wave, characteristic of manifest Wolf–Parkinson–White syndrome. It was the presenting rhythm of an otherwise healthy 18-year-old male seeking wisdom tooth removal under general anesthesia. The patient was referred for further cardiac evaluation.

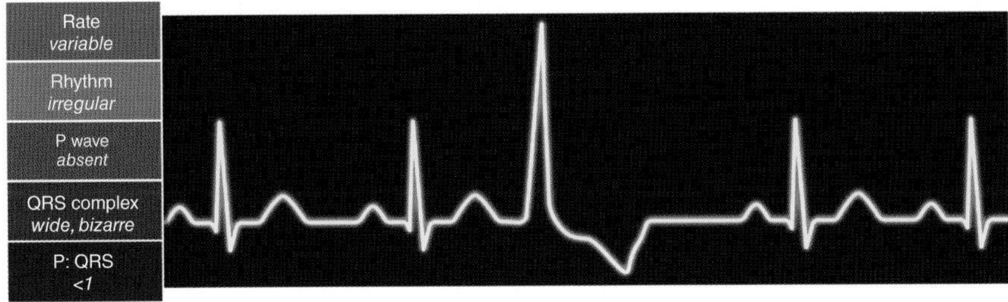

Figure 5.17 Premature ventricular complex.

Table 5.15 Diagnostic features of premature ventricular complexes.

- Premature occurrence
- Absent P wave
- Wide, bizarre QRS (duration > 120msec)
- T wave in the opposite direction of the main QRS vector
- Compensatory pause

Table 5.16 Classification of PVCs.

Simple PVCs	Unifocal (uniform in morphology) Occur AFTER the preceding T wave Are isolated (occur individually) Can be considered normal variant, especially with age
Complex PVCs	Multiformed Occur DURING the preceding T wave (R on T) Occur in pairs, triplets Are never normal

remains, however, that patients with PVCs may be at risk for more sinister dysrhythmias, especially with underlying cardiac disease.

Assessment of PVCs in the general population seeks to rule out coexistent cardiac disease and a quantification of PVC burden with Holter monitoring (Ng, 2006). There is conflicting data concerning the significance of frequent PVCs in patients with apparently normal hearts (Kennedy et al., 1985); however, most studies report an increased mortality in patients with PVCs, yet treatment of PVCs has not been shown to improve mortality (Podrid, 2013).

Non-sustained ventricular tachycardia is characterized by > 3 PVCs in a row, at rates > 100 bpm, but less than 30 seconds in duration and without hemodynamic compromise. In instances of normal cardiac structure and function, this will often resolve spontaneously, rather than deteriorate to ventricular tachycardia.

Bradydysrhythmias

Sinus bradycardia

Sinus bradycardia is regular heart rate less than 60 bpm, originating at the sinoatrial node, thereby displaying identical P waves (Figure 5.18). As expected, the QRS complex is narrow as the impulse originates above the bifurcation of the HIS bundle. Sinus bradycardias can be categorized as physiologic, pathologic, or pharmacologic. Physiologic bradycardia is common in well-trained athletes, where vagal tone predominates at rest. In this instance, parasympathetic input decreases the rate of spontaneous sinoatrial node firing and slows down conduction through the AV node. Slow rates are also considered normal variants during natural sleep, where rates less than 40 bpm, sinus pauses of 2–3 seconds, and junctional rhythms often occur. Parasympathetic tone also increases during vomiting and vagal maneuvers, such as the Valsalva maneuver (forced expiration against a closed glottis) or

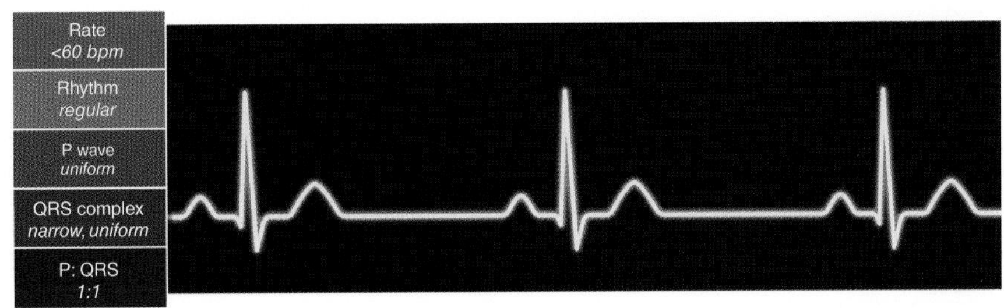

Figure 5.18 Sinus bradycardia.

carotid sinus massage. Pharmacologic sinus bradycardia, as the name implies, is drug induced, and can occur with exposure to systemic β-blockers, timolol eye drops in elderly patients, digoxin, calcium channel blockers, amiodarone, opioids, or succinylcholine (esp. with a repeated dose.) Causes of pathologic sinus bradycardia include hypoxia, infarction, sinus node dysfunction, hypothyroidism, conduction block, and anorexia nervosa, among others. It is important to note that bradycardia can be due to conduction blocks inferior to a normally functioning sinus node; common sites include blocks in the AV node or bundle branches.

Sinus bradycardia, regardless of the etiology, is abnormal when accompanied by symptoms of angina, shortness of breath, exercise intolerance, hypotension, dizziness, syncope, or when it invites ectopy (Mangrum and Dimarco, 2000). Perioperative bradycardia should be closely monitored for new onset ectopic beats or hypotension; possible triggers should be remediated and atropine 0.5 mg IV every 3 to 5 minutes can be considered.

Escape beats

When the SA node fails to initiate a beat, other foci capable of spontaneous discharge can fire, now freed from overdrive suppression. These foci can occur in the atria (atrial escape), the AV node (junctional escape), or in the ventricle (ventricular escape). The escape beat occurs only once or occasionally as compared to an escape rhythm, which occurs when alternate foci continually fire. A lag between beats is often first noticed, with the subsequent appearance of a beat that comes late in the sequence, with an absent or different P wave. The atrial escape beat displays a different P wave, followed by a normal, narrow QRS complex, usually at rates between 60 and 80 bpm, which then leads to overdrive suppression of potential inferior foci. The junctional escape beat displays a normal, narrow QRS complex with variable rates. P waves, if present, are due to retrograde conduction. Atrial and junctional escape beats/rhythms are common during anesthesia. In the absence of hypotension or identifiable triggers, close monitoring is usually all that may be required. Ventricular escape rhythms are ominous, with absent P waves and a widened QRS complex at inherent rates of 20–40 bpm.

Conduction disturbances

Rate-lowering transient or permanent conduction disturbances are classified by location and degree of blockade. Sites of origin include the sinus node, AV node, or the ventricular conduction system. Etiologies include normal variation, syncope, idiopathic fibrosis with advancing age, drug effect, or ischemia secondary to CAD.

Sinus pause (see Figure 5.19)

Sinus pause is a sinus dysrhythmia characterized by the abrupt absence of one or more P waves and associated QRS complexes. The etiology in otherwise healthy hearts can be a failure of impulse generation of the SA node or conduction block from the SA node, due to drug effect or increased parasympathetic tone. When occurrence is isolated and brief, blood pressure is rarely affected. When prolonged, blood pressure will drop. Pathologic causes include ischemia, infarct hyperkalemia, or drug effect, secondary to β-blockers or calcium channel blockers.

Heart block

First degree heart block

First-degree heart block (see Figure 5.20) is characterized by a P–R interval greater than 0.2 seconds, with a P:QRS ratio of 1:1 and normal, narrow QRS complex, signifying a delay in conduction through the AV node. This phenomenon appears at slower heart rates, or as a consequences of aging, ischemia, drug effect, or parasympathetic excess. During anesthesia, it is prudent to avoid drugs or situations that can further slow down the heart rate, which could cause a drop in pressure. First-degree heart blocks do not require treatment if blood pressure is maintained.

Second-degree heart block, Mobitz I

There are two variants of the second-degree heart block. The Mobitz I (Wenchebach) atrioventricular block (Figure 5.21) is characterized by a repetitive and recurring sequence of progressive prolongation of the PR interval culminating in a dropped QRS complex. As a

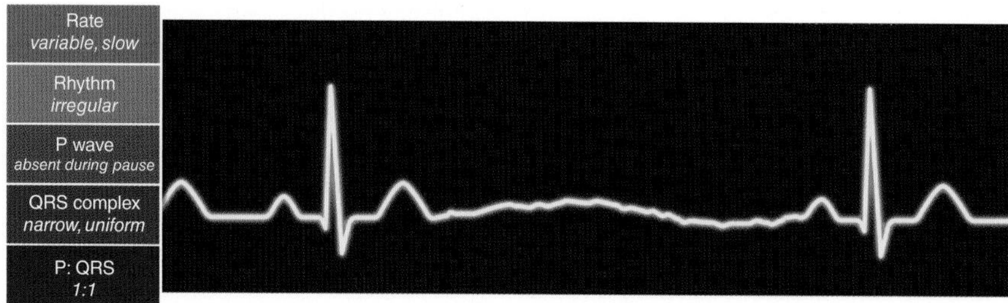

Figure 5.19 Sinus pause.

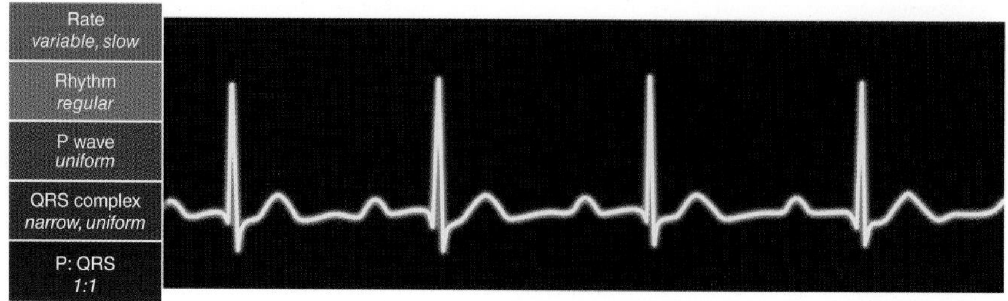

Figure 5.20 First degree heart block.

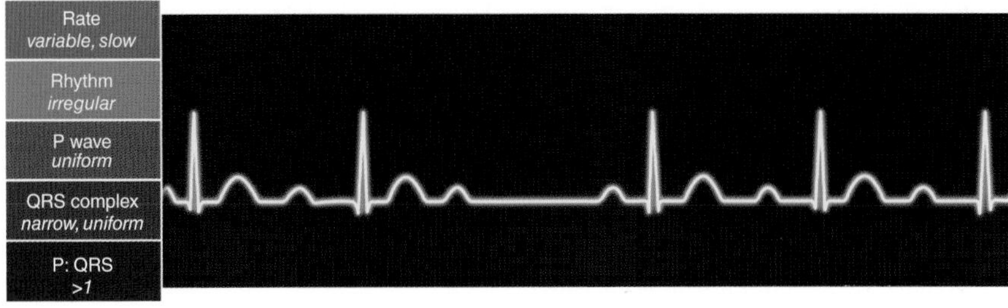

Figure 5.21 Second degree heart block, Mobitz I.

result of delayed conduction, each successive impulse arrives earlier in the relative refractory period until it finally meets absolute refraction, causing the dropped beat. The dropped beat allows ample time for full repolarization, after which the sequence repeats itself. Careful analysis of the ECG tracing reveals a regular atrial rhythm, as seen by identical P–P intervals. This block can be short lived and is usually asymptomatic. Atropine may transiently improve conduction. This block rarely progresses to the Mobitz II block in the absence of structural heart disease.

Advanced heart blocks

The Mobitz II AV block is characterized by a sudden and complete interruption of atrioventricular conduction without progressive PR prolongation, signifying more severe damage to the conduction system. It can be an ominous sign, which can readily progress to complete heart block. Patients demonstrating a second-degree heart block should be triaged appropriately.

Third-degree heart block represents complete atrioventricular dissociation, where atrial impulses do not conduct to the ventricle. Bradycardia, hemodynamic instability, and exercise intolerance often result.

Bundle branch blocks occur at various levels in the HIS–Purkinje system and display a widened QRS complex. The right bundle branch block can be present without cardiac disease and often present without clinical significance in the absence of structural heart disease. Blocks of the left bundle branch are more ominous and are often a marker for serious cardiac disease.

Management decisions

Dysrhythmias occurring during surgery and anesthesia should be promptly identified, evaluated, and triaged as necessary in an orderly sequence. A single-line ECG tracing typically displays 6 seconds of activity, which can make diagnosis of fleeting beats difficult. In that same context, however, fleeting beats usually have little cardiovascular consequence. Once a significant dysrhythmia is identified, the following sequence should be initiated.

1 Stop surgery, check airway, ventilation, and oxygenation.
2 Establish hemodynamic significance:
   (a) Assess blood pressure as compared to baseline.
   (b) Establish origin (ventricular more worrisome than supraventricular).
   (c) Be mindful of duration (transient or prolonged).
   (d) Look for frequency and width of QRS complexes.
3 Identify/remove potential triggers:
   (a) Pain, light anesthesia
   (b) Vasoconstrictor from local anesthetic
   (c) Rule out drug effect – error, interaction
   (d) Possibility of electrolyte disturbance
4 Estimate probability of deterioration, especially with hypotension.
5 Review any underlying patient diseases that may be responsible.
6 Assess patient reserve – ability to tolerate without decompensation.
7 Triage as necessary.

Cardiovascular implanted electronic devices (CIED)

Rapid and significant advances in the durability, reliability, and complexity of CIEDs have led to a plethora of confusing literature and misinformation producing wide communication and knowledge gaps among all heath care providers. These devices include pacemakers, implanted cardiac defibrillators, and devices for cardiac resynchronization therapy (CRT), among others (see figure 5.22). This discussion is limited to pacemakers and implantable cardioverter defibrillators (ICDs), which are used to manage the following enduring conditions, not readily amenable to drug or other therapies: pacemakers for bradycardias (sinus node dysfunction or high-grade (Mobitz II and third degree) AV blocks); ICDs for tachydysrhythmias and biventricular CRT for heart failure.

These devices consist of a pulse generator capable of producing electrical impulses, a lithium-iodide power source (lifespan ~ 10 years), and one or more sensing and pacing electrodes that can be placed in the right atrial or right ventricular endocardium or left ventricular epicardium, when threaded through the coronary

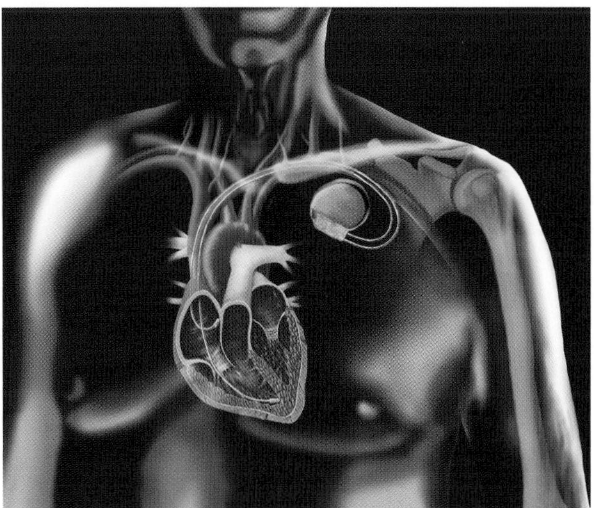

Figure 5.22 This is an illustration of a CIED implanted subcutaneously beneath the left clavicle with electrodes in the right atrium and right ventricle.

sinus. In addition, defibrillators contain a capacitor to allow for more powerful discharges (shocks). Data accumulation (telemetry and storage) is also possible. Some devices are rate-adaptive, which will increase paced rates based on movement (accelerometers) or by transthoracic impedance, in patients who are unable to increase their heart rate in response to activity (chronotropically incompetent).

Patients with these devices periodically report (physically or telemetrically) to a "pacemaker clinic" where information concerning device operation, historical rhythm, shock information, and battery life are monitored.

These devices detect and respond to low-amplitude cardiac electrical events, which are "captured" between the negative pole (active lead) and positive pole of the circuit. Extraneous electromagnetic interference (bipolar electrocautery, TENS units) can be "oversensed" by the device, which can cause inappropriate inhibition of pacing or inappropriate shock therapy.

Adverse events related to device malfunction (esp. ICDs) within the first year after implantation can occur with some frequency – failure to pace or sense, inappropriate therapy, or lead dislodgement.

Pacemakers

A five-letter code describes the pacemaker (Stone et al., 2011).

- Chamber(s) paced – A(atrium), V(ventricle), D (dual – A and V)
- Chamber(s) sensed – O-none, A, V, D
  - If no chamber is sensed, the device functions in an *asynchronous* mode (~70bpm)
- Response to sensed signal – O-none; I-inhibition; T-triggering; D-(both trigger /or inhibit)
  - This implies a *demand* or *synchronous* mode
- Rate responsive – O-no; R-yes
- Multisite pacing – O-no, A, V, D

Asynchronous pacing fires at a fixed rate regardless of inherent underlying rhythm – AOO, VOO, or DOO. This is uncommon for patients with intrinsic ventricular activity, as the R on T phenomenon is possible and can provoke serious dysrhythmias. All other devices provide *synchronous* (non-competitive; demand mode) activity, whereby a given clinical situation will either trigger or inhibit a CIED function. *Single chamber pacing* can stimulate the atrium (AAI) in patients with sinus node disease, but with an intact AV node leading to symptomatic bradycardia. Patients with symptomatic SA or AV node disease can benefit from a VVI, which does not fire if a native R wave is detected. *Dual chamber pacing* (usually DDD or DDI) (see Figure 5.23) is physiologic, as AV synchrony is maintained, facilitating myocardial efficiency. *Cardiac resynchronization therapy* (biventricular) is reserved for drug-refractory heart failure (NYHA III or IV) (see Table 5.17), with a left ventricular ejection fraction less than 35% (nl is ~ 55–70%) and QRS duration greater than 120 msec. In these cases, the underlying electrical dyssynchrony progresses to mechanical dyssynchrony, valvular incompetence, and decreased cardiac output. Pacemaker syndrome is the host of symptoms caused by loss of AV synchony and includes syncope, weakness, and lethargy (forward symptoms), and pulmonary and peripheral congestions (backward symptoms.)

Table 5.17 NYHA heart failure classification.

NYHA Class	Symptoms
I	Cardiac disease, but no symptoms and no limitation in ordinary physical activity, e.g., shortness of breath when walking, climbing stairs
II	Mild symptoms (mild shortness of breath and/or angina) and slight limitation during ordinary activity
III	Marked limitation during less than ordinary activity (e.g., walking short distances) due to symptoms. Comfortable only at rest
IV	Severe limitations. Symptoms at rest. Mostly bedbound patients

Implantable cardioverter defibrillators

In addition to all pacemaker functions, ICDs can detect dysrhythmias (R–R' interval analysis), can cardiovert (1–30j for sustained ventricular tachycardia), can defibrillate (10–30j for sustained ventricular fibrillation), and can result in overdrive suppression of some supraventricular tachycardias. Capacitor energy accumulation and discharge takes approximately 15 seconds from onset of dysrhythmia detection, during which time, hypotension or loss of consciousness can occur. The defibrillating electrode is the titanium case. Patients feel "the kick of a mule on their chest"; a practitioner in physical contact with the patient at this moment will feel the shock but not be hurt.

Indications for ICDs include patients with structural heart disease at risk for or to prevent VT/VF, prior history of resuscitated cardiac arrest or VT, and various channelopathies.

A four-letter code describes the ICD.

- Chamber shocked – O, A, V, D
- Anti-tachycardia pacing chamber – O, A, V, D
- Tachycardia detection mechanism – E (electrogram) or H (hemodynamic)
- Antibradycardia pacing chamber – O, A, V, D

Perianesthetic management of patients with CIEDs

There are special concerns when treating patients with CIEDs, particularly when the use of cautery is anticipated, or when

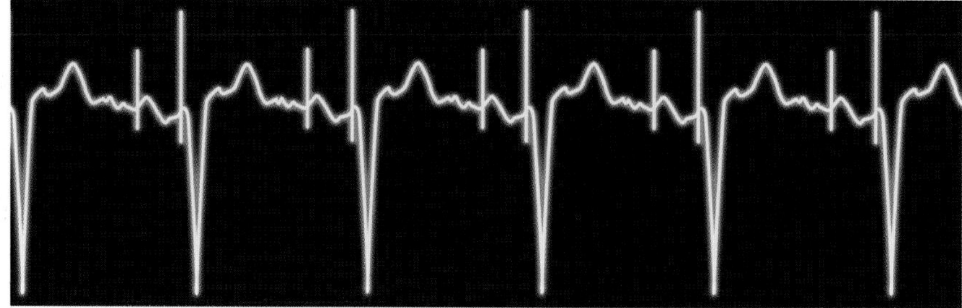

Figure 5.23 Dual chamber pacing.

deeper levels of anesthesia are planned (Rooke and Bowdle, 2013; ASA Practice Advisory, 2011; Crossley et al., 2011). In operating rooms, a 90 gauss donut magnet can be placed in proximity of the device to "blind" it to electromagnetic interference from the cautery. In some instances, pacemakers become asynchronous and ICDs will not defibrillate. However, in the absence of expert consult and knowledge of how the device will behave, "routine magnet placement" has become questionable. If cautery is required, least interference occurs with the use of short bursts of bipolar cutting. The most interference occurs with the use of monopolar coagulation, especially when the return pad location permits the electricity to cross the path of the device. Apex locaters, curing lights, harmonic scalpels, and electrical pulp testers are generally considered to be safe when used in the presence of CIEDs. *Most* ultrasonic dental scalers should also be safe; however, the manufacturer of the ultrasonic unit in question should be contacted regarding the possible interference of their device with CIEDs.

It is difficult to predict the hemodynamic course of patients with CIEDs during light, moderate, or deep sedation. At one end of the spectrum is a patient with sinus node disease with a demand pacemaker, functioning as a "guardian angel" - steadfast in its task of ensuring a heart rate adequate to maintain blood pressure. However, at the other end of the spectrum is an ASA III to IV patient, who requires the ICD to defibrillate recurrent ventricular fibrillation. Consultation with the patient's CIED team is warranted with the ICD patient and can be helpful with the pacemaker patient. In all cases, a thorough device history should be obtained (see Table 5.18). Physical examination should include vital signs, pulmonary auscultation, and a check for ankle edema. A lead II ECG tracing, noting any pacemaker spikes, will aid in determining the degree of device dependence.

Goals of anesthesia are maintenance of ventilation, oxygenation, heart rate, and blood pressure. Backup pacing and defibrillation can be considered. In general, pacing thresholds are not altered by anesthetic agents. Pacing thresholds can be altered by hyperventilation, alterations in serum K+, hypoxia, sympathetic stimulation, and high systemic doses of local anesthetics.

Congestive heart failure

Definition

A normal, healthy heart is able to meet the metabolic requirements of the human body by changing the heart rate and/or SV, thereby changing the cardiac output. Heart failure occurs when the heart cannot pump an adequate amount of blood to the tissues to meet these requirements. The term *heart failure* implies a progressive, complex clinical syndrome that can result from any structural or functional cardiac injury that impairs the ability of the ventricle to fill with blood (diastolic failure) or eject blood (systolic failure) (Jessup and Brozena, 2003). Frequent causes are impaired contractility due to ischemia, cardiomyopathy, dysrhythmia, pressure overload (valvular stenosis, systemic or pulmonary hypertension), or volume overload (valvular regurgitation), among others. Symptoms of heart failure typically include fatigue and shortness of breath, either at rest or during activity. Patients often display lower extremity edema (Figure 5.24), and may have a chronic cough from pulmonary vascular congestion. In spite of optimal medical management, patients can easily slip into decompensation, and can present with a history of frequent hospitalizations.

Heart failure is estimated to affect nearly 6 million Americans and its incidence is expected to increase as populations age and medical advances allow people to survive longer with more severe cardiac conditions (Lloyd-Jones et al., 2009). The prognosis for people with heart failure remains problematic despite medical advances (Konstam, 2000). Studies show that 30–40% of patients die within 1 year of diagnosis and 60–70% will die within 5 years (Parashar et al., 2009). Mortality rates increase with increasing age at diagnosis (Ho et al., 1993). Given the prevalence of this condition, it is likely that many Americans with congestive heart failure will visit the dentist for elective procedures.

Table 5.18 Key elements of history-taking for patients with CIEDs.

- General survey—how do you feel today?
  - weak, tired, short of breath, cough
- Type of device, reason for placement, date of placement
- Is the device functioning as intended?
- Have there been recent shocks?
- Have you been compliant with pacemaker clinic appointments?
- Is the device functioning correctly? Battery status? Results of last interrogation ?

Pathophysiology

Pulmonary circulation should equal systemic circulation, as measured in liters per minute blood flow. Pulmonary circulation is determined by the central venous pressure (preload) and right ventricular function and is the cardiac output from the right side of the heart. Systemic circulation is determined by left atrial filling pressures and left ventricular function and is the cardiac output from the left side of the heart. Failure of the heart to pump either circulation in a forward direction can result in backward congestion in the pulmonary or central venous compartments.

An increase in preload (lying in the supine position, legs elevated above the head, negative pressure inspiration, fluid retention from excess salt intake) increases venous return to the heart. A normal heart would adjust the filling time, SV, and/or heart rate to compensate. A failing heart cannot do this. Venous blood becomes

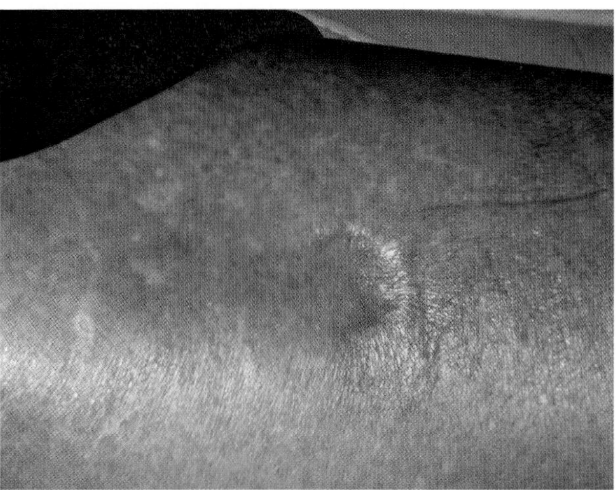

Figure 5.24 Pitting edema. Edema of the lower extremity is termed "pitting" when a depression is left after finger pressure is released.

congested in the lungs and the right heart and pools in the venous circulation.

Three major pathophysiologic processes reflect the fine balance between compensation and decompensation. Compensatory attempts to increase fluid volume and trigger sympathetic stimulation quickly become maladaptive, leading to frequent exacerbation.

1 Excessive sympathetic stimulation – a fall in CO leads to increased sympathetic outflow: increase in inotropy (difficult with pathologic ventricle) and an increase in chronotropy (further decreasing diastolic fill, diastolic coronary perfusion and SV), and so, CO does not change much. Vasoconstriction increases afterload, decreasing CO. Patients are diaphoretic, with pale, cool extremities.
2 Fluid retention – a fall in CO decreases renal perfusion, which triggers Na^+ (and H_2O) retention by the renin – angiotensin – aldo sterone system (RAAS) to restore a perceived decrease in ECV (Colson et al., 1999). The quick fix subsequently leads to pulmonary and systemic congestion due to fluid overload leading to edema.
3 Decrease in CO leads to fatigue, weakness, and exercise intolerance.

Treatment

Patients with well-managed heart failure will often be on several medications, many of which overlap with treatment of other cardiovascular disorders. Typically, a patient will be taking an ACE inhibitor, a diuretic, and a beta-blocker. In some cases, a patient may take a digitalis glycoside called digoxin (Lanoxin™).

Digoxin

Digoxin used to be a mainstay of heart failure treatment until more modern medications were developed. Digoxin works by increasing contractility and is known to slow down the heart rate as well. It does have a very narrow therapeutic window and has mostly been replaced by other medicines except in refractory cases.

Diuretics

In more mild cases of heart failure, a thiazide diuretic such as hydrochlorothiazide may be prescribed. Hydrochlorothiazide reduces circulating plasma volume and is an antihypertensive. In more severe cases, patient may be on furosemide (Lasix™), a loop diuretic. A common consequence of furosemide therapy is hypokalemia. Patients will often take potassium supplements and in some cases take a second, less potent diuretic called spironolactone (Aldactone™), which helps maintain serum potassium levels.

There is no reason to withhold taking any of these medications prior to surgery. Consultation with the patient's cardiologist can be helpful.

Risk assessment

The severity of heart failure is most commonly categorized by the New York Heart Association (NYHA) classification. The NYHA classification is based on functional capacity and symptoms (Klossman, 1964) (Table 5.17).

Functional capacity is very important when evaluating a patient with congestive heart failure prior to an elective dental procedure. A detailed history and physical should be performed with attention to previous diagnoses, recent changes in health, fatigability, dyspnea (at rest, with activity, positional, at night), and functional capacity. The more symptoms or risk factors a patient has, the greater the risk is for heart failure. However, a patient with a functional capacity of 4 METs or greater is likely to tolerate most well managed procedures without a significant increase in cardiopulmonary risk (Fleisher, 2007). In the patient without a diagnosis of heart failure and/or poor overall medical care, a history of symptoms indicating higher risk for heart failure should result in a consultation with a cardiologist and the procedure should be delayed.

Anesthetic concerns

Elective dental procedures should only be performed on heart failure patients who are medically optimized. Medications should be given to minimize the sympathetic stress response and changes in heart rate or blood pressure. Volatile anesthetic agents as well as propofol can be used for anesthetic maintenance but are known cardiac depressants, especially in high doses (Stoelting and Miller, 2007). Nitrous oxide is well tolerated in this population, as it is not known to be a direct cardiac depressant in clinical doses. Etomidate is often favored by anesthesiologists as an induction agent because it offers a stable hemodynamic profile with little variation in heart rate and blood pressure in patients with poor cardiac status. However, it is associated with a higher incidence of post-operative nausea and vomiting, which may decrease patient satisfaction. Of note, if the oral health care professional is considering using any particular anesthetic out of concern for significant hemodynamic variation or instability in a patient with heart disease, referring the patient to a dental practice in a hospital setting may be considered.

Medication circulation time in a patient with heart failure and a reduced ejection fraction is slower when compared to a "healthy" patient. This is important because medication given intravenously may take longer to reach the heart and circulate to its receptor site in the body in a patient with heart failure. The practitioner must recognize that the onset time of intravenous medications (including emergency and vasoconstrictor medications) may be delayed in this patient population. Rapid, frequent dosing of medications can lead to exaggerated responses when the accumulated dose finally reaches its target site. This can result in oversedation and respiratory depression, particularly with narcotic agents. This same concept applies to vasoconstrictor agents and emergency medications such as atropine and epinephrine. Ultimately, careful and deliberate titration of intravenous medications is important.

Alternatively, inhalational agents tend to have a faster onset time in heart failure patients compared to their normal counterparts. This is due to a more rapid accumulation of higher partial pressure of volatile agents in the pulmonary capillary blood. Because of the reduced cardiac output, blood moves slower through the pulmonary circulation from the right ventricle to the left. The partial pressure gradient of a volatile agent, however, remains in favor of diffusion across the pulmonary capillary membrane. Thus, a higher partial pressure of the volatile agent reaches the left ventricle more rapidly and is then distributed to the brain. Given the low solubility and rapid onset of nitrous oxide in healthy patients, this agent may not have a noticeably faster onset in the heart failure population.

Cardiac monitoring is important given that patients with heart failure may be prone to dysrhythmias, such as atrial fibrillation or short runs of ventricular tachydysrhythmias. In fact, patients with heart failure and an ejection fraction less than 35% and falling into NYHA class 2 or 3, are often recommended to have an implanted cardioverter defibrillator (ICD) to prevent sudden cardiac death due to dysrhythmias (Banna and Indik, 2011). Frequent blood pressure monitoring is also important. Sudden increases in afterload create more work for the left ventricle, which may not be able to compensate. This can result in venous congestion, pulmonary edema, and shortness of breath (i.e., worsening of heart failure symptoms) if sustained. Sudden decreases in blood pressure can affect end organ perfusion. Narcotics and volatile agents act as cardiac depressants and may cause hypotension by decreasing cardiac output in high doses. Benzodiazepines may cause hypotension by reducing sympathetic tone. Maintenance of blood pressure should be achieved with vasoconstrictors such as phenylephrine and ephedrine. Extreme bradycardia can be effectively treated with carefully titrated intravenous acetylcholine receptor blocking agents such as glycopyrrolate or atropine.

Induction of general anesthesia with positive pressure ventilation can be challenging. The induction dose of intravenous propofol or etomidate required for the placement of an endotracheal tube or laryngeal mask airway is higher than the maintenance dose and may cause profound hypotension and myocardial depression. Intubation by direct laryngoscopy reverses hypotension and may cause hypertension, which can be detrimental to the patient. Careful titration of induction medications with vasoconstrictors close at hand is as important as is quick and atraumatic intubation by an experienced person (Vacanti, 2011). Positive pressure ventilation is known to decrease pulmonary congestion, which is beneficial in a patient with heart failure. A smooth and careful extubation is important due to the sudden change from positive to negative pressure (spontaneous) ventilation and the resulting increase in venous return to the heart. This increase in filling pressure can worsen heart failure symptoms (Stoelting).

As an alternative to general anesthesia, many dental procedures can be done with local anesthesia and a mild anxiolysis protocol, either with oral agents or with nitrous oxide. Despite the lack of convincing evidence, the use of vasoconstrictors in local anesthetics continues to be discussed in the literature. It is generally accepted that in the patient with heart failure who is stable and well managed by a physician, the amount of epinephrine used in local anesthetics should not exceed 0.04 mg (Rhodus and Falace, 2002; Brown and Rhodus, 2005). This is equivalent to two cartridges (1.8cc/carpule) of lidocaine 2% with epinephrine 1:100,000. It is suggested that in patients with more severe heart failure, or those taking digitalis, epinephrine be avoided due to the possibility of dysrhythmias (Little et al., 2008).

In addition to pharmacologic interventions for patients with heart failure, there are simple ergonomic tools that can greatly increase patient comfort and safety. Many patients with heart failure will note symptoms of dyspnea when supine. When these patients change position from upright to supine, there is a large amount of venous blood in the lower extremities that returns to the heart. The heart, unable to handle the sudden increase in preload, becomes congested, as does the pulmonary circulation. This is the cause for the shortness of breath and is termed *orthopnea.* Positioning the patient in the sitting or semi-recumbent position may prevent orthopnea. Changing from a supine position to sitting or upright positions may cause problems as well. Increased venous capacitance in the lower extremities causes venous pooling. As the blood pools in the legs there is a drop in preload and this may cause syncope. Positional changes should be done slowly in patients with heart failure.

The decision to treat a patient with heart failure in the dental office is multifactorial. Patient functional capacity, the complexity of the procedure to be performed, the ability to monitor and recover the patient, provider and support staff, BLS and ACLS training, the ability to monitor the patient appropriately, and the provider comfort with delivery of the level of anesthesia required are only a few of the factors involved in the decision to treat a patient in the office setting versus referral to a more specialized treatment center. Patient safety should always be a top priority.

Refererences

American Society of Anesthesiologists. Practice advisory for the perioperative management of patients with cardiac implantable electronic devices: pacemakers and implantable cardioverter-defibrillators: an updated report by the American Society of Anesthesiologists Task Force on perioperative management of patients with cardiac implantable electronic devices. *Anesth* **114**: 247–261, 2011.

Attenhofer Jost, C. H., et al. Echocardiography in the evaluation of systolic murmurs of unknown cause. *Am J Med* **108**: 614–620, 2000.

Bader, J. D., et al. Oral and Maxillofacial Surgery. A systematic review of cardiovascular effects of epinephrine on hypertensive dental patients. *Oral Surg Oral Med Oral Pathol Oral Radiol Endod* **93**: 647–653, 2002.

Banna M, Indik J. H.. Risk stratification and prevention of sudden death in patients with heart failure. *Curr Treat Options Cardiovasc Med***13**: 517–527, 2011.

Beckwith, C and Munger, M. A. Effect of angiotensin-converting enzyme inhibitors on ventricular remodeling and survival following myocardial infarction. *Ann Pharmacother* **27**: 755–766, 1993.

Bonow, R. O., et al. ACC/AHA 2006 guidelines for the management of patients with valvular heart disease: a report of the American College of Cardiology/American Heart Association Task Force on Practice Guidelines (writing committee to revise the 1998 Guidelines for the Management of Patients With Valvular Heart Disease): developed in collaboration with the Society of Cardiovascular Anesthesiologists: endorsed by the Society for Cardiovascular Angiography and Interventions and the Society of Thoracic Surgeons. *Circulation* **114**: e84-e231, 2006.

Brown R. S., Rhodus, N. L.. Epinephrine and local anesthesia revisited. *Oral Surg Oral Med Oral Pathol Oral Radiol Endod.* **100**;401–408, 2005.

Cheung, A. T. Exploring an optimum intra/postoperative management strategy for acute hypertension in the cardiac surgery patient. *J Card Surg* **21**: s8–s14, 2006.

Chobanian, A. V., et al. Sevenths report of the Joint National Committee on prevention, detection, evaluation and treatment of high blood pressure. The JNC 7 report. *JAMA* **289**:2560–2572, 2003.

Chiu, A. G., et al. Angiotensin-converting enzyme inhibitor-induced angioedema: a multicenter review and an algorithm for airway managment. *Ann Otol Rhinol Laryngol* **110**: 834–840, 2001.

Colson, P, et al. Renin angiotensin system antagonists and anesthesia. *Anesth Analg* **89**: 1143–1155, 1999.

Coriat, P., et al. Influence of chronic angiotensin-converting enzyme inhibition in anesthetic induction. *Anesthesiol* **81**: 299–307, 1994.

Correll, D. J., et al. Preoperative electrocardiograms: patient factors predictive of abnormalities. *Anesthesiol* **110**: 1217–1222, 2009.

Crossley, G. H., et al. The Heart Rhythm Society (HRS)/American Society of Anesthesiologists (ASA) expert consensus statement on the perioperative management of patients with implantable defibrillators, pacemakers and arrhythmia monitors: facilities and patient management. *Heart Rhythm* **8**: 1114–1154, 2011.

Fleisher, L. A., ACC/AHA 2007 guidelines on perioperative cardiovascular evaluation and care for noncardiac surgery: executive summary: a report on the American College of Cardiology/American Heart Association Task Force on practice guidelines. *J Am Coll Cardiol.* **50**: 1707–1732, 2007.

Greenberg, B. L., et al. Screening for cardiovascular risk factors in a dental setting. *JADA* **138**: 798–804, 2007.

Grines, C. L., et al. Prevention of premature discontinuation of dual antiplatelet therapy in patients with coronary artery stents: a science advisory from the American Heart Association, American College of Cardiology, Society for Cardiovascular Angiography and Interventions, American College of Surgeons, and American Dental Association, with representation from the American College of Physicians. *JADA* **138**: 652–655, 2007.

Goldman, L. and Caldera, D. L. Risk of general anesthesia and elective operation in the hypertensive patient. *Anesthesiol* **50**: 285–292, 1979.

Ho K. K., Anderson K. M., Kannel W. B., Grossman W., Levy D.. Survival after the onset of congestive heart failure in Framingham Heart Study subjects. *Circulation* **88**:107–115, 1993.

Immink, R. V., et al. Impaired cerebral autoregulation in patients with malignant hypertension. *Circulation* **110**: 2241–2245, 2004.

Jessup, M. and Brozena, S. Heart failure. *N Engl J Med* **348**: 2007–2018, 2003.

James, P. A., et al. 2014 evidence-based guidelines for the management of high blood pressure in adults: report from the panel members appointed to the Eight National Committee (JNC8). *JAMA* **311**: 507–20, 2014.

Katzung, B. G.. *Basic and Clinical Pharmacology*. New York: McGraw-Hill, 2001.

Kennedy, H. L., et al. Long-term follow up of asymptomatic healthy subjects with frequent and complex ventricular ectopy. *N Engl J Med* **312**: 193, 1985.

Kodama-Takahashi, K., et al. Myocardial infarction in a patient with severe aortic stenosis and normal coronary arteriograms: involvement of the circumferential subendocardial wall of the left ventricle. *Circulation* **67**: 891–894, 2003.

Kreiner, M., et al. Craniofacial pain as the sole symptom of cardiac ischemia: a prospective multicenter study. *JADA* **138**(1): 74–79, 2007.

Krukemyer, J. J., et al. Comparison of hypersensitivity to adrenergic stimulation after abrupt withdrawal of propranolol and nadolol: influence of half-life differences. *Am Heart J* **120**:572, 1990.

Lessard, E., et al. The patient with a heart murmur: evaluation, assessment and dental considerations. *J Am Dent Assoc* **136**: 347–356, 2005.

Little J. W., Falace D. A., Miller C. S., Rhodus N. L.. *Dental Management of the Medically Compromised Patient*. 7th edn St. Louis: Mosby Elsevier; 2008.

Lloyd-Jones D, et al. Heart disease and stroke statistics: 2009 update—a report from the American Heart Association Statistics Committee and Stroke Statistics Subcommittee. *Circulation* **119**: e21–e181, 2009.

Lockhart, P. B., et al. Dental management considerations for the patient with an acquired coagulopathy, part 2: coagulopathies from drugs. *Br Dent J* **195**: 495–501, 2003.

Klossman, C. *The Criteria Committee of the New York Heart Association. Diseases of the Heart and Blood Vessels: Nomenclature and Criteria for Diagnosis*. 6th edn. Boston: Little, Brown; 1964.

Konstam M. A.. Progress in heart failure management? Lessons from the real world. *Circulation* **102**: 1076–1078, 2000.

Mangrum, J. and Dimarco, J. The Evaluation and Management of Bradycardia. *New Eng J Med* **342**: 703–709, 2000.

Nathanson, M. H. and Gajraj, N.M. The peri-operative management of atrial fibrillation. *Anesthesia* **53**: 665–676, 1998.

Ng, G. A. Treating patients with ventricular ectopic beats. *Heart* **92**: 1707–1712, 2006.

Parashar S., Katz R., Smith N. L. Race, gender, and mortality in adults ≥65 years of age with incident heart failure (from the Cardiovascular Health Study). *Am J Cardiol* **103**: 1120–1127, 2009.

Podrid, P. J. Clinical significance and treatment of ventricular premature beats. UpToDate, 2013. http://www.uptodate.com/contents/clinical-significance-and-treatment-of-ventricular-premature-beats?detectedLanguage=en&source=search_result&search=clinical+significance+of+ventric&selectedTitle=3%7E150&provider=noProvider (Accessed June 25, 2013)

Paulson, O. B., et al. Cerebral Autoregulation. *Cerebrovas Brain Met Rev* **2**: 161–192, 1990.

Prys-Roberts, C., et al. Studies of anesthesia in relation to hypertension I. Cardiovascular responses of treated and untreated patients. *Br. J Anaesth* **43**: 122–127, 1971.

Rhodus NL, Falace DA. Management of the dental patient with congestive heart failure. *Gen Dent* **50**: 260–265, 2002.

Roger, V. L., et al. Heart disease and stroke statistics—2012 update: a report from the American Heart Association. *Circulation* **125**: e2–e220, 2012.

Roizen, M. F. and Fleisher, L. A. Anesthetic implications of concurrent diseases. In Miller, R.D., ed, *Miller's Anesthesia*, 7th edn Philadelphia: Churchill Livingstone Elsevier, 2010.

Rooke, G. A. and Bowdle, T. A. Perioperative management of pacemakers and implantable cardioverter defibrillators: it's not just about the magnet. *Anesth Analg* **117**: 292–294, 2013.

Royster, R. L., et al. Cardiovascular pharmacology. In Kaplan, J. A., et al. *Kaplan's Cardiac Anesthesia: The Echo Era*. St. Louis: Elsevier, 2011.

Sandler G. The importance of the history in the medical clinic and the cost of unnecessary tests. *Am Heart J* **100**: 928–931, 1980.

Sear, J.W. Perioperative control of hypertension: when will it adversely affect perioperative outcome? *Curr Hypertens Rep* **10** :480–487, 2008.

Schaal, S. F. Ventricular arrhythmias in patients with mitral valve prolapse. *Cardiovasc Clin* **22**:307–316, 1992.

Simpson, R. J., Jr., et al. Prevalence of premature ventricular contractions in a population of African American and white men and women: the Atherosclerosis Risk in Communities (ARIC) study. *Am Heart J* **143**: 535, 2002.

Stahmer, S. A. and Cowan, R. Tachydysrhymias. *Emerg Med Clin N Am*, **24**: 11–40, 2006.

Stojiljkovic, L. Renin-angiotensin system inhibitors and angioedema: anesthetic implications. *Curr Opin Anesthesiol* **25**: 1–7, 2012.

Stoelting, RK, Miller RD. *Basics of Anesthesia*. Philadelphia: Churchill Livingstone, 2007.

Stone, M. E., et al. Perioperative management of patients with cardiac implantable electronic devices. *Br J Anaesth* **107**: i16–i26, 2011.

Strandgaard, S. Autoregulation of cerebral blood flow in hypertensive patients. The modifying influence of prolonged antihypertensive treatment on the tolerance to acute, drug-induced hypotension. *Circulation* **53**:720–727, 1976.

Ten Berg, J.M., et al. Antiplatelet and anticoagulant therapy in elective percutaneous coronary intervention. *Curr Control Trials Cardiovasc Med* **2**: 129–40, 2001.

Turnbull, F., et al. Effects of different regimens to lower blood pressure on major cardiovascular events in older and younger adults: meta-analysis of randomized trials. *Br. Med. J* **336**: 1121, 2008.

Vacanti, CA. *Essential Clinical Anesthesia*. New York: Cambridge University Press, 2011.

Valerin, M. A., et al. Relationship between aspirin use and postoperative bleeding from dental extractions in a healthy population. *Oral Surg Oral Med Oral Pathol Oral Radiol Endod* **102**:326, 2006.

Watson, K. T. *Abnormalities of cardiac conduction and cardiac rhythm*. In: Hines, R. L. and Marschall, K. E. *Stoelting's Anesthesia and Co-existing Disease*,6th edn Philadelphia: Saunders, 2012.

Wolfsthal, D.S. Is blood pressure control necessary before surgery? *Med Clin North Am* **77**:349, 1993.

Yost, C.S. Potassium channels. Basic aspects, functional roles and medical significance. *Anesthesiol* **90**:1186–1203, 1999.

6 Anesthetic considerations for patients with respiratory disease

Robert C. Bosack[1] and Zak Messieha[2]
[1]University of Illinois, College of Dentistry, Chicago, IL, USA
[2]University of Illinois at Chicago, Colleges of Dentistry & Medicine, Chicago, IL, USA

Introduction

Respiration involves the ongoing exchange of oxygen and carbon dioxide, which predictably follow concentration gradients. The term respiration refers to three physiologic functions: ventilation (movement of air between the environment and alveoli via periodic bellows movement of the thoracic cage and lungs), diffusion (transfer of gases across the fragile respiratory membrane) and perfusion (continual exposure of blood to alveoli) (see Figures 6.1 and 6.2). Deficiencies in oxygenation (the external administration of oxygen) or any of these three processes interferes with the transport of oxygen from the environment to the erythrocyte, causing both hypoxemia and hypercarbia with attendant sympathetic stimulation. A myriad of diseases are known to alter the effective functioning of the respiratory system; a majority involve alterations in ventilation. Unique to the respiratory system is the fact that disease often progresses insidiously without signs, symptoms or formal diagnosis. This underscores the importance of an accurate history, which many patients typically dismiss as trivial, and physical examination. Familiarity with normal physiology and common pathologies facilitate the ability to efficiently assess and optimize patients prior to anesthetic management. Accrual of this information feeds risk minimization by case refusal or depth of anesthesia limit setting.

Ventilation is the periodic creation of negative and positive intra-pulmonary pressure to move gases by bulk or convective flow to and from the level of the terminal bronchioles. This pathway is lined with mucus producing cells and cilia to trap and expel dust and other inhaled debris to the level of the hypopharynx, where it is either expectorated or swallowed. Distal to the terminal bronchioles, gas instantaneously moves by diffusion, following their individual pressure gradients to the level of the alveolar sacs. As bronchiolar branching proceeds, diameter decreases, cartilage decreases and smooth muscle increases. Bronchiolar smooth muscle controls the diameter of the airway, with a resting autonomic balance favoring parasympathetic vagal tone through the action of acetylcholine on muscarinic receptors. β_2 adrenergic receptors become abundant in the medium and smaller bronchioles, causing bronchiolar dilation when stimulated by endogenous or exogenous catecholamines. H_1 histamine receptors mediate bronchiolar constriction, which would be expected during allergy and anaphylaxis. According to Poiseulle's Law, the resistance to flow is inversely related to the radius^4, such that if the radius is halved, the resistance to flow increases 16 fold, which becomes significant as the diameter of the bronchioles decreases.

The active process of inspiration is mainly due to contraction of the diaphragm, which easily distends the healthy and compliant lung, forcing abdominal contents downward and forward as it moves inferiorly by as much as 12 cm with deep inspiration. Inspiration results in augmented venous return. Negative intrathoracic pressure draws venous blood into the mediastinum, while the increase in intra-abdominal pressure pushes venous blood toward the heart along its valved pathway. Exhalation is a passive process under normal circumstances.

Various lung volumes and capacities (the sum of 2 or more lung volumes) are depicted in Figure 6.3. Functional residual capacity represents the combined respiratory reserve volume and residual volume. This capacity serves as a reservoir for rapidly diffusible oxygen, which can delay the onset of hypoxemia during hypoventilation or apnea. This capacity increases with obstructive disease and decreases with restrictive disease (Figure 6.4). The prudent practice of pre-anesthetic and continuous perianesthetic oxygen administration keeps this capacity enriched with oxygen, which can prolong desaturation with during loss of upper airway tone or deceased ventilator drive. The time to hemoglobin desaturation with apnea is modeled in Figure 6.5, which graphically predicts an earlier onset of desaturation for children and for adults with obesity or illness, as compared to the "normal" adult (Benumof et al., 1997).

Supplemental oxygen administration

Common methods to supplement oxygen during anesthesia without interfering with oral access include the nasal cannula (Figure 6.6), nasal mask (hood) (Figure 6.7), and a tightly sealed nasal mask (Figure 6.8). The simple full face mask and a non-rebreather mask with reservoir (Figure 6.9) cover both the nose and mouth and cannot be used during dental procedures. Normal ventilation consists of 12–15 cycles per minute of inhaling and exhaling 500cc tidal volumes per minute. The duration of a normal inhalation is 2–3 seconds, which infers a flow rate of approximately 10 liters/minute during each breath. If 10 lpm is not available, entrainment of room air results. Depending on quality of

Anesthesia Complications in the Dental Office, First Edition. Edited by Robert C. Bosack and Stuart Lieblich.

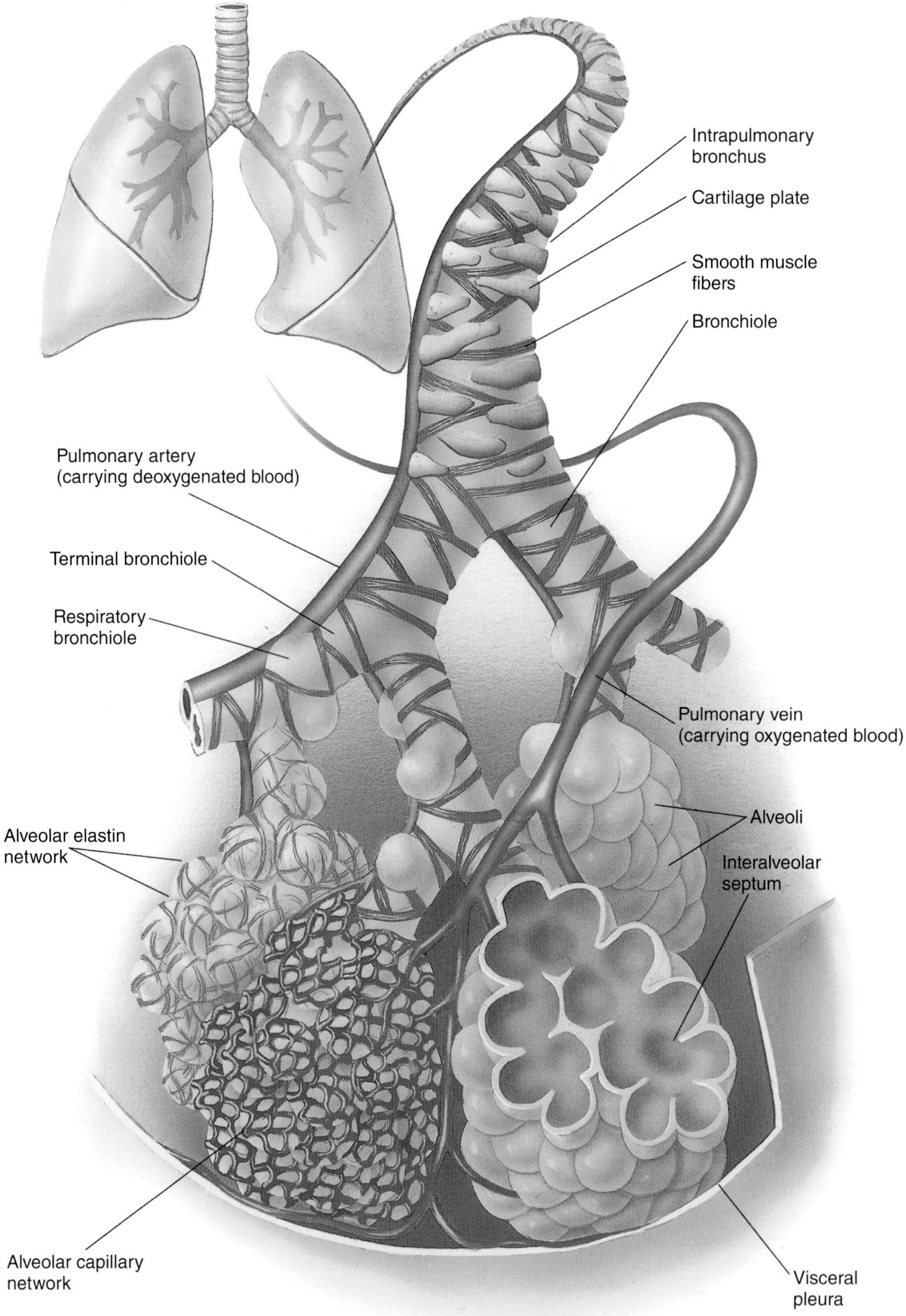

Figure 6.1 The respiratory system macroscopic level (Gartner and Hiatt, 2009) courtesy of Wolters Kluwer, with permission.

seal and the possibility of entraining room air, the efficiency of all nasal devices to deliver oxygen is compromised.

Each of these three methods do not seal the oral cavity. When procedures are not being performed, supplemental oxygen is most efficiently provided with a facemask with O_2 reservoir bag (non-rebreathing mask, "NRB" "non-rebreather"). See Table 6.1 FiO_2 is the fraction of inspired oxygen. Room air, for example provides an FiO_2 of 20%.

The NRB at an oxygen flow rate of 10 LPM or more is the most efficient way to deliver oxygen in an open system.

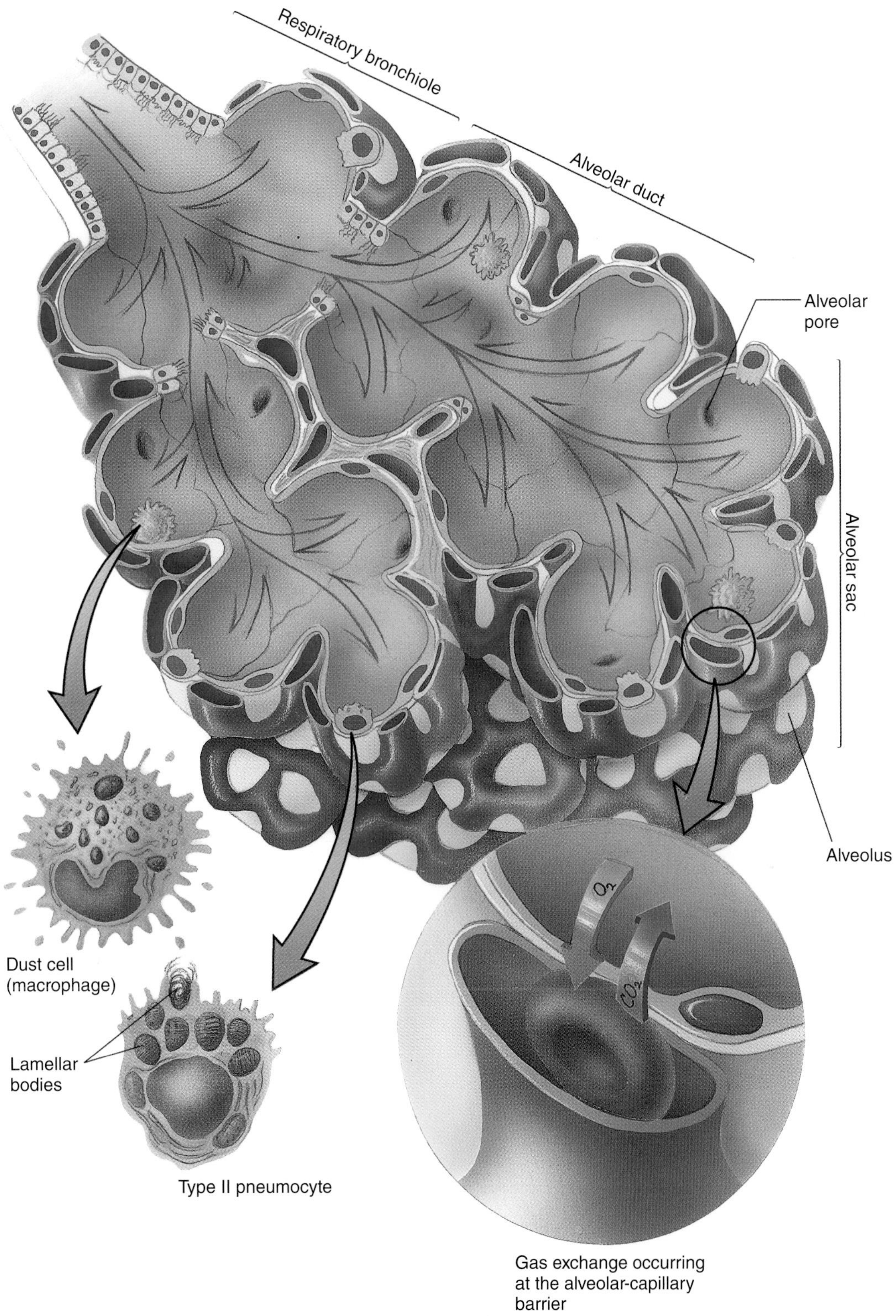

Figure 6.2 The respiratory system macroscopic level, (Gartner and Hiatt, 2009) courtesy of Wolters Kluwer, with permission.

Perianesthetic complications include hypoxemia and hypercarbia, which often are the result of hypoventilation or apnea, atelectasis (alveolar collapse), laryngospasm, bronchospasm, aspiration, pulmonary edema or pulmonary embolism. The risk and severity of these complications often increase with age, underlying chronic lung disease, smoking, poor general health, concomitant upper respiratory tract infections, obstructive sleep apnea and obesity. With ketamine as a notable exception, most sedative, hypnotic, opioid medications decrease ventilation and functional residual capacity, promote atelectasis, reduce upper airway tone, and blunt the ventilatory response to hypercarbia and hypoxia. This is a particular concern in patients with advances stages of obstructive

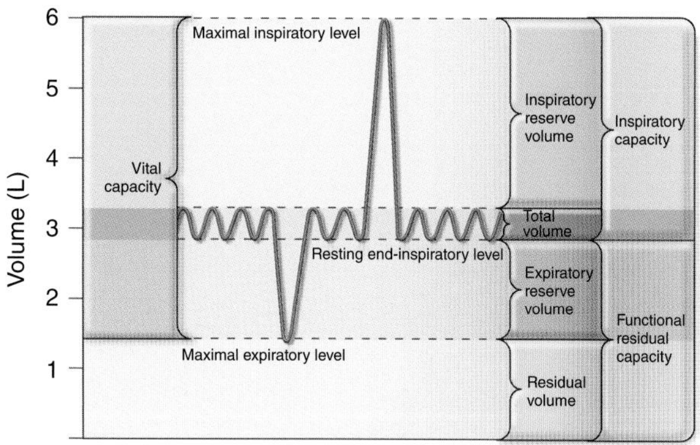

Figure 6.3 Various lung volumes and capacities.

or restrictive disease, where a baseline degree of hypoxia and or metabolically compensated hypercarbia may be present.

Obstructive disease

Obstructive lung disease is a broad clinical term that includes asthma (variable), chronic bronchitis and emphysema (fixed), among other less common diseases. Three common obstructive diseases are compared and contrasted in Table 6.2. The underlying consequence of all obstructive diseases is airway narrowing with resultant limitation of airflow, typically worse on expiration, which leads to air trapping, CO_2 accumulation and subsequent hypoxemia. The variances in lung volumes and capacities caused by obstructive and restrictive diseases are shown in Figure 6.4.

Asthma

Asthma is chronic disease characterized by reversible, variable, recurrent airflow obstruction, bronchiolar hyper-responsiveness and chronic airway inflammation. (Pascual and Peters, 2011) This disease affects approximately 7% of all Americans. (Fanta, 2009) Asthma symptoms are variable and can include cough (especially during nighttime), chest tightness, wheezing and/or shortness of breath. Triggers are categorized as extrinsic (allergic, IgE mediated) or intrinsic (infection, exercise, cold air, strong odors). The common final pathway results in an irritable and inflamed airway leading to bronchospasm, microvascular leakage and mucus secretion. The airway narrowing during an attack is caused by smooth muscle contraction, edema and excessive mucus secretion. Exhalation becomes labored and prolonged, as air gets trapped in and hyper-inflates the lungs (dynamic hyperinflation), compromising future attempts at inspiration. Work of breathing increases and coughing becomes ineffective. If conscious, the patient has a difficult time speaking. If obtunded, the patient may quickly develop hypoxemia.

Asthma is a clinical diagnosis, which is often confirmed by a positive bronchodilator response as measured by spirometry. Well controlled or intermittent disease will often be accompanied by normal spirometry. The disease is categorized as intermittent (mild) or persistent (mild, moderate, severe) based on symptoms and FEV_1 (volume exhaled during the first second of a forced expiratory maneuver started from a maximal inhale, as a percentage of vital capacity)

Treatment includes patient education, trigger avoidance and stepwise pharmacotherapy as needed to control symptoms, prevent attacks, avoid side effects and allow normal daily activity. Patients requiring multiple medications to control symptoms will, by necessity, have more severe disease. Short acting reliever medications

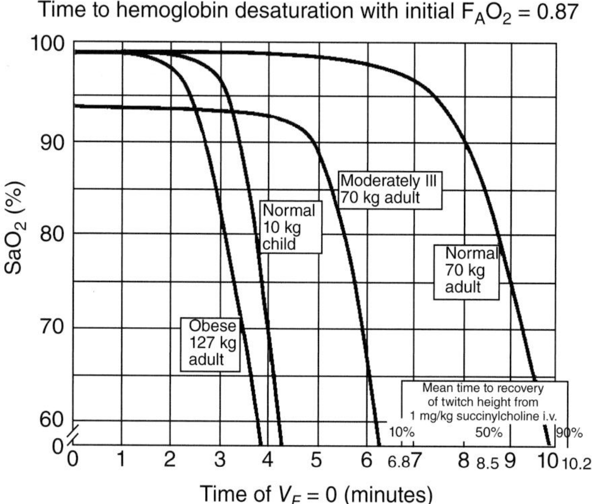

Figure 6.5 Time to hemoglobin desaturation with initial FaO_2 = 0.87. The onset of hemoglobin desaturation with apnea in patients who were completely pre-oxygenated (denitrogenated) is earlier in children and in adults with obesity or illness. (Benumof et al., 1997, with permission.)

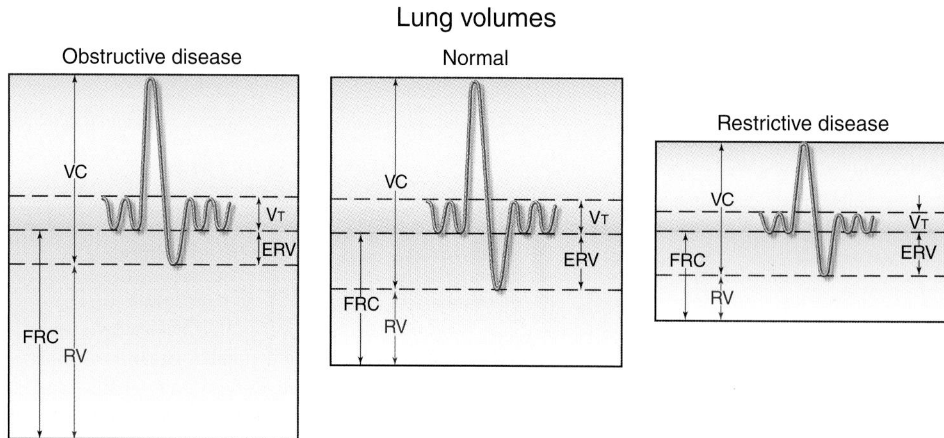

Figure 6.4 A comparison of functional residual capacity in obstructive and restrictive diseases.

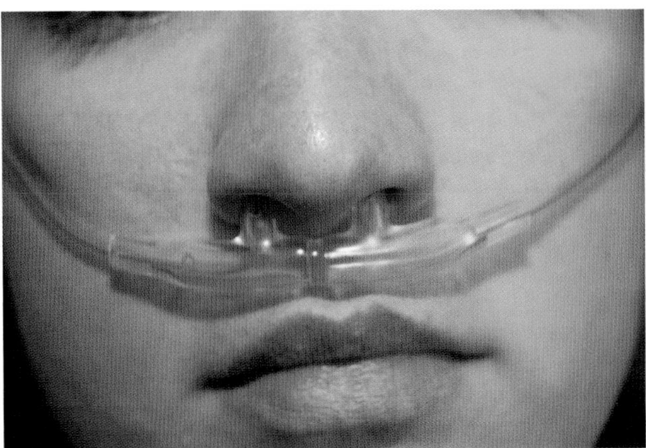

Figure 6.6 Nasal cannula.

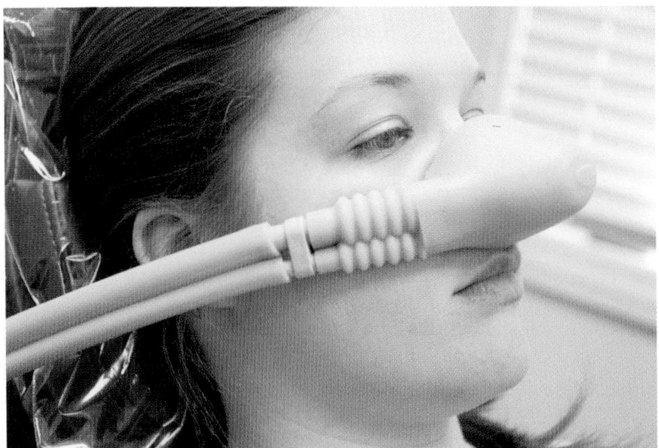

Figure 6.7 Nasal hood with passive fit.

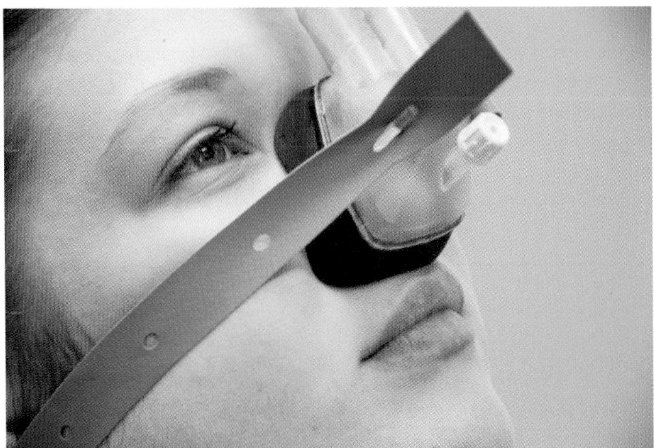

Figure 6.8 Nasal mask with tight fit, courtesy of David Darab, DDS and Anesthesia Innovators, with permission.

include the short acting β_2 agonists (SABAs) and anti-cholinergic medication. Controller medications include long acting β_2 agonists, corticosteroids (oral or inhaled), mast cell stabilizers (cromones), and leukotriene modifiers. Leukotrienes are potent chemical mediators in allergic asthma causing bronchocontriction, mucus secretion and microvascular leakage (See Tables 6.3 and 6.4).

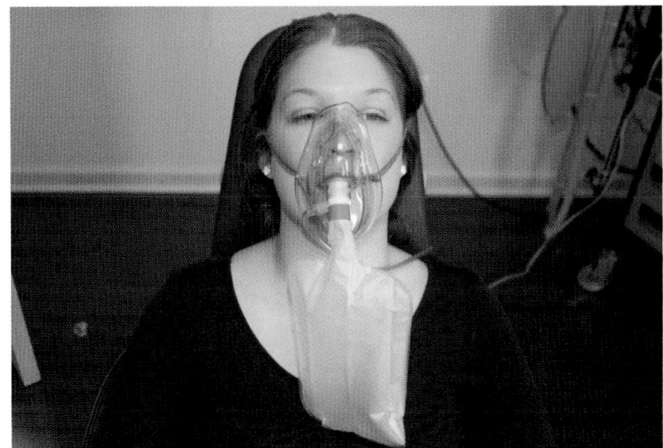

Figure 6.9 Non-rebreather mask with oxygen reservoir.

Table 6.1 Estimates of F_iO_2 with various oxygen delivery systems.

System	100% O2 flow (L/min)	FiO2 (%)
Nasal cannula	2–4	25–35
Nasal hood (with open mouth)	6	35–40
Nasal hood (with closed mouth)	6	35–45
Full face mask	6–10	40–60
Non-rebreather with reservoir	10	95%

Risk assessment

Well-controlled asthma presents no additional risk for the development of complications, provided that airway irritation is minimized. (Ali and Reminick, 2006). Risk assessment for the diagnosed asthmatic patients requires knowledge about the frequency and severity of the symtoms and the recent level of control, including the number, compliance with and efficacy of medications, necessity of oral steroid use and concomitant upper respiratory tract infection. A history of recent attacks can increase the likelihood of further exacerbations as airway hyperreactivity can last up to 6 weeks. Long standing and poorly controlled disease invites the possibility of irreversible airway remodeling, including mucus gland hyperplasia, thickening the alveolar basement membrane, smooth muscle hypertrophy and airway scarring. Exposure to first or second-hand smoke, recent escalation in the use of SABAs, recent exacerbation (within 4–6 weeks), recent hospitalization and a history of perianesthetic respiratory complications are worrisome findings. Physical examination includes observation for respiratory difficulty such as anxiety, tachypnea or substernal retraction. Chest auscultation is performed during vital capacity maneuvers with a wide open mouth. Patients who are wheezing are not optimized, however the silent chest does not preclude the possibility of bronchospasm. Hemoglobin saturation (SpO_2) on room air is a valuable reference prior to anesthesia, but a normal value (>95%) does not necessarily exclude ongoing or suboptimally controlled disease. It is important to note that teenagers or children may attempt to hide warning signs or symptoms. As such, younger patients should be interrogated for the most subtle symptoms, such as (nocturnal) cough, as these patients are generally tolerant to or are readily accommodate bronchiolar constriction without limitation in activity.

Table 6.2 Comparison of common obstructive diseases

Disease	Site	Major changes	Causes
Chronic bronchitis	Bronchus	Hyperplasia and hypersecretion of mucus glands	Smoking, air pollutants
Asthma	Bronchus	Smooth muscle hyperplasia and hyper-reactivity Excessive mucus inflammation	Immunologic or idiopathic
Emphysema	Terminal alveoli	Airspace enlargement and wall destruction	Smoking

Table 6.3 Classification of asthma severity and treatment recommendations.

	Mild intermittent	Mild persistent	Moderate persistent	Severe persistent
Sx frequency	<2/week	>2/week	Daily	Continuous
Exacerbations			>2/week 1 night-time/month	Frequent
Night-time Sx	<2/month	>2/month	<1 night/week	Frequent
FEV_1	>80%	>80%	60-80%	<60%
β adrenergics	Short acting, pm	Short acting, pm	Short acting, pm Can add long acting	Short acting, pm Add long acting
Steroids		Inhaled, low dose	Inhaled, med. dose	Inhaled, high dose Oral steroids
Leukotriene inhibitors	Alternate	YES	YES	YES
Cromolyn		Alternate	PRN	PRN

Table 6.4 Common medications used for the treatment of asthma.

Drug	Examples	Action	Adverse Effects
Inhaled short-acting β_2-agonists (SABA)	Albuterol (Ventolin™ Proventil™) Levalbuterol (Xopenex™)	Rapid and short-lived bronchiolar dilation	Tachycardia, tremor, tolerance, hypokalemia
Inhaled anticholinergics	Ipratropium (short acting)(Atrovent™) Tiotropoium (Spiriva™) (long acting)	Block parasympathetic bronchiolar constriction	Tachycardia, tremor, dry mouth, urinary retention
Inhaled Cromones	Cromolyn (Intal™) Nedocromil (Tilade™)	Stabilize mast cells	Minimal
Long-acting β_2-agonists (LABAs) (supplied together with corticosteroids)	Salmeterol/fluticasone (Advair™) Formoterol/budesonide (Symbicort™)	Long-term bronchodilation	LABAs should not be used as monotherapy
Leukotriene modifiers	Montelukast (Singular™)	Leukotriene receptor antagonist; less effective alternative to ICS	Minimal, hepatic injury possible with other drugs of this class
Corticosteroids - inhaled	Beclomethasone (QVAR™) Budesonide (Pulmicort™) Fluticasone (Flovent™)	Anti-inflammatory Most effective long term control of persistent asthma	Oral candidiasis
Corticosteroids - oral	Methylprednisone, prednisone	Anti-inflammatory Effective for break through attacks	Minimal with intervallic dosage

Drugs for Asthma. Treatment Guidelines from The Medical Letter 10: 11–18, 2012.

Anesthetic concerns

Optimization of the disease, adequate oxygenation and hydration are the sine qua non of anesthetic patient care. Immediate effects of most anesthetic agents include interference with respiratory muscle coordination (Warner, 2011), resulting in a decrease in the functional residual capacity, hypoventilation, atelectasis and impaired cough and laryngeal reflexes (Liccardi et al., 2012). It is important to avoid / prevent bronchoconstriction and induce bronchodilation. Prophylactic preanesthetic administration of an inhaled β_2 agonist is not harmful and will minimize the chance of bronchospasm. Deep general anesthesia or very light anesthetic stages with effective local anesthesia are preferred. Stage II excitement may predispose to laryngospasm and bronchospasm. Drugs that can cause histamine release should be avoided if possible. These include meperidine, morphine, barbiturates and succinylcholine. Propofol, ketamine, sevoflurane, isoflurane and anticholinergics (atropine and glycopyrrolate) are all bronchodilators; however ketamine may increase secretions making it less than an ideal choice. Opioids blunt airway reflexes. Adenosine and non-specific β blockers such as labetolol can cause bronchoconstriction, while desflurane is very irritating to the airway. Aspirin-induced asthma is possible in patients with Samter's syndrome – a triad of asthma, aspirin sensitivity and nasal polyps (Samter and Beers, 1968). These patients can also be sensitive to NSAIDs and cyclo-oxygenase inhibitors. Acetaminophen is considered a safe alternative.

Chronic bronchitis and emphysema

Chronic obstructive pulmonary disease (COPD) is a preventable, treatable (not fully reversible), progressive disease usually due to abnormal inflammatory responses to noxious particles or gases (cigarette smoke, occupational exposure) (Rabe, 2010). COPD includes both chronic bronchitis and emphysema (among others), each with differing pathophysiology, but often occurring together in varying degrees in the same patient. Over 30 million people in the United States have been diagnosed with this disease.

Chronic bronchitis is defined by a chronic, productive cough for three months in each of two successive years in a patient in whom other causes of chronic cough have been excluded (Celli and MacNee, 2004). Pathologic changes are noted in smaller airways consist of enlarged mucus secreting glands, increased number of goblet cells and marked inflammatory infiltrate of the epithelium, which ultimately impairs gas diffusion. Structural remodeling leads to progressive scar tissue narrowing causing a fixed, irreversible airflow obstruction, an increase in collapsibility of the bronchiolar walls and a decrease in the elastic recoil of the lungs. Ciliary dysfunction leads to chronic cough and sputum production, which predispose to infection. Advanced disease can progress to pulmonary hypertension and right sided heart failure (cor pulmonale). Patients classically are noted to be "blue bloaters," tired of the extra work of breathing, edematous from the right sided heart failure, cyanotic and unable to expend the energy necessary to correct the impairment of gas exchange, no matter how hard they try.

Emphysema is defined by an abnormal and permanent enlargement of the airspaces that are distal to the terminal bronchioles (parenchymal damage) (Rennard, 1998) (Figure 6.10). In addition to the pathologic changes noted in chronic bronchitis, patients with "pure emphysema" have destruction of both alveolar septal walls and elastic fibers. As a result, the lung is easier to inflate (more compliant) but more difficult to empty, as the airways close prematurely on necessarily active expiration, leading to gas trapping. The accompanying decrease in the alveolar capillary diffusion area and redistribution of pulmonary blood flow further contribute to hypoxemia (Spieth et al., 2012). Patients classically are noted to be "pink puffers," barely able to keep up with oxygen demand, leaning forward for a mechanical advantage to enable rapid, shallow breaths through pursed-lips to maintain pressure in the distal airways which helps to prevent premature collapse. Breathing in this fashion consumes their awake lives, able to speak only in short phrases and eat small meals, leaving them isolated, exercise-intolerant and cachetic. Suprasternal retraction is easily noted because of the absence of body fat. The typical barrel chest (due to hypertrophy of the accessory respiratory muscles and elevation of the chest cage) encloses hyperinflated lungs.

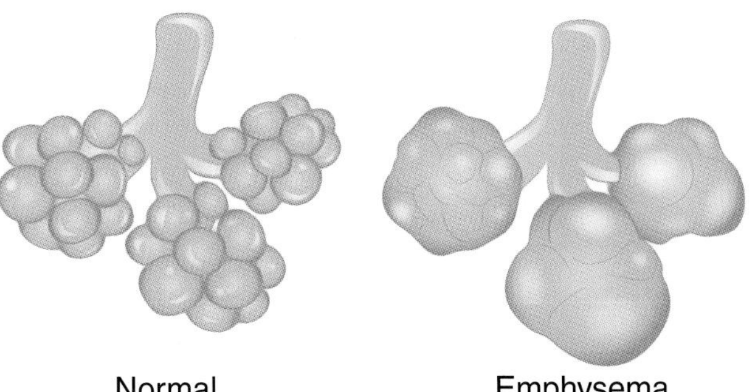

Figure 6.10 A comparison of normal and emphysematous alveoli.

Guidelines for the staging (comparison of the patient's FEV1 against a predicted value) and step-wise treatment of COPD are similar in design to the step-wise treatment of asthma, with the necessity for more drugs as disease severity increases. In contradistinction to asthma, anticholinergics rather than β_2 agonists more effectively treat COPD. Early smoking cessation and oxygen therapy (to maintain SpO_2 above 90%) are the only two therapeutic methods to minimize disease progression. Oxygen therapy improves exercise tolerance and reduces hypoxic pulmonary vasoconstriction with attendant right heart failure. Upper respiratory tract infections take a greater toll on patients with COPD; considerable effort is taken to avoid innoculation and infection, including appropriate vaccination and staying indoors during temperature extremes or local viral outbreaks. Acute exacerbations are managed by antimicrobial therapy, intensification of SABA therapy and corticosteroids (Treatment Guidelines, 2009).

Risk assessment

History and physical examination play a key role in assessing the likelihood of adverse respiratory events or the inability to respond to inadvertent hypoxia during office-based sedation or anesthesia. Questioning focuses on the presence of or recent changes in exercise tolerance, cough or shortness of breath. Recent flu or upper respiratory tract infections should also be noted. Physical examination includes observation of skin color, detection of suprasternal retraction and prolonged expiration as well as chest auscultation. Room air SpO_2 should be measured. Routine use of spirometry is not indicated.

Anesthetic concerns

Regardless of the anesthetic technique, patients should be optimized prior to intervention. As this disease is irreversible, COPD patients have less ability to tolerate hypoventilation, even during supplemental oxygen administration, as they often have a blunted response to hypercarbia. Regional anesthesia is preferred, especially with severe disease. Nitrous oxide can potentially expand and possibly rupture pulmonary bullae with severe emphysema. Opioids blunt respiratory drive, which can predispose to apnea. There is concern of slower metabolism and prolonged action of benzodiazepines in these patients (Hines and Marschall, 2008). Exaggerated respiratory depression should be expected and post-anesthetic observation should be extended as necessary.

Restrictive disease

Restrictive diseases are characterized by variety of pathologic changes that result in the reduction of vital capacity, typically limiting inhalation rather than exhilation (as seen in obstructive diseases). The resultant hypoxemia is due to shunt (perfused, not ventilated portions of the lung) and dead space (ventilated, not perfused portions of the lung), both leading to ventilation perfusion (V/Q) mismatch. Afflicted patients demonstrate shallow but partially compensatory rapid breathing. Most are unable to take a deep breath and relate the common complaint of dyspnea on exertion. Most disorders demonstrate an increase in inward elastic recoil which limits inspiration and decreases compliance (ability of the lung to expand with increased pressure). Acute intrinsic restrictive diseases include pulmonary edema and aspiration pneumonitis. Chronic intrinsic restrictive diseases include conditions which lead to pulmonary fibrosis, including idiopathic disease, radiation injury, sarcoidosis and autoimmune disease. Most intrinsic diseases also interfere with gas diffusion across the respiratory membrane. Extrinsic restrictive diseases (chronic) include conditions that interfere with chest wall expansion, such as advanced pregnancy, obesity, skeletal malformations and neuromuscular disorders (which negatively affect both inspiration and expiration). All of these diseases can severely decrease pulmonary reserve, especially when challenged by depressive actions of anesthetic agents.

Risk assessment

As most restrictive diseases are chronic, history and physical examination are adequate to determine the presence and severity of the various forms of restrictive disease.

Anesthetic concerns

Patients with these diseases are usually diagnosed and optimized prior to presentation for dental care. Increasing disease severity decreases patient reserve. Careful case selection and depth of anesthesia limit setting are prudent to avoid depressed or ineffective ventilation with resultant hypoxemia.

Upper respiratory tract infection

Upper respiratory infections (URI) are common in humans, especially during fall and winter months as viruses move through communities. These viral infection are usually spread by hand to hand contact or inhalation of airborn droplets from a cough or sneeze. Adults usually will get 1–2 "colds" per year, while children will get 5–7 colds/year. Symptom duration in children is approximately 2 weeks. Typically, inflammatory changes of edema, hyperemia and leukocytic infiltration will affect the nasopharyngeal mucosa, slowing mucociliary clearance. Symptoms include sore throat, malaise, fever, anorexia. Secondary bacterial infection is possible, as is extension to the lower airway. An increase in upper and lower airway reactivity/irritability can occur and last for up to 6 weeks after a URI. Respiratory complications (a more rapid oxygen desaturation, breath holding, apnea, bronchospasm, laryngospasm) are more frequent when general anesthesia is administered during or after a recent URI, *especially in children less than 5 years of age* (Cohen and Cameron, 1991). Children (and adults) with asthma and URI can be particularly vulnerable to bronchospasm.

Dental procedures under local anesthesia can usually be accomplished without the risk of significant morbidity. There are currently no generally accepted guidelines regarding the need to cancel IV sedation or general anesthesia WITHOUT INTUBATION in children with an ongoing URI (Tait and Malviya, 2005). Significant nasal and bronchiolar congestion, fever, sore throat, malaise, wheezing and active sputum production may be criteria for cancellation of elective procedures. Clear rhinorrhea and upper airway congestion should not automatically preclude a general anesthetic without planned intubation. In most instances, a two week delay after a URI may be sufficient for general anesthetic cases without planned intubation, while a 6 week delay may be more appropriate for cases where intubation is planned. Decisions regarding suitability and necessity of surgery and anesthesia should be made on a case-by-case basis.

Smoking

Smoking, independent of, or together with COPD has negative consequences for all who choose that lifestyle. Aside from the fact that smoking is an important risk factor for cancer and atherosclerosis, it has a variable, but always negative effect on the pulmonary system. Indirect respiratory risk is related to the underlying respiratory disease it has caused. Direct risk is introduced by insufflation of three major irritants: smoke particles, carbon monoxide and nicotine.

Anesthetic concerns

The incidence of cough, mucous hypersecretion, laryngospasm, bronchospasm, aspiration, breath-holding, hypoventilation and hypoxemia tend to greater in smokers, versus non-smokers (Schwilk et al., 1997). Smoke particles lead to an increase in laryngeal and bronchial reactivity and an increase in the amount and viscosity of mucus. Congestion is made worse as normal ciliary beating is hampered, with subsequent impairment of the mucociliary escalator. The airway lumen is narrowed, airflow obstruction is increased and oxygen diffusion is impaired. Within 1 week of cessation, reactivity diminishes and ciliary activity begins to improve (Egan and Wong, 1992). Effective tracheobronchial clearance can resume after three months of abstinence.

Carbon monoxide has 200 times the affinity for hemoglobin as compared to oxygen; exposure diminishes the oxygen carrying and oxygen releasing capacity of hemoglobin (a left shift in the oxygen-hemoglobin dissociation curve). This leads to arterial hypoxemia and tissue hypoxia. Carbon monoxide also interferes with oxygen utilization at the cellular level. Most pulse oximeters are unable to distinguish carboxyhemoglobin (COHb) from oxyhemoglobin (HbO_2). Oxygen saturation can be overestimated (up to 10%) in patients who have smoked within the past 24 hours (Castleden and Cole, 1974). At rest, the half-life of carbon monoxide in the blood is approximately 6 hours.

Nicotine stimulates the sympathetic nervous system with a resultant increase in heart rate, contractility, blood pressure, peripheral vascular resistance and dysrhythmia frequency. The subsequent increase in myocardial oxygen consumption may be difficult to compensate by coronary vessels, already narrowed by atherosclerosis. The pressor effects of nicotine lasts approximately 30–60 minutes (Ellenhorn and Barceloux, 1988) while significant improvement in the myocardial oxygen supply:demand ratio may require several hours of nicotine abstinence.

There is some evidence smokers may be resistant to the effect of some sedative drugs, perhaps by altering receptor sensitivity or altering the pharmacokinetics of these drugs (Sweeney and Grayling, 2009). Regardless, careful titration of all drugs to desired effect should be done to avoid inadvertent overdose with attendant negative cardiopulmonary effects in patients who are ill-suited to tolerate them. On a positive note, post-operative nausea and vomiting is decreased in smokers.

Smoking cessation should always be recommended prior to any level of anesthesia, even if only for 24 hours in order to diminish carboxyhemoglobin and nicotine levels, improve ciliary beating, and to reduce sympathetic outflow. Patients who stop smoking 1–2 weeks prior to anesthesia may present with more congestion as cough stimulation and bronchial irritation are decreased, while mucus production is not. However, there remains no reason to ever encourage smoking in any patient, at any time (Warner, 2005).

Obstructive sleep apnea

Obstructive sleep apnea (OSA) or more correctly, disordered breathing during sleep, is a complex, chronic disease spectrum characterized by repetitive partial or complete collapse of the upper airway for 5 or more times per hour during sleep. It is accompanied

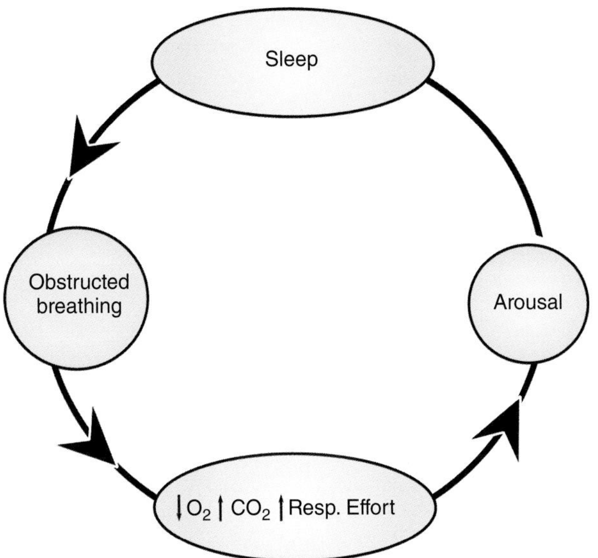

Figure 6.11 The pathophysiologic repetitive cycle of obstructive sleep apnea.

by diminished (hypopnea) or absent (apnea) airflow, usually in spite of continuing ventilatory attempts for a period longer than 10 seconds and resulting in a decrease of SpO_2 by 4% from baseline. Resultant hypoxia (and hypercarbia to a lesser extent) leads to a crescendo increase in sympathetic stimulation and activation of the reticular activating system causing repetitive arousals, sleep fragmentation, daytime sleepiness, poor cognitive functioning and host of other diseases (see Figure 6.11). OSA is diagnosed with polysomnography (sleep study) and is categorized as mild, moderate or severe, depending on the frequent of apneas plus hypopneas per hour of sleep (the AHI, apnea-hypopnea index). 5–15 events per hour is mild disease, 15–30 events per hour is moderate disease and greater than 30 events per hour is severe disease. The prevalence of this notoriously underdiagnosed disease approaches 25% of the population.

To fully appreciate OSA, an understanding of the determinants of upper airway patency is necessary (Figure 6.12). Airway patency is maintained in the awake state by a balance of forces affecting the size of the upper airway. Patency is maintained by position of the mandible and by skeletal muscle tone, including the palatal tensors, pharygneal dilators and genioglossus. Longitudinal traction on the upper airway during inspiration also maintains patency. Collapsing forces include negative intralumenal inspiratory pressure generated by the high resistance created by narrow airways (tonsils, nasal obstruction) and positive extraluminal pressure exerted by the tongue (relative or absolute macroglossia) and lateral pharyngeal fat.

In the awake state, a coordinated activation of the airway dilators occurs just prior to inspiration to splint and stabilize the upper airway against collapse from the drop in intralumenal pressure. Upper airway dilator tone normally decreases during sleep (Dempsey et al., 2010), especially during deep REM (rapid eye movement) sleep. As tone decreases so does airway diameter, which then increases negative intralumenal pressure, causing further collapse, snoring and possible obstruction. Patients with OSA have pathologic anatomy, that is, a smaller, more collapsible airway. The common sites of collapse are retropalatal and retroglossal (Hillman et al., 2010; Eastwood et al., 2002). Patients with OSA can also have concomitant pathologic physiology - altered central nervous system regulation of breathing, which may account for the less than optimal results of many airway altering surgeries (Susarla et al., 2010; Javaheri et al., 2009).

Predisposing factors for OSA include male gender, smoking, African-American, Asian and Hispanic heritage, age >50 years, cervical and central abdominal obesity, increased neck circumference, tonsillar hypertrophy, maxillary constriction, nasal obstruction, relative or absolute macroglossia, retrognathism and diabetes (Young et al., 2004). Unfortunately, elimination of these diseases is not necessarily curative.

The cardiovascular consequences of the large negative swings in intrathoracic pressure are related to the severity of OSA. They include vessel and chamber dilitation leading to arrhythmias and increased cardiac work. Repeated sympathetic discharge can

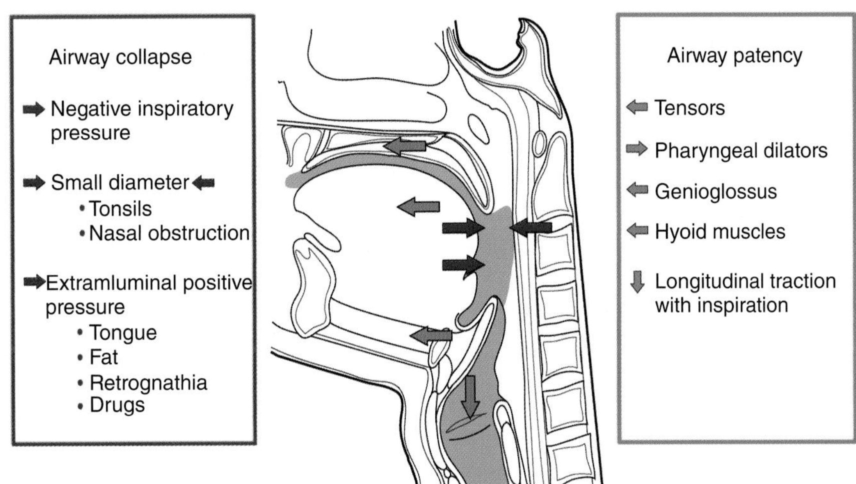

Figure 6.12 Airway patency is determined by net pressures and compliance

lead to endothelial dysfunction, hypertension and premature atherosclerosis (Caples et al., 2007; Peppard et al., 2000). Interestingly, treatment with continuous positive airway pressure (CPAP) has been shown to improve hypertension in patients with OSA. Although true cause and effect relationship is difficult to prove, OSA frequently clusters with obesity, ischemic stroke, insulin resistance and gastro-esophageal reflux disease.

Treatment of OSA decreases daytime sleepiness, improves cognitive function and quality of life, and reduces associated high blood pressure. Modalities include behavior modification (weight loss, smoking cessation, change in sleep position, and alcohol avoidance), nighttime use of positive airway pressure devices (pneumatic upper airway stent), oral repositioning appliances and a myriad of soft and hard tissue anatomy changing surgeries.

Risk assessment

As OSA is underdiagnosed and anesthetic morbidity can be significant, any clinical suspicion of this disease should lead to a presumption of the diagnosis. Chung et al. (2008a) proposed the STOP-BANG screening tool as a highly sensitive for moderate to severe disease (will not miss patients with the disease) but not specific (tends to include patients without the disease), which is totally acceptable for safety reasons. A "yes" response to 3 or more items places respondents at high risk for the disease (see Table 6.5).

In addition to the STOP-Bang questionaire, patients should be questioned concerning concomitant diseases such as hypertension, coronary artery disease, stroke, diabetes, smoking and GERD. Previously diagnosed patients should be questioned regarding severity of disease, results of sleep studies and compliance with recommended treatments. Physical examination is similar to the upper airway evaluation, and seeks to identify retrognathism, nasal obstruction, macroglossia, presence of tonsils, tori or constricted dental arches, Mallampati classification, and oropharyngeal height, width and depth (Tsai et al., 2003) (see Figures 6.13, 6.14 and 6.15). Room air SpO_2 less than 95 per cent should always invite concern.

Anesthetic concerns

There have been significant negative anesthetic outcomes for patients with OSA, with most related to airway difficulty and respiratory arrest. These risks can be mitigated with the use of local anesthesia only. Propofol, benzodiazepines and opioids decrease dilator tone (Norton et al., 2006; Hillman et al., 2009) and promote airway collapse, which may be more severe than anticipated with any given level of sedation (Chung et al., 2008b; Bonara et al., 1985). Patients with OSA are often overly sensitive to the ventilatory suppressant effects of these drugs, resulting in apnea

Table 6.5 The STOP-BANG scoring model (Data from Chung, 2008).

Snoring	Do you snore loudly?
Tired	Do you have daytime sleepiness?
Observed	Has anyone observed you to stop breathing during sleep
Pressure	Do you have high blood pressure
BMI	Is you BMI > 35kg/m^2
Age	Age over 50 years
Neck	Neck circumference > 17 inches
Gender	Male gender

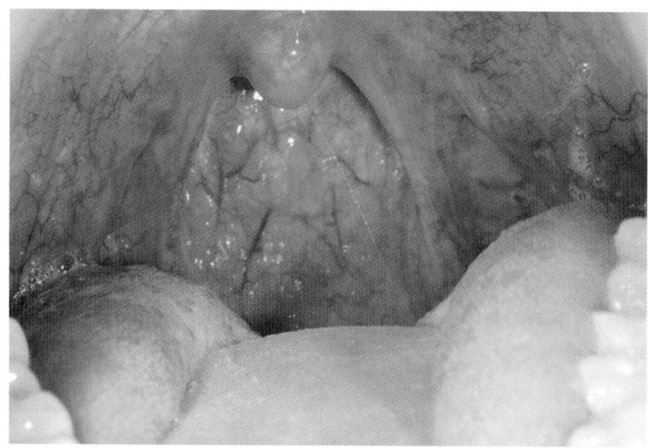

Figure 6.13 Decreased oropharyngeal depth and diameter in this patient who suffers with OSA.

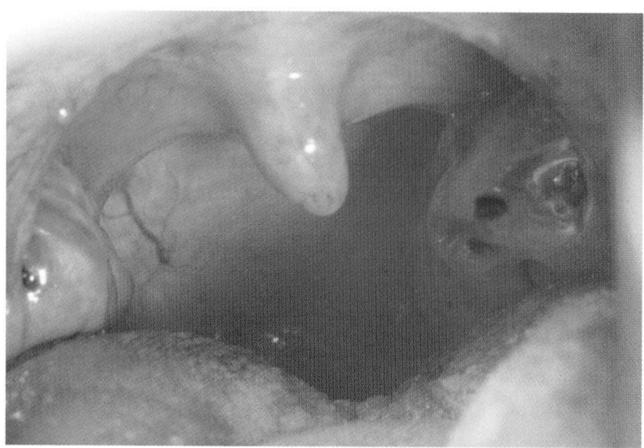

Figure 6.14 A patient with increased oropharyngeal depth and diameter of the oropharynx.

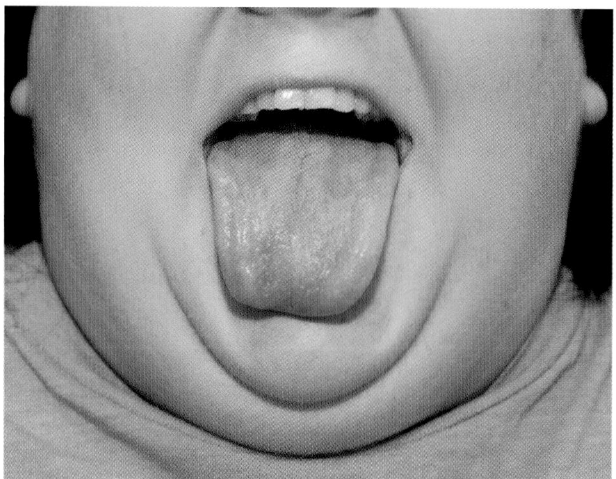

Figure 6.15 Note Mallampati 4 classification in addition to cervical obesity in this patient with obstructive sleep apnea.

and prolonged loss of airway tone (Mickelson, 2007). Anesthetic agents also abolish or blunt the arousal mechanisms necessary to terminate the apnea during sleep. Topical anesthetic agents can also adversely affect the patency of the upper airway, even in sedated patients, as proprioceptive reflexes controlling airway tone can be diminished.

In addition, patients with OSA can have difficult airways. The ASA-OSA practice guideline (Table 6.6) (Gross et al., 2006) aids in determining the suitability for ambulatory anesthesia. Scores are given for A. severity of OSA, B. type of surgery and C. requirement for post-op opioids. If the sum of scores for A + the greater of B or C (subtract 1 if patient is using CPAP) is 5 or greater, consideration should be given to performing anesthesia and surgery in a hospital setting. Use of CPAP up to the night before the procedure is advantageous to avoid post-anesthetic REM rebound and obstruction.

Immediate pre-operative issues include intensive monitoring of those vital parameters most likely to change, to include pulse oximetry, capnography, pre-tracheal auscultation, intervallic blood pressure determinations and continuous ECG. Reversal agents and size appropriate airway adjuncts should be immediately at hand. Supplemental oxygen to maintain saturation of the functional residual reserve volume is key to avoiding desaturations. Nasal hoods are more efficient than nasal prongs in achieving that goal.

Increased sensitivity to and increased duration of drug action should be anticipated. With that in mind, lower doses of shorter acting drugs should be carefully titrated to effect, while entertaining the possibility of narcotic avoidance. Supine posturing should be avoided if possible.

Post anesthetic monitoring should be equally intense. The ASA guidelines suggest monitoring patients who have received sedative agents for 3 hours longer than their non-OSA counterparts, Mickelson (2007) opines that this may be impractical and that a stabilized return to pre-anesthetic condition might be more efficient. Extreme caution should be exercised when prescribing narcotics for home use, as patient deaths have been reported. Supine posturing should again be avoided, while the application of both external and internal ice may help to minimize tissue edema. The immediate return to the use of CPAP is indicated and should be emphasized. CPAP use during "napping" and during the use of narcotic analgesics should also be encouraged. This information must be relayed to both patient AND the caregiver who will assist and continue to monitor the patient at home.

Table 6.6 Risk stratification to aid in determining suitability for ambulatory anesthesia for patients with obstructive sleep apnea (Data from Gross et al., 2006).

	ASA scoring	
A. Severity of OSA	None	0
	Mild	1
	Moderate	2
	Severe	3
B. Type of surgery	Superficial with local	0
	Superficial with sedation/GA	1
	Peripheral with GA	2
C. Requirement for p/o opioid	None	0
	Low dose	1
	High dose	3

References

Ali, R. Y. and Reminick, M. S. Perioperative management of patients who have pulmonary disease. *Oral Maxillofac Surg Clin N Am* **18**:81–94, 2006.

Benumof, J. L., et al. Critical Hemoglobin Desaturation Will Occur before Return to an Unparalyzed State following 1mg/kg Intravenous Succinylcholine. *Anesthesiol* **87**: 979–82, 1997.

Bonara, M., et al. Differential elevation by protriptyline and depression by diazepam of upper airway motor activity. *Am Rev Respir Dis* **131**: 41–50, 1985.

Caples, S. M., et al. Sleep-Disordered Breathing and Cardiovascular Risk. *SLEEP* **30**: 291–304, 2007.

Castleden, C. M. and Cole, P. V Variation in carboxyhaemoglobin levels in smokers. *Br Med J* **4**: 736–38, 1974.

Celli, B. R. and MacNee W., ATS/ERS Task Force. Standards for the diagnosis and treatment of patients with COPD: a Summary of the ATS/ERS paper. *Eur Respir J* **23**: 932, 2004.

Chung, F., et. al. STOP questionnaire: a tool to screen patients for obstructive sleep apnea. *Anesthesiol* **108**: 812–21, 2008a.

Chung, S. A., et al. A Systemic Review of Obstructive Sleep Apnea and Its Implications for Anesthesiologists. *Anesth Analg* **107**: 1543–1563, 2008b.

Cohen M. and Cameron, C. Should you cancel the operation when a child has an upper respiratory tract infection? *Anesth Analg* **72**: 282–288, 1991.

Dempsey, J. A., et al. Pathophysiology of sleep apnea. *Physiol Rev* **90**:47–112, 2010.

Drugs for Asthma. Treatment Guidelines from The Medical Letter 10: 11-18, 2012.

Drugs for Chronic Obstructive Pulmonary Disease. Treatment Guidelines from The Medical Letter 7: 83-88, 2010.

Eastwood, P. R., et al. Collapsibility of the upper airway during anesthesia with isoflurane. *Anesthesiol* **97**: 786–93, 2002.

Egan, T. D., and Wong, K. C. Perioperative smoking cessation and anesthesia. *J Clin Anesth* **4**: 63–72, 1992.

Ellenhorn, M. J. and Barceloux, D. G. Nicotine products. In Ellenhorn, M. J. and Barceloux, D. C., eds. *Medical Toxicology*. New York: Elsevier, 1988, pp 912–921.

Fanta, C. H. Asthma. *New Engl J Med* **360**: 1002–1014, 2009.

Gartner, L. P. and Hiatt, J. L. *Color Atlas of Histtology*. 5th edn. Philadelphia : Saunders Elsevier, 2009.

Gross, J. B., et al. Practice guidelines for the perioperative management of patients with obstructive sleep apnea: a report by the American Society of Anesthesiologist task force on the perioperative management of patients with obstructive sleep apnea. *Anesthesiol* **104**: 1081–1093, 2006.

Hillman, D. R., et al. Evolution of changes in upper airway collapsibility during slow induction of anesthesia with propofol. *Anesthesiol* **111**:63–71, 2009.

Hillman, D. R., et al. Anesthesia, sleep, and upper airway collapsibility. *Anesthesiol Clin* **28**: 443–455, 2010.

Hines, R. L. and Marschall, K. E. *Steolting's Anesthesia and Coexisting Disease*, 5th edn Philadelphia: Churchill Livingstone, 2008, p 172.

Javaheri, S., et al. The prevalence and natural history of complex sleep apnea. *J Clin Sleep Med* **5**: 205–211, 2009.

Liccardi, G., et al. Bronchial asthma. *Curr Opin Anesthesiol* **25**:30–37, 2012.

Mickelson, S. A. Preoperative and postoperative management of obstructive sleep apnea patients. *Otolaryngol Clin N Am* **40**: 877–889, 2007.

Norton, J. R., et al. Differences between midazolam and propofol sedation on upper airway collapsibility using dynamic negative airway pressure. *Anesthesiol* **104**: 1155–64, 2006.

Pascual, R. M. and Peters, S. P.Asthma. *Med Clin N Am* **95**: 1115–1124, 2011.

Peppard, P. E., et al. Prospective study of the association between sleep-disordered breathing and hypertension. *N Engl J Med* **42**: 1378–1384, 2000.

Rabe, K. F., et al. Global strategy for the diagnosis, management and prevention of chronic obstructive pulmonary disease. GOLD executive summary. *Am J Respir Crit Care Med* **176**: 532–555, 2007.

Rennard, S. I. COPD: overview of definitions, epidemiology and factors influencing its development. *Chest* **113**: 235S, 1998.

Samter, M. and Beers, R. F. Intolerance to aspirin: clinical studies and consideration of its pathogenesis. *Ann Intern Med* **68**: 975, 1968.

Schwilk, B., et al. Perioperative respiratory events in smokers and non smokers undergoing general anesthesia. *Acta Anesthesiol Scand* **41**: 348–355, 1997.

Spieth, P. M., et al. Chronic obstructive pulmonary disease. *Curr Opin Anesthesiol.* **25**: 24–29, 2012.

Susarla, S. M., et al. Biomechanics of the upper airway: Changing concepts in the pathogenesis of obstructive sleep apnea. *Int J Oral Maxillofac Surg* **39**: 1149–1159, 2010.

Sweeney, B. P. and Grayling, M. Smoking and anesthesia: pharmacological implications. *Anaesthesia* **64**: 179–186, 2009.

Tait, A.R. and Malviya, S. Anesthesia for the child with an upper respiratory tract infection: Still a Dilemma? *Anesth Analg* **100**: 59–65, 2005.

Tsai, W. H., et al. A decision rule for diagnostic testing in obstructive sleep apnea. *Am J Respir Crit Care Med* **167**: 1427–1432, 2003.

Young, T., et al. Risk factors for obstructive sleep apnea in adults. *JAMA* **291**:20133, 2004.

Warner, D. O. Helping surgical patients quit smoking: why when and how. *Anesth Analg* **101**: 481–487, 2005.

Warner, D. O. *Perioperative management of patients with respiratory disease.* Chicago: ASA Annual Meeting Review Course, 2011.

7 Anesthetic considerations for patients with endocrinopathies

Daniel Sarasin[1], Kevin McCann[2], and Robert Bosack[3]
[1] Private Practice OMFS, Cedar Rapids, IA, USA
[2] Private Practice, Waterloo, Ontario, Canada
[3] University of Illinois, College of Dentistry, Chicago, IL, USA

Patients with diagnosed or suspected endocrine disorders will often present for dental treatment. Even when successfully managed, patients may experience acute changes during and after office-based anesthesia that can lead to adverse and possibly catastrophic outcomes. Complications can be minimized or avoided with an accurate preanesthesia assessment and conservative case selection with appropriate consultations to ensure optimization of the disease process. Close anesthetic monitoring and implementation of preventive and prompt emergent treatment protocols will facilitate desirable outcomes. Focus should similarly be directed toward the presence or extent of endocrinopathy-induced cardiovascular disease and/or negative alterations affecting the upper airway.

Diabetes mellitus (DM)

Diabetes mellitus is a progressive disease of glucose dysregulation and carbohydrate intolerance. Abnormal carbohydrate metabolism that leads to hyperglycemia is due to impairment of insulin secretion and/or peripheral insulin resistance. Glucose that cannot be delivered intracellularly will persist in the blood stream, damaging blood vessels, triggering osmotic diuresis, and causing alterations in metabolic energy production. Diabetes often coexists with cardiovascular disease because of the diffuse vasculopathy that results from oxidative stress associated with chronic hyperglycemia and excessive swings in blood glucose (Moitra and Sladen, 2009; Monnier et al., 2006). Diabetes is the most common endocrinopathy in the world, with the 10% US prevalence expected to increase in concert with the obesity epidemic (AACE, 2009). About 10% of affected patients have type I diabetes mellitus (T1DM), due to autoimmune destruction of insulin-producing pancreatic β-cells. These patients always require insulin to prevent lipolysis and ketoacidosis. The remaining 90% have type II diabetes mellitus (T2DM), characterized by insulin deficiency and/or resistance due to genetic and environmental factors (stress, diet, activity level). T2DM is treated with diet modification, exercise, oral anti-hyperglycemic agents, and insulin as required. DM is diagnosed by the presence of elevated blood glucose levels, further characterized in Table 7.1.

Table 7.1 Abnormal diagnostic findings associated with diabetes mellitus.

- 8-hour fasting plasma glucose level >126 mg/dL
- Random plasma glucose >200 mg/dL Symptoms of polydipsia, polyuria and unexplained weight loss
- 2-hour post oral glucose challenge (75g glucose) >200 mg/dL
- Ketoacidosis

Drugs used to manage hyperglycemia are shown in Tables 7.2 – 7.4 (Treatment Guidelines, 2011). The goal of glycemic control is to replicate normal blood glucose physiology. Basal insulin therapy for type 1 diabetes is provided by subcutaneous injection of longer acting insulin or continuous infusion of short-acting insulin with an infusion pump (Figure 7.1). This therapy is further augmented with adjustable bolus doses of pre-meal short- or rapid-acting insulin.

Optimal daily glucose control is important to delay and possibly prevent long-term complications of hyperglycemia, which can include retinopathy and blindness, nephropathy and renal failure, neuropathy, hypertension, and vascular disease affecting cerebral, coronary, and peripheral vasculature (Table 7.5). These coexisting pathologies must be identified and carefully managed to optimally care for diabetic patients.

Long-term blood glucose control for patients with diabetes is best estimated by measuring glycosylated hemoglobin or Hb_{A1C}. This laboratory value (Table 7.6) provides a "look back" reflection of the degree of hyperglycemia to which RBCs have been exposed, which is a reasonably accurate indicator of average glycemic control for the prior 3 months (average life span of RBC is ~4 months). Normal values are <6%, target goal for DM management is <7%, and levels ≥8% correspond to blood glucose levels above 180 mg/dL, when glucose starts to spill into the urine.

Treatment goals for patients with DM undergoing office-based anesthesia are to (1) identify and manage comorbidities associated with diabetes and (2) minimize hyperglycemia and avoid hypoglycemia (Figure 7.2).

Acute elevations in blood glucose can occur because of the neuroendocrine stress response, triggered by hyperglycemia-inducing epinephrine, norepinephrine, cortisol, and glucagon. Chronic hyperglycemia is worrisome because of the accompanying dehydration (osmotic diuresis), electrolyte abnormalities, ketoacidosis, and prothrombotic state. Hyperglycemia, when severe, can also disrupt autoregulation by blunting compensatory pressure and rate

Anesthesia Complications in the Dental Office, First Edition. Edited by Robert C. Bosack and Stuart Lieblich.

Table 7.2 Commercially available insulin for subcutaneous injection.

Type or duration of action	Preparation	Brand	Onset	Peak	duration
Rapid acting*	aspart lispro glulisine	*Novolog* *Humalog* *Apidra*	10–30 min	.5–3 hours	3–5 hours
Short acting Regular Insulin		*Humulin R* *Novolin R*	30–60 min	2–3 hours	4–12 hours
Intermediate acting	NPH (protamine)	*Humulin N* *Novolin N*	1–2 hours	4–8 hours	10–20 hours
Long acting	detemir glargine	*Levemir* *Lantus*	1–4 hours	Flat No peak	12 - 20 hours 22–24 hours
Premixed	70% NPH + 30% regular 70% aspart protamine + 30% aspart 75% lispro protamine + 25% lispro	*Novolin 70/30 Innolet* *Novolog Mix 70/30 FlexPen* *Humalog Mix 75/25*	30–60 min 10–20 min 10–30 min	2–12 hours 1–4 hours 1–6 hours	18–24 hours 18–24 hours 14–24 hours

*Rapid-acting insulin analogs have a more rapid onset and shorter duration of action compared to regular insulin, and in general are more effective in decreasing A1C. The greatest risk of insulin therapy is hypoglycemia.

Table 7.3 Oral antihyperglycemic agents.

Category	Drug	Brand	Method of action	Comments
Sulfonylureas	Glipizide Glimepiride Glyburide	*Glucotrol* *Amaryl* *DiaBeta, Micronase*	↑ insulin release	Hypoglycemia possible
Meglitinides	Repaglinide Nateglinide	*Prandin* *Starlix*		
Biguanides	Metformin	*Glucophage*	↓ hepatic glucose output, ↑ peripheral glucose utilization	Hypoglycemia rare, lactic acidosis rare in ambulatory patients
α -glucosidase inhibitors	Miglitol Acarbose	*Glycet* *Precose*	↓ CHO breakdown in intestine, delay glucose absorption	"starch blockers" taken before meals
Thiazolidinediones	Pioglitazone Rosiglitazone	*Actos* *Avandia*	↑ insulin receptor sensitivity in fat, muscle and liver	Weight gain and edema possible
Incretin-based agents	Sitagliptin Saxagliptin Linaglilptin	*Januvia* *Onglyza* *Tradjenta*	DPP-4 inhibitors*	↑ incretin levels

*Dipeptidyl peptidase-4 (DPP-4) is an enzyme that degrades incretins. Incretin hormones (GLP-1 glucagon-like peptide and GIP glucose-dependent insulinotropic polypeptide) are released in the stomach after meals are ingested and lead to insulin secretion, decreased glucagon secretion, and increased transit time to soften the glucose spike.

Table 7.4 Non-insulin injectables.

Category	Drug	Brand	Method of action	Comments
GLP-1 analogs	Exenatide Liraglutide	Byetta Victoza	Mimics incretin	Administer SQ prior to meals
Synthetic amylin	Pramlintide	Symlin	Delays gastric emptying, ↑ satiety, ↓ postprandial glucagon and hepatic glucose production	Administer SQ prior to meals

changes. Patients with autonomic instability frequently present with resting tachycardia and orthostatic hypotension.

Signs and symptoms of hypoglycemia usually manifest at blood glucose levels <70 mg/dL. Mild hypoglycemia first manifests as autonomic dysfunction – the classic fight or flight sympathetic response (anxiety, nausea, tachycardia, palpitations, inappropriate sweating, peripheral vasoconstriction (cold, clammy hands), and tremor) (Table 7.7). As blood glucose drops even further, signs and symptoms of *neuroglycopenic* CNS dysfunction appear: cognitive impairment, behavioral changes, slurred speech, seizure, and coma. Notably, patients with long-standing DM are at risk of rapidly developing autonomic failure because of *hypoglycemia unawareness* due to defective glucose counterregulation (Cryer et al., 2009). It is critical to avoid hypoglycemia intraoperatively and

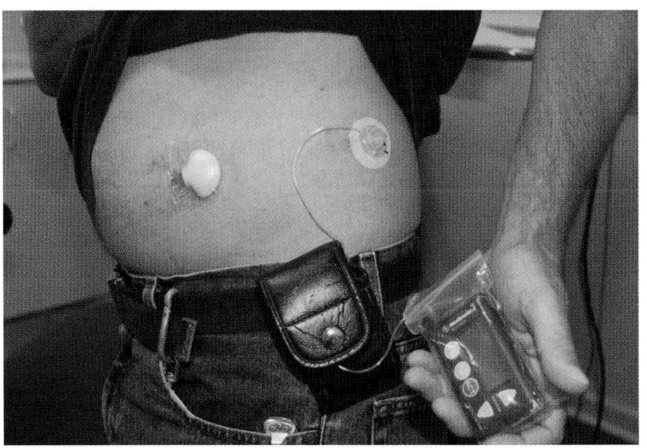

Figure 7.1 Insulin pump (right) and a transcutaneous glucose sensor (left).

Table 7.5 Common diseases that coexist with diabetes mellitus.

Hypertension	Cerebral vascular accident/TIA
Coronary artery disease	Peripheral vascular disease
MI/ silent MI	Nephropathy/renal failure
Cardiac autonomic dysfunction	Gastroparesis
Congestive heart failure	Stiff joint syndrome

Table 7.6 Hemoglobin A1c values.

HbA1c (%)	Mean blood glucose (mg/dL)	Interpretation
4	60	
5	95	Non-diabetic range
6	130	
7	160	Target range for diabetics
8	195	
9	225	Therapy needed
10	260	

postoperatively since its recognition may be blunted and delayed by anesthetics, analgesics, sedatives, β-blockers, and preexisting autonomic neuropathy.

Anesthetic management

A comprehensive evaluation for all patients with DM requires a systematic approach because diabetes affects numerous organ systems. Consultation with the patient's endocrinologist/internist is always helpful, as patients may be unaware of some of the nuances of their disease and responses to therapy.

The Society for Ambulatory Anesthesia (Joshi et al., 2010) has developed a consensus statement (not standard of care) for perioperative glycemic management in patients undergoing ambulatory surgery: these recommendations are based on general principles with a call for further research.

A *thorough preanesthetic evaluation* should always be obtained. Patients should be questioned about drugs, dosing, compliance, and effectiveness. Hb_{AIC} should be noted, with levels >7% inviting suspicion of cardiovascular disease. Thresholds for hypoglycemic symptoms and lability of glycemic control should also be ascertained. Patients who are unable to test their own blood sugar will

Hyperglycemia ⟷ Hypoglycemia

Neuroendocrine stress response
peripheral insulin resistance
hypersecretion of epinephrine, cortisol & glucagon
Inadequate exogenous insulin

Pre-op fast
Excess exogenous insulin

Figure 7.2 Acute changes in blood glucose in the surgical patient.

Table 7.7 Common symptoms of hypoglycemia.

Autonomic	Neuroglycopenic
Sweating	Dizziness
Tremor	Confusion
Palpitations/tachycardia	Difficulty speaking
Anxiety	Headache
Nausea	Inability to concentrate

present more challenges in the postoperative period. Spot blood glucose should be obtained on all patients prior to anesthesia; postponement should be considered when blood glucose values are greater than 250 mg/dL, as the resultant pH and level of dehydration are uncertain due to osmotic diuresis. Attempts to immediately reduce this value in order to proceed with the case may invite hypoglycemia. Although severe hypoglycemia (blood glucose <60 mg/dL) can be immediately corrected, autonomic imbalance may persist and invite hemodynamic instability. NPO times should be verified, as patients with longstanding DM may have delayed gastric emptying resulting in an increased stomach volume, which increases aspiration risk. Increasing the fast for solid food may be warranted in diabetic patients. Particular attention should be given to TMJ and neck mobility as part of the routine airway evaluation – glycosylation of proteins and collagen can lead to hypomobility and difficult airway manipulation. Typically, these patients are short in stature and present with tight, waxy skin.

Morning appointments should be reserved for diabetic patients to reduce NPO time and allow early return to normal dosing and caloric intake.

Oral medication and non-insulin injectables should be withheld on the day of surgery.

Insulin dosing should be kept at basal levels as long as those levels have not been associated with hypoglycemia at night or during normal intervals of no caloric intake. The patient's internist/endocrinologist will have clinical insight into this determination, especially for patients who take intermediate-acting or fixed combination insulins, where dosage is frequently reduced by 25 – 50%.

IV fluids are selected on the basis of preoperative blood glucose levels. Normal saline is appropriate with levels >130 mg/dL, while D5 .45NS can be used if levels are <100 mg/dL. Lactated Ringers solutions will increase sugar as the lactate is converted to glucose.

Blood glucose should be checked prior to discharge and within 2-hour intervals, as determined by surgical time. Acute hyperglycemia is less worrisome than hypoglycemia, which can be quickly remediated.

For patients with poorly controlled diabetes, the blood glucose level should be maintained around the preoperative baseline values rather than temporarily normalizing the levels, if the decision to proceed with surgery is made. Chronically elevated blood glucose levels should not be reduced acutely during anesthesia because the threshold at which patients experience hypoglycemic symptoms or organ impairment is dynamic and varies with their long-term glycemic control. Symptoms of hypoglycemia at normal blood glucose levels may occur in patients with poorly controlled type 2 diabetes secondary to an altered counterregulatory response. In addition, the acute reduction in glucose levels can lead to detrimental biochemical effects including increased oxidative stress response.

Avoidance of postoperative nausea and vomiting (PONV) is important to facilitate early resumption of oral intake and prevent hypoglycemia, especially when antihyperglycemic medication is resumed. Dexamethasone is an attractive option as it not only minimizes postoperative swelling but also has antiemetic properties. Unfortunately, it can increase blood glucose concentration during the first several hours after administration, especially with larger doses. Lowering the dose of dexamethasone to 4 mg often provides adequate PONV prophylaxis while reducing the amount of blood glucose elevation. The use of a long-acting local anesthetic for pain control will help reduce the amount of narcotics postoperatively.

There is no evidence that anesthetic agents or techniques used in the ambulatory setting affects mortality and morbidity in diabetic patients. The combined use of etomidate and opioids for induction and maintenance of anesthesia may reduce hemodynamic stability in patients with DM who have diabetic autonomic neuropathy (DAN) and coronary artery disease. Patients with DAN have blunted heart rate response to atropine and β-blockers.

Hypoglycemia

If symptoms of hypoglycemia are present or suspected, the blood glucose level should be checked. Emergency treatment should not be delayed if blood glucose level cannot be assessed. If the glucose level is at or below 70 mg/dl, treatment for hypoglycemia should be initiated. In the postoperative period, oral glucose tablets or gels should be administered if possible unless severe neuroglycopenic symptoms are present. Symptoms usually subside with oral glucose administration in 10 to 15 minutes. Blood glucose should be rechecked and more oral glucose agents administered to raise serum glucose levels above 100 mg/dl. In the preoperative and perioperative setting, hypoglycemia is treated with intravenous glucose: 25–50 ml (12.5–25 gm) of 50% dextrose solution (0.5–1 gm/kg). The solution is hypertonic and should be diluted prior to slow administration. Intravenous glucose administration is also indicated for patients in the postoperative setting who are unable to tolerate oral glucose agents or those who have severe neuroglycopenic symptoms. The use of intramuscular glucagon (0.5 to 1 mg) is indicated for patients who are extremely uncooperative, combative, or unconscious when intravenous access is not available/or lost. Blood glucose level should be checked after 15 minutes. Hypoglycemia may reoccur after initial treatment, so close monitoring is required.

Thyroid disorders

The thyroid gland is composed of follicles formed by epithelial cells that synthesize, store, and secrete thyroxine (T4) and tri-iodothyronine (T3), in a 10:1 ratio, by actively taking up iodide and attaching it to tyrosine molecules. These molecules are then linked to thyroglobulin and stored in follicles within the gland. When stimulated by thyroid-stimulating hormone (TSH) from the anterior pituitary gland (which itself is stimulated with thyrotropin-releasing hormone (TRH) from the hypothalamus) more T_3 and T_4 are synthesized, and, in addition, stored T3 and T4 are released into the blood. T3 and T4 suppress both TRH and TSH. Small changes in plasma T3 and T4 can lead to large inverse changes in TSH, which is why the TSH titer is the first to be measured. T4 is peripherally converted to T3 (four times more potent) in target tissues. T3 binds to nuclear receptors, resulting in the transcription of a host of cellular proteins and enzymes. The net effect is increased heat and energy production, increased metabolic rate, and increased oxygen consumption, with associated increases in cardiac output, carbon dioxide, and kidney function. T3 is also important for normal growth and development. TSH is often the most sensitive marker for thyroid disease, followed by free T3 and free T4 levels. Symptoms only loosely correlate with blood levels.

Hyperthyroid disease

Hyperthyroid disease results in thyrotoxicosis, a condition where tissues are exposed to increased thyroid hormones. The three most common causes of hyperthyroidism are Graves' disease, where autoantibodies stimulate TSH receptors in the gland, autonomously functioning toxic multinodular goiter, and toxic adenoma (Nayak and Hodak, 2007). There is a female preponderance.

The classic signs and symptoms of thyrotoxicosis (Tables 7.8 and 7.9) are hyperactivity, weight loss, and tremor. It is important to recognize these findings to avoid complications associated with undiagnosed disease. Goiter (enlargement of the thyroid gland) can be characteristic of both hyperthyroidism and hypothyroidism; however, its presence is not necessary to make either diagnosis.

Hyperthyroidism is treated by surgical removal, radioactive iodine destruction, or antithyroid drug therapy. In most cases, the gland function is totally obliterated, and patients take replacement levothyroxine (T4) to achieve a euthyroid state.

Anesthetic management

Anesthetic concerns for the hyperthyroid patient in an office setting include identification through history and physical examination and the delay of elective procedures until a stable, euthyroid state

Table 7.8 Signs of hyperthyroidism.

Cardiovascular	↑ heart rate and contractility, ↑ cardiac output, widen pulse pressures, ↓ systemic vascular resistance, ↓ blood pressure, ectopy, atrial fibrillation, fluid retention
Pulmonary	Dyspnea, ventilatory muscle weakness
Gastrointestinal	Diarrhea, nausea, vomiting
Thermoregulatory	Heat intolerance
Dermatologic	Flushed, warm, moist skin, pretibial myxedema (Graves disease only)
Neurologic	Agitation, tremor, hyperreflexia
Musculoskeletal	Paradoxical fatigue secondary to chronic stimulation
Ocular	Proptosis (Graves' disease only)

Table 7.9 Symptoms of hyperthyroidism.

- Palpitations, rapid heartbeat at rest
- Nervousness, restlessness, irritability
- Insomnia
- Tremor
- Weight loss
- Sweating, heat intolerance

is attained. Patients with even moderate thyrotoxicosis can be extremely sensitive to hypopnea and apnea with sedative, narcotics, or anesthetic agents. Vagolytic drugs such as atropine and glycopyrrolate or sympathomimetic agents such as epinephrine, ephedrine, and ketamine can aggravate cardiovascular stimulation. Phenylephrine would be an acceptable vasopressor if needed. Thyroid storm is characterized by uncontrolled metabolic stimulation including high fever, tachycardia, and delirium. The etiology of this condition is believed to be a shift from protein-bound thyroid hormone to free hormones secondary to circulating binding inhibitors. The mortality rate is 20 to 40%. It is unlikely in the office setting when managing adequately screened patients.

Hypothyroid disease

Hypothyroid disease is characterized by decreased hormonal action at the cellular level, usually due to reduced synthesis and secretion by the thyroid gland in spite of normal or elevated TSH (Devdhar et al., 2007). It is more common than hyperthyroidism, but also shares a female preponderance. Most cases are due to iodine deficiency, ablation of the thyroid gland by drugs or surgery, or autoimmune destruction (Hashimoto's thyroiditis).

Manifestations of hypothyroidism vary considerably, depending on the severity of the disease and age at onset. In adults, hypothyroidism has a slow onset and early stages of this disorder may not be noticed. There is progressive slowing of mental and physical activity as the condition worsens. A reduced β-adrenergic receptor function is anticipated, with resultant α predominance (Kohl and Schwartz, 2010). In later stages of this disorder, hematologic abnormalities such as anemia, platelet and coagulation factor dysfunction, as well as electrolyte imbalances (hyponatremia) and hypoglycemia are common. Signs and symptoms are shown in Tables 7.10 and 7.11. Severe hypothyroidism in adults results in myxedema coma.

Treatment for patients with hypothyroidism is thyroid hormone replacement in the form of levothyroxine (T4). Overdosing remains a concern and patients should be directly questioned about the stability and efficacy of their replacement therapy dose (Devdhar et al., 2007).

Anesthetic management

Anesthetic concerns for the hypothyroid patient in an office setting include identification through history and physical examination and the delay of elective procedures until a stable, euthyroid state is attained. As the half-life of levothyroxine is 7 days, this drug can be missed on the morning of surgery without consequence. Euthyroid patients present with no special anesthetic concerns. A host of undesirable anesthetic consequences can be associated with hypothyroidism, especially with severe disease. Increased sensitivity to anesthetic agents can result from impaired metabolism and reduced volumes of distribution (Farling, 2000). *Upper airway obstruction* can be more likely because of edematous pharyngeal tissue and goiter. *Hypoventilation* can occur because of a reduced ventilatory response to hypercarbia and hypoxia. Increased risk of silent regurgitation and *aspiration* is possible because of delayed gastric emptying. Unstable hemodynamics, especially *hypotension* is facilitated by hypovolemia, abnormal baroreceptor function, reduction in cardiac output, and a slight change in adrenal insufficiency. Careful titration (start low, go slow) of anesthetic agents, full monitoring, and adequate normal saline fluid replacement should result in stable sedation/anesthetic. Hypothyroid patients may be extremely sensitive to the myocardial depressant effects of halogenated inhalation agents. Unresponsive hypotension may require supplemental steroids in addition to ephedrine (Wall, 2008).

Table 7.11 Symptoms of hypothyroidism.

- Weakness, fatigue
- Headache
- Depression
- Cold intolerance
- Anorexia

Obesity and post-bariatric surgery

Obesity has reached epidemic proportions in the United States, and the trend is becoming evident throughout the world (Ogden et al., 2012). Given the medical consequences of obesity (glucose dysregulation, hyperlipidemia, cardiovascular disease and upper airway impingement, among others) weight loss strategies are commonplace. The number of bariatric operations in the United States has plateaued to approximately 125,000 cases per year (Nguyen et al., 2011). Both obese and post-bariatric surgery patients will present with issues that can affect the provision of anesthesia, and it is important that the dental professional be aware of these issues.

Obesity is more than just "being fat." It is a chronic disease similar to hypertension and atherosclerosis (Bray, 2004). The etiology is due to an imbalance in energy of food ingested and the amount of energy expended. The excess energy is stored in fat cells that will increase in size or number. This hyperplasia and hypertrophy of adipose cells is the pathologic entity in obesity. The degree of obesity is often expressed using the body mass index (BMI) (Table 7.12) and is calculated by dividing the weight in kilograms by the square of the height in meters (kg/m^2).

The associated medical consequences of obesity result from both the increased mass of fat tissue and the metabolic changes that arise secondary to the increased fat tissue. Being overweight carries a social stigma, and the obese patient may present with concurrent

Table 7.10 Signs of hypothyroidism.

Cardiovascular	↓ heart rate and contractility, ↓ cardiac output, ↑ blood pressure, narrow pulse pressure, intravascular volume depletion, anemia
Pulmonary	Reduced response to hypercarbia and hypoxia, obstructive sleep apnea
Gastrointestinal	Reduced gastric motility, constipation, weight gain
Thermoregulatory	Decreased sweating
Dermatologic	Dry, pale skin/non-pitting swelling of subcutaneous tissue in face and extremities, coarse, fragile thinning hair
Nervous	Lethargy, hypersomnolence, ataxia, decreased mental acuity, hyporeflexia, peripheral neuropathy
Musculoskeletal	Muscle stiffness

Table 7.12 Adult BMI based on height and weight (kg/m²).

Height	Healthy		Overweight					Obese			
	19	24	25	26	27	28	29	30	35	40	45
	Weight in pounds										
5′0"	97	123	128	133	138	143	149	154	179	205	230
5′1"	101	127	132	138	143	148	153	159	185	212	238
5′2"	104	131	137	142	148	153	159	164	191	219	246
5′3"	107	135	141	147	152	158	164	169	198	226	254
5′4"	111	140	146	151	157	163	169	175	204	233	262
5′5"	114	144	150	156	162	168	174	180	210	240	270
5′6"	118	149	155	161	167	173	180	186	217	248	279
5′7"	121	153	160	166	172	179	185	192	223	255	287
5′8"	125	158	164	171	178	184	191	197	230	263	296
5′9"	129	163	169	176	183	190	196	203	237	271	305
5′10"	132	167	174	181	188	195	202	209	244	279	314
5′11"	136	172	179	186	194	201	208	215	251	287	323
6′0"	140	177	184	192	199	206	214	221	258	295	332
6′1"	144	182	190	197	205	212	220	227	265	303	341
6′2"	148	187	195	203	210	218	226	234	273	312	351
6′3"	152	192	200	208	216	224	232	240	280	320	360

psychological issues. When distressed, many obese patients will turn to food as a temporary coping mechanism, left only to confront a subsequent dysphoric mood (Collins and Bentz, 2009). Substance abuse is not uncommon in such individuals. Diseases of the bones, joints, muscles, and skin are increased in the overweight individual. Osteoarthritis in the weight-bearing joints of the knees, hips, and ankles is a direct result of the trauma associated with excess weight. Osteoarthritis does occur in non-weight-bearing joints suggesting that there are other components of the overweight syndrome that alter bone and joint metabolism (Bray, 2004). Cervical fat deposits can contribute to the loss of airway tone during sleep. Obstructive sleep apnea (OSA), defined as apneic or hypopneic episodes lasting greater than 10 seconds, or resulting in a decrease of oxygen saturation greater than 4% (Brodsky and Lemmens, 2012) is more common among obese patients. Excess abdominal fat can limit diaphragmatic descent and in extreme cases, can result in decreased thoracic volume resulting in a decrease in all pulmonary volumes. This effect is greatest in the supine position. Ventilation–perfusion mismatching can even occur in the awake, seated obese patient (Holley et al., 1967). Problematic tracheal intubation has been found to occur with greater frequency in patients with shorter thyromental distance, increasing neck circumference, increased BMI, and Mallampati score greater than or equal to 3 (Gonzalez et al., 2008). Neligan et al. (2009) and Holmberg et al. (2011) were not able to demonstrate these findings in obese patients, which might underscore the fact that generalized obesity may not affect the oral or pharyngeal spaces with the same degree of severity. Therefore, there appears to be some controversy over the ability to predict difficult intubation in the obese population. OSA alone does not appear to significantly affect successful endotracheal intubation; however, the constellation of physical findings that are often associated with obesity tend to create the "perfect storm" that can deleteriously affect ventilation.

A host of metabolic derangements occur as body weight increases. The "metabolic syndrome" refers to a collection of clinical findings that are frequently associated with obesity (see Table 7.13).

Table 7.13 Criteria for metabolic syndrome (Bray, 2004).

Risk factor	Defining level
Waist circumference – Males	>102 cm (40in)
Waist circumference – Females	>88 cm (35in)
HDL cholesterol – Males	<40 mg/dl
HDL cholesterol – Females	<50 mg/dl
Triglycerides	≥150 mg/dl
Fasting Glucose	≥110 mg/dl
Blood pressure (systolic/diastolic)	≥130/85 mmHg

Adipose tissue was once thought to be an inert storage organ, but the most recent research suggests that it plays a significant role as an endocrine organ and is part of an innate immune system (Rasouli and Kern, 2008). Derangements in this endocrine system give rise to both the insulin resistance seen in type II DM and other manifestations that are associated with the metabolic syndrome. Cardiovascular derangements that are seen with increasing BMI include numerous electrophysiological changes, increases in blood volume, cardiac output, and mild to moderate hypertension (Brodsky and Lemmens, 2012). This cluster of hypertension, dyslipidemia, and insulin resistance are well-known risk factors for the development of atherosclerosis and eventual cardiovascular disease. The inflammatory responses as reported by Rasouli and Kern (2008) contribute to coronary artery disease. As a result of this multisystem involvement, it is easy to appreciate that obesity may be eclipsing tobacco use as the number one killer in North America (Mokdad et al., 2004).

Given the myriad of consequences of obesity, numerous strategies at reducing excess fat storage and hopefully reversing its consequences have been suggested. While obese patients can often lose weight through dieting or enhanced physical activity, the problem is long-term maintenance of the weight loss (Tsai and Wadden, 2005). Non-surgical weight loss is a life-long process with high rates of recidivism and suffering. Bariatric surgery is felt to be the only treatment modality that can produce significant weight loss that is both sustained and long term in patients with severe obesity (Brolin, 2002). Bariatric surgery is indicated in patients presenting with a BMI exceeding 40 kg/m^2 or a BMI greater than 35 kg/m^2 with significant comorbidities such as type II DM, hypertension, OSA, or weight-bearing arthropathy (National Institutes of Health, 1991). The types of bariatric surgical procedures that are in use today can be classified as restrictive or a combination of restrictive and malabsorptive (Christou, 2009).

Restrictive procedures reduce the size of the stomach and are achieved with horizontal or vertical banding, and are most often accomplished laparoscopically. Adjustable gastric banding has become a popular alternative in restrictive procedures that involves the placement of a horizontal band across the proximal portion of the stomach to create a pouch that holds approximately 100 to 200 grams of food (Thompson et al., 2011). Filling of the pouch creates a sensation of satiety earlier, and hence food intake is reduced. The band is both adjustable and removable. The "gold standard" of bariatric surgeries is the malabsorptive procedures that both reduce the size of the stomach and bypass the proximal duodenum, which results in a degree of malabsorption. A vast majority of these procedures are carried out laparoscopically, and demonstrate both high degrees of success and low rates of perioperative mortality (Ashrafian et al., 2008).

Anesthetic management of the obese patient

The prevalence of obesity is high in North America; therefore, the likelihood of such patients presenting for dental treatment and anesthesia is high. It is essential that a thorough history and physical examination be completed to identify the medical consequences and attempt to optimize these conditions prior to the provision of anesthesia or sedation. Airway management is likely to be the most challenging aspect of clinical treatment, and therefore critical assessment is paramount. The availability of airway adjuncts and routine use of ventilation monitors such as capnography will enable a rapid correction of declining ventilatory status. While there does not appear to be an absolute maximal BMI for which outpatient management is contraindicated, evidence does suggest that increased difficulties should be expected once the BMI exceeds 40 kg/m^2. A hospital environment to manage these patient should be considered. The presence of OSA in the obese patient does not always translate into difficulty with airway management; however, when a number of non-reassuring findings are present, the likelihood of difficult airway management should be anticipated.

Procedures that are considered appropriate for surgical management in the outpatient environment are those that are associated with low rates of postoperative complications and allow for postoperative care that is easily provided at home. Duration of surgery and the ability to ambulate post surgery are important considerations that contribute to the incidence of venous thromboembolism, and therefore longer procedures or major bone-grafting cases are not often best suited for the office environment. Due consideration must also be given to the physical environment of the office and the staff available. Wide doorways, chairs that will accommodate the obese patient, and availability of sufficient staff to assist with patient transfers are important considerations. As with any surgical patient, a thorough history and physical examination is required. Attention should be given to any of the consequences of obesity and their degree of control. The challenge however is to identify those patients that are at greatest risk for perioperative events and to employ strategies to mitigate both anesthetic and surgical complications. In general, this risk of complications rises with BMI (Poirier et al., 2009). Reliance solely on BMI has some limitations, as it may overestimate body fat in patients with a muscular build, or underestimate the amount of body fat in older individuals and others who may have lost muscle mass. Patients with an increased BMI, that also report a positive history of dyslipemia, type II DM, smoking, hypertension, and lack of physical activity are at greatest risk of cardiovascular morbidity, and therefore require further investigation, and delay of any non-emergent surgery. A careful review of medications being used and the medications that should be held on the day of surgery is essential. Concurrent use of appetite suppressants that may contain amphetamines can also have anesthetic implications (Fischer et al., 2000). It is important to consider that patients may be reluctant to disclose that they are using appetite suppressants, be they prescription or otherwise.

Perhaps the most important component of the preoperative evaluation is assessment of the airway. The difficult airway is often described as having four dimensions (Walls and Murphy, 2012): difficult laryngoscopy, difficult bag-mask ventilation, difficult extraglottic device placement, and difficult surgical airway. Obese patients will often present with features that affect each of these dimensions. Components of this examination should go beyond the simple Mallampati airway assessment and should include neck circumference, thyromental distance, mandibular space, interincisal distance, tonsil size, and neck mobility. Airway management will likely increase in difficulty as the number of positive, non-reassuring factors increases. Airway management decisions need to be based on how procedures are normally carried out in the office. If an open airway technique is used, careful assessment of the potential challenges to maintaining the airway in a sedated/anesthetized state is essential. If some forms of advanced airways are routinely used such as extra glottic devices or endotracheal tubes, the availability of tools such as video laryngoscopes may turn the difficult airway into a routine airway. As Holmberg et al. (2011) demonstrated, extremes of obesity (BMI > 40 kg/m^2) are associated with increased degrees of difficulty with tracheal intubation in the pre-hospital setting, and therefore extreme caution should be exercised when managing this subset of obese patients. With respect to OSA patients, the anesthesia literature is equivocal on which patients can be safely managed on an outpatient basis (Practice Guidelines, American Society of Anesthesiologists Task Force on Perioperative Management of Patients with Obstructive Sleep Apnea, 2006). Large neck sizes (>40cm) and high Mallampati scores were identified as better predictors of potential difficult intubation by Brodsky et al. (2002). While Neligan et al. (2009) reported that OSA did not influence difficulty with tracheal intubation and laryngoscopy grade, this result should be taken in the context that anesthesia was being provided under optimal conditions with patients in a "ramped" position. These conditions may be difficult to achieve in the outpatient setting and by a practitioner that does not routinely provide tracheal intubation. A crisis plan of action needs to be in place so that if the primary method of airway support fails, alternative methods can be readily accessed. Owing to the decreases in functional reserve capacity (FRC), expiratory reserve volume, and total lung capacity the obese patient has an impaired ability to tolerate periods of apnea (Hines and Marschall, 2008). Hence, airway management tends to become a more dynamic concern with increased time constraints. Pre-oxygenation should be considered as an essential element of anesthetic management.

The second major consideration in the management of the obese patient is drug dosing. Pharmacokinetic parameters of many drugs are related to lean body mass as opposed to total body weight. Lean body weight (LBW) is often calculated using ideal body weight. For males, IBW is estimated by subtracting 100 from the height in centimeters and 105 for females. Lean body weight is calculated with the formula LBW = IBW × 1.3 (Thompson et al., 2011). In the provision of anesthesia, our aim is to provide a balance between hypnosis, muscle relaxation, and analgesia. In the open airway technique that is often used in the oral surgery office, muscle relaxation is not considered, and therefore amnesia and analgesia are the main components of what is often termed a "balanced anesthetic." Benzodiazepines, opioids, and hypnotic agents such as propofol and nitrous oxide are probably the most commonly used agents in the modern oral surgery office. Of the benzodiazepines, midazolam is one of the most extensively used drugs for intravenous sedation and anesthesia. When a single dose of a benzodiazepine is used, its dose should be based on total body weight, but if a continuous infusion is used, the maintenance dose should depend on the ideal body weight (Casati and Putzu, 2005). Fentanyl is likely the most commonly utilized opioid in the oral surgery office, but given some of the benefits of remifentanil, this distinction may soon be lost. Loading doses of both fentanyl and remifentanil should be based on LBW (Barash et al., 2009). Owing to the dependence on plasma cholinesterase to metabolize remifentanil, clearance of remifentanil following an infusion should not be affected by body weight; however, the infusion rate selected may require adjustment based on hemodynamic parameters. Propofol is highly lipid soluble and has a very high hepatic clearance. Induction doses are best based on lean body weight and maintenance infusions based on total body weight (Brodsky and Lemmens, 2012). Dose adjustments during maintenance should be considered if hemodynamic parameters dictate. Newer volatile agents such as sevoflurane and desflurane demonstrate lower lipid solubility compared with older agents. Wash-in and wash-out times for both of these agents are short due to their increased lipid solubility (Hemmings and Egan, 2013). Local anesthetic doses should be based on lean body weight.

Prophylaxis for aspiration is another potential concern in the obese population. Historically, the obese patient was felt to be at a greater risk for a full stomach compared to the non-obese counterpart. While the potential for gastroparesis in the obese patient with type II DM must be considered, there is little evidence to support that special precautions need to be utilized to prevent aspiration (Harter et al., 1998). Consideration of aspiration risk must also take into account the segment of obese patients that have successfully undergone bariatric surgery. Such patients will often achieve substantial improvement in obesity-related diseases including type II DM, hypertension, dyslipidemia, and sleep apnea. Despite these successes, there is little information in the anesthesia literature regarding the safety of anesthesia following successful bariatric surgery. The lone exception is a report by Jean et al. (2008) in which they found that there was a higher risk of pulmonary aspiration in patients who had undergone gastric banding or vertical gastroplasty. No patients in their study had undergone gastric bypass procedures. Gastric bypass procedures by their nature introduce a potential for malabsorption to occur, and therefore the potential for nutritional disturbances following bariatric surgery exist. For patients that have undergone bypass procedures, nutritional deficiencies can arise due to the loss of absorption that results when the duodenum is bypassed. Restrictive procedures can also induce a degree of nutritional disturbances due to the decrease in dietary intake.

Multivitamin supplementation is utilized in all patients regardless of bariatric surgery procedure (Xanthakos, 2009). Micronutrient deficiencies, including iron and vitamins D, B_{12}, E, and C can also occur, and while these may not give rise to complications with the provision of anesthesia, they may affect wound healing.

Adrenocortical insufficiency (AI)

Cortisol release from the adrenal cortex is regulated by the hypothalamic-pituitary-adrenal (HPA) axis, via the respective release of corticotrophin releasing hormone (CRH) and adrenocorticotropic hormone (ACTH). Cortisol, often referred to as the stress hormone, exerts its *permissive action,* which results in increased blood glucose and maintenance of vascular tone by locally facilitating catecholamine effect. As expected, cortisol demand is increased during the stress of anesthesia and surgery. Adrenocortical insufficiency occurs when adrenal cortical output is less than physiologic demand. Signs and symptoms of AI, identified in the early 1950s (Lipset and Pearson, 1956), include the insidious onset of weakness, fatigue, anorexia, nausea, vomiting, abdominal pain, and volume and vasopressor-resistant hypotension. Rapid resolution occurs with the administration of cortisone.

Primary AI (Addison's disease) is due to destruction of the adrenal cortex by tumor, pathologic autoimmunity, infiltration, infection, or hemorrhage. Secretion of both glucocorticoids and mineralocorticoids (aldosterone) is diminished in this uncommon disease. Secondary AI is due to interruption of the HPA axis, which occurs most often by the administration of supraphysiologic doses of exogenous cortisol for the treatment of rheumatoid arthritis, Crohn's disease, and COPD, among others. Even those glucocorticoid formulations that are not intended to have systemic effects (eye drops, inhaled corticosteroids, creams, intra-articular injection) can cause adrenal suppression (Lansang, 2011). Aldosterone secretion is unaffected in patients with secondary AI. The prevalence of secondary AI is unknown; however, given the large number of patients on supraphysiologic corticosteroid therapy, clinicians are likely to see patients with this condition.

Treatment goals for managing patients with adrenocortical hypofunction undergoing ambulatory anesthesia are to (1) identify patients with adrenal insufficiency/those with a high suspicion for developing AI, (2) administer adequate preoperative supplemental corticosteroids if required, and (3) avoid acute adrenal insufficiency/adrenal crisis.

Normal cortisol production of approximately 20 mg/day can increase up to seven-fold, based on the severity and duration of anesthetic and surgical stress (Jabbour, 2001). In patients with varying degrees of adrenal compromise, this protective and necessary increase may not be sufficient. Some degree of adrenal compromise has been long thought to occur in any patient who has received more than the equivalent of 20 mg of prednisone a day for more than 3 weeks, within the previous year (see Table 7.14). A number of drugs can predispose patients to adrenal suppression. Concomitant use of glucocorticoids with inhibitors of CYP3A4 (e.g. itraconazole, diltiazem, mibefradil, and even grapefruit juice), the most abundant drug metabolizing cytochrome P450 enzyme, prolongs the biologic half-life of the glucocorticoids, causing enhanced effect in suppressing adrenal function. The use of some antifungal agents is known to interfere with glucocorticoid synthesis, especially ketoconazole (Bornstein, 2009). It is reasonable to assume that this

Table 7.14 Steroid equivalency chart (Yong et al., 2009).

Glucocorticoid	Equivalent dose (mg)
Hydrocortisone (SoluCortef™)	20
Cortisone	25
Prednisone	5
Methylprednisolone (SoluMedrol™)	4
Dexamethasone (Decadron™)	.5

depression is dose and duration dependent. As a result, a dogma was born requiring that any patient with suspected AI receive a "stress-shielding" pre-surgical dose of steroids to prevent possible adrenal crisis. The corticotropin (ACTH) stimulation test has been used to estimate adrenal cortical functioning. A cortisol level >20 µg/dL any time within an hour of the parenteral administration of 250 µg of Cortrosyn™ (synthetic ACTH cosyntropin) indicates normal adrenal functioning.

The practice of stress shielding patients with presumed AI secondary to steroid usage has recently been questioned (Loriaux and Fleseriu, 2009, Yong et al., 2009). Marik and Varon (2008) concludes from a systematic literature review that patients receiving therapeutic doses of corticosteroids do not routinely require stress dosing, provided they receive their usual dose on the day of surgery. Adrenal function testing in these patients is thought to be overly sensitive and does not predict the occurrence of adrenal crisis. Patients with primary diseases of the HPA axis will still require supplemental doses in the perioperative period. The practice of tapering steroids is used to ameliorate signs and symptoms of steroid withdrawal, which include lethargy, muscle ache, nausea, vomiting, abdominal pain, and postural hypotension.

Anesthetic management

A comprehensive history (including time, duration and dose of steroid exposure) and physical examination prior to anesthesia is essential to avoid intraoperative and postoperative complications associated with AI.

Decision to administer supplemental corticosteroids preoperatively and perioperatively is based on the diagnosis of AI or suspicion of adrenocortical hypofunction by history and physical findings, the acuity of care, type and depth of anesthesia, and severity of the dental/surgical treatment. As indicated above, for minor dental/oral surgical procedures under ambulatory anesthesia, there is no consensus on the guidelines for preoperative supplemental steroid administration in patients with known or suspected adrenal suppression or AI. Some authors suggest doubling or tripling the usual steroid dose the day of surgery and 1 to 2 days postoperatively while other authors recommend administering the patient's baseline dosage of glucocorticoids plus intravenous supplementation in the intraoperative period (25 mg of hydrocortisone). No benefit has been determined for excessive dosing and/or prolonged duration of supplemental therapy.

When administering more than 100 mg/day of hydrocortisone, substituting with methylprednisolone should be considered due to less mineralcorticoid effects in order to avoid fluid retention, edema, and hypokalemia (Wall, 2008).

Patients with untreated AI should not be operated upon in an ambulatory dental anesthesia setting, due to the need for aggressive management with invasive monitoring and fluid and electrolyte resuscitation. There is no specific anesthetic agent or technique recommended in the anesthetic management of patients with medically treated AI or at risk of developing AI, except for supplemental glucocorticoid administration, which was discussed previously. Etomidate should be avoided because it inhibits the synthesis of cortisol and may precipitate acute AI.

References

American Association of Clinical Endocrinologists and American Diabetes Association Consensus statement on inpatient glycemic control. *Diabetes Care* **32**:1119–1131, 2009.

Ashrafian, H., et al. Effects of bariatric surgery on cardiovascular function. *Circulation* **118**: 2091–2102, 2008.

Barash, P. G., et al. *Clinical Anesthesia*, 6th edn. Philadelphia, Lippincott Williams & Wilkins, 2009, pp. 1230–1246.

Bornstein S. R. Predisposing factors for adrenal insufficiency. *N Engl J Med* **360**: 2328–2339, 2009.

Bray, G. A. Medical consequences of obesity. *J Clin Ednocril Metab* **89**: 2583–2589, 2004.

Brodsky, J. B., et al. Morbid obesity and tracheal intubation. *Anesth Analg* **94**: 732–736, 2002.

Brodsky, J. B. and Lemmens, H. J. M. (eds): Preoperative considerations. *in Anesthetic Management of the Obese Surgical Patient*. Cambridge: Cambridge University Press, 2012, pp. 12–23.

Brolin R. E. Bariatric surgery and long-term control of morbid obesity. *JAMA* **288**: 2793–2796, 2002.

Casati, A. and Putzu, M. Anesthesia in the obese patient: pharmacokinetic considerations. *J Clin Anesth* **17**: 134–145, 2005.

Chan, J. M., et al. Obesity, fat distribution, and weight gain as risk factors for clinical diabetes in men. *Diabetes Care* **17**: 961–969, 1994.

Christou, N. V. Impact of obesity and bariatric surgery on survial. *World J Surg* **33**: 2022–2027, 2009.

Collins, J. C. and Bentz, J. E. Behavioral and psychological factors in obesity. *J Lancaster Gen Hosp* **4**: 124–127, 2009.

Cryer, P. E., et al. Evaluation and management of adult hypoglycemic disorders : an Endocrine Society clinical practice guideline. *J Clin Endocrinol Metab* **94**: 709–728, 2009.

Treatment Guidelines Drugs for type 2 diabetes treatment guidelines. *Med Lett* **9** (108): 47–54 2011.

Devdhar, M., et al. Hypothyroidism. *Endocrinol Metab Clin N Am* **36**: 595–615, 2007.

Farling, P. A. Thyroid disease. *Br J Anaesth* **85**: 15–28, 2000.

Fischer, S. P., et al. General anesthesia in a patient on long-term amphetamine therapy: is there a cause for concern?. *Anesth Analg* **91**: 758–759, 2000.

Gonzalez, H., et al. The importance of increased neck circumference to intubation difficulties in obese patients. *Anesth Analg* **106**: 1132–1136, 2008.

Harter, R. L., et al. A comparison of the volume and ph of gastric contents of obese and lean surgical patients. *Anesth Analg* **86**: 147–152, 1998.

Hemmings, H. C. and Egan, T. D. (eds): *Pharmacology and Physiology for Anesthesia: Foundations and Clinical Application*. Philadelphia: Elsevier Saunders, 2013, pp. 43–57.

Hines R. L. and Marschall K. E. (eds): *Stoelting's Anesthesia and Co-Existing Disease*, 5th edn. Philadelphia, Churchill Livingstone, 2008, pp. 297–322.

Holley, H., et al. Regional distribution of pulmonary ventilation and perfusion in obesity. *J Clin Invest* **46**: 475–481, 1967.

Holmberg, T. J., et al. The association between obesity and difficult prehospital tracheal intubation. *Anesth Analg* **112**: 1132–1138, 2011.

Jabbour, S. A. Steroids and the surgical patient. *Med Cllin N Am* **85**: 1140–1147, 2001.

Jean, J., et al. The risk of pulmonary aspiration in patients after weight loss due to bariatric surgery. *Anesth Analg* **107**: 1257–1259, 2008.

Joshi, G. P., et al. Society for ambulatory anesthesia consensus statement on perioperative blood glucose management in diabetic patients undergoing ambulatory surgery. *Anesth Analg* **111**: 1378–1387, 2010.

Kohl, B. A. and Schwartz, S. How to manage perioperative endocrine insufficiency. *Anesthesiol Clin* **28**: 139–155, 2010.

Lipset, M. B. and Pearson, O. H. Pathophysiology and treatment of adrenal crisis. *New Engl J Med* **254**: 511–514, 1956.

Loriaux, D. L. and Fleseriu, M. Relative adrenal insufficiency. *Curr Opin Endocrin Diab Obes* **16**: 392–400, 2009.

Marik, P. E. and Varon, J. Requirement of perioperative stress doses of corticosteroids: a systematic review of the literature. *Arch Surg* **143**: 1222–1226, 2008.

Moitra, V. and Sladen, R. N. Monitoring endocrine function. *Anesthesiol Clin* **27**: 355–364, 2009.

Mokdad, A. H., et al. Actual causes of death in the united states. *JAMA* **291**: 1238–1245, 2004.

Monnier L., Mas R. E., Ginet C., et al. Activation of oxidative stress by acute glucose fluctuatin compared with sustained chronic hyperglcemia in patients with type 2 diabetes. *JAMA* **295**: 1681–1687, 2006.

National Institutes of Health, NIH Gastrointestinal Surgery for Severe Obesity: National Institutes of Health Consensus Development Conference Statement. Available at: http://consensus.nih.gov/1991/1991GISurgeryObesity084html.htm 1991

Nayak, B. and Hodak, S. Hyperthyroidism. *Endolcrinol Metab Clin N Am* **36**: 617–656, 2007.

Neligan, P. J., et al. Obstructive sleep apnea is not a risk factor for difficult intubation in morbidly obese patients. *Anesth Analg* **109**: 1182–1186, 2009.

Nguyen, N. T., et al. Trends in use of Bariatric surgery, 2003 – 2008. *Am Coll Surg* **213**: 261–266, 2011.

Ogden, C. L., et al. *Prevalence of obesity in the United States, 2009 – 2010*. NCHS data brief, no 82. Hyattsville, MD: National Center for Health Statistics, 2012.

Rasouli, N. and Kern, P. A. Adipocytokines and the Metabolic Complications of Obesity. *J Clin Endocrinol Metab* **93**: S64–S73, 2008.

Poirier, P., et al. Cardiovascular evaluation and management of severely obese patients undergoing surgery: a science advisory from the American Heart Association. *Circulation* **120**: 86–95, 2009.

American Society of Anesthesiologists Task Force on Perioperative Management of Patients with Obstructive Sleep Apnea, Practice guidelines for the perioperative management of patients with obstructive sleep apnea: a report. *Anesthesiology* **104**: 1081–1093, 2006.

Thompson, J., et al. Anesthesia case management for bariatric surgery. *AANA J* **79**: 147–160, 2011.

Tsai, A. G. and Wadden, T. A. Systematic review: an evaluation of the major commercial weight loss programs in the United States. *Ann Intern Med* **142**: 56–66, 2005.

Wall R. T. *Endocrine. in* Hines R. A., Marschall K. E. (eds): Stoeling's Anesthesia and Co-existing Disease, 5th edn. Philadephia: Churchill Livingstone, 2008.

Walls, R. M. and Murphy, M. F. (eds): *Manual of Emergency Airway Management*, 4th edn. pp. 9–21, Philadelphia, Lippincott Williams & Wilkins, 2012.

Xanthakos, S. A. Nutritional deficiencies in obesity and after bariatric surgery. *Pediatr Clin N Am* **56**: 1105–1121, 2009.

Yong, S. L., et al. Supplemental perioperative steroids for surgical patients with adrenal insufficiency (review). *Cochrane Database Syst Rev* 4: 1–16, 2009.

8 Anesthetic considerations for patients with psychiatric illness

Daniel L. Orr[1], Robert C. Bosack[2], and John Meiszner[3]
[1]UNLV School of Dental Medicine and University of Nevada School of Medicine, Las Vegas, NV, USA
[2]University of Illinois, College of Dentistry, Chicago, IL, USA
[3]Private Practice in General and Addiction Psychiatry, Orland Park, IL, USA

Introduction

Psychiatric illness is among the most common of all human afflictions, and ranges from simple personal distress and anxiety to disorders of mood, eating, thought, personality, emotion, and behavior. Substance abuse, epidemic in many communities, must also be included in this spectrum. Most patients who suffer from these conditions are able to either manage without treatment or adequately function within social norms with the aid of therapy and/or medication. There are, however, a significant number of patients who remain undiagnosed, mismanaged, or who are habitually noncompliant with their psychotropic medication. This puts them at risk for problems associated with office-based anesthesia. Effective screening for both undiagnosed and diagnosed conditions, as well as adequacy of treatment is paramount to safe anesthetic care in the dental office. Many of these patients either cannot or will not communicate adequately with the anesthesia provider, who must subsequently make decisions relating to medication issues, drug interactions, and psychological challenges that may occur during treatment, sedation/anesthesia, or during early recovery.

Problematic psychogenic issues during dental or surgical procedures are generally not a frequent concern for most practitioners, until they manifest. Relative to airway, pulmonary, and cardiovascular emergencies, more difficult psychogenic matters, although rare, demand immediate and expert attention to avoid a wide range of morbidity and possibly mortality. These reactions may or may not be related to practitioner interaction or administered drugs. These reactions range from mild stress-induced hyperventilation to acute psychosis occurring either during the procedure or in the early postoperative period. The goal of this chapter is to familiarize the practitioner with some of the more common syndromes and treatments, providing knowledge to fuel appropriate clinical decision-making when treating patients with psychogenic challenges.

Overview of psychiatric disease

Psychiatric illness is fraught with fear, disbelief, and superstition, which supports a stigma that incessantly separates it from tangible, medical, and physical illness, in spite of the fact that many core psychiatric diseases have been shown to be associated with changes in both brain structure and function. Resolution of organic versus psychological theories is aided by the hypothesis that most mental disorders represent a disease spectrum, treatable with both drugs and psychological therapy.

Abnormal behavior (thought and actions) represents a continuum that is relative to value judgments based on cultural norms. It can involve atypical (deviant) behavior, which is disturbing to the values or beliefs of a given society. In a different sense, it can be harmful or maladaptive whereby patients are unable to adjust to society, becoming a pervasive interference with life activities. As such, it often leads to situational difficulties and subjective stress.

In 2013, the American Psychiatric Association published its most recent version of the *Diagnostic and Statistical Manual of Mental Disorders, Fifth Edition*, to categorize mental disorders reflecting the overall ability of a patient to function satisfactorily in society. Axis I disorders include major psychiatric disorders reflecting the current clinical problem. Axis II includes personality disorders (paranoid, antisocial, schizoid, narcissism) and mental retardation. A partial list of the axis I disorders included in this chapter are listed in Table 8.1. Disorder is the terminology used to reflect behavioral, psychological, or biologic dysfunction. An understanding of these disorders will aid in patient management in the perianesthetic period. Diagnostic criteria can be fluid and differential diagnosis is as much an art as it is a science.

Anxiety disorders

It is normal to experience bouts of stress and anxiety and treatment is indicated if symptoms interfere with normal societal functioning. Preexisting anxiety disorders by themselves, or aggravated by impending dental treatment, may be the reason for the administration of office-based sedation/anesthesia.

Common symptoms of anxiety, due in large part to sympathetic stimulation, are listed in Table 8.2. Panic attacks, by comparison, are unprovoked, intense but short-lived surges of anxiety, accompanied by an increase in sympathetic tone. This is in contradistinction to long-term low level continuous anxiety, which manifests as social or stress-related anxiety, phobias, or post-traumatic stress disorder (PTSD). Anxiety can also be a component of underlying medical illness, such as hypoglycemia, mitral valve prolapse, myocardial ischemia, hyperthyroidism, or cardiac arrhythmias. Amphetamines, appetite suppressants, albuterol, caffeine, steroids,

Anesthesia Complications in the Dental Office, First Edition. Edited by Robert C. Bosack and Stuart Lieblich.

Table 8.1 Select Axis I psychiatric disorders.

Anxiety disorders
- Panic attacks (without provocation), general anxiety, post-traumatic stress disorder, obsessive–compulsive disorder, phobias

Mood disorders
- Depression, dysthymia (mild depression)
- Bipolar illness

Thought disorders
- Psychosis
- Schizophrenia (disorders of thought, perception, and emotion)

Eating disorders

Substance abuse

Data from American Psychiatric Association, 2013.

Table 8.2 Symptoms of anxiety.

- Nervousness
- Restlessness, trembling, feeling shaky
- Shortness of breath
- Palpitations
- Tachycardia
- Sweating
- Lightheadedness, dizziness
- Impaired attention and concentration

and cocaine are among many drugs that share anxiety as a frequent side effect. Treatment of anxiety includes psychotherapy, stress management, exercise, biofeedback, and medications, including benzodiazepines, β-blockers, venlafaxine, clomipramine, SSRIs, and MAOIs, among others. As with most psychotropic medication, symptomatic improvement may take several weeks. Abrupt discontinuation of these medications can lead to withdrawal symptoms. Benzodiazepines are synergistic with drugs used to induce sedation/anesthesia, whose doses should be adjusted accordingly.

Patients with PTSD (military combat veterans, rescue workers, law enforcement, etc.) who have witnessed an incidence that resulted in psychological trauma may require vigilant care both during anesthesia and in the perianesthesia time frame. The incidence of PTSD is surpassed only by substance use and depression, which can also be present in the PTSD patient (Fullerton and Ursano, 2004). PTSD patients will occasionally warn providers that they have been diagnosed with PTSD and, at times, relate histories about successful or unsuccessful post-PTSD anesthetic or surgical experiences. Such patients may not be truthful about additional self-prescribed premedication, such as ethanol or cannabis, taken in an attempt to cope with anticipated stress. A major concern with PTSD patients is "sedative-facilitated" disinhibition (transient psychosis) triggered by traumatic memory. In addition, patients can interpret the anesthetic and/or surgical procedure itself as traumatic and such an experience can initiate new or enhance preexisting PTSD.

Mood disorders

Depression is the most common psychiatric disorder. Prominent features of depression are listed in Table 8.3. A familial pattern is often traced and depression is more common in women. It is more severe and longer lasting than reactive sadness or grief, as would be expected following interpersonal loss. The pathophysiology of depression is not fully elucidated; however, dysregulation of neurotransmitters (norepinephrine, serotonin and dopamine) at any number of receptors is a possibility. Depression can be a side effect of many medical illnesses, notably hypothyroidism, chronic pain, and diseases of aging. Drugs such as benzodiazepines, antihypertensives, corticosteroids, and alcohol, among others, can cause depression as a side effect. Aside from general concerns about patient well-being, depression rarely interferes with office anesthesia/sedation. There are some caveats that should be observed concerning the medications used in the management of depression.

Table 8.3 Features (when persistent) that can characterize depression.

- Depressed mood (de novo or due to psychological trigger)
- Apathy, low motivation, loss of energy, social withdrawal
- Irrational erosion of self-esteem, a feeling of worthlessness, or guilt
- Increasing impairment of normal functioning (work, school, intimate relationships)
- Change in sleep, appetite, sex drive
- Appearance of atypical physical complaints
- Suicidal ideation

As with most psychiatric illness, treatment of depression often extends beyond medication. There are four major categories of drugs used to manage depression: tricyclic antidepressants (TCA), selective serotonin reuptake inhibitors (SSRI), atypical agents, and monoamine oxidase inhibitors (MAOI). A partial list of drugs in these classes is included in Table 8.4 to aid in recognition. Medications are generally started at lower doses and gradually titrated up. The appearance of side effects is often sufficient for noncompliance in depressed patients, who grow impatient without immediate clinical improvement. Although biochemical changes are thought to occur immediately, clinical improvement frequently takes much longer, on the order of weeks to months.

SSRI increase synaptic serotonin concentration. As the most frequently prescribed class of antidepressant medication, SSRIs enjoy a wide therapeutic index. However, agitation, tremor, headache, and sexual dysfunction are common side effects. Notably, they are devoid of the autonomic side effects seen with TCAs. Many patients experience "activation"—a transient increase in anxiety, restlessness, or insomnia during the first few weeks of treatment or dose escalation (Preston and Johnson, 2012). Some SSRIs, notably fluoxetine (Prozac®), are potent inhibitors of the CYP 450 enzymes, which can lead to increased plasma levels of drugs such as benzodiazepines, warfarin, phenytoin, and TCAs. Although rarely encountered in an office setting, serotonin syndrome is a potentially fatal toxic reaction from increased synaptic serotonin in the central nervous system, a result of gross overdose or interaction with drugs that also increase serotonin activity, including MAOIs, TCAs, meperidine, tramadol, and dextromethorphan. The syndrome presents with behavioral changes (agitation, confusion), increased motor activity (rigidity, hyperreflexia and clonus), and autonomic instability (hyperthermia, tachycardia, labile blood pressure and diarrhea). SSRIs should not be used with MAOIs or TCAs.

The tricyclic antidepressants, once widely used for the treatment of depression, have been replaced to a large extent with SSRIs. They are also used for the management of chronic pain syndromes. TCAs competitively block the reuptake of norepinephrine and serotonin

Table 8.4 Drugs useful for managing depression (generic - trade name®)

- Selective serotonin reuptake inhibitors
  - Citalopram – Celexa
  - Escitalopram – Lexapro
  - Fluoxetine – Prozac / Serafem
  - Fluvoxamine – Luvox
  - Paroxetine – Paxil / Pexeva
  - Sertraline - Zoloft
- Tricyclic antidepressants
  - Amitriptyline – Elavil
  - Clomipramine – Anafranil
  - Desipramine – Norpramin
  - Doxepin – Sinequan
  - Imipramine – Tofranil
  - Maprotiline – Ludiomil
  - Nortriptyline – Pamelor
  - Protriptyline – Vivactil
- Monoamine oxidase inhibitors
  - Isocarboxazid – Marplan
  - Tranylcypromine – Parnate
  - Phenelzine – Nardil
  - Pargyline Eutonyl
  - Selegiline – Emsam
  - Selegiline - Eldepryl
  - Moclobemide - Aurorix
- Atypical agents
  - Bupropion – Wellbutrin /Zyban
  - Desmethylvenlafaxine - Pristiq
  - Duloxetine – Cymbalta
  - Venlafaxine - Effexor
  - Mirtazapine – Remeron
  - Nefazodone – Serzone
  - Trazodone - Desyrel

(5-HT) from the synaptic cleft, thereby flooding the synapse with these mediators and increasing serotinergic and adrenergic activity. Side effects, related to variable blockade of muscarinic, histaminergic, and α-adrenergic receptors, include xerostomia, blurred vision, orthostatic hypotension, and sedation. TCAs are highly protein bound and can increase the effect of other highly protein-bound drugs by displacement, such as benzodiazepines. An increased pressor response can be anticipated with concomitant use of epinephrine or ketamine at sufficient doses. Anticholinergics should be avoided, benzodiazepines should be carefully titrated (start low and go slow), and ECG should be carefully monitored during sedation/anesthesia.

The monoamine oxidase inhibitors (MAOI) are usually reserved for the last line treatment of depression because of a long list of possible adverse side effects. In addition to CNS accumulation of norepinephrine, serotonin, and dopamine, they permanently deacti vate monoamine oxidase, preventing the deamination and breakdown of these monoamine neurotransmitters, thereby increasing their availability and presynaptic buildup. The sympathomimemtic vasopressor ephedrine, with both direct and indirect action, is contraindicated in patients taking MAOIs, as the indirect action stimulates the release of abundant stores of norepinephrine causing an exaggerated hypertensive response. Direct-acting sympathomimetics, such as epinephrine, phenylephrine, or levonordefrin do not share this worrisome interaction. The deactivation of tyramine (a precursor of norepinephrine) is also inhibited by monoamine oxidases, leading to a significant increase in blood pressure when tyramine-containing foods (cheese, wines, processed meats) are consumed. Possible side effects of this drug class include orthostatic hypotension, sedation, and blurred vision. Phenylzine decreases plasma cholinesterase, which prolongs the action of succinylcholine. MAOIs can adversely interact with meperidine, resulting in serotonin syndrome (Boyer and Shannon, 2005).

Atypical agents comprise of group of heterogeneous drugs with similar clinical actions. In addition to other drug effects, buproprion, venlafaxine, and duloxetine inhibit norepinephrine synaptic reuptake. Unlike other agents in this group, trazodone can both cause and enhance sedation when used in conjunction with other sedative drugs. Venlafaxine may contribute to opioid-induced rigidity (Roy and Fortier, 2003).

Bipolar illness involves episodes (cycles) of depression, alternating with bouts of mania: periods of elevated, expansive, or irritable moods characterized by grandiosity, decreased need for sleep, and reckless involvement in goal-oriented activity with high potential for adverse consequences. Disease variation includes bipolar disease with mild mania (hypomania) and rapidly cycling disease, where patients can shift moods on weekly or even daily basis. Use of antidepressants for depression in undiagnosed bipolar patients can precipitate a shift into mania or cycle acceleration. Treatment of bipolar disease can be frustrating as it involves both reduction of current symptoms and prevention of recurrence in patients who may not be "engaged" in their therapy. As with other psychiatric diseases, bipolar disorder should be viewed as a biologic disorder, and not a moral weakness or character flaw.

Bipolar patients usually need life-long medication treatment to avoid relapse. Lithium remains a mainstay for treatment of bipolar disorder, especially for acute mania, maintenance therapy, and reduction in suicide. Side effects of lithium include sedation, tremor, and weakness. Unfortunately, lithium has a narrow therapeutic index; even a slight elevation in blood concentration can lead to signs of toxicity, including nausea, vomiting, diarrhea, dysrhythmias, hypotension, confusion, agitation, and seizures. Therefore, lithium levels should be monitored on a regular basis. An elevation of lithium blood levels is seen with renal dysfunction, dehydration, concomitant use of NSAIDs, and low salt intake. Long-term side effects of lithium therapy include hypothyroidism and goiter. Lithium can prolong the action of muscle relaxants and can reduce anesthetic requirement.

Other antimanic agents are often used alone or in conjunction with lithium to improve treatment success including mood-stabilizing anticonvulsants and second-generation neuroleptic agents. (See Table 8.5)

Thought disorders

Psychosis is a condition characterized by the inability to accurately perceive reality. It can include disturbances in emotion, cognition (confusion, delusion, hallucination), and/or behavior (impairment in judgment or reason). Psychosis can also be due to somatic diseases such as CNS pathology, lupus, hypercortisolism, or hypoadrenalism, among many others. Schizophrenia is a psychotic disorder that presents with a heterogeneous group of positive, negative, and cognitive symptoms (see Table 8.6) Similarly to other psychiatric disorders, psychoses can result from medical diseases and drug effect (illicit drugs, steroids, anticholinergics, among others). Patients with psychotic symptoms will have significant

Table 8.5 Drugs useful for managing bipolar disease (generic – trade name®)

- Mood-stabilizing anticonvulsants
  - Lamotrigine-Lamictal
  - Valproate-Depakote
  - Carbamazepine-Tegretol
  - Oxcarbazepine-Trileptal
  - Leveteracetam-Keppra
- Atypical Neuroleptics
  - Olanzapine-Zyprexa
    - Olanzapine + fluoxetine = Symbyax
  - Risperidone-Risperdal
  - Paliperidone-Invega
  - Ziprasidone-Geodon
  - Quetiapine-Seroquel
  - Aripiprazole-Abilify

Table 8.6 Symptoms of Schizophrenia.

Positive Symptoms (excess or distortion of language, perception, thought, or behavior)
- Delusion, hallucination
- Disordered thought
- Disorganized behavior, incoherent speech
- Severe anxiety, agitation

Negative Symptoms (diminution of function, emotion, behavior)
- Apathy
- Social withdrawal
- Blunted affect
- Anhedonia
- Poverty of thought
- Failure of initiation in goal-oriented behavior

Cognitive Symptoms
- Impairment in attention
- Difficulty in information processing
- Defective memory formation and recall

difficulty with dental therapy, regardless of the level of anesthesia. Further complicating treatment is the extensive list of adverse side effects associated with antipsychotic medication (Reilly and Kirk, 2007).

Antipsychotic medication should be started early to avoid social or physical harm often associated with more severe psychotic episodes. As schizophrenia is a chronic disorder, life-long treatment is usually required to avoid relapse. Antipsychotic medications (major tranquilizers) are more correctly termed *neuroleptics*, as many of these drugs have clinical usefulness in disorders other than psychoses. Neuroleptics are divided into the older, first-generation "typical antipsychotics" and the newer second-generation "atypical antipsychotics" with less propensity for extrapyramidal side effects. The method of action of all neuroleptics is interference with central dopaminergic transmission by nonselective blockade of the D2 dopamine receptor in the CNS; selectivity is improved with atypical drugs. Potency refers to the ability of the drug to bind to dopamine receptors, and does not describe the effectiveness of the drug. High potency drugs are more effective in D2 blockade at lower doses, while low potency drugs require higher doses for similar effectiveness, thereby inviting a greater degree of anticholinergic, antihistaminergic, and anti-α-adrenergic effects. Many of the

Table 8.7 Neuroleptic drugs (generic – trade name®).

- Typical, "first-generation" neuroleptics
  - High potency
    - Fluphenazine - Prolixin
    - Haloperidol - Haldol
    - Droperidol - Inapsine
    - Perphenazine - Trilafon
    - Pimozide - Orap
    - Thiothixene - Navane
    - Trifluoperazine - Stelazine
  - Mid potency
    - Loxapine - Loxitane
    - Molindone - Moban
  - Low potency
    - Chlorpromazine - Thorazine
    - Mesoridazine - Serentil
    - Thioridazine - Mellaril
    - Prochlorperazine – Compazine
- Atypical, "second-generation" neuroleptics
  - Clozapine – Clozaril
  - Aripiprazole - Abilify
  - Olanzapine – Zyprexa, Zydis
  - Quetiapine - Seroquel
  - Paliperidone - Invega
  - Risperidone - Risperdal
  - Ziprasidone - Geodon

atypicals also block serotonin receptors, which can improve the negative symptoms of schizophrenia. QT prolongation is possible with second-generation drugs. A partial listing of neuroleptics is depicted in Table 8.7. Clozapine deserves special note. Unlike most first-generation drugs, clozapine is useful for treating both positive and negative symptoms of schizophrenia. Secondly, there is no risk of developing extrapyramidal side effects. Seizures and agranulocytosis are rare but significant side effects of this efficacious drug, often used in "treatment-resistant" cases. Of note, clozapine can cause sialorrhea (Davydov and Botts, 2000).

Antipsychotic medications have five categories of possible side effects that can affect both compliance with medication and delivery of anesthesia. These side effects categories are anticholinergic, antihistaminic, α-1 blockade, extrapyramidal effects, and weight gain/metabolic effects.

Anticholinergic effects include dry mouth, blurred vision, constipation, tachycardia, agitation, delirium, and exacerbation of acute narrow-angle glaucoma. It is important to avoid/limit the use of drugs that can intensify these effects. In addition to antipsychotics, drugs with central anticholinergic properties include benzodiazepines, atropine, first-generation antihistamines (diphenhydramine and hydroxyzine), and TCAs. Clinicians should be mindful of the possibility of central anticholinergic syndrome in patients who become agitated, combative, or delirious when sedated or during prolonged recovery (see Table 8.8). Treatment includes "waiting it out," maintaining oxygenation, use of flumazenil to reverse larger doses of benzodiazepines, or physostigmine, a centrally acting anticholinesterase to increase the amount of acetylcholine in the CNS. The addition of peripheral-acting glycopyrrolate should be considered to avoid symptoms of cholinergic rebound including severe bradycardia, hypersalivation, seizures, nausea, and vomiting (see Chapter 36).

Table 8.8 Classic signs of central anticholinergic syndrome.

- Dry as a bone
  - Absence of sweating and salivation
- Blind as a bat
  - Loss of accommodation
- Hot as hell
  - No sweating
- Red as a beet
  - Cutanous vasodilation "atropine flush"
- Mad as a hatter
  - Delirium

Table 8.9 QT prolongation.

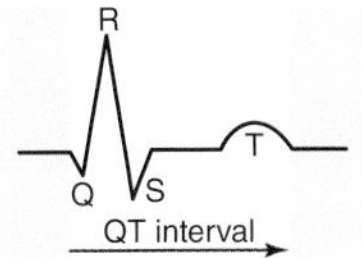

QT prolongation
QT interval - time segment from the onset of ventricular depolarization (Q wave) to the termination of ventricular repolarization (T wave), with a normal QTc (corrected for rate changes) < 450msec. As this interval gets longer, so does the possibility of serious ventricular arrhythmias, including torsades de pointes, a polymorphic ventricular tachycardia. Congenital prolonged QT syndrome is a disorder of ventricular repolarization due to mutations in cardiac ion channels. Acquired prolonged QT syndrome is usually secondary to drug therapy (possibly in genetically susceptible patients) including (especially at higher doses) (Ray et al., 2009) antipsychotic agents, TCAs, methadone, and drugs that can cause hypokalemia, among many others (Booker et al., 2003). Providers should carefully consider risks and benefits prior to managing patients' diagnosed prolonged QT syndrome when contemplating the use of parenteral agents in an office setting. Patients who take drugs that can prolong QT intervals should be carefully screened for a history of structural heart disease, arrhythmia, or syncope prior to the administration of parenteral agents. Otherwise, these patients should be handled with the same care and precautions as other patients, avoiding hypoxia, sympathetic stimulation, and swings in heart rate. The dentist should also be aware of possible electrolyte imbalances (K^+, Mg^{++}, and Ca^{++}).

Anti-histaminic effects include sedation, drowsiness, and hypotension, which are potentiated by benzodiazepines and narcotics.

α1-blockade exacerbates postural hypotension, often times leading to dizziness or light-headedness. Reflex tachycardia can be anticipated. There is some sedation associated with α1-blockade.

Adverse metabolic effects include agranulocytosis, possible prolongation of the QTc interval (see Table 8.9), and weight gain (with the notable exception of ziprasidone or aripiprazole), which can be a contributing factor to the development of type II diabetes.

Non-specific D2 blockade will also affect the extrapyramidal system, which modulates reflexes, locomotion, complex movements, and postural control. There are four classes of extrapyramidal symptoms: acute akathisia, acute dystonia, chronic Parkinson-like effects, and tardive dyskinesia. Akathisia is a feeling or sense of restlessness. Acute dystonias are prolonged, painful, spasmodic muscular contractions, usually of the head or neck. Parkinson-like side effects include muscular rigidity, tremor, and bradykinesia (slow motor response). These movement disorders are often managed with anticholinergics (benzotropine, trihexyphenidyl), β-blockers, diphenhydramine, or benzodiazepines. Tardive dyskinesia (Kane et al., 1988) is a serious, often irreversible, late onset extrapyramidal side effect causing involuntary sucking or smacking of the mouth and lips. This choreoathetotic movement disorder can also affect the extremities. Frequency worsens as treatment duration increases, and may slowly improve over time with cessation of the antipsychotic medication (Correll and Schenk, 2008).

Eating disorders

The American culture is obsessed with weight loss, which undoubtedly affects impressionable youth, leading to a grossly underestimated incidence of eating disorders. Anorexia nervosa is an intense fear of becoming obese and a distorted perception of body weight and shape that leads to a refusal to maintain appropriate body weight and amenorrhea. Bulimia nervosa includes recurrent episodes of binge eating accompanied by inappropriate behavior to prevent weight gain (DSM-V, 2013). These diseases are more common in females between the ages of 15 and 30; however, males and middle-aged females are also vulnerable. Other psychiatric problems are common in patients with eating disorders, including depression and substance abuse.

Similar to substance abuse, denial is near-universal, as these "self-imposed" disorders are associated with shame and guilt due to an apparent failure of will. Questioning should proceed in an understanding, non-judgmental manner. Similar to other undiagnosed or hidden illnesses, clinical suspicion should clinch the diagnosis when managing patients with eating disorders for office-based sedation/anesthesia.

Medical complications common to both anorexia and bulimia include low body mass, cardiac abnormalities (repeated vomiting and use of ipecac), bradycardia and heart block, hypotension, hypoglycemia, dehydration, hypokalemia, low serum proteins, muscle wasting and myalgia, seizures, and delayed gastric emptying (Mitchell and Crow, 2006). Anorexic patients will appear cachectic, while bulimic patients may not. Self-induced vomiting can be more frequent with bulimic patients, possibly increasing the risk of silent aspiration. Signs of repeated vomiting include dental erosion and palatal petechiae.

Successful long-term management of both disorders remains elusive, and includes both psychotherapy and pharmacotherapy (Sigman, 2003).

There are four major anesthetic concerns for patients with eating disorders (Seller and Ravalia, 2003). Preexisting hypotension due to blunted autonomic reflexes and hypovolemia is exacerbated with the use of anesthetic agents. Bradycardia due to blunted autonomic reflexes and excess parasympathetic tone is exacerbated by narcotics and can contribute to hypotension. Exaggerated drug response is anticipated because of decreased plasma proteins (decreased binding increases concentration of the free, active drug), hypovolemia (reducing the volume of distribution, hastening and magnifying drug action), and decreased muscle mass (magnifying drug action). Electrolyte disturbances (hypokalemia and hypocalcemia) can contribute to cardiac conduction abnormalities: PACs, PVCs, and heart block, among others. Hypokalemia is worsened with hyperventilation and the use of glucose-containing solutions.

Every attempt should be made identify and medically optimize patients with eating disorders prior to anesthetic intervention. Careful case selection, assurance of appropriate preanesthetic fast, adequate hydration with isotonic crystalloids, and slow titration of small doses will minimize adversity.

Substance abuse

It is difficult to argue against the statement that the worldwide prevalence of substance abuse is both underestimated and escalating. It is a condition that is oblivious to age, race, sex, occupation, or financial status. Managing patients who abuse drugs is extremely difficult and fraught with complications for several reasons. Patients are often less than forthcoming (denial, understatement) concerning specifics of their habit (drugs, dose, frequency, route of ingestion) and have little knowledge of the accurate composition of the drugs because of a totally unregulated market. Anesthesia providers who are understandably reticent to treat patients with recent drug use may unwittingly expose their patients and themselves to complications associated with acute drug withdrawal. These complications include irritability, seizures, autonomic instability (wide swings in blood pressure and heart rate), tremor, and fever. Other concerns relate to problems associated with the drug-abusing lifestyle. These include decreased appetite, infection, upper airway irritation, cardiovascular inflammation, premature atherosclerosis, difficult vascular access, hepatitis, and HIV infection.

Drug tolerance refers to a progressive decline in drug activity with chronic use, increasing the dose requirement to achieve the initial effect. Physiological drug dependence refers a condition where a drug is required to maintain normal physiologic function and avoid signs and symptoms of withdrawal with drug depletion. Psychological dependence occurs when drug use for non-medical reasons persists despite problems related to the use of the substance. Drug addiction is the compulsive use of drugs, despite negative or dangerous effects.

Alcohol abuse is a chronic disorder marked by episodes of acute intoxication, which are obvious in most instances and should lead to postponement of all but emergency procedures. Acute alcohol exposure is heralded by a characteristic breath odor. In this case, patients should be asked to verify that there is alcohol on their breath, versus the question "are you drunk?" Anesthetic concerns with chronic alcohol exposure include hypertension, cardiac arrhythmia and failure, liver disease, decreased plasma proteins, electrolyte disturbances, coagulopathy, prolonged bleeding time, and enzyme induction (Chapman and Plaat, 2009).

Marijuana use, similar to the use of all other illicit drugs, often results in an unpredictable clinical picture. Classic effects include relaxation, euphoria, and emotional instability. The substance is often diluted with contaminants or spiked with other drugs. Marijuana is referred to as the *gateway drug*, as users frequently go on to experiment with other drugs.

Increased sympathetic tone occurs at moderate doses, but hypotension and bradycardia predominate at higher doses. Duration of activity is dose dependent and on a scale of minutes to hours; elimination T1/2 of this highly lipid soluble drug ranges from days to weeks. Cross tolerance with barbiturates, opioids, and benzodiazepines is possible; however, the drug can also be additive with benzodiazepines (Hernandez et al., 2005).

Cocaine affords its users a powerful, but short-lived euphoria and stimulation that ends in irritability and fatigue. Cocaine interferes with the uptake of sympathomimetic amines and floods the synapse with norepinephrine, serotonin, and dopamine (Carrera et al., 2004). The risk of acute myocardial infarction is elevated 23 times over baseline in the first 60 minutes after use; this elevated risk decreases rapidly thereafter (Mittleman et al., 1999). The intense stimulation increases cardiac oxygen consumption by increasing blood pressure, heart rate, and contraction while decreasing coronary perfusion by vasoconstriction of epicardial vessels. Cocaine also has prothrombotic effects. Patients who test positive for cocaine, but are "non-toxic" (hemodynamically stable), present no greater risk than comparable ASA and age-matched drug-free patients (Hill et al., 2006; Granite et al., 2007).

Opioid abuse is particularly rampant because of wide availability, low cost, and propensity for addiction. The analgesia and euphoria afforded by drugs such as hydrocodone (Vicoden®), oxycodone (Oxycontin®), and heroin make them attractive for abuse. Hypotension, bradycardia, and respiratory depression add to the risk of opioid abuse. Several treatment options for opioid addiction are available. The long-acting opioid receptor antagonist naltrexone (Revia®, Depade®, Vivitrol®) is intended to block the effects of illicit opioids. Methadone and buprenorphine are longer acting opioid agonist substitutes for heroin, which are prescribed only from specialized addiction clinics. Both drugs occupy the opioid receptor to reduce craving, decrease euphoria, withdrawal, and other side effects to facilitate return to society. Methadone is particularly attractive as it also inhibits serotonin and norepinephrine synaptic reuptake, while antagonizing NMDA receptors. Physical dependence persists, while disruptive behavior does not. In higher doses, methadone can prolong the QT interval in a small percentage of patients. Suboxone® and Zubsolv®(sublingual formulation) are both combinations of buprenorphine and naloxone (to prevent IV abuse) with less prescribing limitations. Several caveats emerge concerning office-based anesthetic management of opioid-addicted patients. Opioids should not be administered to patients taking antagonists (naltrexone or Suboxone®) for obvious reasons. Agonist–antagonist combinations (pentazocine (Talwin®), nalbuphine (Nubain®), and butorphanol (Stadol®) should be avoided in addicted patients to avoid withdrawal symptoms and in those taking methadone or buprenorphine. Sedation providers should be aware of the synergistic effect that benzodiazepines share with methadone or buprenorphine, and the risk of deeper than intended anesthesia that is possible even without additional opioid administration. Finally, although opioid-addicted patients may be tolerant to the effect of opioids, they may not be as tolerant to side effects including hypotension, bradycardia, and respiratory depression.

Amphetamines stimulate the release and block the reuptake of norepinephrine, dopamine, and serotonin. As expected, drugs of this class cause hyperactivity, anxiety, insomnia, anorexia, sweating, mydriasis, tachycardia, palpitations, arrhythmias, and hypertension. Ecstacy (3,4 methylenedioxmethamphetamine, MDMA) is both a hallucinogen and a stimulant that causes prolonged, intense euphoria, augmented sensual awareness, and increased emotional energy (Greydanus and Patel, 2003).

Patient management

It is a well-established fact in all of medicine, regardless of specialty, that the rapport between patient and treater has powerful prognostic implications. It is crucial that the patient have confidence and trust in the doctor, which is possible only if the doctor is able to embrace the patient in a non-judgmental healing spirit. This is especially important when dealing with "psychiatric patients," and even more so when dealing with substance abusers, for these people often appear culpable for their own misery. Regrettably, though understandably, it is often difficult to embrace them as "sick" in the same way one would embrace a medically ill individual.

Accordingly, when dealing with these patients it is important to check one's own attitude. If the treater's heart is not in the right place (i.e., judgmental attitude), his ministrations, no matter how expert, are much less likely to yield a positive result. People in psychic distress, and addicts in particular, are often hyper-aware of the treater's attitude, almost as if they had a "sixth sense." So, it is highly recommended that, before dealing with this patient population, one do a "gut check." If, in fact, one has a strongly negative opinion of them, for whatever reason, it is important to be aware of it and keep it in check. In some cases, it may be better for all concerned to deflect than to treat them with covert contempt. The first admonition of the Hippocratic Oath is "First, do no harm."

Anesthetic management of patients with psychiatric disease in an office setting begins with an accurate medical history, screening for diagnosed or undiagnosed (Ansseau et al., 2004) psychiatric problems, as they relate to the patient's ability to understand, choose, and safely undergo the planned procedure with both office and home recovery, regardless of the level of anesthesia. As psychiatric labels tend to dehumanize patients, it is important to develop and maintain rapport with a non-judgmental perspective when gathering this history. Elevated concern is warranted for patients who "don't feel good," who are unable to live independently, or who have lost driving privileges. Once the diagnosis is identified, the adequacy of control should be questioned, including the recent addition or cessation of medication/dose, ongoing side effects of medication, and compliance (engagement) with dosing.

The possibility of medication side effects should be ascertained to rule out drug toxicity or withdrawal states (Smith et al., 2008). All psychotropic agents can be continued into the perianesthetic period (De Baerdemaeker et al., 2005), as abrupt discontinuation can lead to a variety of short-lived (days to weeks) withdrawal symptoms, including nausea, abdominal pain, diarrhea, malaise, sleep disturbance (insomnia, nightmares), somatic symptoms (headache, sweating, lethargy, phantom nerve pain), and affective symptoms (depression, anxiety, irritability). Relapse of the condition for which the drugs were taken (with a possible notable exception of lithium for bipolar disorders, Cavanagh et al., 2004), usually takes a longer time than the duration of the withdrawal symptoms.

As the list of medications used to treat psychiatric disorders is extensive and frequently changing, it is impossible to be mindful of each and every action, interaction, and side effect. In general, these side effects include hypotension or hypertension, tachycardia, and sedation. Cardiovascular stability should be maintained with adequate sedation, analgesia, local anesthesia, isotonic fluid replacement, and careful use of vasoconstrictors (especially in patients taking TCAs). Deeper than intended levels of anesthesia are possible, and sedative drugs should be careful titrated. Ephedrine should be avoided in patients taking MAOIs. Meperidine and atropine are best avoided in patients taking psychotropic medication. Atropine is additive with psychotropic anticholinergic effects and can also exacerbate tachycardia, while meperidine can enhance tachycardia and adversely interact with MAOIs. The use of ketamine can be questioned because of its possible psychomimetic side effects.

Macrolide antibiotics, antifungals, and antivirals are medications often used by the dental profession. These drugs should be avoided, if possible, as they are potent cytochrome P450 inhibitors, which can lead to toxicity of those psychotropic agents (TCAs) that are metabolized by these enzymes.

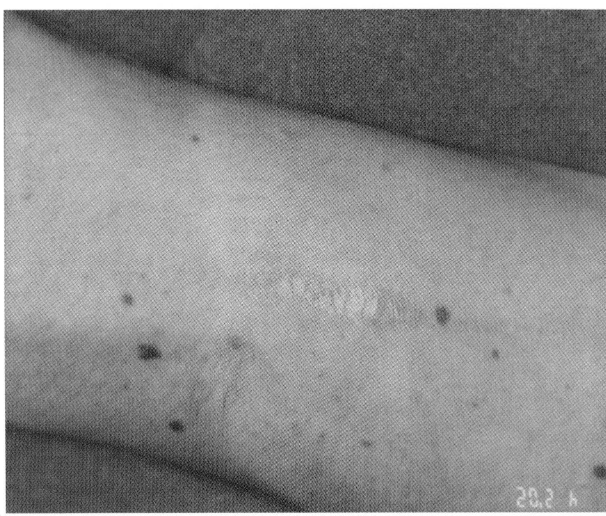

Figure 8.1 Needle track from repeated vascular access and inflammation.

Management of patients with substance abuse problems can be more problematic, as identification can be obscure and difficult. History and physical examination are the only mechanisms to identify drug abuse. Acute exposure is often obvious and should lead to postponement. Rapport, privacy, and a non-judgmental, non-threatening demeanor are necessary to encourage even a moderate degree of truthfulness. Casual physical exam (without overt search for signs of drug abuse) notices agitation, withdrawal, fleeting ideas, rapid speech, sluggishness, and overly dilated or constricted pupils and explores the arms for absence of superficial veins, needle tracts (scarred veins from repeated percutaneous access and infection) (Figure 8.1), and small, circular scars after subcutaneous injections. Urine drug screening panels rapidly detect the presence of amphetamines, cocaine, opiates, and marijuana; however, positive tests may not indicate acute intoxication, as elimination half-lives are greater than clinical effects.

It is impossible to predict dose requirements for patients who abuse drugs. Recent use of stimulants or chronic use of depressants often increases anesthetic requirements, while acute use of depressants will decrease anesthetic requirements. Moderate sedation providers should be wary about unintentional overdosing and loss of airway or respiratory depression. Providers of general anesthesia should be aware of cross tolerance and the possibility of inadequate dosing, especially with respect to opioids. Cardiovascular stability should be maintained with careful and vigilant use of sympathomimetics, ketamine, vagolytics, local anesthetics, and systemic analgesics.

References

American Psychiatric Association. *Diagnostic and Statistical Manual of Mental Disorders*, 5th edn., Washington, DC: American Psychiatric Association, 2013.

Ansseau, D. M., et al. High Prevalence of mental disorders in primary care. *J Affect Disord* **78**: 49–55, 2004.

Booker, P. D., et al. Long QT syndrome and anaesthesia. *Br J Anaesth* **90**: 349–366, 2003.

Boyer, E. W. and Shannon, M. The serotonin syndrome. *N engl J Med* **354**: 1112–1120, 2005.

Carrera, M.R., et al. Cocaine pharmacology and current pharmacotherapies for its abuse. *Bioorg Med Chem* **12**: 5019–5030, 2004.

Cavanagh, J., et al. Relapse into mania or depression following lithium discontinuation: a 7-year follow-up. *Acta Psychiatr Scand* **109**: 91–95, 2004.

Chapman, R. and Plaat, F. Alcohol and anaesthesia. *Continuing Education in Anesthesia, Critical Care and Pain* **9**: 10–13, 2009.

Correll, C. U. and Schenk, E. M. Tardive dsykinesia and new antipsychotics. *Curr Opin Psychiatry* **21**: 151–156, 2008.

Davydov, L. and Botts, S. R. Clozapine-induced hypersalivation. *Ann Pharmacother* **34**: 662–665, 2000.

De Baerdemaeker, L. D., et al. Anaesthesia for patients with mood disorders. *Curr Opin Anaesthesiol* **18**: 333–338, 2005.

Fullerton, C.S. and Ursano, W. Acute stress disorder, posttraumatic stress disorder, and depression in disaster or rescue workers. *Am J Psychiatry* **161**: 1370–1376, 2004.

Granite, E. L., et al. Parameters for treatment of Cocaine-positive patients. *J Oral Maxillofac Surg* **65**: 1984–1989, 2007.

Greydanus, D. E. and Patel, D. R. Substance abuse in adolescents: a complex conundrum for the clinician. *Pediatr Clin N Am* **50**: 1179–1223, 2003.

Hernandez, M., et al. Anesthetic management of the illicit-substance-using patient. *Curr Opin Anaesthesiol* **18**: 315–324, 2005.

Hill, G. E., et al. General anaesthesia for the cocaine abusing patients. Is it safe? *Br J Anaesth* **97**: 654–657, 2006.

Kane, J. M., et al. Tardive dyskinesia: prevalence, incidence and risk factors. *J Clin Psychopharmacol* **8**: 52S, 1988.

Mittleman, M. A., et al. Triggering of Myocardial Infarction by Cocaine. *Circ* **99**: 2737–2741, 1999.

Mitchell, J. E. and Crow, S. Medical Complications of anorexia nervosa and bulimia nervosa. *Curr Opin Psychiatry* **19**: 438–443, 2006.

Preston, J. and Johnson, J. *Clinical Psychopharmacology made ridiculously simple*, 7th edn. Miami: MedMaster, 2012.

Reilly, T. H. and Kirk, M. A. Atypical antipsychotics and newer antidepressants. *Emerg Med Clin N Am* **25**: 477–497, 2007.

Ray, W. A., et al. Atypical Antipsychotic drugs and the risk of sudden cardiac death. *N Engl J Med* **360**: 225–235, 2009.

Roy, S. and Fortier, L. P. Fentanyl-induced rigidity during emergence from general anesthesia potentiated by venlafexine. *Can J Anaesth* **50**: 32–35, 2003.

Seller, C. A. and Ravalia, A. Anaesthetic implications of anorexia nervosa. *Anaesth* **58**: 437–443, 2003.

Sigman, G. S. Eating disorders in children and adolescents. *Pediatr Clin N Am* **50**: 1139–1177, 2003.

Smith, F. A. et al. Medical complications of psychiatric treatment. *Crit Care Clin* **24**: 635–656, 2008.

9 Anesthetic considerations for patients with neurologic disease

Joseph A. Giovannitti
University of Pittsburgh School of Dental Medicine, Department of Dental Anesthesiology, Pittsburgh, PA, USA

The major function of the nervous system is to receive information and then process and transmit it to other cells. Information is received from peripheral sensory systems and interpreted centrally. Impulses are then transmitted via peripheral motor neurons to elicit an appropriate response, or via the autonomic nervous system for an appropriate visceral or endocrine reaction. Disturbances in receipt, processing, or transmission will result in significant disturbances in neurologic and neuromuscular functioning.

These neuronal signals are transmitted electrically along axons by a wave-like series of action potentials. When a nerve is at rest its membranes are hyperpolarized by the action of the $Na^+ - K^+$ ATPase pump, which maintains a higher concentration of sodium ions outside of the nerve membrane relative to the inside. Gated channels are located within the nerve membrane which, when activated, allow the passage of sodium ions into the nerve in exchange for potassium ions along a concentration gradient. This is known as *depolarization*. These channels are activated by the presence of certain excitatory and inhibitory neurotransmitters that induce conformational changes in the channel to allow the influx of sodium ions (Table 9.1). Impulses traveling along smaller, unmyelinated nerve fibers, such as a-delta and c-fibers that commonly transmit painful stimuli, are conducted by a rolling wave of depolarization that travels along the nerve. Larger, myelinated nerve fibers, such as large motor neurons, conduct impulses rapidly by a process known as saltatory conduction in which impulses jump rapidly from one Node of Ranvier to another as the membranes located there are depolarized.

When there is a dysfunction or disruption of the nervous system, abnormal and pathological responses may result. These may be excitatory or inhibitory depending upon the areas involved and the mechanism behind the involvement. Abnormalities may include excesses or deficiencies in neurotransmission and/or motor function, and may occur peripherally or centrally. This chapter reviews some of the commonly encountered nervous system disorders and makes recommendations for the safe anesthetic management of patients so afflicted.

Motor neuron disease

Motor neuron diseases are primarily caused by progressive degeneration of motor nerve fibers in the anterior horn of the spinal cord. As they degenerate, these fibers may fire spontaneously, producing clinically evident twitching. Two major motor neuron diseases, spinal muscular atrophy and amyotrophic lateral sclerosis (ALS), are considered.

Spinal muscular atrophy

Spinal muscular atrophy is a genetic disorder of degenerating lower motor neurons, which may manifest in childhood or early adulthood (Monani, 2005.) It is caused by mutations in the Survival of Motor Neuron 1 (SMA1) gene and occurs in 1:6000 births. Spinal muscular atrophy type I, or Werdnig–Hoffman disease, develops during the first 3 months of life and progresses aggressively until death occurs around the age of 3. Spinal muscular atrophy type II also occurs early in life, but progresses more slowly and patients may survive into early adulthood. Spinal muscular atrophy type III, or Kugelberg–Welander disease, is also a slowly progressive form in which limb muscles are primarily affected. Patients with type III disease usually have a normal life span. This disease progresses with further degeneration characterized by severe scoliosis, respiratory muscle weakness, frequent and recurrent pulmonary infections, and respiratory failure.

Amyotrophic lateral sclerosis

ALS, also known as Lou Gehrig's disease after the famous Yankee slugger who famously succumbed to this disease, develops between the ages of 30 and 60 years. It is characterized by progressive deterioration of the corticospinal tract, brainstem, and upper and lower motor neurons (Hardiman et al., 2011). Diagnosis is made initially by limb weakness followed by eventual difficulties in swallowing, eating, speaking, and breathing. Dementia may be an eventual consequence of the disease. It is usually fatal within 3–5 years after diagnosis, most often from pneumonia or respiratory failure. The cause of ALS is unknown and there is no known effective treatment.

Anesthetic considerations

Patients with spinal muscular atrophy and ALS are vulnerable to hyperkalemia following the administration of succinylcholine for intubation. Hyperkalemia is known to produce cardiac dysrhythmias and arrest. There may also by sensitivity to the nondepolarizing muscle relaxants, resulting in a prolongation of effect. These motor neuron diseases make patients susceptible to aspiration during anesthesia, including non-intubated moderate and deep sedation. Care must be taken to ensure the NPO status

Anesthesia Complications in the Dental Office, First Edition. Edited by Robert C. Bosack and Stuart Lieblich.

Table 9.1 Excitatory and inhibitory neurotransmitters.

Excitatory	Site of action
Glutamate	Brain and spinal cord
Acetylcholine	Brain, neuromuscular junction, autonomic nervous system
Dopamine	Brain, autonomic nervous system
Norepinephrine	Brain, spinal cord, autonomic nervous system
Serotonin	Brain, gastrointestinal system
Inhibitory	**Site of action**
GABA	Brain
Glycine	Spinal cord

of the patient, and aspiration precautions, such as a rapid sequence induction with cricoid pressure, must be considered. When the patient is not intubated, aspiration of aerosolized water spray from a handpiece or ultrasonic scaler may seed the lungs and produce postoperative aspiration pneumonia. Patients with spinal muscular atrophy and ALS are prone to excessive salivation, and may require antisialogogues such as glycopyrrolate to reduce salivary flow. Autonomic dysfunction may make patients susceptible to hypotension and hypothermia during anesthesia.

Parkinson disease

Parkinson disease is a disorder of the central nervous system characterized by clinical signs of resting tremor, muscle rigidity, lack of spontaneous movement (akinesia), slowness of movement (bradykinesia), and problems with walking or postural instability. Parkinsonism may be familial or secondary to chronic exposure to antidopaminergic drugs such as phenothiazines and butyrophenones, among others. Pathophysiologic changes include degeneration of dopaminergic neurons in the substantia nigra of the basal ganglia (Navailles and De Deurwaerdère, 2012). Dopamine is an inhibitory neurotransmitter that helps modulate the excitatory activity of acetylcholine in the brain. The resulting overactivity of acetylcholine produces the tremor of parkinsonism. Dopamine also inhibits GABA transmission. When dopamine is depleted as in Parkinson disease, GABA effects become clinically evident as akinesia and bradykinesia, which can become disabling. Treatment of Parkinson's disease is usually two-pronged, combining dopaminergic and anticholinergic drugs. Levodopa is useful in increasing dopamine levels and restoring the balance with acetylcholine. Ergotamine derivatives such as bromocriptine and pergolide may also be used in the treatment of Parkinson disease because they are dopaminergic. Other agents such as amantadine and selegiline increase dopamine levels and may be useful management tools. Anticholinergics and antihistaminics are also used to antagonize the effects of acetylcholine.

Anesthetic considerations

Treatment of Parkinson disease with levodopa results in systemic cardiovascular system effects that may have anesthetic consequences. Levodopa not only increases the levels of dopamine in the central nervous system but also in the systemic circulation. Dopamine is a vasoactive drug that has positive inotropic and chronotropic effects. The chronic administration of levodopa may result in depletion of norepinephrine stores in the autonomic nervous system. Depletion of norepinephrine may sensitize adrenergic receptors to the effects of exogenously administered catecholamines such as epinephrine administered with local anesthetics, resulting in an increase in blood pressure. This hypertension can be further exacerbated by the vasoconstrictive effects of high concentrations of dopamine. Drugs such as ketamine, which have significant sympathetic effects, may be relatively contraindicated. Low systemic concentrations of dopamine can increase renal blood flow and increase urine output. The renin–angiotension system is also inhibited by dopamine. These renal effects may result in reduced intravascular fluid volume and make patients susceptible to intraoperative and/or orthostatic hypotension. Patients may be especially at risk for the development of hypotension during the induction of general anesthesia. The provider must be prepared to rapidly restore the blood pressure with fluids or vasopressors. A side effect of levodopa is nausea and vomiting. Prophylaxis or treatment of postoperative nausea and vomiting should include dexamethasone, 5-HT_3 receptor antagonists such as ondansetron, or transdermal scopolamine. Traditional antiemetics such as phenothiazines (promethazine) and butyrophenones (droperidol) are dopaminergic blockers, which may worsen the patient's condition.

Myasthenia gravis

Myasthenia gravis is an autoimmune disorder of neuromuscular acetylocholine transmission that affects primarily small motor muscles including the ocular, oropharyngeal, and flexor and extensor muscles of the head and neck. Patients with myasthenia gravis present with characteristic eyelid droop and difficulty in maintaining an erect head position. Autoantibodies at the postsynaptic portion of the neuromuscular junction result in a 70%–90% reduction in functioning nicotinic receptors, decreasing the ability of the neuromuscular end plate to transmit an impulse (Meriggioli and Sanders, 2009). Myasthenia gravis can be associated with other autoimmune disorders such as hyperthyroidism, rheumatoid arthritis, system lupus erythematosis and pernicious anemia, and thymic disease.

Treatment of myasthenia gravis focuses on increasing the amount of acetylcholine available at the neuromuscular junction and by inhibiting the extent of autoimmune destruction of nicotinic receptors. Cholinesterase inhibitors, such as edrophonium and pyridostigmine, prevent the hydrolysis of acetylcholine and increase the amount of this neurotransmitter. Improved muscle function is the result. Plasmapheresis, corticosteroids, and immunosuppressants may also be effective in reducing the level of autoantibodies. Thymectomy produces remission of the disease in about one-third of affected patients.

Anesthetic considerations

Preanesthetic assessment of patients with myasthenia gravis should start with a thorough history, including the severity of the disease process with specific attention to respiratory muscle strength, which may be significantly impaired as the disease progresses. Pulmonary function tests may also be warranted. Premedication with benzodiazepines, opioids, or other sedatives may have an additive effect on respiratory depression and should potentially be avoided in susceptible patients. Since hyperthyroidism is prevalent in patients with myasthenia gravis, pre-treatment thyroid function testing may be indicated. If muscle relaxation is needed, a baseline train-of-four should be obtained for reference prior to the administration of non-depolarizing muscle relaxants, as these patients may be exquisitely sensitive to these drugs (Itoh et al., 2002). Patients undergoing general anesthesia should be made aware of the potential to remain intubated postoperatively for ventilatory support.

Patients with myasthenia gravis do, however, exhibit resistance to depolarizing muscle relaxants such as succinylcholine. This may be attributed to a smaller number of acetylcholine receptors available to produce the desired agonist effect of succinylcholine. Long-acting muscle relaxants should be avoided in these patients and intermediate and short-acting relaxants should be used conservatively and with careful monitoring of neuromuscular transmission.

In patients receiving general anesthesia, induction should be done with short-acting intravenous anesthetics. A combined intravenous and inhalation anesthetic induction will allow for enough indirect muscle relaxation to avoid the use of muscle relaxants to facilitate intubation. Maintenance of anesthesia with a slightly higher level of volatile agent or total intravenous anesthetic will often provide adequate muscle relaxation. Should additional muscle relaxation be needed, the initial dose of nondepolarizing muscle relaxant should be decreased and the responses followed closely by the use of a nerve stimulator. Reversal of a nondepolarizing muscle relaxant block with cholinesterase inhibitors should be done cautiously since the relative increase in acetylcholine may lead to a desensitization of the nicotinic receptor and produce a depolarizing block similar to that seen with succinylcholine. This is known as a cholinergic crisis. It may be prudent to allow a nondepolarizing block to resolve spontaneously to avoid this issue.

Aminoglycoside antibiotics, such as gentamycin, kanamycin, streptomycin, and neomycin, should be avoided in patients with myasthenia gravis. These drugs inhibit calcium entry into the nerve terminal and reduce acetylcholine release, exacerbating the patient's muscle weakness.

Muscular dystrophy

Muscular dystrophy is an X-linked recessive genetic disease that results in progressive skeletal muscular weakness and degeneration. The most significant type is known as pseudohypertrophic, or Duchenne muscular dystrophy. It occurs in 1 in 3500 males, starting at a young age and becoming progressively debilitating with age (Hayes et al., 2008). The cardiac muscle also progressively degenerates, which leads to decreased myocardial contractility and congestive failure. Defects of the cardiac conduction system are also possible. Weakness of the respiratory muscles causes a loss of pulmonary reserve; the ability to clear secretions and the cough reflex are diminished, and functional residual capacity is reduced. Pulmonary infections may become commonplace. Kyphoscoliosis results from weakness of postural muscles and the resultant restricted lung expansion further decreases pulmonary function residual capacity. Plasma creatine kinase levels are elevated significantly in Duchenne muscular dystrophy as a reflection of muscle destruction and membrane instability. Most patients succumb to respiratory failure, pneumonia, and/or congestive heart failure. Becker muscular dystrophy progresses slower than does Duchenne; however, cardiac involvement is still possible (Hermans et al., 2010; Hsu, 2010).

Anesthetic considerations

Patients with Duchenne muscular dystrophy are primarily at risk when general anesthesia is administered. There is a propensity for the development of malignant hyperthermia when triggering agents such as succinylcholine and potent inhalational agents are used (Hayes et al., 2008). When general anesthesia is required, total intravenous anesthesia is the technique of choice. Succinylcholine should be avoided, not only because of its potential for malignant hyperthermia but also because it may trigger potassium release from permeable skeletal muscle membranes. The resultant hyperkalemia can produce difficult to manage cardiac dysrhythmias and/or cardiac arrest. Volatile inhalational anesthetics have also been implicated in the production of rhabdomyolysis, which may resemble acute malignant hyperthermia. Patients may have increased sensitivity to nondepolarizing muscle relaxants, and they should be used judiciously and in decreased dosages. Patients must be monitored well into the postoperative period for the development of respiratory insufficiency following reversal of non-depolarizing muscle relaxants, even when recovery is deemed adequate. Close attention must be paid to the patient's NPO status since gastric emptying is delayed. These patients must be considered to be aspiration risks regardless of anesthesia type.

Multiple sclerosis

Multiple sclerosis is an acquired autoimmune disease of young adults that is characterized by the demyelination of corticospinal tract neurons in the brain and spinal column (Compston and Coles, 2008). It does not affect the peripheral nervous system. The etiology is unknown, but has been associated with genetic and viral factors. More women are affected than men. Patients may manifest with visual disturbances, gait disturbances, limb weakness, urinary incontinence, and sexual dysfunction. Disconjugate gaze, nystagmus, skeletal muscle spasticity, and a positive Lhermitte's sign (electric shock sensation down the back and into the legs upon neck flexion) may also be present. Typically, patients experience symptoms of demyelination followed by periods of remission. Residual symptoms may persist during remission. Diagnosis is based upon clinical presentation, but immersion in hot water may invoke symptoms by blocking conduction in demyelinated nerves. Corticosteroids may be used to manage acute symptoms, but there is no cure. Emotional stress, fatigue, and temperature changes may exacerbate or induce symptoms. Patients with multiple sclerosis may also be at risk for the development of seizure disorders.

Anesthetic considerations

The stress of anesthesia and surgery may exacerbate or provoke symptoms of multiple sclerosis. The choice of drugs or technique will not influence the overall outcome as much as the stress of the procedure or the increases in body temperature. If general anesthesia is used, hyperkalemia may occur after succinylcholine administration similar to that seen with muscular dystrophy, and resistance to nondepolarizing muscle relaxants may result. Care must be taken to prevent elevations in body temperature during treatment to prevent acute symptoms of demyelination. The ability to cough, exhale deeply, or clear secretion can contribute to airway risk in these patients. Hemodynamic instability may result from autonomic dysregulation.

Cerebral palsy

Cerebral palsy is a group of non-progressive neuromuscular disorders caused by brain damage sustained during the prenatal or perinatal period, or during infancy, affecting 2 in 1000 patients (Odding et al., 2006). The classifications of cerebral palsy is listed in Table 9.2. Spastic and dyskinetic palsies are the most common,

Table 9.2 Major types of cerebral palsy.

Spastic	Most common manifestation
Dyskinetic	Twitching, jerking, uncontrolled limb, head, and eye movement
Ataxic	Tremors, poor sense of balance
Mixed	Combination of above

characterized by uncontrollable muscle spasticity, including uncoordinated limb, head, and eye movements. Intellect can be normal, but many patients with cerebral palsy present with mental retardation and seizure disorders. Gastroesophageal reflux is common in cerebral palsy, and patients are at risk for aspiration and pulmonary infections.

Anesthetic considerations

Although patients with cerebral palsy have skeletal muscular degeneration, it is not a motor neuron disease. As such, patients do not exhibit a hyperkalemic response to succinylcholine administration. If desired, succinylcholine may be used safely for endotracheal intubation in these patients. Obtaining vascular access is a major challenge in patients with cerebral palsy due to uncontrolled spasticity, rigidity, or joint contractures. Induction of anesthesia may require inhalation of nitrous oxide or volatile anesthetic gases, and/or intramuscular ketamine. Owing to the significant aspiration risk, endotracheal intubation should be considered in cases where significant bleeding or water spray is anticipated. Drugs such as phenytoin or carbamazapine for seizure control may induce liver enzymes producing unwanted metabolic drug interactions. In patients taking clonazepam for control of seizures, reversal of benzodiazepines with flumazenil may precipitate frank seizure activity. Generally speaking, patients with cerebral palsy tolerate sedation and general anesthesia well, but recovery is sometimes prolonged due to a propensity to develop intraoperative hypothermia.

Seizure disorders

Seizures are caused by the paroxysmal, abnormal synchronous firing of cerebral cortical neurons resulting in transient cognitive impairment, loss of consciousness, and/or tonic–clonic muscle contractions. Epilepsy is characterized by recurrent seizures and may be idiopathic (75%), genetic, or the result of brain injury or metabolic causes. During normal brain function, neurons are activated and inhibited in a non-synchronous manner to allow the propagation of signals throughout the brain. When the activity becomes synchronized in a focal area, seizures occur. The type of seizure depends upon the degree of signal propagation and spread throughout the brain. Seizures remain focal if the activity is confined to a prescribed area, or may be generalized if the activity spreads to other parts of the brain such as the thalamus or brainstem. The majority of new onset seizures occur in children, most are idiopathic, but some are due to trauma. When new onset seizures occur in adults, causes such as brain injury due to trauma, stroke, brain lesions, or metabolic causes should be investigated.

Seizures are classified as either partial (focal) or generalized (Table 9.3). Partial seizures are usually caused by focal brain damage or disease, so underlying causes should be examined. They may be simple seizures characterized by motor, sensory, or psychic symptoms. They may be complex in nature, accompanied by an aura, impaired consciousness, involuntary movement, and confusion. Generalized seizures are categorized as either absence or tonic–clonic in nature. Patients with absence seizures encounter brief alterations in consciousness without loss of posture. The episodes are short-lived and consciousness is not impaired afterward. Tonic–clonic seizures are the characteristic seizure with sudden loss of consciousness, and tonic and clonic muscle contractions, shaking and twitching. These seizures are usually self-limiting, lasting from 1 to 2 minutes, followed by several minutes of unconsciousness and a prolonged period of depressed consciousness. Patients actively seizing should be managed with airway support and with an attempt to prevent self-injury. Status epilepticus, or sustained tonic–clonic seizure activity, should be managed with airway support, oxygen, and parenteral midazolam.

Treatment of seizure disorders is geared toward the use of drugs that inhibit ion transmission through sodium and potassium channels, or drugs that increase GABA, a major inhibitory neurotransmitter. Useful anticonvulsants are listed in Table 9.4.

Table 9.3 Seizure classification.

Partial seizures
Simple (Jacksonian)
Complex (Psychomotor and temporal lobe)
Generalized seizures
Tonic–clonic (Grand mal)
Absence seizures (Petit mal)
Myoclonic seizures
Atonic seizures

Table 9.4 Useful anticonvulsants.

Barbiturates	Phenobarbital
Hydantoins	Phenytoin
Carboxylic acids	valproic acid
Iminostilbenes	Carbamazepine
Succinimides	Ethosuximide
Benzodiazepines	Diazepam and Midazolam

Anesthetic considerations

Patients with a seizure disorder history should be evaluated to determine the type of seizure, the frequency of occurrence, and precipitating factors. Patients should be followed up regularly by their physician to ensure adequate degree of control with therapeutic blood levels of anticonvulsant drugs. Anticonvulsants such as phenytoin, carbamazepine, and phenobarbital induce the liver enzyme, CYP 3A4, which is involved in the metabolism of many drugs, especially benzodiazepines. When using benzodiazepines such as diazepam and midazolam during anesthesia, the practitioner should be aware of a potential drug interaction in which the metabolism of the administered benzodiazepine would be accelerated, resulting in an incomplete, inadequate, or lessened effect.

An old-line drug, methohexital, once the mainstay of dental sedation, is seeing a clinical resurgence due to sporadic propofol shortages. This oxybarbiturate has been shown to activate excitable foci and induce seizure activity in patients with epilepsy (Loddenkemper et al., 2007). Its use is therefore relatively contraindicated in patients with seizure disorders. Ketamine activates both excitatory and inhibitory centers in the brain and produces some tonic–clonic muscle activity. However, ketamine may be used safely in patients with seizure disorders (Corssen et al., 1974). Obviously, benzodiazepines are useful for sedation and anesthesia due to their strong anticonvulsant properties. Opioids, propofol, muscle relaxants, and potent inhalational anesthetics may also be used safely in these patients.

Consideration must be given to patients taking clonazepam for control of their seizure disorder. Clonazepam is a benzodiazepine, and as such is reversed by flumazenil. Flumazenil reversal of a benzodiazepine overdose during anesthesia could therefore potentially trigger a seizure in these patients.

Developmentally impaired disorders

Down syndrome

Down syndrome is the result of a deviation from the normal chromosome complement in which there is an extra copy of chromosome 21. Also known as trisomy 21, Down syndrome occurs in 1:800 births (Abanto et al., 2011). The incidence increases with advancing maternal age and accounts for approximately one-third of cases of intellectual disability. Approximately 50% of patients have congenital heart defects, the most common being atrioventricular septal defects, followed by atrial-septal defects, patent ductus arteriosis, ventricular septal defects, and tetralogy of Fallot (Abanto et al., 2011). Patients with Down syndrome also have increased incidences of obesity, respiratory infections, seizures, hematological and immunological problems, hypothyroidism, gastroesophageal reflux disease (GERD), musculoskeletal problems, obstructive sleep apnea, diabetes, and Alzheimer's disease (Abanto et al., 2011).

Anesthetic considerations

The provision of anesthesia and sedation to patients with Down syndrome is complicated by the various anatomic and physiologic deficiencies that may be present. Airway maintenance and security is a major issue due to anatomical changes related to the syndrome. Patients are frequently obese, with a short, thick neck, and a large protruding tongue. Mallampati Class IV airways are common. There is a midface deficiency with a high, vaulted and constricted palate. Malocclusions are common as well as skeletal class II profiles. Hypotonia and ligament laxity make these patients prone to airway obstruction as they relax during sedation. Nasal passages are narrow and patients often require the insertion of airway adjuncts such as a nasopharyngeal airway during treatment. Excessive hyperextension or flexion of the neck should be avoided in patients with Down syndrome due to an increased propensity for atlantoaxial subluxation of the cervical spine. These maneuvers could result in severe spinal cord injury resulting in paralysis or death. Atlantoaxial instability should be suspected if patients have a history of declining physical activity and the onset of a sedentary lifestyle. Cervical spine films should be reviewed if any question exists as to the presence of instability. Cervical collars should be considered for neck support, and to prevent hyperextension or flexion in these patients. In severe cases, the airway should be secured with the aid of video or fiberoptic laryngoscopy.

A cardiologist should evaluate patients with unrepaired congenital heart defects and testing should include a 12-lead electrocardiogram, echocardiography, and evaluation of the patient's exercise capacity. Consideration should be given for the provision of care in a hospital setting. Medical consultation should also be considered for patients with repaired cardiac defects. Sedation is advisable in these patients to reduce stress on the cardiovascular system. Antibiotic prophylaxis is recommended for patients who meet the American Heart Association Guidelines for prophylactic coverage.

When Down syndrome patients present with severe behavioral problems secondary to mental retardation or dementia, deep levels of sedation may be preferable to control aberrant behavior. This presents a challenge in regard to airway maintenance as described above. Obstructive sleep apnea is a growing problem in these patients and presents a particular management challenge. Owing to the ease of airway obstruction in these patients, moderate levels of sedation are usually advisable. However, this may not be practical if the behavior is unmanageable. In this case, general anesthesia with the security of endotracheal intubation is advisable.

GERD provides another challenge for anesthetic management. Since patients or their caregivers may not always be aware of this condition, the teeth should be examined for the presence of excessive wear or erosive loss of enamel. The existence of GERD makes patients susceptible to perioperative passive regurgitation or active vomiting. Aspiration of gastric contents thus becomes a risk, so care must be taken to ensure the patient's NPO status. The presence of GERD along with airway hypotonia makes Down syndrome patients prone to aspiration of oral secretions as well. Fine aerosolized spray, as found in dental handpieces or ultrasonic scalers, may be inhaled by the patient during sedation and may produce a postoperative respiratory infection that could become severe.

If patients have particularly difficult management issues, the practitioner should be prepared with several options for induction of anesthesia. Oral premedication with midazolam may be particularly effective and should be considered if the patient is compliant. Intramuscular induction with ketamine may be necessary if the patient is not cooperative for venipuncture. Inhalation induction with potential volatile agents may be a last resort if all else fails. The practitioner should be aware, however, that patients with Down syndrome are prone to the development of profound bradycardia during inhalation induction.

Autism

Autism is a pervasive developmental disorder, a clinical diagnosis of what we see, and not a biological diagnosis. Patients begin to develop normally, but regress at 18–24 months of age. The clinical presentation is similar among different cultures and ethnic groups, 80% have some form of mental impairment, sleep disorders are common, and 40% develop seizure disorders. The core deficits of autism include problems with communication, social interaction, and behavior. Communication problems include the inability to express oneself clearly, altered or non-existent speech patterns, developmental delay, and/or mental retardation. Social interaction issues include difficulty understanding social situations, trouble regulating emotions, and the inability to relate to people and events. Behavioral problems are characterized by difficulties in sensory processing, an altered response to stimuli, a high need for predictability, repetitive behaviors, and self-abuse. Patients with autism have much concomitant comorbidity such as anxiety, attention-deficit hyperactivity disorder, Tourette syndrome, obsessive–compulsive disorder, depression, bipolar disorder, and epilepsy (Levy et al., 2010).

Treatment strategies in autism include extensive patient preparation, the use of visual aids, social stories, and reinforcement. Patient preparation means giving the patient structure. Each appointment must appear to be the same to the patient. The same treatment team must be involved each time, and the same treatment room must be utilized. Appointments must be short, frequent, and punctual. The appointment atmosphere must be calm, there should be no small talk, and the operatory should be visually unimpressive, i.e., plain, free from clutter or extraneous objects and equipment.

The practitioner should speak with the parents or caregivers without the patient being present to determine things such as how the patient usually communicates. Is he or she accustomed to visual communication using pictures, words, or symbols? How does the patient respond to touch, are rewards used, and what works and what does not? Many patients with autism are visual learners. To take advantage of this, one should use picture support in the development of a scrapbook or social story that can be individualized for the patient. Each phase of the appointment, from the outside of the building to the treatment area can be documented in pictures and words for the patient to review over and over again in the weeks leading up to the appointment. When the patient encounters the situations presented in the social story, he or she will be more likely to comply with treatment.

Anesthetic considerations

Despite the potential for non-pharmacological treatment interventions, 77% of children with autism were frightened and uncooperative at their initial visit to the dentist, and 50–65% of patients with autism were uncooperative during dental appointments (Loo et al., 2008). Owing to a myriad of behavioral problems in patients with autism, they recommended that long and involved treatment be performed under general anesthesia. As in other patients with profound mental or behavioral disabilities, multiple anesthetic induction plans must be readily available. Oral premedication is helpful if the patients will comply with administration of the drug. Benzodiazepines such as lorazepam, triazolam, and midazolam are particularly useful. If the patients are not compliant with venipuncture, intramuscular ketamine should be considered. Maintenance of anesthesia should be with deep levels of sedation or general anesthesia in order to adequately control aberrant behaviors. Airway adjuncts are often necessary. The use of intravenous dexmedetomidine to prevent emergence delirium is extremely beneficial when a stormy recovery is anticipated.

Alzheimer's disease

Alzheimer's disease accounts for more than 50% of cases of dementia (Blennow et al., 2006). It is characterized by a progressive decline in intellectual function resulting in a loss of social independence. Patients with Alzheimer's disease have amyloid plaques forming in the cerebral cortex and blood vessels. This results in an initial impairment of learning and recent memory loss. Other functions such as spatial orientation, judgment, and decision-making may also be affected, leading to the eventual inability to provide self-care. Patients may develop hallucinations or become paranoid or delusional. Typically, Alzheimer's disease begins insidiously after the age of 65 and the course of the disease plays out over a 5–10 year period. Thus, patients with Alzheimer's disease are often medically complex. Patients may have concomitant cardiovascular or cerebrovascular disease, kidney disease, and chronic obstructive pulmonary disease, and be prone to aspiration and respiratory infections. Their behavior is frequently defiant and combative, making routine dental care a difficult challenge. They may require sedation in order to complete an examination and formulate a treatment plan. This is, however, not without risk due to underlying medical conditions and debilitation.

Anesthetic considerations

The anesthetic challenges of Alzheimer's disease have to do with behavioral and complex medical issues. Patients with severe behavioral problems may not comply with venipuncture, but premedication either orally or intramuscularly may not be feasible due to the patient's debilitated condition. Gentle restraint, with caregivers being present may be preferable to safely induce sedation or anesthesia. Protective stabilization, if used, should be carefully reviewed with the caregiver prior to treatment, and appropriate consent must be obtained. Moderate levels of sedation are the preferred anesthetic option to ensure behavior control while maintaining a patent airway and minimizing stress to the patient's cardiovascular system. If underlying medical conditions significantly compromise treatment, consideration should be given to hospitalization for proposed treatment. Medical consultation is necessary to accurately ascertain pertinent details of the patient's medical condition. Dexmedetomidine should be considered for maintenance of sedation in these patients since it does not produce respiratory depression and has a stabilizing effect on the cardiovascular system (Ramsay and Luterman, 2004).

References

Abanto, J., et al. Medical problems and oral care of patients with Down syndrome: a literature review. *Spec Care Dentis* **31**, 197–203, 2011.

Blennow, K., et al. Alzheimer's disease. *Lancet* **368**: 387–403, 2006.

Compston, A. and Coles, A. Multiple sclerosis. *Lancet* **372**, 1502–1517, 2008.

Corssen, G., et al. Ketamine and epilepsy. *Anesth Analg* **53**: 319–333, 1974.

Hardiman, O., et al. Clinical diagnosis and management of amyotrophic lateral sclerosis. *Nat Rev Neurol* **7**, 639–649, 2011.

Hayes, J., et al. Duchenne muscular dystrophy: an old anesthesia problem revisited. *Pediatr Anesth* **18**: 100–106, 2008.

Hermans, M. C. E., et al. Hereditary muscular dystrophies and the heart. *Neuromuscul Disord* **20**: 479–492, 2010.

Hsu, D. T. Cardiac manifestations of neuromuscular disorders in children. *Paediatr Respir Rev* **11**: 35–38, 2010.

Itoh, H., et al. Sensitivity to vecuronium in seropositive and seronegative patients with myasthenia gravis. *Anesth Analg* **95**(1): 109–113, 2002.

Levy, S. E., et al. Autism spectrum disorder and co-occurring developmental, psychiatric, and medical conditions among children in multiple populations of the United States. *J Dev Behav Ped* **31**(4): 267–265, 2010.

Loddenkemper, T., et al. Seizures during intracarotid methohexital and amobarbital testing. *Epilepsy Behav* **10**(1), 49–54, 2007.

Loo, C.Y., et al. The caries experience and behavior of dental patients with autism spectrum disorder. *JADA* **139**, 1518–1524, 2008.

Meriggioli, M. N. and Sanders, D. B. Autoimmune myasthenia gravis: emerging clinical and biological heterogeneity. *Lancet Neurol* **8**: 475–490, 2009.

Monani, U. R. Spinal muscular atrophy: a deficiency in a ubiquitous protein; a motor neuron-specific disease. *Neuron* **48**: 885–96, 2005.

Navailles, S. and De Deurwaerdère, P. Imbalanced dopaminergic transmission mediated by serotonergic neurons in L-DOPA-induced dyskinesia. *Parkinson's Dis* 2012, 323686, **2012**.

Odding, E., et al. The epidemiology of cerebral palsy: incidence, impairments and risk factors. *Disabil Rehabil* **28**: 183–191, 2006.

Ramsay, M. A. E. and Luterman, D. L. Dexmedetomidine as a total intravenous anesthetic agent. *Anesthesiology* **101**(3): 787–790, 2004.

10 Anesthetic considerations for patients with hepatic disease

Jeffrey Miller[1] **and Stuart Lieblich**[2]

[1] University of Connecticut Health Center, Department of Oral and Maxillofacial Surgery, Farmington, CT, USA

[2] University of Connecticut, Department of Oral and Maxillofacial Surgery, Farmington, CT, USA

Introduction

The liver is the largest organ in the body. It receives dual blood supply from both the hepatic artery (25%) and the portal vein (75%), with each vessel contributing 50% of the oxygen supply because of the respective differences in oxygen content of the blood carried in each vessel. Significant hypotension reduces the portal venous flow, which is compensated by an increase in hepatic artery flow in the normal liver to maintain perfusion and avoid hypoxic injury (Muilenburg et al., 2009). The liver processes dietary nutrients, making it the major metabolic and detoxification center in the body. It plays a significant role both in the synthesis, storage, and release of glucose and glycogen and in the metabolism of protein and fat. As the liver also metabolizes drugs and produces enzymes and proteins, it significantly affects both hemostasis (the liver is involved with the synthesis of all clotting factors, with the exception of Factor VIII) and the pharmacokinetic behavior of anesthetic drugs. Bile is produced in the liver with bilirubin (a breakdown product of red blood cells). Unconjugated (indirect) bilirubin is conjugated (direct) in the liver to make it water soluble, which is then excreted in the bile to emulsify fats in the gastrointestinal tract to facilitate absorption. Disruption of this process elevates bilirubin leading to jaundice, where the sclerae and skin turn yellow (icterus) (see Figure 10.1). Normal total bilirubin concentration is <1 mg/dL. Jaundice appears at levels >3 mg/dL. It is important to note that an elevation in bilirubin can also occur with increased production, as seen in hemolytic diseases.

Identification and classification of liver disease

Liver injury can occur from a variety of acute or chronic pathologic insults. Acute liver failure (ALF) refers to the rapid development of severe acute liver injury with impaired synthetic function and encephalopathy in a patient who had a previously normal liver or well-compensated liver disease. ALF can result from a wide variety of causes, most commonly due to viral infection or exposure to toxins, especially high doses of acetaminophen (Ostapowicz et al., 2002). Common causes of chronic liver disease are alcohol abuse, viral infection (especially hepatitis C), and non-alcoholic fatty liver disease (NAFLD). Other parenchymal diseases include hemochromatosis (abnormal iron elevation), alpha-1-antitrypsin deficiency, and neoplasms, among others. All of these diseases can lead to elevations in liver enzymes, jaundice, and eventually cirrhosis in severe or prolonged cases.

The responses to hepatic injury include inflammation (hepatitis), cellular necrosis, regeneration, and/or fibrosis. Liver failure can lead to jaundice (inability to conjugate and secrete bilirubin), fasting hypoglycemia (decreased gluconeogenesis), coagulopathy, muscle wasting, and decreased plasma protein production, which can enhance and prolong anesthetic drug action. Cirrhosis is a result of chronic, repeated injury causing progressive parenchymal damage with resultant nodular regeneration and fibrous band formation. Normal hepatic architecture is disrupted, leading to progressive occlusion of the portal vein, resulting in portal hypertension, ascites (fluid accumulation in the abdomen), and shunting of the portal and arterial blood away from the liver. Hepatocyte function is impaired as a result of hepatic blood flow (Schuppan and Afdhal, 2008). Drugs, toxins, and nitrogenous waste accumulate due to decreased metabolism. A hyperdynamic circulation results from splanchnic engorgement, where heart rate and cardiac output increase, yet blood pressure and systemic vascular resistance decrease—a condition called *functional hypovolemia*. Autonomic compensation eventually fatigues, leaving these patients intolerant to dehydration or hemorrhage. Proximal vessels dilate often, resulting in variceal hemorrhage (GI bleeding). In most patients, 80 to 90% of liver parenchyma must be destroyed before liver failure becomes clinically manifest (Heidelbaugh and Bruderly, 2006).

Liver function can be measured by a variety of laboratory tests, most of which are nonspecific for liver disease. Early Hepatocellular injury is accompanied by spillage of hepatic enzymes, which is reflected by increased plasma levels of two transaminases: AST (aspartate aminotransferase) and ALT (alanine aminotransferase). Alkaline phosphatase can be elevated with hepatic injury, as well as in biliary disease, instances of high bone turnover, and pregnancy. Liver function (ability to synthesize proteins) is assessed by albumin levels and prothrombin time (INR). The liver continually synthesizes albumin, whose half-life is on the order of weeks. Hypoalbuminemia is not specific for liver disease, as low levels are seen with both decreased production and increased loss. Acidic and neutral parenteral anesthetic drugs bind to albumin in

Anesthesia Complications in the Dental Office, First Edition. Edited by Robert C. Bosack and Stuart Lieblich.

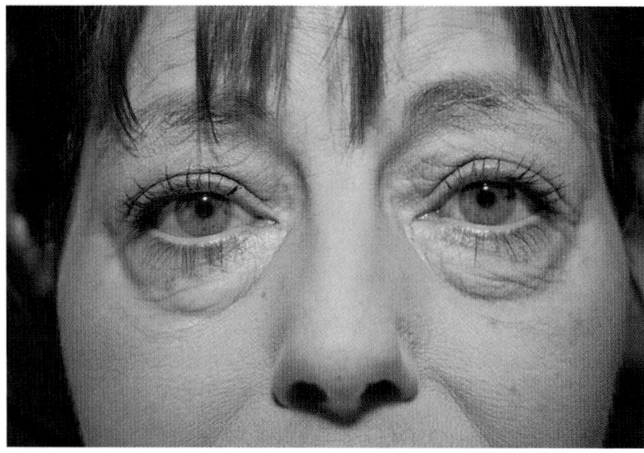

Figure 10.1 Scleral icterus. Note obvious yellowish hue of the sclera and periorbital soft tissue, visible in spite of heavy make-up and vigorous denial of liver problems.

varying degrees; the less bound the drug is, the more efficiently it traverses cell membranes and attaches to receptors. Proteins, such as albumin, also serve as an additional reservoir for drugs, which can extend the duration of action. The prothrombin time is dependent on levels of I (fibrinogen), II (prothrombin), V, VII, and IX. As these factors are all synthesized in the liver, patients with diminished liver function can present with a clotting deficiency. Of note, however, is that significant liver disease must be present before altered hemostasis or INR is seen as most clotting factors require only 25% of their normal levels for adequate clot formation. However, due to the short half-life of multiple factors, altered coagulation time (vis-à-vis clinical bleeding) is likely to be seen in patients with acute liver dysfunction. Synthesis of factors II, VII, IX, and X is vitamin K dependent, a process that is antagonized by warfarin, leading to elevation of the INR. As malnutrition often accompanies severe liver disease, vitamin K intake is often deficient. Bleeding risk is further exacerbated by thrombocytopenia, due to platelet sequestration from portal hypertension and splenomegaly.

Risk assessment

Patients with liver disease are at a greater risk for anesthetic complications when compared to patients with normal liver function. Chronic liver disease and cirrhosis may not be clinically obvious, as most affected patients remain asymptomatic until decompensation occurs. While some patients may present with an established diagnosis of liver disease, it is still important to perform a thorough history and physical evaluation, as appropriate in the dental office, to help identify patients with undiagnosed disease. A history of illicit drug use, excessive alcohol consumption, acetaminophen overdose, or prior blood transfusions should raise suspicion of hepatic disease. For diagnosed patients, consultation with the patient's gastroenterologist can be helpful to determine the extent of the disease and comorbid conditions, such as malnutrition, coagulopathy, renal or cardiovascular dysfunction, and fluid and electrolyte imbalance.

The Child-Turcotte-Pugh score serves as a tool for risk stratification of patients with liver disease undergoing surgery (Table 10.1). A Child's Class A (low risk) is 5–6 points, while the Child's Class C risk is >10 (high risk). Class B (7–9) represents an intermediate risk. The utility of this score in the office setting has not been established.

Table 10.1 The Child–Turcotte–Pugh risk stratification for patients with liver disease.

Points	1	2	3
Ascites	Absent	Present	Severe
Bilirubin (mg/dL)	<2.0	2–3	>3
Albumin (g/dL)	>3.5	2.8–3.5	<2.8
INR	<1.7	1.7–2.3	>2.3
Encephalopathy	None	Moderate	Severe

Anesthetic concerns

Acute intoxication or acute liver disease prompts postponement of all but the most emergent cases, which are seldom encountered in the dental office setting. Intravenous fluids should be administered cautiously in these cases to avoid further fluid overload. Chronic liver disease invites concerns regarding fluid and electrolyte disturbances (especially hypokalemia), with sodium and water retention resulting in ascites and peripheral edema. Ascites causes increased upward pressure on the diaphragm, especially with supine or semi-Fowler's positioning, decreasing lung volumes and promoting hypoxemia and atelectasis, more pronounced with deeper levels of sedation. Ascites can also lead to increased gastric volume and delayed emptying. Significant ascites, similar to pregnancy, can interfere with venous return, leading to hypotension during supine posturing. Fasting hypoglycemia due to diminished gluconeogenesis is also a possibility in patients with liver disease. As mentioned previously, coagulopathy secondary to decreased clotting factors, vitamin K deficiency, and thrombocytopenia is also a concern.

The hyperdynamic circulation accompanying portal hypertension leads to a higher risk of hypotension, often accompanied by a decreased response to exogenous or endogenous vasoconstrictors. The liver serves as a reservoir of blood, which (in healthy patients) can transfer up to 1 liter of whole blood to the systemic circulation within 30 seconds of sympathoadrenal activation. This reservoir is compromised in patients with liver disease (Mushlin and Gelman, 2010); therefore, even mild decrease in intravascular volume can result in hypotension, such as can occur with prolonged NPO periods, or on days with high ambient temperatures, accelerating insensible water loss. Cirrhotic patients often demonstrate a decreased therapeutic effect of β-adrengeric antagonists, possibly due to a decrease in the density of β-adrenergic receptors.

Pharmacokinetic behavior of most parenteral anesthetic agents is altered in patients with liver disease. Decreased plasma proteins and albumin (malnutrition and decreased synthesis) increase the free (unbound) fraction of administered drugs, amplifying their effect. The increased volume of distribution tends to delayed onset and prolonged duration. Decreased CYP450 enzymes delay metabolism and clearance. As such, a low and slow protocol is advisable when administering parenteral agents. Redosing of drugs such as diazepam or midazolam can lead to unpredictable action. Metabolism of oxazepam or lorazepam is not affected as they undergo extrahepatic metabolism (Verbeeck, 2008). The pharmacodynamics of fentanyl and remifentanil is thought to be unaltered by liver diseases (Muilenburg et al., 2009). Propofol may be helpful in these patients, due to rapid onset and short duration of action. After a single IV bolus dose, cirrhotic patients do not have significantly different total body elimination and elimination half-life compared to those with normal liver function (Servin et al., 1988).

A 50% dose reduction should be entertained when administering drugs orally. Most oral sedatives have a high hepatic extraction ratio (first pass metabolism) which is bypassed in the liver patient because of shunting of portal blood to the central circulation. As a result, these drugs display a faster onset, increased profundity, and increased duration of action. Meperidine, morphine, and midazolam are known to have a two-fold increase in bioavailability after oral administration in cirrhotic patients.

Amide local anesthetics are metabolized by enzymatic degradation in the liver. As such, only 2 – 3% is excreted unmodified by the kidneys (Orlando et al., 2004). Both lidocaine and bupivacaine have a high extraction ratio and are therefore sensitive to alterations in liver function. With advanced liver disease leading to prolonged clearance and elevated blood levels, a dose reduction of 50% should be entertained.

Pseudocholinesterase concentration is decreased in patients with liver disease, which may prolong the action of succinylcholine, a depolarizing muscle relaxant often used to break laryngospasms during deeper levels of sedation.

Summary

Patients with liver disease who require surgical interventions are at a greater risk for surgical and anesthetic complications compared to those with a healthy liver. To determine a patient's ability to safety tolerate a procedure, one should start by determining the patient's CTP class. Baseline liver enzymes should be obtained prior to the procedure, and in general these values should be stable prior to proceeding. Fluid status should be closely monitored to assure adequate hydration or diuresis as needed. Optimization of electrolytes and nutrition is important prior to proceeding with any surgical intervention. Bleeding risk needs to be ascertained, with correction of coagulopathy, thrombocytopenia and anemia as needed. Patients with current alcohol use will require adjustments in their pre-operative and anesthetic management. Anesthetic medication management will need to be modified in patients with liver failure, avoiding hepatotoxic agents, choosing agents that are least effected by liver dysfunction and adjusting dosage as needed based on the degree of liver failure.

References

Heidelbaugh, J. L. and Bruderly, M. Cirrhosis and chronic lever failure: Part I. Diagnosis and evaluation. *Am Fam Physician* **74**: 756 – 762, 2006.

Muilenburg, D. J., et al. Surgery in the patient with liver disease. *Med Clin N Am* **93**: 1065 – 1081, 2009.

Mushlin, P. S. and Gelman S. Hepatic physiology and pathophysiology. In: Miller, R. D. *Miller's Anesthesia*, 7th edn. Philadelphia: Elsevier, 2010.

Orlando, R. et al. Cytochrome P450 1A2 is a major determinant of lidocaine metabolism in vivo: effects of liver function. *Clin Pharmaco Ther* **75**: 80 – 88, 2004.

Ostapowicz, G., et al. Results of a prospective study of acute liver failure at 17 tertiary care centers in the United States. *Ann Intern Med* **137**: 947 – 954, 2002.

Schuppan, D. and Afdhal, N. H. Liver cirrhosis. *Lancet* **37**: 838 – 851, 2008.

Servin, F., et al. Pharmcokinetics and protein binding of propofol in patients with cirrhosis. *Anesthesiol* **69**: 887 – 891, 1988.

Verbeeck, R. K. Pharmacokinetics and dosing adjustment in patients with hepatic dysfunction. *Eur J Clin Pharmacol* **64**: 1147 – 1161, 2008.

11 Anesthetic considerations for patients with renal disease

Marci H. Levine[1] and Andrea Schreiber[2]

[1]New York University College of Dentistry, Department of Oral and Maxillofacial Surgery, New York, NY, USA

[2]New York University College of Dentistry, Department of Oral and Maxillofacial Surgery, New York, NY, USA

Introduction

The kidneys regulate fluid, electrolyte, and acid–base balance; eliminate metabolic wastes; excrete both water-soluble and metabolized drugs; modulate blood volume and vascular tone; and regulate hematopoiesis and bone metabolism. It is easy to appreciate how renal disease can have devastating effects on the cardiovascular and hematological systems. Effective management of patients with renal disease will reduce the overall morbidity and mortality associated with the delivery of anesthesia.

The anatomy of the nephron, one of 1 million such functional units contained in the normal adult kidney, is depicted in Figure 11.1. The efferent arteriole feeds the tuft of capillaries (glomerulus) surrounded by Bowman's capsule, which subsequently drains to an efferent arteriole. Changes in the tone of these two vessels determines the glomerular filtration rate (GFR) (normally 125 ml/min or 180 L/day in the adult) and the formation of the filtrate. A majority of the filtrate including glucose, amino acids, and Na^+ (water passively follows Na^+) is actively transported back into the plasma.

Similarly to the heart and the brain, the kidney is adept at autoregulation – the intrinsic ability to maintain steady and adequate perfusion over a wide range of blood pressures – typically between a mean arterial pressure (MAP) of 50 and 150 mmHg. This process is regulated by the juxtaglomerular apparatus, a group of cells that lies close to the afferent arteriole, near the distal convoluted tubule. In response to hypotension or sympathetic stimulation, these cells secrete renin, which catalyzes the hydrolysis of angiotensinogen to angiotensin I. Angiotensin I is subsequently cleaved to form angiotensin II (a potent vasoconstrictor) by the angiotensin-converting enzyme (ACE). Angiotensin II also maintains GFR by constricting the efferent arteriole. Aldosterone release is also stimulated, which enhances Na^+ and water resorption in the distal convoluted tubule.

GFR provides the best estimate of kidney function, and is *estimated* from creatinine levels in the blood (Jones and Lee, 2009). Creatinine is the end product of skeletal muscle metabolism and is present in a fairly constant concentration in the plasma. It is freely filtered, not resorbed, and is secreted only in small amounts. When GFR decreases by more than 50%, creatinine production exceeds its limit to be filtered and serum concentration will rise. Since the absolute value of serum creatinine is related to skeletal muscle mass, the trend of this value is more important than the value itself, which typically ranges between 0.5 and 1.2 mg/dL.

Classification of kidney disease

Pathologic destruction of nephrons will eventually overcome the compensatory "adaptive hyperfiltration" of the remaining functional nephrons. Azotemia, which is characterized by abnormally high blood levels of nitrogen-containing compounds such as urea, creatinine, and waste products, will result. Pre-renal azotemia results from hypoperfusion of the kidney, usually secondary to hypovolemia or vascular disease (Carlisle, 1995), and is characterized by a BUN:Cr > 20, as creatinine (in addition to being filtered) is also secreted by the proximal convoluted tubule. Effective volume depletion causes a decrease in renal perfusion and is common in both congestive heart failure and cirrhosis. Renal azotemia is characteristic of acute renal failure, which prevents urea resorption, resulting in a BUN:Cr < 15. The etiology of renal azotemia spans a wide range of pathology, most commonly hypertension, diabetes, exposure to nephrotoxic drugs, infection, lupus, ischemia, and polycystic kidney disease. Post-renal azotemia is usually due to a ureteral blockage (compressive tumor, urinary stones) leading to an increase in back pressure with increased urea resorption, resulting in a BUN:Cr > 15. To summarize, all forms of azotemia are characterized by a decrease in GFR, an increase in blood urea nitrogen (BUN), and an increase in serum creatinine (Cr) concentrations. With further urea accumulation, the signs and symptoms of uremia appear. These include lethargy, anorexia, nausea, vomiting, platelet dysfunction, cramps, reduced body temperature, and insulin resistance, among others.

Chronic kidney disease (CKD) is the progressive, irreversible loss of renal function that persists for more than 3 months due to damage to the glomerular or tubule-interstitial apparatus. CKD is staged per Table 11.1. CKD is most often caused by hypertension and diabetes, but can be due to many other causes including polycystic kidney disease, urinary obstruction, glomerulonephritis, lupus, and amyloidosis (USRDS, 2001). Afflicted patients lose the ability to excrete

Anesthesia Complications in the Dental Office, First Edition. Edited by Robert C. Bosack and Stuart Lieblich.

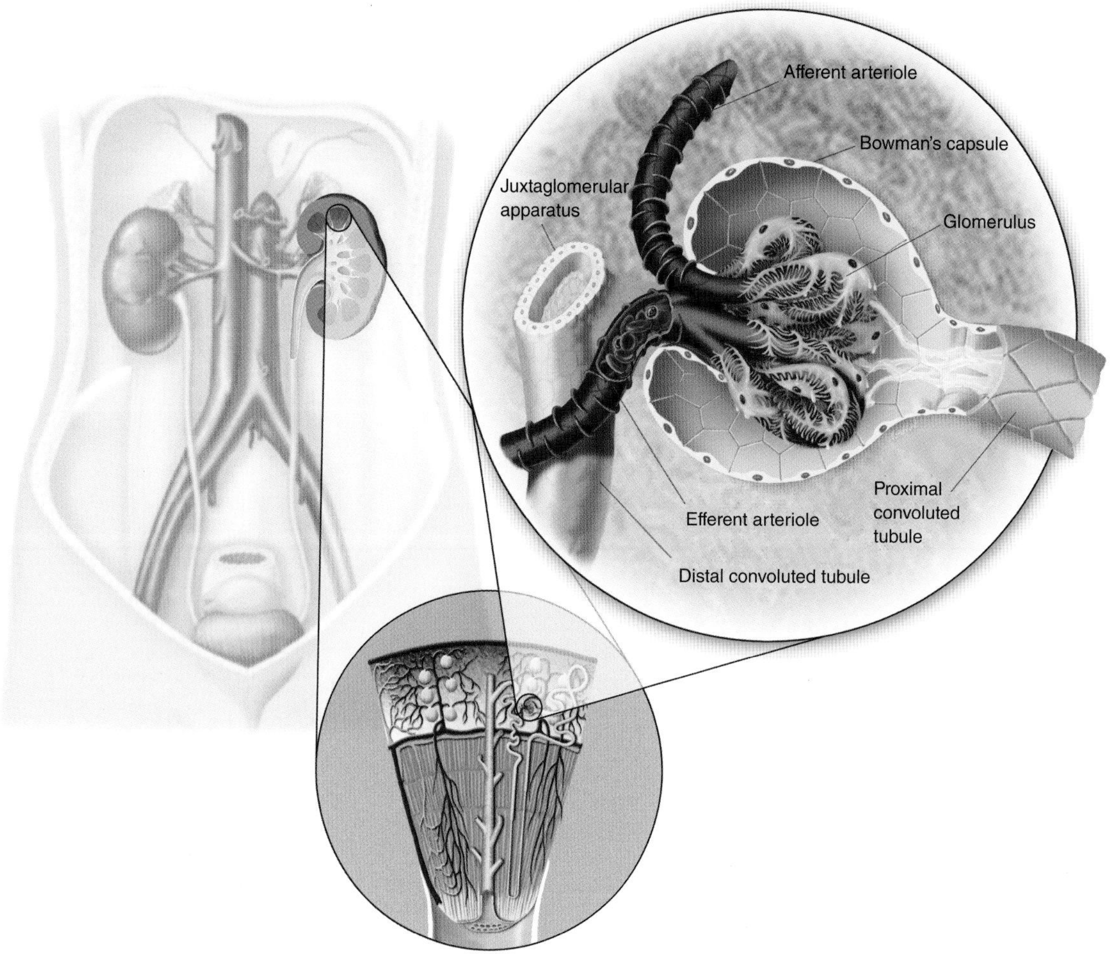

Figure 11.1 Anatomy of the nephron.

Table 11.1 Stages of chronic kidney disease (Jones and Lee, 2009).

Stage	Description	GFR (mL/min/1.73 m²)
1	Kidney damage with normal or ↑ GFR	≥90
2	Kidney damage with mild ↓ in GFR	60–89
3	Moderate ↓ in GFR	30–59
4	Severe ↓ in GFR	15–29
5	Kidney failure	<15 (or dialysis)

nitrogenous waste and become unable to regulate fluid and electrolyte balance.

Comorbidities

The pathophysiologic changes associated with CKD are listed in Table 11.2. Frequent comorbidities include hyperkalemia, fluid overload, angina, hypertension, anemia, and bleeding. Anemia in renal disease is due to decreased synthesis of erythropoietin. Ideal hemoglobin ranges between 11 and 12 g/dL (NKF-K/DOQI, 2000). Therapy is contemplated for patients with advanced stages of CKD and hemoglobin levels less than 8–10 g/dL. Iron and erythropoietin are often the first choice therapies if time permits, prior to transfusions. These present inherent risks including the development of hyperkalemia from cell breakdown and the production of antibodies that can complicate future transplantation efforts. Severe anemia, with preexisting cardiac failure, may worsen myocardial ischemia.

Excessive bleeding can be due to several factors including platelet dysfunction, uremia, or decreased levels of vWF (Wagener and Brentjens, 2010). Patients with prolonged bleeding can be managed by transfusion, exogenous Epogen® administration, DDAVP, or cryoprecipitate. Certain medications including diphenhydramine, NSAIDs, antiplatelet drugs, chlordiazepoxide, and cimetidine can increase the risk of intraoperative bleeding in patients with ESRD and should therefore be avoided (Steiner et al., 1979).

Secondary hypertension can be exacerbated by excessive fluid volumes associated with fluid retention as well as increased sympathoadrenal discharge (Carrasco et al., 2006). The neuroendocrine stress response associated with surgery can further aggravate this pressure elevation.

Metabolic acidosis results from the accumulation of sulfates, phosphates, and uric acid. Altered enzyme activity exacerbates hyperkalemia (upper limits of normal are 5–5.5 mmol/L), secondary to impaired renal excretion of potassium. The ECG findings of hyperkalemia are best seen in precordial leads and can include bradycardia, PR prolongation, AV block, QRS widening, and peaked T waves (Figure 11.2) (Hollander-Rodriguez and Calvert, 2006). Hypokalemia is a risk after dialysis due to excessive removal

Table 11.2 Pathophysiologic changes associated with chronic kidney disease.

- Cardiovascular
  - Hypertension, ischemic heart disease
- Endocrine
  - Diabetes mellitus
- Gastro-intestinal
  - Delayed gastric emptying
- Nervous System
  - Peripheral neuropathy, autonomic dysfunction
- Renal
  - Inability to excrete nitrogenous waste – uremia
- Fluids and electrolytes
  - Inability to correct volume overload – peripheral and pulmonary edema
  - Altered pharmacokinetics of analgesic medication due to proteinuria
  - Inability to excrete water soluble drugs or water soluble metabolized drugs resulting in accumulation
  - Metabolic acidosis
  - Hyperkalemia
- Hematologic
  - Anemia
  - Bleeding tendency due to uremic platelet dysfunction

of potassium. The ECG findings of hypokalemia can include flattened or inverted T waves, prominent U waves, ST depression, and tachycardia. Patients with CKD are usually tolerant to modest changes in potassium levels.

Patients with kidney disease and type I diabetes mellitus are at an increased risk of perioperative hyperglycemia and ketosis. Preoperative fasting, perioperative stresses associated with surgery, and intraoperative anesthetics, which induce the release of glucagon, growth hormone, cortisol, epinephrine, and norepinephrine, can all contribute to insulin deficiency and resistance (Carrasco et al., 2006). Preoperative glucose levels should be checked. Patients with uremia and diabetes should ideally maintain glucose levels between 150 and 200 mg/dL during surgery to avoid hypoglycemia. Postoperatively, levels should range between 120 and 180 mg/dL. Glycemic control is critical to avoid fluid overload, electrolyte disturbances, delayed wound healing, and infection.

Treatment

The primary goal of managing renal disease is to halt its progression. As all forms of CKD are associated with dysfunction of the renin–angiotensin–aldosterone system, angiotensin converting enzyme inhibitors (ACEI) or angiotensin receptor blockers (ARB) are recommended, irrespective of whether hypertension is present or not. These drugs can decrease proteinuria, slow the progression of renal dysfunction, and reduce overall mortality due to this disease. Anemia is prevented or corrected as stated earlier. Renal replacement therapy, usually in the form of hemodialysis (vs. peritoneal dialysis), is indicated when GFR < 15 mL/min/1.73 m^2. This process becomes necessary to remove waste and excess water from the blood and to correct electrolyte imbalance, when the kidneys are unable to do so. A fistula (direct surgical anastomosis between an artery and vein) is created to bypass capillary beds to improve blood flow, minimize thrombosis, and allow for more effective hemodialysis. Renal transplantation may also be a viable

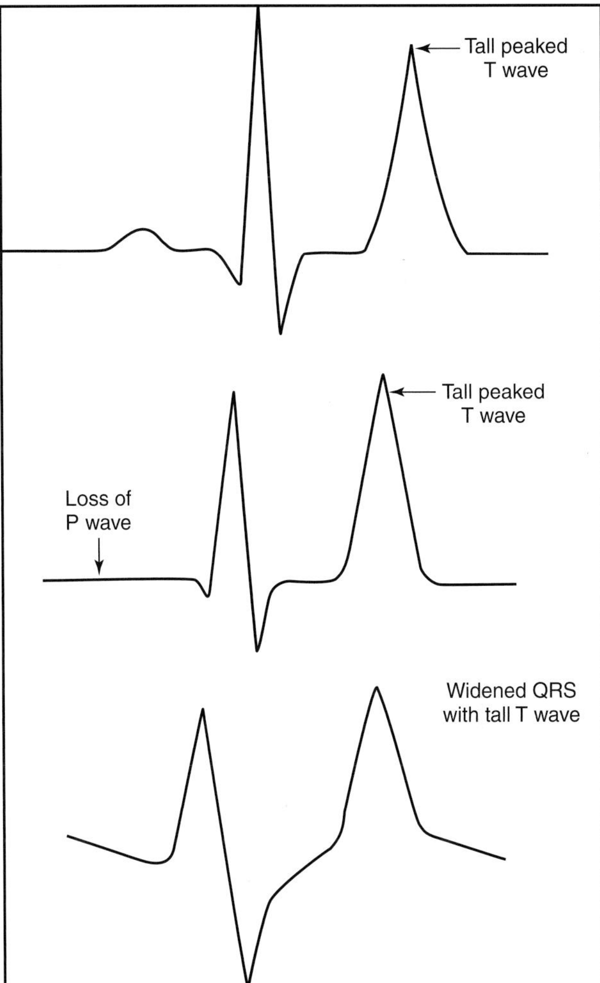

Figure 11.2 ECG changes often seen with hyperkalemia.

option in some patients. Diagnosis and medical management of comorbidites remain a priority.

Risk assessment

Patients with CKD are usually aware of their condition. Consultation with their nephrologist can be helpful in determining the extent of the disease and the current level of management. Comorbid conditions, including hypertension, diabetes mellitus, anemia, and electrolyte imbalance can also be identified. Renal insufficiency, by itself, is considered a "clinical risk factor" according to the 2007 ACC/AHA guidelines on perioperative cardiovascular evaluation, which does not impact decision-making for low risk surgery (Fleisher et al., 2007).

Functional capacity is difficult to ascertain in patients with CKD for many reasons. Dialysis-induced weakness and anemia will limit exercise tolerance regardless of cardiovascular status. As fluid retention is ameliorated at every dialysis treatment, the severity of heart failure cannot be clinically assessed. Blood pressure control should be optimized and fluid and electrolyte balance should be stable. Patients with hyperkalemia (>5.5 mmol/L) should have treatments deferred.

Typically, removal of excess fluid and metabolic waste via dialysis should be performed on the day prior to anesthesia to avoid an overly depleted intravascular volume and residual heparinization used in the hemodialysis circuit, and to avoid possible hypokalemia from excessive removal by dialysis. Ideally, the patient should be normovolemic and normotensive prior to the administration of any anesthetic agent.

Prophylactic antibiotics prior to invasive dental procedures in non-infected areas have not been recommended (Baddour et al., 2003), irrespective of whether a fistula is present or not. Consultation regarding the necessity for prophylactic antibiotics, especially with immature fistulas, can be considered on an individual basis.

Knowledge of recent laboratory test results can be helpful, including a complete blood count, metabolic panel to include electrolytes and glucose, bleeding time, INR, aPTT, and ECG, among others.

Anesthetic concerns

In general, medications should be continued into the anesthetic period. Controversy exists regarding the continuation of ACEI or ARBs, as they may exacerbate hypotension during anesthetic induction (Rang et al., 2006). Comfere et al. (2005) has recommended that these drugs be avoided for 10 hours prior to anesthesia to avoid that circumstance. The possibility of hypotension in a carefully titrated sedation may be less likely in a hemodynamically stable patient.

As in other medically compromised patients, local anesthesia is often the most physiologically stable choice, followed by light sedation and then deeper levels of anesthesia. The actions of local anesthetics can be altered in renal patients due to their underlying acid–base derangements. Increases in perfusion and systemic acidosis can cause a reduction in the overall duration of the local anesthetic. Although it has been shown that patients with renal failure have no greater complication rates with regional anesthetics when compared to general anesthetics, these patients are at increased risk for complications from increased free plasma concentrations, such as seizures and enhanced cardiotoxicity (Carlisle, 1995).

Intravascular access may be challenging in these patients, and the arm with the present or future fistula site should be avoided. Blood pressure cuffs should also not be placed on arms that have surgically created fistulas. Choice of fluids remains controversial, as lactated Ringer's solution contains potassium that may be unnecessary, while normal saline can lead to hyperchloremic acidosis. The hourly rate of milliliter volume replacement is estimated as weight (in kg) + 40, with an anticipated deficit in the range of 80 to 100 mL/hour of NPO status for an average-sized adult. These numbers are likely overestimated in a patient with CKD. Inadequate fluid replacement invites hypotension, while over-replacement can lead to pulmonary and peripheral edema.

Protein deficits are likely, which will enhance the availability and action of protein-bound anesthetic agents. Slow titration with small doses is recommended, as most sedative agents will decrease systemic vascular resistance, contractility, and cardiac output, which will attenuate the normal response to hypovolemia, a response already challenged in patients with kidney disease. Drugs with water-soluble metabolites, including morphine, codeine, meperidine, and NSAIDs should be avoided. The pharmacokinetics of all inhalational agents, propofol, and remifentanil are not significantly altered in patients with CKD; however, redosing of longer acting intravenous agents should be avoided when possible. Succinylcholine can exacerbate preexisting hyperkalemia.

References

Baddour, L. M., et al. Nonvalvular cardiovascular device-related infections. *Circ* **108**: 2015–2031, 2003.

Carrasco, L. R., et al. Perioperative management of patients with renal disease. *Oral Maxillofacial SurgClin NA* **18**: 203–212, 2006.

Carlisle, A. S. Anesthesia and renal failure. *Semin Anesth* **14**: 187–192, 1995.

Comfere, T., et al. Angiotensin system inhibitors in a general surgical population. *Anesth Analg* **100**: 636–644, 2005.

Fleisher, L. A., et al. ACC/AHA 2007 guidelines on perioperative cardiovascular evaluation and care for noncardiac surgery: executive summary: a report on the American College of Cardiology/American Heart Association Task Force on practice guidelines (writing committee to revise the 2002 guidelines on perioperative cardiovascular evaluation for noncardiac surgery) *Circ* **116**: 1971–1996, 2007.

Hollander-Rodriguez, J. C., and Calvert, J. F. Hyperkalemia. *Am Fam Physician* **15**: 283–290, 2006.

Jones, D. R. and Lee, H. T. Surgery in the patient in renal dysfunction. *Anesthesiol Clin* **27**: 739–749, 2009.

NKF-K/DOQI. Clinical practice guidelines for chronic kidney disease, evaluation, classification, and stratification. *Am J Kidney Dis* **37**: S1–S266, 2000.

Rang, S. T., et al. Anaesthesia for chronic renal disease and renal transplantation. *EAU-EBU Update Series* **4**: 246–256, 2006.

Steiner, R. W., et al. Bleeding time in uremia: a useful test to assess clinical bleeding. *Am J Hematol* **7**: 107–117, 1979.

U.S Renal Data System, USRDS 2001 Annual Data Report: Atlas of End-Stage Renal Disease in the United States, National Institutes of Health, National Institute of Diabetes and Digestive and Kidney Diseases, Bethesda, MD, 2001.

Wagener, G. and Brentjens, T. E. Anesthetic concerns in patients presenting with renal failure. *Anesthesiol Clin* **28**: 39–54, 2010.

12 Anesthetic considerations for pediatric patients

Michael Rollert[1] and Morton Rosenberg[2]

[1]Private Practice, Denver, CO, USA

[2]Tufts University School of Dental Medicine and Tufts University School of Medicine, Boston, MA, USA

Introduction

Pediatric patients who are in need of dental or oral surgical treatment, especially those between the ages of 1 and 5 years, are often difficult to manage due to the presence of pain and anxiety coupled with the inability to understand the nature of and reason for the treatment. Children are not simply 'small adults,' but have many unique and constantly changing anatomic, physiologic, pharmacologic, and psychological differences. These differences make the child more susceptible to airway obstruction (with faster oxygen desaturation) and bradycardia (which rapidly compromises organ perfusion). Understanding these differences that gradually disappear with age is the first step in providing safe sedation and anesthesia. The pediatric patient is defined in this discussion as a child 1 year old to puberty.

The pediatric airway (see Figure 12.1)

The upper airway anatomy of the pediatric patient is different from that of an adult, especially at younger ages. Small nares, especially during preferential nasal breathing, limit airflow and worsen negative airway pressure, promoting airway collapse on inspiration. A comparatively large tongue compounded by decreased muscle tone can cause passive airway obstruction (Wheeler et al., 2007), especially with enlarged tonsils and adenoids. Children have a large head, yet a short neck, leading to neck flexion and airway obstruction when lying supine. The epiglottis can be long, narrow, and often angled posteriorly. The vocal cords are inclined, with the anterior attachments more inferior than the posterior attachments. The larynx is higher than in the adult, and funnel shaped, with the narrowest portion located below the vocal cords. These factors hamper direct laryngoscopy and can complicate removal of foreign bodies, which may wedge beneath the cords. Finally, the pediatric airway is typically much more reactive to stimuli such as secretions or foreign bodies than the adult airway (Cohen et al., 1990). These factors can present significant challenges during airway management. However, the differences become less important as the child grows. By approximately 8 years of age, the upper airway of the child assumes many of the characteristics of the adult airway.

The pediatric pulmonary system

The lower airway anatomy of the pediatric patient also differs significantly from that of the adult. It is both smaller in diameter and shorter in length. The pediatric patient relies heavily on the muscles of the diaphragm for breathing as the accessory muscles develop (Rosenberg and Phero, 1995). There are fewer alveoli available for oxygen exchange. A relative lack of elastin causes the collapse of terminal airways to occur earlier. The resultant small tidal volume makes barotrauma more likely with aggressive positive pressure ventilation. Until the lung size increases significantly, the pediatric patient has a markedly decreased functional residual capacity. This decrease in the "oxygen reserve tank" coupled with a higher per kilogram oxygen consumption rate results in a more rapid desaturation and onset of hypoxemia during upper airway obstruction or apnea. Any event that leads to airway obstruction (e.g., soft tissue obstruction, laryngospasm, foreign body, or bronchospasm) resulting even in a 1% drop in oxygen saturation must be immediately recognized and rapidly addressed.

The relative smaller diameter of the trachea and bronchioles renders the pediatric airway susceptible to exponential increases in airway resistance with even minor mucus secretion or bronchospasm. The resistance to flow is inversely related to the 4th power of the radius. Circumferential edema of 1mm or mucus in an airway with a 2mm radius will decrease the radius by 1/2, causing a 16× increase in resistance, while 1 mm of edema or mucus in an airway with 4 mm radius will decrease the radius by only 1/4, causing a 3× increase in resistance. The importance of this concept makes it imperative that preexisting conditions, such as asthma, be optimized as much as possible prior to sedation/anesthesia.

The pediatric cardiovascular system

As compared to the adult, on a per kilogram basis, the pediatric heart has less muscle mass and a lower strength of contraction leading to an invariant stroke volume. Because of the higher oxygen consumption, cardiac output per kilogram is twice that of the adult. This makes any decrease in oxygen delivery life threatening in the smallest pediatric patients. Although cardiac output can be maintained over a wide range of preloads and rates without failing, young pediatric patients rely almost solely on heart rate to maintain blood pressure, as stroke volume cannot be changed. Confounding this

Anesthesia Complications in the Dental Office, First Edition. Edited by Robert C. Bosack and Stuart Lieblich.

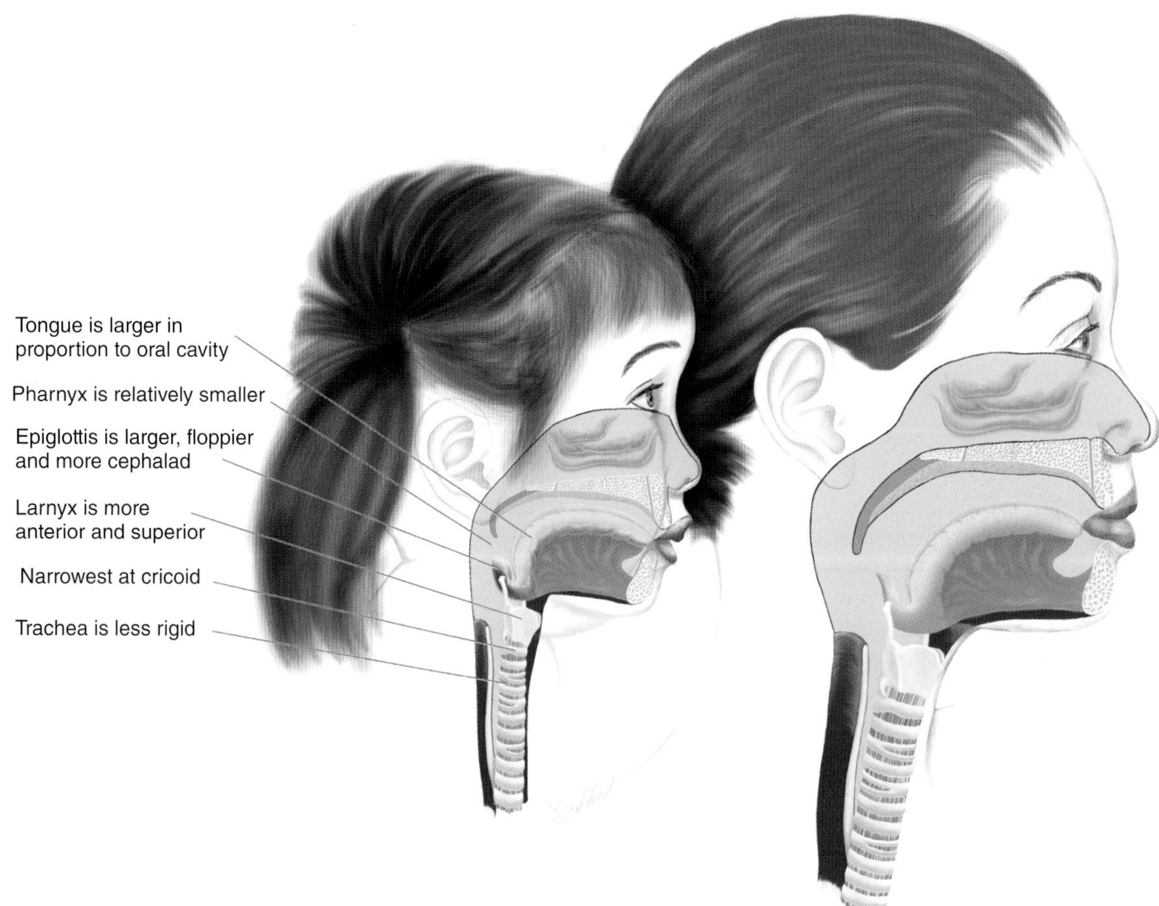

Figure 12.1 Comparison of the pediatric and adult airway.

Heart rate ↑	Blood pressure ↓
Respiratory rate ↑	Functional residual capacity ↓

Figure 12.2 Normal pediatric values as compared with the adult.

rate-dependent cardiac output is profound parasympathetic hypertonia, which leads to bradycardia and hypotension especially when triggered by hypoxia. Bradycardia is an ominous sign during any pediatric emergency and must be immediately detected and corrected. On reviewing cases of cardiac arrest during pediatric sedation/anesthesia, the single most common causative factor was found to be an untreated respiratory event degenerating to cardiac arrest (Morray et al., 2000). This only reinforces the importance of airway management in the sedative/anesthetic care of the pediatric patient (Figure 12.2).

Table 12.1 Factors affecting drug activity in pediatric patients.

Factors increasing drug activity	Factors decreasing drug activity
↑ Cardiac output - delivers more drug, more rapidly to CNS receptors ↓ Plasma proteins - increases (active drug) ↓ Redistribution to inactive spaces (less fat and muscle stores) ↓ Metabolic enzymes - prolong drug activity	↑ Total Body Water – ↑ Vd – drug is diluted prior to binding to CNS receptors ↓ Plasma protein – ↑ Vd

Pediatric pharmacodynamics

It is difficult to estimate volumes of distribution, protein binding, receptor sensitivity, or hepatic enzyme activity in pediatric patients (See Table 12.1). Administration of any sedative/anesthetic drug, in any dose and by any route, can result in a wide variety of patient responses, which often do not follow the arbitrary divisions associated with each level of sedation. It is for these reasons that all central nervous depressants (sedatives/anesthetics) should be carefully titrated to effect when targeting an open airway technique.

Preoperative evaluation

Pediatric evaluation begins with a psychological assessment addressing the child's temperament, attachment to parent or caregiver, and ability to regulate emotions (Kain, 2005; Lopez and Mellick, 2005). The flexible child is positive and able to quickly adapt, while the cautious child may be slow or unable to adapt and require the security of the parent. Difficult children may be active and moody, but most importantly, may be distractible. Children under the age of 5 years are usually incapable of reason and are

Table 12.2 Age-specific concerns and management techniques.

Age	Fears	Useful techniques
1–3 (toddler)	Brief separation/pain	Keep in parents lap, allow some choices, maintain verbal communication, reinforce good behavior
3–5 (pre-school)	Long separation Pain, disfigurement	Allow expression, questions; encourage fantasy and play, encourage participation in care, distraction, provide detail
5–10 (school age)	Disfigurement, loss of function, death	Explain procedures, what and why, project positive outcome, enable child to master situation, distract
10–19 (adolescence)	Loss of autonomy, loss of peer acceptance, death	Allow choices and control, stress acceptance by peers, respect autonomy, privacy

Data from Lopez and Mellick (2005), Chiang (2012) and Behrman et al. (2000).

unable to express themselves other than through crying or withdrawal. In all instances, the practitioner should keep the child at the center of attention, and should speak directly to the child, even though information may come from the parent. Timing, format, and content of information are very important variables when trying to gain cooperation and trust from the pediatric patient (Chiang, 2012). Table 12.2 provides an overview of age-specific concerns and management techniques.

The initial evaluation of the pediatric patient is unique for several reasons. The history is derived almost completely from the caregiver, and rarely from the patient. Systemic diseases and prescription medications can be uncommon, and past anesthetic experiences are often rare. Instead, a family history of allergies and familial condition such as sickle cell anemia and malignant hyperthermia are of great import. Past anesthetic experiences, if they have occurred, can be helpful in developing the appropriate anesthetic plan. The history of a recent cold, asthma attack, snoring, or concealed neuromuscular disorders should be obtained. The targeted physical examination should always consist of an airway examination and an evaluation of the heart and lungs. Fever, mucopurulent nasal discharge, audible wheezing, or productive cough, especially with an asthmatic history, should prompt further evaluation and optimization prior to anesthesia, as these conditions often predispose to laryngospasm and accelerated oxygen desaturation (Rolf and Cote, 1992). Because of the pediatric patient's more reactive airway, it is important to confirm the presence of an upper respiratory infection at the time of the anesthetic (or in the recent past) and verify the presence of any loose teeth, which may become an airway concern (Tait and Malviya, 2005). Some dental practitioners may be able to appreciate murmurs of cardiac origin. In general, soft, systolic crescendo–decrescendo murmurs are usually benign, while loud, harsh, or diastolic murmurs, especially with bounding pulses are always pathologic. The presence of a new cardiac murmur should be evaluated completely before proceeding.

Recording of vital signs is an important component of the physical examination. All pediatric patients should be weighed prior to drug dosage selection. Unfortunately, the incidence of pediatric obesity is mirroring the pandemic of adult obesity in the United States. Therefore, a computation of the patient's body mass index (BMI) is appropriate for the obese child. Obese children have the same risk factors as their adult counterparts, especially airway issues including a more rapid oxygen desaturation when coupled with anatomic factors, the presence of obstructive sleep apnea, and the difficulty of obtaining intravenous access (Hedley et al., 2004). Fasting guidelines for pediatric patients about to undergo sedation/anesthesia are changing, with the most current ones allowing for a light meal 6 hours, breast milk 4 hours, and clear fluids 2 hours prior to surgery.

Sedative/anesthetic techniques

The sedative/anesthetic goals for pediatric patients are safety, cooperation, elimination of pain, reduction of anxiety, and control of behavior and movement to allow completion of the planned intervention. Above all, a risk/benefit analysis should be tailored to the individual patient, proposed surgical procedure, and the training, preparation, and comfort of the surgical/anesthesia team.

Sedation/anesthesia can be achieved through both nonpharmacologic and pharmacologic methods. Oral, nasal, rectal, intramuscular, intravenous or inhalation routes of drug administration are available to the dental practitioner. Minimal and moderate sedation may be inadequate for many children less than 6 years of age, with deep sedation or general anesthesia being the only alternative. The risks of an adverse respiratory event do increase if deep sedation or general anesthesia is required (Cote et al., 2000). It is beyond the scope of this chapter to discuss specific anesthetic drug regimens or techniques in any depth; however, oral and nasal midazolam, intramuscular and intravenous ketamine, nitrous oxide, narcotic analgesics, sevoflurane, and dexmedetomidine have all been used successfully in oral surgical practice by the trained practitioner (Karlis et al., 2010; Todd, 2013) Preoperative oral midazolam (~0.5–0.75 mg/kg, 20 mg maximum dose) is often successful to gain cooperation, and can often assist in parental separation. Oral sedative medications should only be given to children monitored by direct visual observation by a health care professional and all dosages should be individualized based on weight, response to medications, past anesthetic experiences, and the duration of the procedure. All anesthetic techniques in the dental office depend upon effective local anesthesia, intra- and postoperatively. The practitioner should be familiar with recommended maximal dose, especially local anesthetics. Airway management can vary from the "open" spontaneously breathing child maintained on nasal airways, nasal hood to the insertion simple airway adjuncts of nasal/oral airways to the advanced use of laryngeal mask airways or endotracheal tubes.

Controversies

Although sedative/anesthetic care is often necessary for pediatric patients needing surgical intervention, there are concerns whether anesthetics by themselves pose a risk to their later intellectual development. Although some clinical trials assessing the effects of anesthesia on pediatric development are ongoing, definitive data will likely require numerous studies over many years. At this time, there is not enough information to draw any firm conclusions between anesthetic administration and subsequent disabilities (Rappaport et al., 2011).

Intravenous access prior to administration of an anesthetic is the usual course for the adult patient. However, during pediatric anesthesia, many factors may prevent this. These include the uncooperative, anxious child requiring restraint or an anesthetic plan for an extremely short case utilizing intramuscular or inhalational induction. In these cases, unless the procedure will take less time than it takes for the experienced practitioner to obtain vascular access, then intravenous access should be strongly considered after induction of general anesthesia. The introduction of intraosseous techniques is an important adjunct to emergency vascular access.

There is a wide range of opinion among anesthesia providers regarding the importance of parental presence during the induction of pediatric anesthesia. Although there is evidence that adequate premedication and child comfort are more effective in reducing anxiety than the presence of the parent during induction, the presence of a parent during anesthetic administration is the decision of the anesthesia provider (Kain et al., 1998). Whatever the decision, it is important that the anesthesia provider effectively communicate the reasons for the decision to the parent.

Safety in pediatric anesthesia

Safety, irrespective of the depth of anesthesia, is the goal of pediatric care. This begins with the experienced and educationally qualified health professional and his/her support team. Being current and a practicing pediatric advanced life support (PALS) is the foundation of acute medical emergency care for children (Chamedies et al., 2011). Adherence to meticulous preoperative evaluation and application of appropriate monitoring will guide the practitioner as to the choice of technique and the most suitable environment, office versus hospital, for the child. Intraoperative and postoperative monitoring is instrumental in detecting situations early enough for corrective interventions. Determining the anesthetic drug dosages and possible emergency drug dosages based on lean body weight prior to the case is an indispensable aid to preparing the team.

References

Behrman, R., et al. *Nelson Texbook of Pediatrics*, 16th edn. Philadelphia: W. B. Saunders Co., 2000: pp. 32–57.

Chiang, V. W. Procedural sedation: let's review the basics - the pediatrician's perspective. In: Mason, K. P. *Pediatric Sedation Outside of the Operating Room*. New York: Springer, 2012.

Chamedies L, et al. *Pediatric advanced life support provider manual*. American Heart Association, 2011.

Cohen, M. M., Cameron C. B., Duncan P. G. Pediatric anesthesia morbidity and mortality in the perioperative period. *Anesth Analg* **70**: 160–167, 1990.

Cote, C. J., et al. Adverse sedation events in pediatrics: a critical analysis of contributing factors. *Pediatrics* **105**: 805–814, 2000.

Hedley, A., et al. Prevalence of overweight and obesity among US children, adolescents and adults. 1999-2002. *J Am Med Assoc* **23**: 291–294, 2004.

Kain Z. L. Preoperative psychological preparation of the child for surgery : an update. *Anesth Clin N Am* **23**(4): 591–614, 2005.

Kain, Z. L., et al. Parental presence during induction of anesthesia versus sedative premedication: which is more effective? *Anesthesiol* **89**: 1147–56, 1998.

Karlis V, et al. Pediatric outpatient anesthesia and sedation. *Selected readings in Oral Maxillofac Surg* **18**: 1–4, 2010.

Lopez, M. and Mellick, L. B. Pearls and pitfalls of pediatric assessment: secrets for approaching children in the Emergency Department. American Health Consultants Emergency Medicine Reports, Nove. 2005.

Morray, J. P., et al. Anesthesia-related cardiac arrest in children: initial findings of the pediatric perioperative cardiac arrest (POCA) registry. *Anesthesiol* **93**: 6–14, 2000.

Gross J. B., Bailey P. L., Connis R. T., et al. Practice guidelines for sedation and analgesia by non-anesthesiologists. Anesthesiol **96**: 1004–1017, 2002.

Rappaport, M. D., et al. Defining safe use of anesthesia in children. *N Engl J Med* **364**: 1387–1389, 2011.

Rolf, N. and Cote, C. J. Frequency and severity of desaturation events during general anesthesia in children with and without upper respiratory tract infections. *J Clin Anesth* **4**: 200–203, 1992.

Rosenberg, M. B. and Phero, J. C. Resuscitation of the pediatric patient. *Dent Clin North Am* **39**: 663–676, 1995.

Tait, A. R. and Malviya, S. Anesthesia for the child with an upper respiratory tract infection: still a Dilemma? *Anesth Analg* **100**: 59–65, 2005.

Todd, D. W. Pediatric sedation and anesthesia for the oral surgeon. *Oral Maxillofacial Clin North Am* **25**: 467–478, 2013.

Wheeler, D. S., et al. Assessment and management of the pediatric airway. In: Wheeler, D. S., et al., eds. *Pediatric Critical Care Medicine. Basic Science and Clinical Evidence*. New York: Springer, 2007.

13 Anesthetic considerations for geriatric patients

Andrea Schreiber[1] **and Peter M. Tan**[2]
[1]New York University College of Dentistry, Department of Oral and Maxillofacial Surgery, New York, NY, USA
[2]Mid-Maryland Oral and Maxillofacial Surgery, P.A. Frederick, MD, USA

Introduction

In the United States, population projections indicate that by the year 2030 over 20% of the population (70 million) will be over 65 years of age (Lamster, 2004). Dental professionals will be challenged with meeting the surgical and anesthetic needs of this growing portion of the population, since functional edentulism will not be as acceptable to this generation as it has been to its predecessors. Geriatric patients may also present with conditions unrelated to the dentition, including maxillofacial trauma resulting from gait disturbance, neuromuscular disease, or, unfortunately, elder abuse. Benign or malignant pathology may also be present in the partially or fully edentulous geriatric population, and they should be screened accordingly. The Surgeon General's report on Oral Health in America estimates that more than 20% of homebound or institutionalized elderly require emergency dental care annually (U.S. Department of Health and Human Services, USDHHS, 2000).

As geriatric medicine and anesthesiology become more complex, practitioners must appreciate the implications of age and related comorbidities to insure the safe management of these patients. These include the deterioration of the elderly patient's ability to handle surgical/anesthetic stress and the natural incidence of age-related diseases and organ failure (Schreiber et al., 2010). This chapter focuses on preoperative assessment and anesthetic management of elderly patients, which includes risk stratification, physiologic and cognitive assessment, recognition of factors that can complicate administration of anesthesia to the elderly, and strategies to minimize complication frequency.

The effects of aging on major organ systems

The universal, heterogeneous, and unpredictable responses to aging are complex. Although not fully understood, a steady decline in organ function does occur with advancing age, which eventually increases the risk of mortality (see Table 13.1). In many instances, this decline goes unnoticed, as it insidiously imposes limitations on daily activity, such as stair climbing and walking long distances. These variable and subtle decreases in organ reserve, which are difficult to quantify, can manifest at inopportune times, when elderly patients become unable to respond appropriately to the stress of surgery or anesthesia (Forrest et al., 1992, Tonner et al., 2003). Examples include the inability to increase heart rate or vasoconstrict when challenged with a hypotensive episode, the inability to maintain protective laryngeal reflexes, or the inability to augment ventilation during hypoxia. These issues are further compounded by the presence of comorbid diseases and the complex medical regimes that result. Makary et al., (2010) introduce the concept of frailty as a means to assess vulnerability to adverse events, which is characterized by unintentional weight loss (greater than 10 pounds), weak hand grip, exhaustion with and limitation of activity, and slow walking speed.

Chronologic age often does not predict physiologic age, as variation exists among different patients and even among different organ systems in the same patient. What remains unclear is whether old age, in and of itself, can be considered an independent risk factor (Tiret et al., 1986).

Central nervous system

Aging is accompanied by a variable reduction in total nervous system mass, cerebral blood flow, neuronal density, and concentration of neurotransmitters (notably acetylcholine and serotonin) and receptors (Muravchick 2003; Zakriya, 2007). This may contribute to pharmacodynamic changes resulting in altered sensitivity to medications such as midazolam, opioids, and drugs with anticholinergic properties. While some memory decline is to be expected in patients over the age of 65, senile dementia is observed in a small percentage of the population at that age, which increases with advancing years. Dementia should not be confused with cognitive impairment and needs to be diagnosed by an appropriately trained clinician. Acute changes in cognition in the perioperative period needs to be evaluated, and other causes of dementia, such as hypoxia, hypotension, hypoperfusion, electrolyte imbalance, drug intoxication, or infection—specifically urinary tract infections in the nursing home population, should be considered (Corey-Bloom et al., 1995).

Age-related changes in the autonomic system include a reduced β-adrenergic responsiveness and moderate decrease in parasympathetic tone, both of which reduce the tachycardic response to exercise or hypotension. Delayed gastric emptying and impaired temperature regulation are other possibilities.

Anesthesia Complications in the Dental Office, First Edition. Edited by Robert C. Bosack and Stuart Lieblich.

Table 13.1 Expected physiologic changes in the geriatric population.

GENERAL
↓lean muscle mass
↑fat stores
↓blood volume
CNS
Cerebral atrophy: cognitive impairment, confusion, dementia
Autonomic impairment: labile BP, impaired thermoregulation, delayed gastric emptying
Neurotransmitter deficiencies: Parkinson's and Alzheimer's
CARDIOVASCULAR
CHF/CAD
Atrial fibrillation
Hypertension and changes in arterial elasticity (stiffness)
PULMONARY
Diminished functional reserve: ↓ VC, flattened diaphragms, weak muscles
Blunted response to ↑CO_2 or ↓O_2
Loss of protective coughing and swallowing reflexes
RENAL
↓GFR and blood flow to the kidneys
Fluid and electrolyte imbalance
↓capacity to excrete drugs and metabolites
HEPATIC
↓blood flow to the liver
↓ability to metabolize drugs with high E ratio
↓albumin and protein binding

Cardiovascular system

Anatomic changes in the aging cardiovascular system profoundly affect cardiovascular functioning. These changes are best characterized by a progressive stiffening (loss of elasticity) in both the myocardium and vasculature due to loss of elastin and increased collagen deposition. The accumulation of lipid plaques exacerbates this stiffening and decreases lumen diameter, which limits blood flow. The impedance to blood flow increases systolic blood pressure (afterload), which contributes to left ventricular hypertrophy. Ventricular compliance (stretch) is decreased, which limits passive diastolic fill and systolic contraction, causing a decrease in cardiac output and organ perfusion. The loss of the atrial "kick" augmenting diastolic ventricular filling in cases of atrial fibrillation often contributes to hypotension. The loss of vessel compliance contributes to systolic hypertension, which characteristically widens pulse pressures in the elderly. Fibrotic infiltration (among other causative factors) of the cardiac conduction pathway contributes to the development of bradydysrhythmias and vulnerability to ectopic premature or escape beats.

These changes, in addition to the blunting of the baroreceptor reflex (White et al., 1994), hypovolemia from the preanesthetic fast, and exaggerated sensitivity to anesthetic medications, make the elderly patient both prone to hypotension and unable to compensate for it. As systolic hypertension also plagues the elderly, labile changes in blood pressure during the administration of anesthetic drugs can be common occurrences. Orthostatic hypotension should be anticipated when elderly patients first rise from the dental chair to assume an upright posture. Given the above, it becomes easy to share the frustration of managing systolic hypertension in the elderly.

Respiratory system

Age-related structural change insidiously decreases efficiency of the respiratory system, which predisposes to upper airway obstruction and rapid onset of hypoxemia.

Upper airway changes common in the elderly that often lead to obstruction during sedation or open airway general anesthesia include large neck circumference (cervical obesity) and diminished range of neck motion, hampering the ability to open the airway with a chin-lift, jaw-thrust maneuver. Male gender, age greater than 50 years, BMI $> 28\,kg/m^2$, hypertension, and a history of snoring are other risk factors for obstructive sleep apnea that are or can be present in the elderly patient (Chung and Elsaid, 2009). Suspicion of this diagnosis is sufficient to plan for its presence. A loss of the gag reflex due to a decrease in protective laryngeal reflexes and a diminished cough reflex may predispose the elderly to aspiration.

Restrictive changes that negatively impact pulmonary expansion include spinal cord deformities, calcification of costochondral cartilage, diaphragmatic flattening, barrel-shaped and stiffer chest walls, and diminished intercostal muscular strength. Work of breathing is increased and fatigue interferes with efficient ventilation, especially in longer cases.

Parenchymal changes with advancing age mimic those seen in emphysema: reduction of elasticity, passive recoil, and surface area for gas exchange (Sprung et al., 2006). Air trapping and hypercarbia result along with this pathologic increase in residual volume.

The result of all of these changes is obvious: most anesthetic agents, especially narcotics, can easily cause apnea in the elderly, even in low doses. Severe hypoxemia and hypercarbia can rapidly develop. Diminished activity in peripheral CO_2 receptors and CNS responsiveness blunt the expected compensatory hyperventilation in this situation, which will prolong the insult, thereby increasing the severity and promoting further adversity.

Renal system

Aging is accompanied by a gradual decrease in functioning glomeruli, blood flow to the kidneys, and renal mass. The process is a slow one, with the estimation of a loss of ~1% of function/year after the age of 40, and up to 10% of blood flow to the kidney/decade. This translates into a compromised ability of the kidneys to conserve and/or excrete electrolytes and to excrete drugs and their metabolites. As the body loses the capacity to conserve sodium there is a tendency toward sodium depletion. Similarly, an inability to excrete potassium occurs, and hyperkalemia is frequently observed. Responses to fluid imbalances are also diminished in the elderly and both fluid overload and dehydration may be encountered. This may be due to changes in electrolyte balances or aldosterone levels or due to self-imposed fluid restrictions for a variety of reasons, which may include incontinence or prostate hypertrophy (Lamb et al., 2003).

Pharmacologic considerations

Both pharmacokinetics (relationship between administered dose and concentration in various tissues) and pharmcodynamics (relationship between drug concentration at the receptor site and intensity of effects) (Rivera and Antognini, 2009) are altered in geriatric patients. These changes are due to alterations in body composition, CNS receptor activity, and the ability to metabolize and excrete drugs.

In the geriatric population, the practitioner may expect an increase in the length of time that a drug is active due to changes in body compartments, protein binding, metabolism, and elimination of the agent, and altered sensitivity to the drug due to changes in the CNS. The increase in body fat increases the volume of the slow equilibrating compartments, which results in increasing the volume of distribution and prolonging the drug half-life. The loss of muscle mass and a proportional increase in fat are responsible for the prolonged anesthetic effects observed. The decrease in blood volume, total body water, and muscle mass decreases the volume of rapidly equilibrating compartments, which impairs initial drug distribution, causing a transient, yet clinically significant elevated initial drug concentration, especially with bolus or rapid administration. Protein binding is less efficient with age, and less albumin is produced, which results in more active drug being available for clinical effect. As the GFR decreases with age, so does the elimination of water-soluble agents. Finally, reduced hepatic blood flow with age results in slower elimination of high extraction drugs – specifically ketamine, fentanyl, morphine, etomidate, and lidocaine. These are agents that have a high E or extraction value, meaning that they are dependent on blood flow for clearance (Rivera and Antognini, 2009).

The depletion of neurotransmitters in the brain with no change in receptor sensitivity, the development of cerebral atrophy with age, delayed homeostatic mechanisms, and the reduction of cerebral blood flow with age, all impact upon the pharmacodynamics of drugs that are administered to elderly patients.

As a result of all of these factors, a practitioner should plan for reduced dosage requirements and expect longer elimination half times when treating elderly patients. Increased sensitivity to anesthetic agents carries the implication of increased sensitivity to their side effects, often leading to decreases in heart rate, blood pressure, cardiac output, ventilatory drive, and upper airway patency (Vuyk, 2003).

Preanesthetic evaluation

Obtaining a complete and correct medical history often requires time and patience, especially when dealing with geriatric patients, who may have difficulties hearing or processing questions or who may just simply forget important information. Determination of a geriatric patient's mental status is essential as confusion may be commonly encountered both pre and postoperatively. Furthermore, an individual's preoperative mental status may have important medicolegal ramifications in addition to the clinical consequences. Distinctions between dementia, delirium and postoperative cognitive deficit are sometimes subtle, which makes documentation of the preoperative condition essential. A mini-mental status examination is easily administered chairside (Folstein et al., 1975). If responses to orientation (time and place), registration (naming and repeating 3 objects), calculation (serial 7's), language (following a 3 stage command or repeating a sentence), or recall (remembering the 3 objects named earlier) are noted to be impaired – referral to a specialist for further delineation may be indicated.

Assuming normal mental status, further key information includes approximations of the effects of aging on the cardiac, respiratory, hepatic, and renal systems, and the presence and level of management of comorbid diseases. A thorough drug history (names, dose, and compliance) is also necessary, as the likelihood of adverse drug reactions increases with the number of medications taken. Consultation may be necessary to complete this history or entertain further optimization of disease states.

The level of exercise tolerance is easy to estimate with a 4 MET functioning level (light housework, one flight of stairs without rest, or shortness of breath) considered normal. This history informs the estimate of the patient's ability to handle the combined stress of both anesthesia and surgery, notably the ability to mount or tolerate stress-induced tachycardia or the ability to increase depth of ventilation (Fleisher et al., 2007).

Physical examination includes vital signs (with pulse check for regularity and room air SpO_2), airway assessment with particular attention to cervical mobility and vertebral column deformity, and auscultation of the lungs. Visual examination of skin and extremities for signs of edema, pallor, or cyanosis may be useful in determining the extent of respiratory or cardiovascular diseases.

Anesthetic management

It is difficult to quantify or differentiate levels of risk with levels of anesthesia (local only, light, moderate, deep sedation or general anesthesia.) With case refusal as a viable option in the dental office, both patient selection and type/level of anesthesia become elective. Continuous supplemental oxygen and robust monitoring are the sine qua non of optimal care. Table 13.2 reflects the time proven adage – "start low and go slow."

Medications with central anticholinergic properties (see Table 13.3) should be avoided or limited, as they may worsen an already decreased cholinergic reserve with aging, especially when administered with other agents with similar properties, such as psychotropic agents. Cholinergic deficiency can be particularly debilitating in the elderly. Signs include sedation, cognitive dysfunction, delirium, fever, impaired vision, tachycardia, xerostomia, and elevated heart rate.

Table 13.2 Anesthetic modifications for the geriatric population.

REDUCE DOSAGES and administer slowly
↓ blood volume and ↓ muscle mass → ↑ initial drug concentration
↓ protein binding→ ↑ free drug available for effect
↓ muscle mass, ↑ fat → prolonged effect as drug is released from fat stores

INCREASE INTERVAL BETWEEN DOSES
Limit total doses
Consider changes in receptor sensitivity, pharmacokinetics and pharmacodynamics
↓ hepatic and renal function → ↓ability to metabolize and excrete drugs

PRUDENT AGENT SELECTION
Short half life
Minimal side effects
Few active metabolites

Table 13.3 Select medications that have central anticholinergic properties (Tune, 2001).

- Atropine
- Antihistamines
- Codeine
- Diazepam
- Dexamethasone
- Meperidine

Perioperative complications

Although it is difficult to extrapolate medical data to ambulatory anesthesia in the dental office, it is prudent to consider advancing age, frailty, and comorbid disease as risk factors for anesthetic morbidity. This underscores the importance of assessment and optimization of these patients in the non-emergent setting. Studies of patients over 100 years of age undergoing surgery have shown that age alone is not a good predictor of risk, as the surgical cohort survival was equal to the non-surgery group after 1 year. Not surprisingly, a substantial proportion of cardiovascular complications occurs in patients who presented with preexisting cardiovascular disease. Approximately 7% of octogenarians develop postoperative pulmonary complications, and most frequently this occurs among those with preexisting pulmonary, cardiovascular, or neurologic disease (e.g. Parkinson's) history (Liu, 2000).

Airway patency is continuously challenged in the elderly due to the increased prevalence of obstructive sleep apnea, limitation of cervical range of motion, increased fat, and decreased muscle tone. Aspiration can occur because of preexisting reflux disease, neuromuscular disease, or decreased laryngeal and cough reflexes (Muder 1998; Terpenning et al., 2001). Improving oral hygiene with physical means and pre-treatment chlorhexidine rinses can diminish the bacterial load of aspirates and thus diminish the risk of subsequent bacterial pneumonia, even with subclinical aspiration.

Hypoventilation with subsequent hypoxemia is a very real risk after the administration of anesthetic agents, irrespective of whether it is due to unintentional drug overdose (rapid administration or too much drug), diminished hypercarbic respiratory drive, or inability to increase depth of ventilation because of obesity or stiff chest walls as discussed above. The duration of hypoventilation increases the severity of its consequence - hypoxemia, which is poorly tolerated by a compromised cardiovascular system.

Cardiovascular complications include hypotension, bradycardia, ectopy, and a diminished ability to respond to these challenges. Small changes in venous return can cause large changes in blood pressure with a noncompliant, slowly beating ventricle. Leg elevation can be a rapid and effective treatment to augment venous return and correct hypotension. Preexisting systolic hypertension can worsen with poor anesthetic technique, and possible triggers should be remediated prior to the administration of a venodilator that can have profound and exaggerated hypotensive effects.

Prolonged recovery should be anticipated in all elderly patients, who are already prone to orthostatic hypotension and neuromuscular weakness, which can both result in falls that can have disastrous results.

Postoperative cognitive deficit or decline (POCD) is a condition that has been long recognized and equally long been questioned and disputed in the anesthesia and neurology literature. Controversy exists over whether it actually exists, how to define it, and how to definitively test for it. There is, however, no controversy over what it is not – which is to say, delirium or dementia. Delirium is also observed postoperatively in some patients. It is characterized by fluctuating levels of consciousness and is often observed in patients previously diagnosed with dementia. Dementia is a preexisting persistent impairment of cognitive and emotional abilities that interferes with the individual's ability to perform activities of daily living. Despite the limited knowledge on the subject, those who believe that POCD does exist state that it is characterized by changes in memory, attention, planning, speed of information processing, and social disinhibition of the subject. This behavior is frequently reported to occur shortly after an anesthetic event. Reports of incidence and recovery from POCD vary from 5–33% (Cryns et al., 1990). Liu noted POCD in 25% of patients 1 week postoperatively, which dropped to 9% at the 3 months postoperative point. No particular anesthetic technique has been identified as being a greater risk, although inhaled anesthetic agents are sometimes implicated. Several hypotheses for the development of POCD exist including cholinergic failure of the CNS, hypotension, hypoxia, or intraoperative emboli. Clinical recommendations include minimizing agents and avoiding hypercarbia and hypoxemia. Anecdotal experience seems to support that the fewer the variety of agents administered, the swifter the recovery with less incidence of POCD.

A recent study (Avidan et al., 2009) seems to contradict the conventional wisdom about the effect of surgery and general anesthesia on precipitating or exacerbating Alzheimer's disease. In a study of over 500 patients, it was concluded that there was no evidence of long-term effect on cognitive function of surgery or major illness in progression in patients without an initial diagnosis of dementia.

Finally, there are two equally important but less often discussed factors to consider when making decisions about anesthesia and the elderly patient. They both involve the "human" aspect of care and are discussed last not because of diminished importance, but for added emphasis. The first element to consider is the level of administrator skill and experience in dealing with the particular set of challenges presented by elderly patients. This requires introspection on the part of the practitioner, which may result in case referral to a different practitioner or management in a different environment. The second element is that the surgeon/anesthesiologist must be aware of the patient's social/living situation – assisted living, nursing home, living alone or with family, and the level of postanesthetic care and monitoring that is expected to be available during routine or emergency situations. Considerations must be given to anesthetic techniques that will cause the least disruption to an elderly patient's daily routine, as those are the best tolerated. Technique modification to local anesthesia supplemented by mild or moderate sedation, or in some cases, treatment as an inpatient may need to be considered depending on the answers to these questions.

The take-home message is simply this: the octogenarian sitting in your operatory is likely to be someone's grandparent; treat them as if they were your own, with patience, respect and care.

References

Avidan, M. S., et al. Long term cognitive decline in older subjects was not attributable to noncardiac surgery or major illness. *Anesthesiology* **111**: 964–970, 2009.

Chung, F. and Elsaid, H. Screening for obstructive sleep apnea before surgery: Why is it important? *Curr Opin Anaesthesiol* **22**: 405–411, 2009.

Corey-Bloom J., et al. Diagnosis and evaluation of dementia. *Neurology* **45**: 211–218, 1995.

Cryns, F. F. et al. Effects of surgery on the mental status of older persons. A meta-analytic review. *J Geriatr Psychiatry Neurol* 3: 184–191, 1990.

Fleisher, L. A., et al. ACC/AHA 2007 guidelines on perioperative cardiovascular evaluation and care for noncardiac surgery: executive summary: a report on the American College of Cardiology/American Heart Association task force on practice guidelines (writing committee to revise the 2002 guidelines on perioperative cardiovascular evaluation for noncardiac surgery) *Circulation* **116**: 1971–1996, 2007.

Folstein, M. F., Folstein, S. E., McHugh, P. R. Mini mental status state: a practical method for grading the cognitive state of patients for the clinician. *J Psychiatr Res* **12**: 189–198, 1975.

Forrest, J. b., et al. Multicenter study of general anesthesia. III. Predictors of severe perioperative adverse outcomes. *Anesthesiology* **76**: 3–15, 1992.

Lamb, E. J., O'Riordan, S. E., Delaney, M. P. Kidney function in older people: pathology, assessment and management. *Clin Chim Acta* **334**: 25–40, 2003.

Lamster, I. B. Oral health care services for older patients: a looming crisis. *Am J Public Health* **94**: 699–702, 2004.

Liu L. L. Predicting adverse post-operative outcomes in patients aged 80 years or older. *J Am Geriatr Soc* **48**: 405–412, 2000.

Makary, M. A., et al. Frailty as a predictor of surgical outcomes in older patients. *J Am Coll Surg* **210**: 901–908, 2010.

Muder, R. R. Pneumonia in residents of long-term care facilities: epidemiology, etiology, management, and prevention. *Am J Med* **150**: 319–330, 1998.

Muravchick, S. Physiological changes of aging. *ASA Refresh Courses Anesthesiol* **31**: 139–150, 2003.

Rivera, R., Antognini, J. F. Perioperative drug therapy in elderly patients. *Anesthesiology* **110**: 1176–1181, 2009.

Sadean, M. R. and Glass, P. S. A. Pharmacokinetics in the elderly. *Best Pract Res Clin Anaesthesiol* **17**: 191–205, 2003.

Schreiber, A., et al. Geriatric Dentistry: Maintaining Oral Health in the Geriatric Population, *in* Fillit, H. M., Rockwood, K., Woodhouse, K. (eds): *Brocklehurst's Textbook on Geriatric Medicine and Gerontology* 7th edn. Saunders Elsevier, 2010, pp. 599–607.

Sprung, J., et al. Review article: age related alterations in respiratory function - anesthetic considerations. *Can J Anaesth* **53**: 1244–1157, 2006.

Tiret, L., et al. Complications associated with anaesthesia: a prospective study in France. *Can Anaesth Soc J* **33**: 336–344, 1986.

Tonner, P. H., et al. Pathophysiologic chages in the elderly. *Best Pract Res Clin Anaestehsiol* **17**: 163–177, 2003.

Tune, L. W. Anticholinergic effects of medication in elderly patients. *J Clin Psychiatry* **62**: 11–14, 2001.

Terpenning, M. S., et al. Aspiration pneumonia: dental and oral risk factors in an older veteran population. *J Am Geriatr Soc* **49**: 557–563, 2001.

U.S. Department of Health and Human Services (USDHHS). *Oral Health in America: SA Report of the Surgeon General*. Washington, DC: U.S. Department of Health and Human Services, 2000.

Vuyk, J. Pharmacodynamics in the elderly. *Best Pract Res Clin Anaesthesiol* **17**: 207–218, 2003.

White, M., et al. Age-related changes in beta-adrenergic reuroeffector systems in the human heart. *Circulation* **90**: 1225–1238, 1994.

Zakriya, K. J. Central/Peripheral Nervous System, *in* Sieber, F. E. (eds): Geriatric Anesthesia. New York: McGraw-Hill, 2007, pp. 21–30.

14

Anesthetic considerations for patients with bleeding disorders

O. Ross Beirne
Department of Oral and Maxillofacial Surgery, University of Washington, Seattle, WA, USA

The surgical and anesthetic management of patients with inherited or acquired bleeding disorders requires careful presurgical planning based on a clear understanding of the pathophysiology of bleeding disorders (Jaffer, 2009; Chassot, 2010; Levy and Azran, 2010; Vandermeulen, 2010; Hall and Mazer, 2011). The severity of the bleeding disorder and the location and complexity of the surgery will determine whether systemic interventions, in addition to routine or special local measures, will be necessary to control anticipated or unanticipated hemorrhage during or after surgery.

Normal hemostasis following vascular injury involves three phases (Norris, 2003; Donegan et al., 2007). The immediate *vascular phase* is vasoconstriction, which slows blood loss and facilitates formation of the *platelet plug* (second phase), which involves platelet aggregation at the site of exposed subendothelial collagen. Platelet activation is followed by the release of platelet granule proteins that further enhance the third and final *amplification or coagulation phase.* Coagulation is triggered by the traumatic release of a tissue factor (thromboplastin), followed by a complex and highly interwoven cascade of simultaneous or sequential enzyme activations, ultimately resulting in the formation and cross-linking of fibrin. If any one of these phases is abnormal, patients can develop uncontrollable bleeding with trauma or surgery. Figure 14.1 provides a concise, simplified scheme of these events, and depicts the locations of the multiple opportunities to medically disrupt this process.

Presurgical evaluation of all patients includes questions relating to past surgery and injuries to determine if a possible bleeding disorder exists. The patient's current list of medications should be screened for recent ingestion of aspirin, NSAIDs, and herbals such as ginkgo biloba, garlic, and ginseng, among others.

Patients with platelet disorders will often present with unmanageable bleeding immediately during or after surgery. This is in contrast to patients with coagulopathies, who typically will have uncontrolled bleeding several hours after surgery or injury. Depending on the density of the nearby tissue, blood pressure, and vessel caliber, continuous and prolonged bleeding can result in anatomic distortion, airway compromise, and hemodynamic instability. The strategy for managing excessive and continuous bleeding is determined by the nature of the underlying abnormality.

Laboratory testing of hemostasis

There are several laboratory tests that are useful for screening patients and evaluating the efficacy of antithrombotic therapy (Gupta et al., 2007; Donegan, 2007). Prothrombin time (PT), activated partial thromboplastin time (aPTT), bleeding time, thrombin time, platelet count, and platelet function analysis 100 (PFA-100) are tests that are commonly used to evaluate hemostasis.

Prothrombin time (PT) tests the extrinsic and common coagulation pathway and includes factors X, VII, V, prothrombin, and fibrinogen. Because three of the factors (prothrombin, VII, and X) are vitamin K dependent, PT is useful for monitoring patients receiving warfarin therapy. The interlaboratory variability of PT is standardized using the international normalized ratio (INR). The INR is the ratio of the patient's PT to the control PT that is standardized to a World Health Organization control that corrects for laboratories using different reagents and thromboplastins to assay the PT. Because the INRs are standardized, the results from different laboratories are essentially equivalent. The normal value of the INR is 1.

Activated partial thromboplastin time (aPTT) tests the intrinsic coagulation pathway (factors VIII, IX, XI, and XII) and common coagulation pathway (factors V, X, prothrombin, and fibrinogen). The aPTT will be prolonged in patients that have factor deficiencies in the intrinsic and common pathways. The aPTT can be used to identify patients that have hemophilia (deficiency in factors VIII and IX) and to monitor patients that are anticoagulated with heparin or direct thrombin inhibitors. The normal value of aPTT is 22–34 seconds. Both PT and aPTT show poor correlation with bleeding risk; rather, they are helpful in monitoring the effect of anticoagulants or the severity of end-stage liver disease.

Bleeding time is measured by the time until bleeding stops after a "standardized" 1 mm slit is made in the skin. The normal time for the bleeding to stop ranges between 7 and 9 minutes. Because of several uncontrollable variables associated with this test, sensitivity, specificity, and predictive information are limited to some extent.

Thrombin time measures the conversion of fibrinogen to fibrin by thrombin. Heparin prolongs thrombin time, while warfarin has little effect. Normal values are less than 10 seconds.

Platelets function is evaluated using the platelet count, bleeding time, and platelet function analysis 100 (PFA-100) (Donegan et al., 2007; Favaloro, 2008). The platelet count identifies patients with thrombocytopenia, but is not indicative of platelet function. As mentioned above, bleeding time can be unreliable and is not a good predictor of perioperative bleeding. However, it is sometimes used to screen for qualitative defects in platelets. PFA-100 can be used to quantitatively measure platelet function. PFA-100 closure time can screen for the effect of aspirin and test for von Willebrand's disease (vWD). PFA-100 testing is currently insensitive to clopidogrel.

Anesthesia Complications in the Dental Office, First Edition. Edited by Robert C. Bosack and Stuart Lieblich.

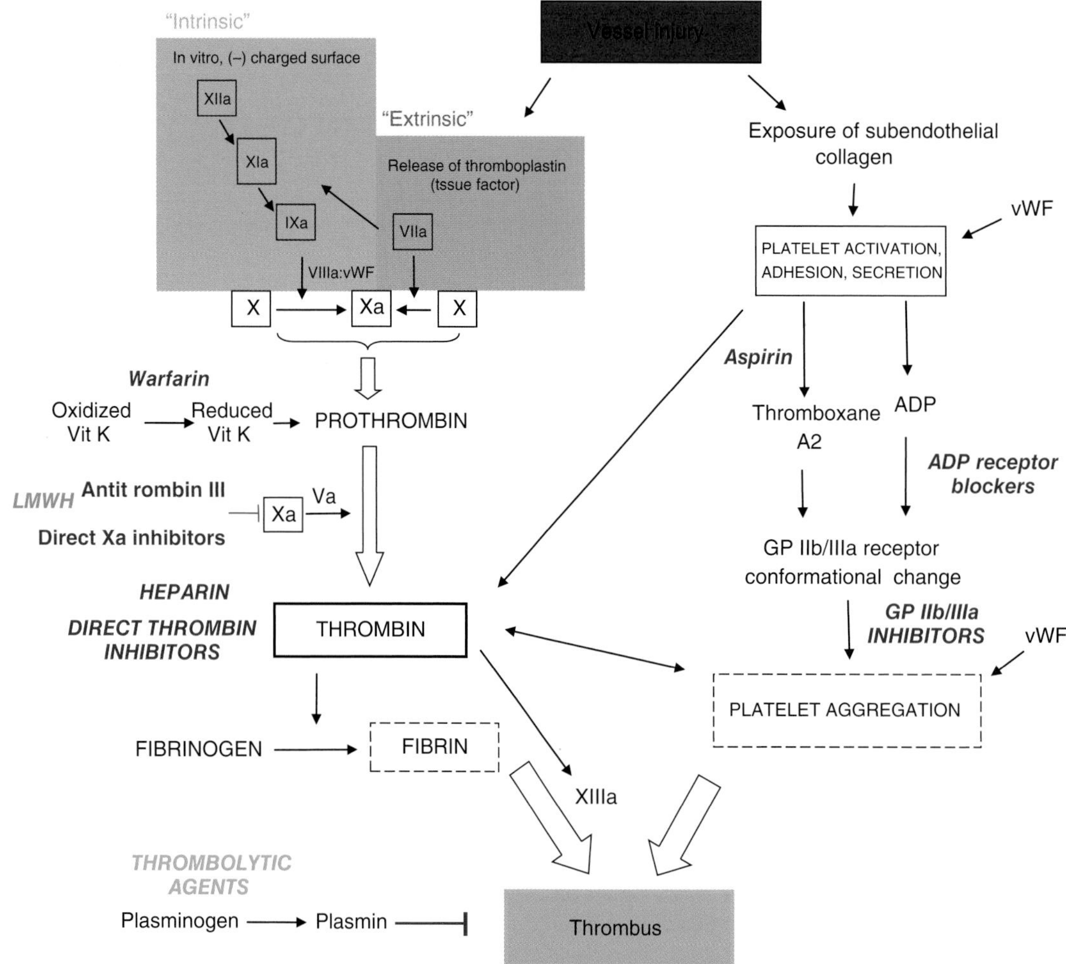

Figure 14.1 Pathways to thrombus formation and sites of drug intervention.

Common bleeding disorders

Von Willebrand's disease

Von Willebrand's disease is an inheritable mutation or drug- or disease-induced condition, which leads to the impairment of synthesis or function of von Willebrand factor (vWBF), which is necessary for satisfactory platelet and factor VIII function (Mannucci, 2004; Yawn et al., 2009). It is the most common bleeding disorder, affecting up to 1% of the population, most of whom remain asymptomatic. There are three types of vWD that present with wide clinical variability. Type I vWD, which is the most common, is an autosomal dominantly inherited disease with a partial quantitative vWBF deficiency. Type III, which is extremely rare, is an autosomal recessively inherited disease, and the patient develops significant bleeding due to a total quantitative deficiency of vWBF. Type II disease is an autosomal dominantly inherited disease that involves a qualitative deficiency of vWBF. Because vWBF normally slows down the turnover of factor VIII, these patients can have symptoms characteristic of hemophilia A in addition to their platelet disorder. Typically, patients with platelet disorders present with immediate, prolonged bleeding of the skin and mucous membranes (oropharyngeal, nasopharyngeal, gastro-intestinal, and uterine) and petechiae, while patients with coagulopathies characteristically present with hemarthroses, muscle hematomas, and expansive ecchymosis.

Treatment is based on disease type and symptom severity, and does not aim to normalize bleeding time, which does not correlate well with disease severity. Desmopressin (1-desamino-8-D-arginine-vasopressin, DDAVP) promotes the release of vWBF from endothelial storage sites, which increases the levels of both vWBF and VIII (vWBF slows factor VIII turnover and prolongs its activity) and can be effective in type I and some type II variants (not 2B). It is ineffective in type III disease. Because DDAVP has an indirect action, tachyphylaxis will occur with repeated dosing. Desmopressin can be administered intravenously or subcutaneously, 0.3 mcg/kg, or intranasally, 300 mcg for patients heavier than 50 Kg and 150 mcg for patients less than 50 Kg. Desmopressin has its peak effect 90 minutes following intravenous administration. Water retention is usually not a problem but diuretics may increase the risk of hyponatremia in patients receiving desmopressin. Because the response to desmopressin is not the same for every patient, the patient's reaction to the desmopressin should be tested before using it to control surgical bleeding. In addition to increasing circulating factor levels, patients with vonWillebrand's disease can be given antifibrinolytic drugs. The release of plasminogen activator by DDAVP mandates consideration of the use of a fibrinolysis inhibitor such as epsilon aminocaproic acid or tranexamic acid.

Patients with type 2 and type 3 disease are usually managed with vWF replacement. All the available vWF replacements are plasma derived from human plasma and all contain factor VIII. The three FDA-approved replacements for vWF are Humate P, Alphanate (not approved for patient with type 3 disease having major surgery), and Wilate. (Table 14.1) A single dose of vWF is administered before tooth extraction and the patients are given antifibrinolytic therapy starting before the extractions and continued for 5–7 days after surgery. Local measures should be applied to prevent bleeding during healing. The initial dose of vWF is 50 units/kg body weight. The half-life of vWF is 12 hours and if repeat dosing is planned the patient should receive half the loading dose every 12–24 hours.

The ristocetin cofactor activity, which measures blood levels of vWF, can also be used to guide vWF dosing. The desired ristocetin cofactor level is subtracted from the patient's blood ristocetin cofactor level and then multiplied by half the patient's body weight. For example, if the patient has a ristocetin cofactor level of 10 IU/dl (10%) and 100 IU/dl (100%) is the target level, the calculated loading dose for vWF in a 70 kg adult would be $(100 - 10\ \text{IU/dl}) \times 70\ \text{kg}/2 = 3150$ units.

If repeat dosing of vWF replacement is planned, factor VIII levels should be measured because repeating doses can cause abnormally high levels of factor VIII (Mannucci, 2004). These high levels develop because factor VIII is included in the vWF replacement and infusion of normal vWF stimulates the patients' production of their own normal factor VIII. Increased levels of factor VIII can trigger thrombosis.

Table 14.1 Coagulation factor replacement products.

Factor	Product	Source
VIII	Hemofil M	Human plasma
	Monoclate P	Human plasma
	Alphanate	Human plasma
	Koate-DVI	Human plasma
	Advate	Recombinant
	Recombinate	Recombinant
	Kogenate FS	Recombinant
	Helixate	Recombinant without human protein
	Xynthia	Recombinant without human protein
IX	Bebulin	Human plasma
	Mononine	Human plasma
	Alphanine	Human plasma
	BeneFIX	Recombinant without human protein
vWF	Wilate	Human plasma
	Humate P	Human plasma
	Alphanate	Human plasma
Activated factor IX Complex	FEIBA	Human plasma
	Autoplex-T	Human plasma
Activated Factor VII	NovoSeven	Recombinant

Antifibrinolytic agents can also be used to prevent dissolution of the hemostatic plug that is formed, especially at mucous membranes, where there is a naturally high fibrinolytic activity. These drugs help prevent bleeding by inhibiting plasminogen activation and slow the breakdown of the fibrin clot. Tranexamic acid (Cyklokapron® and Lysteda®) or epsilon-aminocaproic acid (Amicar®) is started before surgery and continued for 5 to 7 days following surgery. Tranexamic acid can be given intravenously, 10 mg/kg, or orally, 25 mg/kg, followed by the same dose every 6 to 8 hours. Epsilon-aminocaproic acid can be given orally or intravenously. The initial adult oral or intravenous dose is 50 mg/kg, and the maximum dose is 5 gm, before surgery followed by 50 mg/kg every 6 hours for 5–7 days.

Tranexamic acid or epsilon aminocaproic acid can also be used as an oral rinse to control bleeding from tooth extractions (Patatanian and Fugate, 2006; Gupta et al., 2007; Aldridge and Cunningham, 2010). A 10 ml 5% solution of tranexamic acid or epsilon aminocaproic acid is held in the mouth for 2 minutes every 2 hours. The rinse is started just before the extraction of the teeth and repeated for a total of 6-10 doses. Instead of every 2 hours, the 2-minute rinse can be used every 6 hours starting just before the surgery and continued for 5 days after the extraction.

In addition to using an antifibrinolytic agent, topical therapy, which is described at the end of this chapter, can be used to control superficial bleeding.

Hemophilia A and B

Hemophilia A and B are sex-linked recessively inherited bleeding disorders (Gupta et al., 2007; Sahu et al., 2011; Wong and Recht, 2011). Hemophilia A is caused by a defect in factor VIII and hemophilia B is caused by a defect in factor IX. Because both factors are needed to activate factor X, the clinical presentation of hemophilia A and B is identical. Approximately 80% of patients with hemophilia have hemophilia A and 20% have hemophilia B. The majority of patients with hemophilia that present for surgery know that they have a bleeding disorder. However, some children or patients with mild disease and no family history of bleeding problems may be naive to their disease.

Hemophilia A or B can be classified as severe, moderate, or mild. Patients with severe disease have less than 1% factor function, while those with moderate disease have 1–5% factor function and those with mild disease have 6–25% factor function. Individuals with greater than 30% factor usually have normal hemostasis. Individuals with severe disease have spontaneous bleeding and are the most challenging to manage when they need minor or major surgery. Bleeding following tooth extraction in patients with mild, moderate, or severe hemophilia can be difficult to control.

Factor replacement is required for patients with severe hemophilia undergoing major abdominal, thoracic, head and neck, and orthopedic surgery. Factor is replaced before surgery and the factor level is usually maintained for 5–7 days following surgery. Factor is commonly replaced using a dose that increases plasma levels to 80–100% of normal. Factor VIII's half-life is 8–12 hours and after surgery, patients are given half the initial loading dose of factor VIII every 12 hours to maintain the level between 40–80%. Factor IX's half-life is 18–30 hours and patients with hemophilia B are given half the initial loading dose of factor IX every 24 hours instead of every 12 hours.

Bleeding in patients with mild or moderate hemophilia A is sometimes managed using desmopressin (1-desamino-8-D-arginine-vasopressin, DDAVP). Desmopressin does not increase circulating factor IX plasma levels and is ineffective when given to patients with hemophilia B. A single dose of desmopressin will cause a 3–6 fold increase in factor VIII. Because the response to repeated doses of desmopressin decreases with each administration, it cannot be used to increase factor VIII levels for prolonged periods. Desmopressin can be administered intravenously or subcutaneously, 0.3 mcg/kg, or intranasally, as noted in the above protocol for von Willebrand's disease. Water retention is not usually a problem but diuretics may increase the risk of hyponatremia in patients receiving desmopressin. Because the response to desmopressin is not the same for every patient, the patients' reaction to the desmopressin should be tested before using it to control surgical bleeding. In addition to increasing circulating factor levels, patients with hemophilia can be given antifibrinolytic drugs.

Unlike a major maxillofacial surgery, tooth extraction in patients with hemophilia does not usually require repeated dosing of factor. For patients with mild or moderate hemophilia A, a single dose of desmopressin is given before removal of the teeth and tranexamic acid or epsilon-aminocaproic acid is started just before surgery and continued for 5 to 7 days. Local measures, which will be discussed at the end of the chapter, are used to prevent bleeding during healing of the extraction sites.

Factor replacement is needed to prevent bleeding when extracting teeth in all patients with hemophilia B or in patients with severe hemophilia A. A dose of Factor VIII or Factor XI and tranexamic acid or epsilon-aminocaproic acid is administered before removal of teeth. Antifibrinolytic agents are continued for 5–7 days following the surgery. Local measures are also used to prevent bleeding during healing. If the patients have an episode of bleeding after the extraction that cannot be controlled with local measures, another dose of factor can be administered.

Local anesthesia using the inferior alveolar nerve block for packing and suturing bleeding extraction sites before giving another dose of replacement factor is not recommended (Gupta et al., 2007). Without factor replacement, injury to a blood vessel might cause bleeding, which results in swelling and life-threatening obstruction of the airway. Infiltration anesthesia is safer and 4% articaine may be more effective than other local anesthetics because it may have greater bone penetration (Skjevik et al., 2011).

Cryoprecipitate and factor IX concentrates isolated from human blood donors were previously given to increase plasma factor levels and to stop or prevent bleeding (Wong and Recht, 2011). These products controlled bleeding, but they transmitted infectious diseases. Because of the disease transmission, cryoprecipitate and factor IX concentrates have been replaced with safer factor replacements. Recombinant DNA technology as well as improved purification methods with patient screening and viral inactivation of human blood products has produced factor VIII and IX that are much less likely to transmit disease than cryoprecipitate and untreated factor concentrates (Table 14.1).

Improved donor screening and virus inactivation have improved the safety of the replacement factors purified from human blood (Kauffman, 2011; Wong and Recht, 2011). Such methods for concentrating factor VIII and inactivating viruses have produced Hemofil M, Monoclate P, Alphanate, and Koate-DVI. Recombinant DNA technology has been used to produce factor replacements that do not require the use of human blood products. Recombinant factor VIII has been produced through stabilization with human proteins—Advate, Recombinate, and Kogenate FS–and without human proteins–Helixate and Xyntha. There are fewer choices for the replacement of factor IX. Bebulin, Mononine, and Alphanine are plasma-derived factor IX concentrates and BeneFIX is a recombinant factor IX replacement without human proteins (Table 14.1).

Administration of the same dose of factor VIII and factor IX do not produce the same increase in plasma factors (Wong and Recht, 2011). A dose of 1 unit of factor/kg body weight will cause a 2% increase in factor VIII and the same dose of factor IX will produce a 1% increase in factor IX. A single dose of factor that increases factor level to 100% of normal combined with local measures and antifibrinolytic therapy will usually control surgical and post-surgical bleeding associated with minor oral surgery. If a 70-kg patient with hemophilia A has less than 1% circulating factor and 100% replacement is planned before surgery, the calculated dose is the patient's weight in kg/2 × % increase in factor (70 kg/2 × 100% = 3500 units). If the patient will need repeated doses every 12 hours, half of the loading dose or 1750 units would be given to the 70-kg patient.

If a 70-kg patient with hemophilia B has less than 1% factor and 100% replacement is planned before surgery, the calculated dose is the patient's weight in kg X increase in factor (70 kg × 100%= 7000 units). Half the loading dose, 3500 units, would be given every 24 hours if repeated doses are needed to maintain factor IX following surgery.

Hemophilia and inhibitors

Patients with hemophilia can develop inhibitors (Wong and Recht, 2011). Inhibitor levels are measured in Bethesda units (BU). These inhibitors are immunoglobulins that develop in patients that have received multiple doses of factor. Inhibitors develop in approximately 20% of patients with hemophilia A and less than 5% of patients with hemophilia B. The presence of inhibitor should be suspected in patients with hemophilia who develop uncontrolled bleeding following tooth extraction or surgery, which does not respond to repeated factor replacement therapy.

Management of hemophilia patients with inhibitors can be difficult. Before surgery, the inhibitor levels must be measured. Patients that have inhibitor levels of less than 5 BU that do not increase with repeated doses of factor are low responders. Patients with inhibitor levels greater than 5 BU that increase with repeated doses of factor are high responders. Low responders can usually be managed with higher doses of factor replacement. High responders must be managed with factor bypass agents (Table 14.1).

Factor VIIa (Novoseven) is a bypass agent that is produced using recombinant DNA technology (Kauffman, 2011). It is started at a low dose of 30 mcg/kg and increased to 90 mcg/kg every 2–3 hours until bleeding is controlled. FEIBA (factor VIII inhibitor bypassing activity) is an activated prothrombin complex that is produced from human blood for use in hemophilia patients with inhibitors. A dose of 50–100 units/kg is administered every 6–8 hours until bleeding is controlled. No more than 200 units/kg should be administered in 24 hours. Porcine factor VIII can sometimes be used in patients with inhibitors. However, some patients' immunoglobulins cross-react with porcine factor VIII and inactive it.

Thrombocytopenia

Thrombocytopenia is caused by insufficient production or destruction/sequestration of platelets (Donegan et al., 2007; Gupta et al., 2007). Patients with bone marrow suppression from tumors or receiving chemotherapy for malignancy can develop thrombocytopenia. Because the spleen sequesters platelets, patients with enlarged spleens can develop very low levels of circulating platelets.

If the platelet counts are greater than 50,000/mcL, patients will usually have normal hemostasis. However, if the platelet count is below 50,000/mcL, platelet transfusion may be needed to prevent bleeding.

There are two sources for platelets (Marwaha and Sharma, 2009). Platelets can be pooled from individual donors or obtained from a single donor using apheresis. Platelets isolated from six donors are usually combined to make a "six pack" of platelets for transfusion. Transfusion of apheresis platelets from a single donor or a "six-pack" will increase the platelet count to 30,000–60,000/mcL in a 70-Kg patient. A single transfusion will usually be adequate to control surgical bleeding.

Apheresis platelets are considered safer to transfuse than the "six-pack." It is easier to type and cross-match the platelets from a single patient than a pooled sample from six different patients. There is less chance for transmission of infection from single donors than from multiple donor pooled platelets. However, apheresis platelets are more expensive than the pooled packs of platelets.

Antithrombotic therapy

Patients take anticoagulants for a variety of reasons. Inherited coagulopathies include factor V Leiden mutation, protein C or S deficiency, or antithrombin III deficiency. "Acquired" hypercoagulable diseases include atrial fibrillation, immobility, heart failure, atherosclerosis, prosthetic cardiac valves, pregnancy, surgery (especially on legs or pelvis), and malignancy, among others. In general, platelet inhibitors are used to reduce the risk of arterial thrombi, while factor inhibitors are used to prevent venous thrombi.

The management of dental patients taking long-term antithrombotic therapy who need surgery is determined by estimating the balance of risk between the likelihood of significant post-surgical hemorrhage versus the likelihood of a devastating thromboembolic event (Du Breuil and Umland, 2007; Donegan et al., 2007; Thachil et al., 2008; Jaffer, 2009; Vandermeulen, 2010; Aldridge and Cunningham, 2010). Uncomplicated tooth extraction is considered a low risk for bleeding. Extensive, office-based oral surgery, including multiple tooth extractions and surgery near the floor of the mouth, are most often considered an intermediate risk for bleeding. In both situations, the surgical site is usually superficial and exposed, lending itself to topical pressure and medications. There is little evidence to support the discontinuation of therapeutic levels of either antithrombotic, INR $\leq$ 3.5 (Little, 2012), or antiplatelet medications prior to dental surgery (Firriolo and Hupp, 2012). Justifiable concern persists, however, regarding administration of a mandibular block in patients with an INR at the 2.5–3.5 range, as inadvertent vessel injury may occur leading to airway compromise from uncontrollable bleeding in the pterygomandibular space. Thromboembolic risk stratification is shown in Table 14.2. Patients with malignancy and those receiving chemotherapy are also at increased risk of pathologic thrombosis.

If bleeding risk is low, or easily controlled using local measures, antithrombotic therapy is usually continued without interruption

Table 14.2 Thromboembolic risk stratification.

- High Risk
  - Atrial Fibrillation
    - With a prosthetic heart valve in any position
    - With any history of stroke or TIA
    - With rheumatic mitral valve disease
  - Thromboembolism
    - Recurrent (2 or more) thromboembolic events
    - Any thromboembolic event with hypercoagulopathy
    - Any thromboembolic event within 3 months
  - Prosthetic heart valve
    - Any valve placed within 3 months
    - Older style (single leaflet (Bjork-Shiley) or ball in cage (Starr-Edwards)) in mitral position
    - Aortic single leaflet
    - >1 prosthetic heart valve
- Intermediate risk
  - Atrial fibrillation
    - Without history of cardiac embolism, but with risk factors*
  - Thromboembolism
    - Any thromboembolic event within 6 months but no sooner than 3 months
    - two or more strokes or TIAs without risk factors for cardiac embolism
  - Prosthetic heart valve
    - Newer type (bi-leaflet, St. Jude) in the mitral position
    - Older mechanical valves in aortic position
    - Aortic valve and >2 risk factors for cardiac embolism
- Low Risk
  - Atrial fibrillation
    - Without risk factors
  - Thromboembolism
    - Prior events more than 6 months prior
    - Cardiovascular disease and risk factors without prior events
  - Prosthetic heart valve
    - Newer type valve in aortic position

*Risk factors - heart failure, age > 75 years, diabetes mellitus, any history of stroke or TIA.

for all risks of thromboembolism. If significant bleeding is anticipated in low risk patients, therapy can be interrupted by the primary care physician without bridging. If significant bleeding is anticipated in moderate to high risk patients, the possibility of short-term anticoagulation dose reduction or bridging therapy (Table 14.2) can be entertained. For patients at intermediate risk of bleeding and low or intermediate risk of thromboembolism, antithrombotic therapy can be diminished or stopped with or without bridging. Before changing antithroboembolism therapy, the dentist must consult with the patient's primary care provider to coordinate bridging or alterations in the antithrombotic medications.

Antiplatelet therapy

Long-term antiplatelet therapy is given to prevent stroke, MI, and thrombosis of metal and drug-eluting coronary stents (Donegan, 2007; Jaffer, 2009; Chassot, 2010, Aldridge and Cunningham, 2010; Vandermeulen, 2010; Hall and Mazer, 2011). Dual therapy with aspirin and clopidogrel (Plavixl®) is recommended for a minimum of 6 weeks after insertion of a bare metal stent and for 12 months after insertion of a drug-eluting stent. All elective surgery should be delayed for patients with stents until they have completed the recommended course of treatment, to avoid risk of re-thrombosis.

The perioperative management of patients that take long-term continuous antiplatelet therapy is based on the relative risks of bleeding and thrombosis.

Aspirin irreversibly inhibits platelet cyclooxygenase, which decreases thromboxane A2 synthesis and reduces platelet activation and vasodilatation. Onset of action is rapid at 30 minutes for non-enteric coated aspirin. The thienopyridines (clopidogrel (Plavix™) and prasugrel (Effient™) irreversibly inhibit platelets by blocking ADP-induced platelet aggregation. The effects of aspirin and thienopyridines can only be reversed with platelet administration or bone marrow production of platelets. Because the half-life of platelets is 7–10 days, bone marrow production of platelets requires 4 to 7 days to reverse the inhibition of aspirin and thienopyridines.

Glycoprotein (GP) IIb/IIIa receptor inhibitors including abciximab (Reopro®), tirofiban (Aggrastat®), and eptifibatide (Integrilin®) are sometimes used for antiplatelet therapy. The effects of these agents are not as prolonged as aspirin and thienopyridines because the effects of GP IIb/IIIa inhibitors are reversible. Inhibition by abciximab significantly decreases 12–24 hours after discontinuing the medication and the effects of eptifibatide and tirofiban are reversed 4–8 hours after stopping the drugs.

Because anticoagulants are not as effective as antiplatelet therapy for the prevention of thrombosis in coronary stents, GP IIb/IIIa inhibitors, instead of heparin, have been used as bridging therapy for aspirin and thienopyridines (Chassot, 2010; Morrison et al., 2012). Aspirin and thienopyridines are stopped beginning 5 days before surgery and a GP IIb/IIIa inhibitor such as eptifibatide is started 3 days before surgery. The eptifibatide is stopped 6–12 hours before surgery and then aspirin and clopidogrel are started the day after surgery with or without restarting eptifibatide. Bridging avoids prolonged discontinuation of antiplatelet therapy and prevents thrombosis especially in patients taking antiplatelet drugs to prevent a recurrence of coronary thrombosis and in patients with coronary stents that have not completed the recommended period of antiplatelet therapy. Although there are no reports of using GP IIb/IIIa inhibitors for bridging therapy in patients having teeth removed, they theoretically could be used for patients taking aspirin and/or clopidogrel.

There are no well-controlled clinical trials that have established the risks of bleeding and thrombosis with continuing or stopping antiplatelet therapy for minor or major oral and maxillofacial surgery (van Diermen et al., 2009). However, antiplatelet therapy is usually continued for minor oral surgery and local measures are applied to control surgical and post-surgical bleeding. If local measures cannot control the bleeding, stopping the drugs with or without platelet transfusion may be required.

Anticoagulation agents

Patients with atrial fibrillation, mechanical heart values replacements, and thrombotic disorders such as factor V Leiden, or deficiencies of antithrombin III, protein C, or protein S (regulators to limit the extent of coagulation) require life-long anticoagulation therapy to prevent thrombosis (Donegan, 2007; Du Breuil, 2007; Jaffer, 2009; Levy, 2010; Vandermeulen, 2010). There are several drugs that are used to prevent thrombosis. The surgical management of patients taking anticoagulants is determined by the mechanism of action of the drugs, the risk of life-threatening bleeding, and the risk of thrombosis with discontinuing the therapy.

Heparin is a mixture of low and high molecular weight disaccharide fragments that binds antithrombin III and inhibits factor Xa and thrombin. Low dose heparin is used to prevent deep vein thrombosis and high dose intravenous heparin is used to treat deep vein thrombosis and pulmonary emboli. The half-life of intravenous heparin is 1 to 2 hours and the duration of its effects are short. Since heparin has unpredictable binding to plasma proteins, the anticoagulant effect needs to be monitored. The activated partial thromboplastin time (aPTT) is used to monitor high dose heparin, and the therapeutic goal is an aPTT that is 2 times the control value. If a patient receiving heparin needs surgery, intravenous high dose heparin can be stopped 4 hours before surgery and restarted 6–12 hours after surgery. If the patient has uncontrolled bleeding protamine sulfate can be used to reverse the effects of heparin. One mg of protamine neutralizes approximately 100 units of heparin.

Because heparin can cause heparin-inducted thrombocytopenia (HIT), the platelet count should be monitored in patients that are to receive unfractionated heparin for several days. HIT is caused by an immune response to the heparin. Heparin must be stopped immediately if a patient develops HIT.

Unlike high dose heparin treatment, low dose heparin is administered subcutaneously every 8–12 hours before and after surgery to prevent thrombosis. Low dose subcutaneous heparin can effectively prevent deep vein thrombosis and pulmonary embolism associated with surgery without risk of significant bleeding during surgery.

Low molecular weight heparins (LMWHs) are prepared by depolymerizing unfractionated heparin and purifying the smaller fragments. These smaller fragments inhibit Xa more than thrombin. The LMWHs have a longer half-life than unfractionated heparin and the dose is based on the patient weight. Laboratory testing is not required to monitor the LMWHs, whose pharmacokinetics are more predictable than that of heparin.

Enoxaparin (Lovenox®), dalteparin (Fragmin®), and tinazparin (Innohep®) are LMWHs that are administered subcutaneously once or twice a day. Low dose LMWHs are used to prevent deep vein thrombosis and, similarly to low dose heparin, are given immediately before surgery and continued after surgery. High dose LMWHs are used to treat deep vein thrombosis and pulmonary emboli. High dose LMWHs that are administered once a day are stopped on the day of surgery and restarted the day after surgery. If the LMWH is used twice a day, it is stopped on the day of surgery and restarted on the evening of surgery or the day following surgery.

The synthetic Xa inhibitor fondaparinux (Arixtra®) is given subcutaneously once daily and does not require laboratory monitoring. It is used as an anticoagulant in patients with HIT who cannot be given heparin or LMWHs. The elimination half-life is 18–21 hours in patients with normal renal function and 36–42 hours in patients with compromised kidney function. Fondaparinux must be stopped 2–3 days before surgery to reverse its effects. If the risk of bleeding is low, fondaparinux can be continued in patients with high risk for thromboembolism. However, if local measures do not control the bleeding, there are no agents that can immediately reverse fondaparinux.

Other direct factor Xa inhibitors including lepirudin (Refludan®), bivalirudin (Angiomax®), and argatroban (Argatroban®) are given intravenously. These are used for prophylaxis of venous thromboembolism after orthopedic procedures and for patients with HIT. The aPTT can be used to monitor these agents. The half-life for these drugs is less than 2 hours. Therapy can be stopped 4–8 hours before surgery and restarted 2 hours following surgery.

Rivaroxaban (Xarelto™) is an oral Xa inhibitor used for the treatment and prevention of deep vein thrombosis and pulmonary embolism and prevention of deep vein thromboses in patients undergoing hip or knee replacement surgery. It is administered once daily, with an onset of 3 hours and a half-life of 12 hours. The half-life of rivaroxaban is short and if necessary in patient with low or intermediate risk of thrombosis, therapy can be stopped with the recommendation of the patient's primary care physician the day before surgery and restarted the day following surgery (Schulman, 2012). There is no direct reversal agent for rivaroxaban; however, FEIBA, which is used to stop bleeding in hemophiliacs with inhibitors, may stop uncontrolled bleeding in patients taking rivaroxaban (Marlu et al., 2012).

Warfarin (Coumadin®) interferes with the synthesis of the vitamin-K-dependent coagulation factors by inhibiting vitamin K epoxide reductase, which converts vitamin K to vitamin K epoxide. Vitamin K epoxide is needed for the carboxylation of factors II, VII, IX, and X and proteins C and S. Because of numerous drug and dietary interactions and a narrow therapeutic index, patients taking warfarin must have frequent monitoring of the prothrombin time (PT). INR is used to monitor warfarin therapy because it standardizes the interlaboratory variability of the PT assay. Because warfarin interferes with synthesis of several factors, a delayed onset following drug initiation and a delayed offset after drug cessation can be expected. Both metronidazole and macrolide antibiotics can enhance the action of warfarin.

The target INR for prevention of venous thromboembolism and pulmonary embolism is 2–3. The target INR for prevention of thromboembolism in atrial fibrillation is also 2–3. The prophylaxis target in patients with mechanical heart values is a slightly higher INR, 2.5–3.5. The INR must be monitored closely to maintain it within the therapeutic range. The INR is monitored every 4–8 weeks after the dose has been established because changes in diet and drugs including antibiotics can interfere with warfarin.

Minor oral surgery can be done without stopping or altering warfarin therapy. INR should be measured within 24 hours of the surgery and if it is in the therapeutic range, 3.5 or less, surgery can be done. Local (topical) measures should be used to control bleeding. These patients do not develop life-threatening bleeding but will sometimes require treatment for slow oozing of blood that will not stop with pressure.

Because patients having minor oral surgery and continuing warfarin therapy may develop minor bleeding following oral surgery, they should be treated early in the day and at the beginning of the week. Clear post-operative instructions describing the use of local pressure with moistened gauze, no rinsing for 24 hours, no spitting, and no drinking with straws must be given to the patient. Rinsing with 5% solutions of tranexamic acid or epsilon-aminocaproic acid as described for patients with von Willebrand's disease can be used to prevent fibinolysis in anticoagulated patients. Phone numbers to call for help if bleeding occurs after clinic hour should be given to the patient.

Warfarin can be reversed with fresh frozen plasma (FFP) and prothrombin complex concentrates if bleeding cannot be controlled with local measures. Vitamin K can be used to reverse warfarin but the onset of action of the vitamin K is slower than with FFP or prothrombin complex because it takes a few hours for the patient's liver to produce adequate concentrations of factors. If the bleeding is not life-threatening, 1 mg of vitamin K can be administered intravenously. If the patient has a major bleed, FFP or prothrombin complex concentrates and high dose intravenous vitamin K, 5–10 mg, can be given.

If a patient taking warfarin requires surgery with a high risk of bleeding, the warfarin must be stopped. Because it will take several days for the INR to return to normal and because of the possible hypercoagulation condition that may occur when stopping warfarin, bridging with heparin or LMWHs is recommended (Table 14.3). Warfarin is stopped 5 days before surgery and heparin or LMWH is started 3 days before surgery. The INR is measured on the day of surgery and should be less than 1.5. Heparin is stopped 4–6 hours before surgery and restarted 6–8 hours after surgery. LMWHs are stopped 12–24 hours before surgery and restarted 12–24 hours following surgery. The warfarin is restarted 12–24 hours after surgery and the LMWHs are stopped when the INR is in the therapeutic range.

Table 14.3 Example of bridging warfarin therapy using low molecular weight heparins (LMWH).

Days	Medications
4–5 days before surgery	Stop warfarin with INR at 2–3
2–3 days before surgery	Start dalteparin, 100 IU/Kg BID (Dalteparin can be given once a day, 200 IU/Kg) or Start enoxaparin, 1 mg/Kg SQ BID
Day of surgery	Hold AM dose of the LMWH Confirm that the INR < 1.5 Restart dalteparin, 100 IU/Kg, in the evening (Once /day dosing of dalteparin should be restarted the day after surgery, 200 IU/Kg) or Restart enoxaparin, 1 mg/Kg, in the evening
Day after surgery	Restart patient's normal dose of warfarin Continue the Dalteparin once per day or BID or Continue the enoxaparin BID Stop the LMWH when the INR is therapeutic (2–3)

Oral dabigatran (Pradaxa®) is a specific, reversible inhibitor of both free and fibrin-bound thrombin (van Ryn et al., 2010). It is currently used for prevention of cardiac thromboembolic events in patients with non-valvular atrial fibrillation. Dabigatran's predictable pharmacokinetic profile includes an onset of action at 2–4 hours with a half-life of 12–17 hours. Unlike warfarin, dabigatran does not require laboratory monitoring; however, aPTT and TT will be altered by this drug. The adult dose is 150 mg once or twice daily. There is no antidote for dabigatran; however, FEIBA may overcome the effects of dabigatran in patients with life-threatening bleeding (Marlu et al., 2012). A decision to hold dabigatran is made by the primary care physician. Reversal of the drug depends on renal function because termination of the drug's effect relies on renal excretion. If a decision to withhold this drug is made, a 1-day abstinence is recommended with creatinine clearance > 80mL/min (van Ryn, 2010).

There are no studies examining dabigatran and tooth extraction. However, for patients requiring minor oral surgery, dabigatran can be continued and local measures used to control bleeding. If the patients develop bleeding that cannot be controlled with local measures, dabigatran can be stopped and its effects will be reversed in 1–2 days, depending on renal function.

Local (topical) hemostatic measures

There are several local treatments that have been used to control bleeding from tooth extractions and minor surgical wounds (Gupta et al., 2007; Perry et al., 2007; Aldridge and Cunningham, 2010; Ogle et al., 2011). Injection of local anesthesia with vasoconstrictor causes vasoconstriction and slows bleeding. Applying pressure with moist gauze over the extraction socket or wound will stop bleeding and aid coagulation. The wounds can be packed with various resorbable materials that will control bleeding. Tannic acid in tea is a well-established hemostatic agent that stimulates vasoconstriction.

Porcine-derived gelatin sponges (Gelfoam®) that stabilize the clot and resorb in 3–7 days can be placed into tooth extraction socket. Gelfoam can also be used to carry activated thrombin into extraction sockets. Recombinant human thrombin or bovine-activated thrombin is reconstituted to a concentration of 1000 U/ml and absorbed into the Gelfoam and placed into the extraction site. The thrombin in the Gelfoam converts fibrinogen into fibrin, the last step in coagulation before cross-linking of the fibrin.

Oxidized methylcellulose (Surgicel®) is derived from plants. Similarly to Gelfoam®, Surgicel® stabilizes the clot. Surgicel® is acidic and stimulates platelet aggregation. It cannot be used as a carrier for thrombin because the acidity of the material may inactivate the thrombin. Surgicel® resorbs slowly but does not need to be removed.

Bovine collagen (Colla-Plug®, Avitene®) is available in various forms for application to wounds and extraction sockets. Microfibrillar collagen and collagen sponges can be placed in extraction sites. The collagen stabilizes the clot and attracts platelets and triggers aggregation. Collagen should not be used as a carrier for thrombin because it can inactivate the thrombin.

Gelatin–thrombin combinations (Floseal®, Gelfoam Plus®) can be inserted into tooth extraction sites or placed over a bleeding wound. Gelatin is bovine derived and the thrombin is concentrated from human blood products. The gelatin seals the bleeding wound and the thrombin converts the fibrinogen at the surgical site to fibrin.

Chitosan sponges (HemCon®), which are a polysaccharide composed of D-glucosamine and D-acetyl-glucosamine that is derived from the exoskeleton of shell fish, can be used to control bleeding (Ogle, 2011). Negatively charged red blood cells bind to the positively charged chitosan, creating a hemostatic plug. The chitosan does not require an intact coagulation pathway to control bleeding. HemCon® has been approved by the United States Food and Drug Administration for insertion into extraction sites to control bleeding. Chitosan sponges are biocompatible and biodegradable.

Topical application of fibrin sealants (Tisseel®, Evicel®, Crosseal®, Artiss®) can control bleeding. Fibrin sealants are formed by using human blood-derived thrombin and fibrinogen. The thrombin and fibrinogen are concentrated from human blood. The concentrates are treated to inactivate viruses to prevent transmission of infectious diseases. The two components, fibrinogen and thrombin, are supplied in separate syringes that are connected to a single needle. As the two components are injected through the single needle, the thrombin and fibrinogen are combined and will form a fibrin seal, which directly controls bleeding at the surgical wound.

The efficacy of the various topical hemostatic agents has not been established for patients with bleeding disorders. The agents have different mechanisms of action. Some agents stabilize the clot while others bypass normal hemostasis or directly form fibrin. Agents such as chitosan create a plug that stops bleeding without forming fibrin. Selection of local hemostatic agents is based on the surgeon's experience and understanding of the mechanism of action of the agents.

Summary

Patients with bleeding disorder that require surgery are challenging to manage. Patients with deficient coagulation factors can sometimes be treated using only local measures. If local measures do not control bleeding the deficient factor must be replaced. Ideally, the factors should be replaced with recombinant products to avoid transmission of infections and reaction to contaminants in factors concentrated from human blood.

For patients on antithromboembolic therapy, the risk of bleeding must be balanced against the risk of thrombosis. For minor oral surgery, antithromboemobolic therapy can be continued with the aggressive use of topical hemostatic agents and antifibrinolytic medications. If the risk of bleeding is high, bridging therapy is sometimes required to minimize the time that the patient is not receiving antithromboembolic therapy. The surgeon and the patient's primary care physician must work together to develop a plan to avoid complications in patients receiving antithromboembolic therapy.

References

Aldridge, E. and Cunningham, L.L. Jr., Current thoughts on treatment of patients receiving anticoagulation therapy. *J Oral Maxillofac Surg* **68**: 2879–2887, 2010.

Chassot, P.G., et al. Perioperative antiplatelet therapy. *Am Fam Phys* **82**: 1486–1489, 2010.

Donegan, E., et al. In: (eds.) R.K. Stoelting & R.D. Miller *Basics of Anesthesia* 5th edn pp 331–346. Philadelphia: Churchhill Livingstone, 2007.

Du Breuil, A. L. and Umland, E.M. Outpatient management of anticoagulation therapy. *Am Fam Phys* **75**: 1032–1042, 2007.

Favaloro, E.J. Clinical utility of the PFA-100. *Semin Thromb Hemost* **34**:709–733, 2008.

Firriolo, F. J. and Hupp, W. S. Beyond warfarin: the new generation of oral anticoagulants and their implications for the management of dental patients. *Oral Surg Oral Med Oral Pathol Oral Radiol* **113**: 431–441, 2012.

Gupta, A., et al. Bleeding disorders of importance in dental care and related patient management. *J Can Dent Assoc* **73**:77–83, 2007.

Hall, R. and Mazer, C.D. Antiplatelet drugs: A review of their pharmacology and management in the perioperative period. *Anesth Analg* **112**: 292–318, 2011.

Jaffer, A.K. Perioperative management of warfarin and antiplatelet therapy. *Cleve Clin J Med* **76** (Suppl. 4), S37–S44, 2009.

Kauffman, J. Recombinant infusion therapies indicated for bleeding disorders. *J Infus Nurs* **34**: 29–35, 2011.

Levy, J.H. and Azran, M. Anesthetic concerns for patient with coagulopathy. *Curr Opin Anaesthesiol* **23**: 400–405, 2010.

Little, J. W. New oral anticoagulants: will they replace warfarin? *Oral Surg Oral Med Oral Pathol Oral Radiol* **113**: 575–580, 2012.

Mannucci, P.M. Treatment of von Willebrands' disease. *New Engl J Med* **351**: 68–694, 2004.

Marlu, R., et.al. Effect of non-specific reversal agents on anticoagulation activity of dabigatran and rivaroxaban: a random crossover ex-vivo study in healthy volunteers. *Thromb Heomost* **108**:217–224, 2012.

Marwaha, N. and Sharma, R.R. Consensus and controversies in platelet transfusion. *Tranfus Apheresis Sci* **41**: 127–133, 2009.

Morrison, T.B., et al. Bridging with glycoprotein IIb/IIIa inhibitor for periprocedural management of antiplatelet therapy in patients with drug eluting stents. *Cathet Cardiovas Intervent* **79**(4), 575–582, 2012.

Norris, L.A. Blood coagulation. *Best Pract Res Clin Obstet Gynaecol* **17**:369–383, 2003.

Ogle, O. E., et al. Hemostatic Agents. *Dent Clin N Am* **55**: 433–439, 2011.

Patatanian, E. and Fugate, S.E. Hemostatic mouthwashes in anticoagulated patients undergoing dental extraction. *Ann Pharmacother* **40**: 2205–2210, 2006.

Perry, D.J., et al. Guidelines for the management of patients on oral anticoagulants requiring dental surgery. *Brit Dent J* **203**: 389–393, 2007.

Sahu, S., et al. Revisiting hemophilia management in acute medicine. J Emerg Trauma Shock **4**:292–298, 2011.

Schulman, S, and Crowther, M.A. How I treat with anticoagulants in 2012: new and old anticoagulants, and when and how to switch. *Blood* **119**:3016–3023, 2012.

Skjevik, A.A., et al. Intramolecular hydrogen bonding in articaine can be related to superior bone tissue penetration: a molecular dynamic study. *Biophy Chem* **154**: 18–25, 2011.

Thachil, A., et al. Management of surgical patients receiving anticoagulation and antiplatelet agents. *Br. J Surg.* **95**: 1437–1448, 2008.

Vandermeulen, E. Regional anaesthesia and anticoagulation. *Best Pract Res Clin Anaesth* **24**: 121–131, 2010.

van Diermen, D.E., et al. Dental management of patients using antithrombotic drugs: critical appraisal of existing guidelines. *Oral Surg Oral Med Oral Patholol Oral Radiol Endodont* **107**: 616–624, 2009.

van Ryn, J. et al. Dabigatran etexilate - a novel, reversible, oral direct thrombin inhibitor: Interpretation of coagulation assays and reversal of anticoagulant activity. *Thrmob Haemost* **103**: 1116–1127, 2010.

Wong, T. and Recht M. Current options and new developments in the treatment of haemophilia. *Drugs* **71**:305–320, 2011.

Yawn, B.P., et al. Diagnosis and management of von Willibrand disease: Guidelines for primary care. *Am Fam Physician* **80**: 1261–1268, 2009.

15 Anesthetic considerations for patients with cancer

Andrea M. Fonner[1] and Robert C. Bosack[2]
[1]Private Practice, Seattle, WA, USA
[2]University of Illinois, College of Dentistry, Chicago, IL, USA

Introduction

Cancer is the uncontrolled growth of cells that have sustained genetic mutation, usually, but not always, due to considerable exposure to carcinogens such as tobacco, alcohol, and sunlight in a susceptible host. Invasive spread typically follows pathways of least resistance (often lymphatics), as these cells are capable of evading normal immunologic destruction. Cancer is the second leading cause of death in the United States after cardiovascular disease, but its prevalence is increasing with a growing elderly population (American Cancer Society, 2012). Patients with malignancy often require palliative dental care because of (understandable) neglect, complications of the disease, or complications from the treatment of the disease. Sedation or general anesthesia can serve as an appropriate way to keep patients with cancer comfortable during a dental procedure. A growing number of patients successfully overcome their cancer, but may still be left with permanent side effects of therapy. Notably, survivors of Hodgkin's lymphoma may carry a risk of coronary artery disease, stroke, valvulopathy, and thyroid disease (Oeffinger, 2006).

Classification and treatment of malignancy

Most malignant tumors are solid masses, which can compress, distort, invade, or interfere with the blood flow of organs. Many lead to a hypercoagulable state because of higher levels of cytokines, clotting factors, and cancer procoagulant A (Gouin-Thibault, 2001). A host of qualitative and/or quantitative disorders of blood elements are also possible.

The extensive variety of cancers can compromise every major organ system. The most common types of cancer affect the lung, breast, prostate, and colon. *Lung cancer* is the leading cause of cancer deaths in men and women and accounts for nearly one-third of all cancer-related deaths in the United States despite the over 400,000 lung cancer survivors. Treatment includes surgery, radiation therapy, and chemotherapy, based on the type, size, location, patient factors, and tumor behavior. The 5-year survival rate for all stages combined is only 16% (Howlander, 2011). *Breast cancer* is the most frequently diagnosed cancer in women and is the second leading cause of cancer death in women (after lung cancer). Treatment usually involves a lumpectomy or mastectomy and typically removal of some underarm lymph nodes. When full axillary node dissection is necessary, it is important to consider placement of blood pressure cuffs and intravenous catheters in the contralateral arm if possible for fear of aggravating or causing lymphedema, which can be difficult to resolve. The 5-year survival rate for breast cancer has improved considerably within the last several decades, and is now approaching 90%. *Prostate cancer* is the most frequently diagnosed cancer in men aside from skin cancer and is the second leading cause of cancer death in men. Treatment options vary depending on age, stage, and grade of cancer, as well as other medical conditions. Over the past 25 years, the 5-year survival rate for all stages combined has increased from 68% to almost 100%. *Colorectal cancer* is the third most common cancer in both men and women and accounts for 9% of all cancer deaths. Surgery is the most common treatment for colorectal cancer and can be curative if the disease has not spread. The 5-year survival rate for all stages is 64%. At least 50% of the above patients will develop metastatic disease (Schottenfeld, 2000).

Common cancer therapies

Cancer represents a disruption of the body's homeostasis, and the common therapies available for cancer treatment can disrupt this even further. Treatment risk includes damage to healthy tissues, which may or may not be clinically evident (Latham and Greenberg, 2010a). Common therapies for the management of cancer include chemotherapy, surgery, and radiation or often a combination therapy of the three.

Chemotherapy

Chemotherapeutic agents act by disrupting cell proliferation by inhibiting RNA, DNA, or protein synthesis, in a manner that preferentially maximizes the destruction of cancer cells while minimizing damage to normal tissues. Adverse side effects are both expected and tolerated. Residual effects of chemotherapy can cause unpredictable or life-threatening perioperative complications. Two types of chemotherapeutic agents deserve special attention from the anesthesiologist – anthracyclines and bleomycin.

The anthracycline class of chemotherapeutic agents includes daunorubicin (Cerubidine®), doxorubicin (Adriamycin®), and epirubicin (Ellence®). FDA-approved uses of these agents include the treatment of breast cancer, lung cancer, sarcoma, leukemia, or lymphoma. Cardiac toxicity is rare with some agents, but may occur in >20% of patients treated with anthracyclines. These agents

Anesthesia Complications in the Dental Office, First Edition. Edited by Robert C. Bosack and Stuart Lieblich.

have the ability to cause cardiotoxic effects that can manifest as decreased cardiac performance, which can endure for years after therapy. These changes include coronary vasospasm, rhythm and pressure disturbances, thrombosis, reduced systolic left ventricular function, and congestive heart failure. Electrocardiographic changes such as dysrhythmias and QT prolongation are a common sign of post-anthracycline cardiotoxicity. These symptoms can occur immediately or can be delayed by months and sometimes years, possibly only to manifest during the unintended stress of anesthesia. (Huettemann and Sakka, 2005).

Bleomycin is typically used to treat testicular cancer, lymphoma, squamous cell carcinoma, and malignant pleural effusions. Significant, but often clinically silent lung injury such as pulmonary fibrosis can be seen in 2–40% of patients that receive this drug. In addition to the adverse pulmonary effects, bleomycin has been implicated in the causation of rapidly progressive severe pulmonary oxygen toxicity to patients on high inspiratory oxygen fractions (F_iO_2) during anesthesia. The current recommendation for patients that have received bleomycin is to assess for possible risk factors prior to anesthesia. These factors include evidence of preexisting bleomycin pulmonary damage, bleomycin exposure within the previous 1–2 months, or a total bleomycin dose >450 mg. Single breath CO diffusing capacity (DLCO) is the most sensitive indicator of subclinical damage. A fall of 10–15% should be considered significant. Patients with no major risk factors appear to be at negligible risk from hyperoxia exposure and can be managed accordingly. Patients with one or more risk factors should be maintained on the lowest F_iO_2 to maintain $SpO_2 > 90\%$. When using a nasal cannula at 2–3 liters per minute, the F_iO_2 is estimated to be between 29–33%. The formula to calculate F_iO_2 for a nasal cannula or simple mask is $F_iO_2 = 21\% + [4 \times \text{flow rate (in lpm)}]$.

Radiation

Radiation is an integral part of cancer treatment and is commonly used in combination with chemotherapy and surgery. Permanent tissue fibrosis resulting in trismus and limited tongue, pharyngeal, and neck mobility can occur in patients who have had radiation to the head and neck region. A normal airway examination does not preclude intubation difficulty. Delayed onset mucositis is a familiar finding. Radiation to the mediastinum poses a potential risk of damage to both myocardium and coronary arteries, resulting in accelerated coronary artery disease, conduction abnormalities, and valvular fibrosis. This risk increases when radiation therapy is combined with the use of any anthracycline chemotherapeutic agents. Pulmonary fibrosis can also be expected. Radiation to the abdomen can lead to nausea, vomiting, diarrhea, adhesions, and stenotic lesions.

Surgery

Over 90% of patients diagnosed with cancer will undergo some sort of surgical procedure related to their diagnosis. While some may have the tumor completely removed, others may have surgical procedures done to help with life-saving therapy (i.e. intravenous port inserted) or to improve their quality of life.

Pathophysiological changes associated with malignancy

Chronic and acute pain

Pain is one of the most common symptoms associated with cancer. It occurs in 25% of patients with newly diagnosed malignancies and in 75% of those with advanced disease. A frequent cause of pain is the metastatic spread of the cancer, particularly to bones. These patients are frequently on chronic opioid therapy, which should be continued in the perioperative period. As expected, opioid tolerance is possible, which may necessitate larger doses to minimize surgical stress. Ketamine is an excellent adjunct for pain control in these patients as it works at the N-methyl-D-aspartate receptor rather than at the opioid receptors, and it is analgesic in subanesthetic doses. At the other end of the spectrum, unintentional narcotic overdosage is possible in patients who have not disclosed the use of fentanyl patches, especially when placed in the immediate past.

Psychological distress and depression

Chronic and acute pain issues can lead to psychological distress and depression. Current research is investigating the role that psychological distress and depression play in the overall prognosis for cancer therapy. Tricyclic antidepressant drugs are recommended for those patients who remain depressed despite improved pain control. Careful consideration of drug interactions must be contemplated prior to administering sedation or anesthetic medications.

Vascular access

Vascular access can be difficult in patients with cancer, and special consideration must be given to the location of the intravenous catheter. If patients are currently undergoing chemotherapy, a central line or peripherally inserted central catheter (PICC) might be in place (Figure 15.1). These ports are ideal for the administration of intravenous medication, once patency is confirmed with saline.

Drug metabolism

Most of the drugs we use for sedation in dentistry, such as benzodiazepines, opioids, and local anesthetics, are biotransformed by the cytochrome P450 enzyme system. Many chemotherapeutic agents can inhibit these enzymes, resulting in overdosage or delayed recovery, especially with orally administered medication (Beijnen and Schellens, 2004).

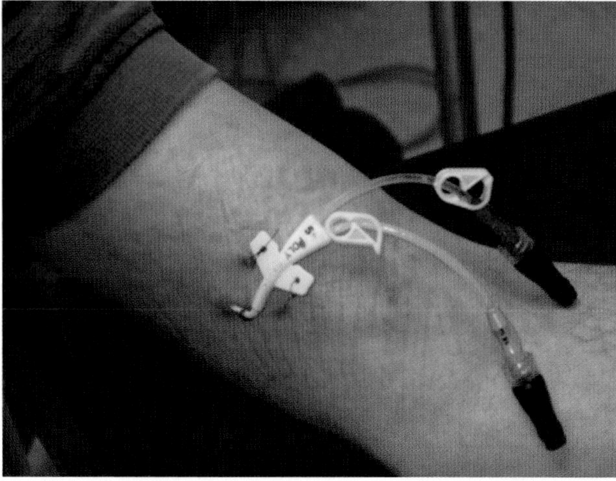

Figure 15.1 Peripherally inserted central catheters (PICC) are large-bore intravenous catheters whose tips lie near the heart. This serves as an ideal route for any intravenous medication, including sedatives and pain medication.

Cardiac toxicity

Cardiac toxicity can occur with certain chemotherapeutic agents such as anthracyclines or patients that have received radiation to the chest, resulting in conduction defects, radiation-induced myocardial ischemia, anthracycline and radiation-induced cardiomyopathy, peripheral vascular disease, and pericardial disease. Delayed cardiac toxicity (years after chemotherapy) has been seen only after anthracycline therapy. For this reason, a cardiology consultation is advisable prior to the sedation or anesthesia.

Pulmonary toxicity

Adverse pulmonary reactions such as acute non-cardiogenic pulmonary edema are likely to occur in 5–10% of patients undergoing chemotherapy (McDonald et al., 2000). Another 5–20% of patients undergoing radiation are likely to develop radiation pneumonitis. More commonly, a late-onset bleomycin-related pulmonary fibrosis can occur. Symptoms of pulmonary fibrosis include dyspnea or non-productive cough. If suspected, maintaining a low F_iO_2 is suggested to prevent hyperoxia.

Hematologic considerations

Anemia, neutropenia, thrombocytopenia, and platelet dysfunction are possible in cancer patients as a result of chemotherapy or malignancy involving these cells, affecting bone marrow function. Bleeding and increased susceptibility to infection can result. Deep vein thrombosis is also a concern for patients with cancer, with risk approaching 30%, especially in patients with obesity or advanced age.

Renal and hepatic failure

Kidney dysfunction can be a direct complication from tumor invasion or can be a result of chemotherapy, especially cisplatin or high dose methotrexate or damage from tumor products. It can also occur as a result of inadequate renal perfusion from dehydration or cardiac failure. Care must be given when using nonsteroidal anti-inflammatory agents to patients receiving nephrotoxic chemotherapy, as it could precipitate acute renal failure. Liver failure also remains a possibility, increasing the spectrum and severity of coagulopathy and malnutrition.

Gastrointestinal considerations

Nausea, vomiting, diarrhea, and enteritis and vomiting are common side effects of cancer treatment. The resultant dehydration, electrolyte imbalance, and malnutrition, aggravated by decreased appetite and malabsorption will have a significant effect on anesthetic technique. Albumin levels <3g/dL are significant (Smetana et al., 2006). Approximately half of all cancer patients will develop cachexia. Symptoms include weight loss, anorexia, muscle atrophy, fatigue, weakness, significant loss of appetite, and impaired immune function. Patients with cachexia have a reduced quality of life, lower activity level, and a reduced survival time.

Nervous system considerations

Reversible autonomic neuropathies are possible, leading to cardiovascular instability, such as orthostatic hypotension. Chronic steroid therapy can lead to non-specific myopathies affecting balance and respiration (Holt, 2012).

Metabolic imbalances

Hyponatremia (low serum sodium) can be a complication of brain tumors, a toxic side effect of medication, or the result of poor oral intake during the end stages of cancer. Symptoms can include malaise, fatigue, confusion, delirium, and seizures. Hypercalcemia (high serum calcium) occurs in up to 5% of all cancer patients. Symptoms can be nonspecific as they include fatigue, nausea, abdominal pain, constipation, depression, and delirium.

Airway considerations

Radiation or chemotherapy-induced mucositis and mucosal friability increase the likelihood of hemorrhage when instrumenting the upper airway. Radiation-induced fibrosis can limit mobility of the mouth, tongue, neck, and pharyngeal structures, which can increase the difficulty with mask ventilation and/or intubation. Advanced airways adjuncts, such as the video laryngoscope, can be very useful in managing the unintentional lost airway.

Anesthetic concerns

A comprehensive patient assessment (Table 15.1) is crucial to understanding critical anesthesia considerations. The accrual of this information is challenging by the sheer number of treating physicians and ancillary medical caregivers, rapidly changing conditions of the patient, and complex medical and chemotherapeutic regimes. Because there are no set guidelines available to determine the course of treatment for cancer patients, it is important to determine the severity of the cancer, chemotherapeutic exposure, radiation exposure, and comorbid non-malignant diseases (Smetana et al., 2006). As there is insufficient data to recommend any routine pre-anesthetic testing, a history-driven focused laboratory investigation can be helpful (Latham and Greenberg, 2010b) Consultation with the oncologist is most valuable for patient assessment. Blood dyscrasias, electrolyte abnormalities, anemias, coagulopathies, and nutritional deficiencies should be optimized or corrected prior to sedation or anesthesia.

There is insufficient evidence to favor any one anesthetic technique (Arain and Buggy, 2007). The use of effective local anesthesia in appropriate doses rarely leads to systemic complications. Systemic use of benzodiazepines, opioids, and possibly hypnotics is often necessary for optimal patient care, but can invite untoward complications when used inappropriately. A fully monitored, "low and slow" protocol is prudent because of the possibility of decreased protein binding, decreased volume of distribution (dehydration and decreased muscle and fat stores), and inhibition of cytochrome enzymes. In general, cancer patients, especially the elderly, are assumed to have a decreased physiologic reserve so vitally necessary in instances of hypoxia, tachycardia, or hypotension. Supplemental

Table 15.1 Patient assessment points.

1 Type, severity, stage, behavior, and past/current treatment of cancer
  (a) Treatment side effects
2 Comorbid disease, level of optimization
3 Current list of medications, including narcotics
4 Exercise tolerance, results of recent stress tests
5 Shortness of breath, cough
6 Level of immunosuppression / bone marrow suppression, nutritional status
  (a) CBC, hemostasis, electrolytes, liver and kidney function, albumin, glucose
7 Vital signs, ECG, pulmonary function tests
8 Upper airway exam

oxygen is always appropriate to maintain oxygen saturation above 90%, to prolong the oxygen saturation in patients with an unexpected compromised airway. A prolonged apneic response to succinylcholine should be anticipated in patients who have been treated with cyclophosphamide, as this drug is known to inhibit plasma cholinesterase.

References

American Cancer Society. *Cancer facts & figures*. Atlanta, GA: American Cancer Society, 2012.

Arain, M. R. and Buggy, D. J. Anaesthesia for cancer patients. *Curr Opin Anaesthesiol* **20**: 247–253, 2007.

Beijnen, J. H. and Schellens, J. H. Drug interactions in oncology. *Lancet Oncol* **5**: 489–496, 2004.

Gouin-Thibault, I., et al. The thrombophilic state in cancer patients. *Acta Haematol* **106**: 33–42, 2001.

Holt, N. F., Cancer, *in* Hines, R. L. and Marschall, K. E. (eds): *Stoelting's Anesthesia and Co-Existing Disease*, 6th edn. Philadelphia: Saunders Elsevier, 2012.

Howlader, N., et al. *SEER Cancer Statistics Review, 1975-2008*, Bethesda, MD: National Cancer Institute, 2011.

Huettemann, E. and Sakka, S. G. Anaesthesia and anti-cancer chemotherapeutic drugs. *Curr Opin Anaesthesiol* **18**: 307–314, 2005.

Latham, G. J. and Greenberg, R. S. Anesthetic considerations for the pediatric oncology patient – Part 2: systems-based approach to anesthesia. *Pediatr Anesth* **20**: 396–420, 2010a.

Latham, G. J. and Greenberg, R. Anesthetic considerations for the pediatric oncology patient – Part 3: pain, cognitive dysfunction and per-operative evaluation. *Pediatr Anesth* **20**: 479–489, 2010b.

McDonald, S., et al. Pulmonary Complications, *in* Abeloff, M. D., et al. (eds): *Clinical Oncology*, 2nd edn, New York: Churchill Livingstone, 2000.

Oeffinger, K. C., et al. Chronic health conditions in adult survivors of childhood cancer. *N Engl J Med* **355**: 1572–1582, 2006.

Sahai, S. K. and Zalpour, A. Preoperative evaluation of the oncology patient. *Anesthesiol Clin* **27**: 805–822, 2009.

Schottenfeld, D. Epidemiology, *in* Abeloff, M. D., et al., (eds): *Clinical Oncology*, 2nd edn. New York: Churchill Livingstone, 2000.

Smetana, G. W., et al. Preoperative pulmomary risk stratification for noncardiothoracic surgery: systematic review for the American College of Physicians, *Ann Intern Med* **144**: 581–595, 2006.

16 Anesthetic considerations for pregnant and early postpartum patients

Robert C. Bosack
[1]University of Illinois, College of Dentistry, Chicago, IL, USA
[2]Private Practice Oral, Maxillofacial and Implant Surgery, Chicago, IL, USA

Pregnant patients will occasionally present for dental/oral surgical treatment, usually on an emergent basis. The physiologic and anatomic changes that accompany pregnancy and early postpartum introduce many variables that can lead to complications during office-based anesthesia. These complications can be minimized through an accurate preanesthetic evaluation, appropriate consultation with the patient's obstetrician, and judicious use of anesthetic agents.

All females of childbearing years should be questioned about possible pregnancy. A small percentage of female patients, who are naïve to their pregnancy, will be exposed to surgery and general anesthesia (Reitman and Flood, 2011, Hennrikus et al., 2001.) Although the risk of miscarriage cannot be ruled out, the absence of reports of birth defects in these cases suggests that anesthesia is well tolerated during the first trimester (Cohen-Kerem et al., 2005). Currently, there is no regulatory group that mandates routine pregnancy testing. Any possibility of pregnancy should be resolved with blood or urine testing prior to elective procedures. Pregnancy awareness has been shown to improve with the manner of questioning. "As far as you know, this morning, are you pregnant?" is more predictive of discovering pregnancy versus "Are you pregnant?" (Milles, 2008)

Anxiety and pain should be minimized to avoid increases in endogenous catecholamines with attendant tachycardia, increase in oxygen utilization, and a decrease in vital capacity. Hyperventilation decreases uterine blood flow and impairs oxygen transport. Changes associated with pregnancy often render the pregnant patient more sensitive to the actions of narcotics and may decrease local anesthetic and sedative requirements. As with all patients, the minimal amount (both number of drugs and dose of drugs) of anesthesia necessary to complete the procedure safely and comfortably is the amount that should be used. It is easy (but time consuming) to carefully titrate and give more medication as needed; however, it is difficult to remove or counteract the medication once it has been given.

Concern over the increased morbidity for the pregnant patient and developing fetus usually centers on the severity and duration of the underlying disease process requiring anesthesia and not on the one-time use of anesthetic agents, which, at worst, alters maternal and fetal physiology for only a short period of time. Current practice is to avoid elective surgery during pregnancy and defer necessary treatment to the second trimester to minimize risks of teratogenicity, spontaneous miscarriage, and preterm labor. Consultation with the patient's obstetrician is prudent. Despite the fact that no anesthetic agent has been proved to be teratogenic in humans (Fisher et al., 2008), local anesthesia remains preferable to general anesthesia, using the least necessary amount of drugs with good safety records.

The risks of anesthesia *to the pregnant patient* are hypoxemia, acidosis, and alterations in blood pressure. The risks of anesthesia *to the developing fetus* are drug teratogenicity, hypoxemia, and triggering of premature labor. (Rosen, 1999).

Maternal concerns

Maternal physiologic and anatomic changes accommodate the developing fetus and adapt the mother to withstanding the growing metabolic demands of pregnancy and delivery. All organ systems are affected; changes in the respiratory, cardiovascular, gastrointestinal, and central nervous systems are most relevant to anesthetic management. (Mhuireachtaigh and O'Gorman, 2006) These changes persist into the early postpartum period—a time soon after delivery when the patient with dental needs will seek immediate treatment.

Respiratory system

Upper airway management during sedation becomes more challenging with advancing gestational age, including the ability maintain an upper airway, the ability to achieve adequate mask ventilation, and the ability to intubate. Reasons include excessive weight gain, upper airway mucosal edema (hormonal mediated vascular engorgement), and an increase in total body water. Upper airway secretions can also be increased, which increases the likelihood of upper airway obstruction. Mucosal edema can make emergent intubation more difficult and traumatic, requiring a smaller sized endotracheal tube to be used. Gentle instrumentation with tonsillar suctioning and/or laryngoscopy minimizes trauma and bleeding in the upper airway.

An *increase in oxygen consumption* is satisfied by an *increase in minute ventilation*, mostly due to an increase in tidal volume (and not ventilatory rate) This increase in minute ventilation leads to quicker induction of anesthesia with inhalational agents.

Anesthesia Complications in the Dental Office, First Edition. Edited by Robert C. Bosack and Stuart Lieblich.

Hyperventilation leads to a modest hypocarbia, compensated by a decrease in plasma bicarbonate levels.

The gravid uterus exerts upward pressure on the diaphragm, especially when supine. This leads to a *decrease in the functional residual capacity* (FRC, oxygen reserve) of approximately 20%. The increase in oxygen consumption combined with a decrease in FRC often leads to quicker desaturation with upper airway obstruction, in spite of seemingly adequate preoxygenation. The consequences of transient hypoxia are worsened during pregnancy, since it can lead to a decrease in fetal pH and can become additive to other undetected problems, such as toxemia (pre-eclampsia.) An acidotic baby tends to sequester and accumulate drugs.

Cardiovascular system

Pregnancy is accompanied by an *increase in blood volume*, up to one liter at term, which is greater than the increase in RBC, leading to a relative *dilutional anemia*. Plasma proteins also become diluted, decreasing osmotic pressure and possibly leading to dependent edema. An increase in volume of distribution and decrease in plasma protein binding will alter the pharmacokinetic profile of all nonvolatile drugs.

Cardiac output increases by 30–50% during the first trimester, and then stabilizes at that level for the duration of pregnancy, mostly due to an increase in stroke volume, with a minor contribution from a modest increase in resting heart rate. A generalized decrease in peripheral vascular resistance modulates the anticipated increased in blood pressure due to the increase in cardiac output. These changes tend to ensure adequate oxygen delivery to the developing fetus.

Hypotension is a concern in the pregnant female. Since uterine blood flow is not autoregulated, any decrease in maternal blood pressure diminishes oxygen delivery to the fetus, as shown in the following.

$$\text{Uterine blood flow} = \frac{\text{Uterine artery pressure} - \text{uterine venous pressure}}{\text{Uterine vascular resistance}}$$

Uterine perfusion becomes more critical as gestational age increases. Uterine artery pressure is decreased with supine hypotension or maternal hypotension of any etiology (including the administration of most anesthetic agents.) Uterine venous pressure is increased with seizures, valsalva maneuvers, or venacaval compression. Uterine vascular resistance is increased with endogenous or stress-induced exogenous catecholamines. Increases in maternal blood volume and decreases in systemic vascular resistance occur to safeguard uterine perfusion.

The gravid uterus can compress both the abdominal aorta and the inferior vena cava, especially when the patient is supine, causing *supine hypotensive syndrome.* (Bamber and Dresner, 2003). Inferior vena cava compression interferes with venous return (hence preload), causing a decrease in blood pressure, cardiac output, and uterine blood flow. Abdominal aorta compression can result in a decrease in uterine blood flow, although this may not cause any maternal symptomatology. These phenomena can start as early as 20 gestational weeks, and become more pronounced with the increasing weight of the uterus and the occasional significant weight gain in the mother. This decrease in blood pressure may not necessarily be compensated by a tachycardia. Treatment consists of the propping up of the right hip with a wedged pillow (left lateral tilt) to shift the weight of the uterus to the left. Hypotension is always treated aggressively with early recognition, appropriate positioning (Trendelenburg, left lateral decubitus), and rapid administration of isotonic crystalloid solution (lactated Ringers or 0.9% normal saline.) If necessary, ephedrine or phenylephrine can be used (Reitman and Flood, 2011).

Hypertension is similarly a concern in the pregnant female. *Preeclampsia* is characterized by the development of hypertension (BP > 140/90 in a previously normotensive pregnant female) and proteinuria after the 20th gestational week. The appearance of headache, visual disturbance, abdominal pain, and rapid weight gain (edema) heralds the onset of eclampsia. Eclampsia is defined as convulsions and/or coma *in addition to* preeclampsia, and is not caused by coincidental neurologic disease. It is important to note that the onset of preeclampsia can develop between obstetric appointments or be missed because of patient noncompliance. Blood pressure should be carefully monitored in all pregnant patients.

Gastrointestinal system

All pregnant females should be considered full stomachs when anesthetized, secondary to a progesterone-mediated *decrease in motility* of the gastrointestinal tract and an *increase in acid production* (placental influence.) The *lower esophageal sphincter tone is diminished* and the intragastric pressure is elevated due to compression by the enlarging uterus. It is understandable that these changes will place pregnant females at an increased risk for regurgitation and aspiration. A tendency toward nausea and vomiting is noted in pregnant females, especially during the first trimester.

Central nervous system

Pregnant patients often demonstrate an increased sensitivity to most general anesthetic agents, which results in an up to 30% decrease in minimum alveolar concentration of inhaled agents. An increased sensitivity to local anesthetic agents also occurs, which would reduce both toxic and therapeutic doses.

During the first trimester, an increased vagal tone usually occurs together with decreased baseline sympathetic activity. The autonomic imbalance reverses as pregnancy progresses to maintain placental circulation and to compensate for aortocaval compression. (Kuo et al., 2000)

Fetal concerns

Fetal hypoxemia is always a concern. This can be triggered by reduced uterine blood flow, maternal hypotension, maternal hypoxia, and/or depression of the fetal cardiovascular system by anesthetic agents. Strategies to minimize fetal hypoxemia include the avoidance of maternal hypoxia, hypotension, and hypoventilation (by reducing venous return and decreasing cardiac output) and avoidance of atropine or beta blockers, which could affect the fetal heart rate.

The *first trimester* (weeks 1–12) is the period of organogenesis. If possible, only truly emergent surgery/anesthesia should be performed during this period to minimize the potential risks of teratogenicity or fetal death. Organ development can be affected by the long-term administration of anesthetic drugs, although the one-time administration of the same agents has never been conclusively shown to be detrimental.

The *second trimester* is a period of organ development and is generally regarded as the safest time to perform needed dental or surgical work. The fact that the patient is truly in the second trimester needs to be clearly documented for obvious reasons. Risk of teratogenicity or premature labor is minimal during the second trimester.

The *third trimester* brings with it the possibility of maternal–fetal hypotension, because of decreased venous return by compression of the inferior vena cava (and aorta) by the gravid uterus when the patient is placed in a semi-Fowlers (lounging) or supine position. Tilting the patient to her left side and propping the right hip up tends to take pressure off of the vena cava and minimize the frequency and severity of this event. The risk of preterm labor and delivery also occurs during the third trimester. Studies are unclear or silent with respect to the possibility of anesthesia and/or surgical stress triggering premature labor and delivery. The relatively noninvasive nature of dental procedures and the one-time dose of anesthetic medication would tend to distance them as probable causes of preterm labor. The highest risk period for preterm labor and delivery appears to be from 6 1/2 to 7 1/2 months.

Medications

Pharmacokinetic profiles are altered in pregnancy and all drugs should be titrated accordingly. MAC of volatile agents is reduced by 30%. The increase in blood volume causes a physiologic hypoalbuminemia, which increases the unbound, active form of the drug.

The fetus is exposed to all drugs administered to the mother by simple diffusion. The amount of drug seen by the fetus is less than the amount delivered. This occurs because a significant portion of blood delivered to the fetus is first exposed to hepatic metabolism and is subsequently diluted with drug-free blood from the lower extremities. Minimizing the amount of drug used decreases fetal exposure, with its attendant concerns of cardiovascular and central nervous system depression.

All drugs have been shown to have some degree of teratogenicity in some species under specific circumstances and at some specific stage of gestational development; however, no anesthetic agents, as yet, have been identified as definite human teratogens. (Kuczkowski, 2004, Fisher et al., 2008, Koren et al., 1998, Cheek and Baird, 2009.) Furthermore, there is no anesthetic technique that has been shown to be optimal (Reitman and Flood, 2011). Studies of human teratogenicity are nonexistent due to ethical concerns, so most information comes from retrospective analyses in other species, where issues such as dose, time, or duration of exposure and fetal susceptibility are difficult to measure. Furthermore, mechanisms of teratogenicity are not fully elucidated.

Once a decision is made to proceed with anesthesia during pregnancy, one should strive to use the least amount of the safest drugs. The Food and Drug Administration has published a rating system (Table 16.1) in an attempt to classify or stratify risk associated with the use of various medications.

The choice of agent/technique is secondary to the overall management of the pregnant female, namely, providing adequate pre-oxygenation, avoiding hypoxia, and maintaining cardiovascular stability. Use of anesthetic drugs should be guided by the maintenance of blood pressure rather than effect on uterus.

It is understandable that few clinicians or scientific publications espouse the absolute safety of anesthetic medications when used during pregnancy. Most anesthetic agents are category B or C; none are currently regarded as absolute definitive human teratogens.

Table 16.1 FDA pregnancy risk categories.

A – Controlled studies in humans show no fetal risk. Adequate, well-controlled studies in pregnant women have failed to demonstrate risk to the human fetus in the first trimester (or latter trimesters).
B – No evidence of fetal risk in humans Either animal findings show risk (but human findings do not) or, if inadequate human studies have been done, animal findings are negative.
C – Risk cannot be ruled out Human studies are lacking and animal studies are either positive for fetal risk or lacking as well. However, potential benefits may justify the potential risk.
D – Positive evidence of fetal risk Investigational or postmarketing data show risk to the human fetus. Nevertheless, potential benefits may outweigh the risk.
X – Contraindicated in pregnancy or in patients who may become pregnant Studies in animals or humans, or investigational or postmarketing reports have shown fetal risk which clearly outweighs any possible benefit to the patient.

Local anesthetics (Fayans et al., 2010)

All local anesthetics freely cross the placental barrier. Protein binding decreases during pregnancy, which increases the activity of the administered dose. Local anesthetics (and other basic drugs) will accumulate in fetal circulation during periods of fetal acidosis (ionized form is favored), which restricts the diffusion away from the fetus. This should not be a concern with "normal" pregnancies. Higher blood levels of lidocaine, such as those seen with rapid, intravascular, or high dose administration can lead to uterine vasoconstriction. Lidocaine and prilocaine are category B, while mepivicaine and bupivacaine are category C.

Vasoconstrictors

There is concern that high blood levels of vasoconstrictors may lead to decreased uterine blood flow. Hemodynamic significance depends on the duration and severity of the insult and the susceptibility of the fetus, all of which are unknown in clinical practice. The least amount of vasoconstrictor necessary is the amount that should be used, with appropriate care to avoid intravascular injection and increased plasma levels. The vasoconstrictive response may be exaggerated in patients who are pre-eclamptic, whereby the mechanisms that control vascular tone may be altered. A second area of concern is the use of vasopressors for the treatment of maternal hypotension. Hypotension during deep sedation or general anesthesia should be treated (in order) by left lateral supine positioning, fluid challenge, decreasing the depth of anesthesia, and finally by the use of an indirect acting vasopressors such as ephedrine, which is viewed as the vasopressor of choice in hypotensive pregnant females. The ß adrenergic increase in cardiac output compensates for its mild α adrenergic vasoconstriction. It has been thought that α-adrenergic agents such as phenylephrine might lead to direct uterine vasoconstriction with a decrease in fetal oxygen delivery; however, its use is currently considered safe (Reitman and Flood, 2011).

Benzodiazepines

Concern remains over the possibility of fetal clefting if benzodiazepines are used on a chronic basis during the first trimester. There are no studies to prove this concern. Category D has been used because of the possibility of floppy baby syndrome at the time of delivery (Dolovich et al., 1998).

Sedatives and hypnotics

Sedatives and hypnotics tend to cause a decrease in maternal systemic blood pressure, which can lead to a reduction in uterine blood flow. Using too small a dose can lead to light anesthesia, increased endogenous catecholamine release, and subsequent decrease in uterine blood flow. Unlike with most other agents, the dose of propofol needed for unconsciousness does not decrease with pregnancy. Maternal hypotension remains a risk, especially with rapid bolus infusion. Both propofol and barbiturates are classified as category B.

Ketamine

Ketamine can increase uterine tone by stimulating the release of epinephrine and norepinephrine. Low doses have little effect on fetal cardiovascular status. It has been assigned category B.

Opioids

Fentanyl and its cogeners have been assigned a category C rating, while meperidine is category B. Respiratory depression with subsequent hypoxia remains a concern.

Nitrous oxide

Nitrous oxide has been shown to oxidize cobalamin (vitamin B_{12}) in rats, which inhibits methionine synthase activity, possibly leading to alterations in DNA production and myelin deposition, among others. (Dolovich et al., 1998) Although the human clinical significance of this finding is questionable, and studies fail to demonstrate adverse outcomes to patient or fetus (Mazze and Kallen, 1989), it is reasonable to avoid the use of nitrous oxide during the first trimester. If nitrous oxide is used during the latter two stages of pregnancy, pretreatment with folic acid may be of some benefit. When used in the absence of other inhalational agents, nitrous oxide can lead to uterine vasoconstriction. On the other hand, if nitrous oxide is not used, a greater concentration of inhalational agents may be necessary, resulting in a drop in maternal blood pressure. (Warner and Warner, 2008) An FDA category rating has not been assigned.

References

Baden, J. M., et al. Effects of nitrous oxide on day 9 rate embryos grown in culture. *Br J Anaesth* **66**: 500–503, 1991.

Bamber, J. H. and Dresner, M. Aortocaval compression in pregnancy: the effect of changing the degree and direction of lateral tilt on maternal cardiac output. *Anesth Analg* **97**: 256–258, 2003.

Cheek, T. G. and Baird, E. Anesthesia for nonobstetric surgery: maternal and fetal considerations. *Clin Obstet Gynecol* **52**: 535–545, 2009.

Cohen-Kerem, R. et al. Pregnancy outcome following non-obstetric surgical intervention. *Am J Surg* **190**:467–473, 2005.

Dolovich, L. R., et al. Benzodiazepine use in pregnancy and major malformations or oral cleft: meta-analysis of cohort and case-control studies. *Br Med J* **317**: 839–843, 1998.

Fayans, E., et al. Local anesthetic use in the pregnant and postpartum patient. *Dent Clin North Am* **54**: 697–713, 2010.

Fisher, B., et al. Principles and practice of teratology for the obstetrician. *Clin Obstet. Gynecol* **51**:106–118, 2008.

Hennrikus, W. L., et al. Prevalence of positive preoperative pregnancy testing in teenagers scheduled for orthopedic surgery. *J Pediatr Orthop* **21**; 677–679, 2001.

Koren, G. G., et al. Drugs in pregnancy. *N Engl J Med* **338**: 1128–1137, 1998.

Kuczkowski, K. M. Non-obstetric surgery during pregnancy: What are the risks of anesthesia? *Obstet Gynecol Surv* **59**: 52–56, 2004.

Kuo, C. D., et al. Biphasic changes in autonomic nervous activity during pregnancy. *Br J Anaesth* **84**: 323–329, 2000.

Mazze, R. I. and Kallen, B. Reproductive outcome after anesthesia and operation during pregnancy: a registry study of 5405 cases. *Am J Obstet Gynecol* **161**: 1178–1185, 1989.

Milles, M. Pre-operative pregnancy testing data in a large urban hospital clinic. Scientific poster session, AAOMS annual meeting, 2008.

Mhuireachtaigh, R. N. and O'Gorman, D. A. Anesthesia in pregnant patients for nonobstetric surgery. *J Clin Anesth* **18**:60–66, 2006.

Reitman, E. and Flood, P. Anaesthetic consideration for non-obstetric surgery during pregnancy. *Br J Anaesth* **107**: i72–i78, 2011.

Rosen, M. A. Management of Anesthesia for the pregnant surgical patient. *Anesthesiology* **91**: 1159–1163, 1999.

Warner, D. S. and Warner, M. A. Biologic Effects of Nitrous Oxide. *Anesthesiology* **109**: 707–722, 2008.

SECTION 4

Review of anesthetic agents

17 Clinical principles of anesthetic pharmacology

Richard C. Robert
University of California at San Francisco, Department of Oral and Maxillofacial Surgery, San Francisco, CA, USA

For the induction and maintenance of anesthesia, the site of action for agents is the central nervous system. Although neuroscience defines more of the action of drugs and their specific site of activity, the exact mechanism by which a patient "goes to sleep" is not well defined. Various centers of the brain are involved with components of memory and wakefulness and therefore by definition, the anesthetic agents must modify or act in these regions.

Various investigators have identified areas of the prefrontal cortex, amygdala, thalamus, and hypothalamus as responsible for the experience and expression of emotion. Clinically, the agents that have the most profound effect on these areas of the brain are the benzodiazepines, which play a major role in overcoming anxiety and fear. Patients also hope to have no recall of the procedure, that is, that they be amnestic for their procedure. The hippocampus plays a pivotal role in declarative memory, and is in close proximity and has multiple connections to the amygdala. These pathways are also profoundly affected by the benzodiazepines, which make significant contributions to amnesia.

The reticular activating system

As in the case of the limbic system, the reticular activating system is the area of the brain that controls consciousness, a state of wakefulness and awareness. This system includes the reticular formation itself as well as adjacent areas of the cortex and thalamus, which are rich in gamma-aminobutyric acid (GABA) receptors. It is these receptors that are most profoundly affected by the intravenous anesthetic agents including benzodiazepines, barbiturates, and propofol that render patients unconscious (Antognini and Carstens, 2003). The thalamus is an integral part of this system and functions as a "relay station" for sensory impulses. Impulses through these pathways are inhibited by ketamine, which produces a state in which the patient is dissociated from his environment (Angel, 2003).

Central opioid receptors

Investigations in the 1970s disclosed the presence of three receptors, the mu (μ) receptor, the delta (δ) receptor, and the kappa (κ) receptor. From an anesthetic standpoint, the most important of these is the μ receptor. Agents such as fentanyl, alfentanil, and remifentanil that target this receptor are the opioids most successfully employed as components of a balanced anesthetic. The functions of the μ receptor include analgesia, sedation, and euphoria, but also include respiratory depression and modulation of hormone and neurotransmitter release.

Mechanism of action of anesthetic agents

The receptor concept

The action of drugs is due to the binding of drug molecules to protein molecules ("receptors"). The term *receptor* is used to designate any cellular macromolecule capable of binding a drug, thereby initiating its effect. An essential characteristic of a drug and its interaction with the receptor is the spatial arrangement of its functional groups that leads to the drug's biological activity. An example is the opioid receptor, which binds with both natural opioid agents and synthetic opioids such as meperidine, drugs that share spatial molecular similarities.

The extent to which a drug binds to the receptor is its *affinity* and its tendency to actually activate the receptor is its *efficacy*. There are several relationships that exist between the drug and its targeted receptor site. When the binding between the drug and its receptor site elicits a maximal response, it acts as a *full agonist*, and when the response is less than maximal, the drug is denoted as a *partial agonist*. When a drug binds to a receptor site and does not activate it, but instead prevents an agonist from binding to the site, the drug is termed a *receptor antagonist* (Rang et al., 2011).

Conduction of the impulse and $GABA_A$ and NMDA receptors

On a molecular basis, all intravenous and inhalation agents share a common mechanism of action: they affect the movement of ions through ion channels in neuronal membranes. Axon voltage-gated channels allow passage of ions into the neurons, producing depolarization and generation of an action potential (Becker, 2012).

Anesthetic agents exert their effects by enhancing, inhibiting, or mimicking the action of the neurotransmitters, which modify conduction through the synapse. Two of the most important neurotransmitter-activated ion channels affected are the inhibitory gamma-aminobutyric acid channel ($GABA_A$) (see Figure 17.1), which is enhanced by drugs such as propofol and benzodiazepine, and the excitatory N-methyl D-aspartate (NMDA) receptor

Anesthesia Complications in the Dental Office, First Edition. Edited by Robert C. Bosack and Stuart Lieblich.

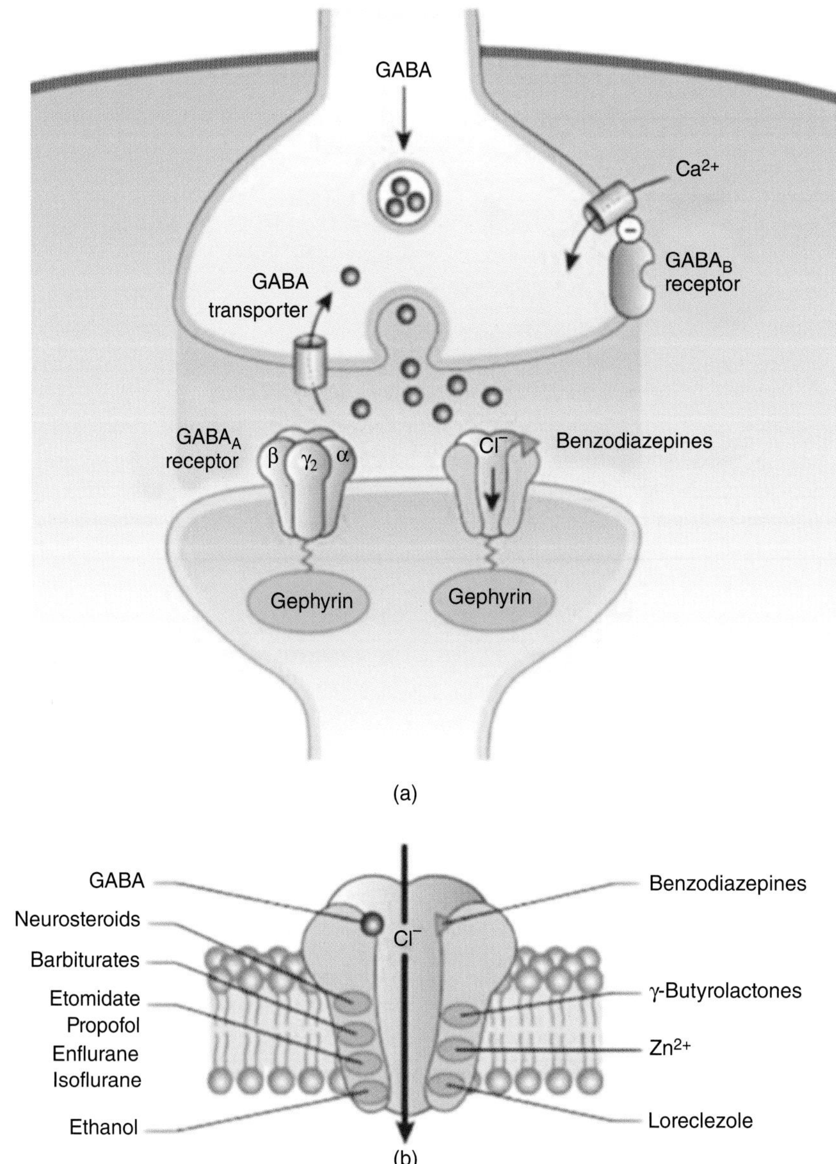

Figure 17.1 The $GABA_A$ receptor.

channel, which is inhibited by ketamine and nitrous oxide (see Figure 17.2). Although both benzodiazepines and propofol enhance GABA binding on the $GABA_A$ receptor ("GABA-ergic"), propofol also can directly open the chloride channels ("GABAmimetic"). It is this mechanism that accounts for the more profound effect of propofol to induce deeper levels of anesthesia. Benzodiazepines are limited in effect since they only facilitate the binding of GABA, and since the amount of GABA is limited, deeper levels of sedation/anesthesia may not occur even with very high doses.

Pharmacodynamics and pharmacokinetics

Pharmacodynamics can be defined as what the drug does to the body (results of receptor binding), and pharmacokinetics represents what the body does to the drug (absorption, distribution, biotransformation, metabolism and elimination). Both are important factors that should be taken into account in the selection and administration of anesthetic drugs.

Pharmacodynamics

There are several pharmacologic parameters that should be considered in selecting and administering anesthetic drugs. The first of these is drug *efficacy*, which is a measure of the extent to which the drug produces the desired effect, and in large part determines its practical clinical use. The second parameter is drug *potency*, which refers to the dose of a drug required to produce 50% of the drug's maximal effect. Thus, if one drug produces 50% of maximal effect at a dose of 10 mg while a second drug produces the same effect with a dose of 5 mg, the second drug is twice as potent as the first. A third important parameter is *dose response* over time. A drug that produces a desired effect over a short interval of time is considered to have *rapid onset* (Schnider and Minto, 2004).

Pharmacokinetics

The two basic parameters in the pharmacokinetic profile of a drug are volume of distribution and drug clearance. *Volume of distribution* is a measure of the apparent space in the body that is available

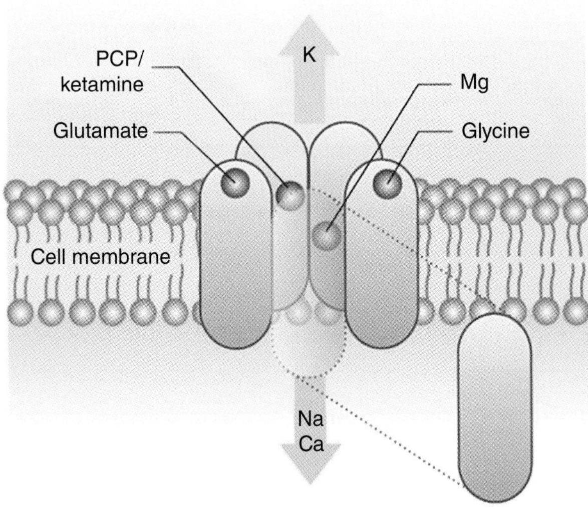

Figure 17.2 The NMDA receptor.

to contain the drug. *Clearance* is a measure of the ability of the body to eliminate the drug. The primary processes of pharmacokinetics are a drug's absorption, its distribution, its biotransformation, and its final elimination from the body.

Compartments and distribution

There are a number of routes by which drugs can be administered, and each has its advantages and disadvantages. The clinician's primary concern is the extent to which the dose of the drug reaches its site of action, which is termed *bioavailability*. Bioavailability is greatest for intravenously administered drugs and lowest for those administered by the *enteral* (intestinal) route.

The enteral route, *oral ingestion*, is usually considered to be the safest and most convenient route. Its disadvantages include limited absorption of some drugs because of their physical characteristics, irritation of the gastrointestinal mucosa, and destruction of the drug by enzymes or low gastric pH. Furthermore, drugs administered by the oral route may be metabolized by gastrointestinal enzymes or hepatic enzymes before they gain access to the general circulation (the *first-pass* effect). Other "oral" routes that are not technically enteral (intestinal) include the *sublingual* route, which relies on transmucosal and vascular absorption in the floor of the mouth, thereby circumventing the first pass metabolism. The *transmucosal* route, which is widely used in dentistry, is utilized with the application of topical anesthetics prior to local anesthetic injection.

The three most commonly used *parenteral* (literally "not by the intestinal route") routes are those requiring injection. These include the *intravenous* route (IV), the *intramuscular* route (IM), and the *subcutaneous* route (SQ). The intravenous route provides 100% bioavailability, the most rapid onset, and the ability to deliver large volumes. However, it carries increased risks of adverse effects due to rapid administration as well as possible tissue damage from irritating substances. Absorption of *aqueous* solutions of drugs via the intramuscular route is relatively rapid but is somewhat unpredictable due to a variety of reasons including body habitus and gender. Subcutaneous injection frequently provides relatively slow and constant absorption, which enables a more sustained effect. This can be advantageous in certain situations such as the administration of epinephrine for allergic reactions.

A final route of administration is that of *inhalation* of volatile gases. The large surface area of the lungs allows for rapid access of the agent to the systemic circulation. However, a major disadvantage is the fact that some inhalation agents are irritating to the pulmonary epithelium and the mucous membranes of the remainder of the respiratory tract.

After the drug reaches the circulation, it can either be bound to plasma proteins (bound, inactive) or circulate in an unbound (free, active) form. Acidic drugs bind largely to plasma albumin, while basic drugs preferentially bind to α_1-acid glycoprotein. In the case of anesthetic agents, the extent of protein binding varies considerably from 12% for ketamine up to 98% for propofol. When there is a decrease in plasma protein due to age or comorbidities such as anorexia or substance abuse, the amount of freely circulating drug is increased, which increases drug effect.

Once a drug has been absorbed into the systemic circulation, it diffuses to its receptor site of action as well as to other tissues of distribution. Drugs are not distributed uniformly throughout the body. The speed with which a drug reaches a given tissue type is primarily dependent on the local blood flow. Similar tissue types are frequently grouped together, based on the extent of blood flow as a percentage of cardiac output into entities termed *compartments* – places to where drugs are capable of diffusing (see Table 17.1) Drugs distribute to various compartments based on blood flow to that compartment as well as on the affinity for variable tissue types. The central compartment is plasma. A lipid-soluble drug that is widely distributed may have a central compartment, a vessel-rich compartment, as well as a vessel-poor compartment (Roberts and Freshwater-Turner, 2007) (Figure 17.3).

A highly lipid-soluble drug such as propofol or fentanyl will tend to cross lipid membranes rapidly and have a very high *volume of distribution*. Volumes of distribution, designated V_d, are theoretical and are based upon the volume that would be necessary for a drug to be fully distributed at equilibrium; they are expressed as liters per kilogram. However, a highly ionized drug such as glycopyrrolate that does not readily cross lipid membranes has a low volume of distribution.

Since intravenously administered drugs are delivered into the central compartment by injection, their primary obstacle in reaching the brain to exert their effects is the blood brain barrier (BBB), a dynamic and complex interface between the blood and the central nervous system. The barrier is predominantly defined by the specialized microvasculature of the brain, which consists of a single layer of polarized endothelial cells interconnected by complex tight junctions that limits permeability. The sites prevent the movement of large molecules and favor the passage of those of small size such as propofol and methohexital.

Table 17.1 Body Tissue compartments.

Compartment	Tissue type	Blood flow (% of cardiac output)
Vessel-rich compartment	Brain Heart Kidney Liver	75
Muscle compartment	Skeletal muscle	19
Fat compartment	Adipose tissue	5
Vessel-poor compartment	Bone	1

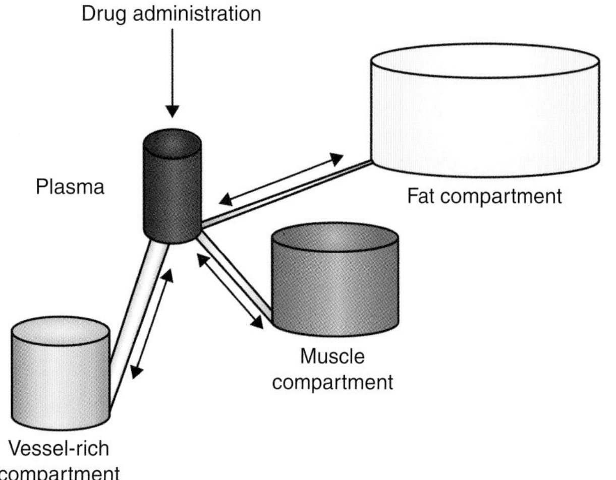

Figure 17.3 Tissue compartments.

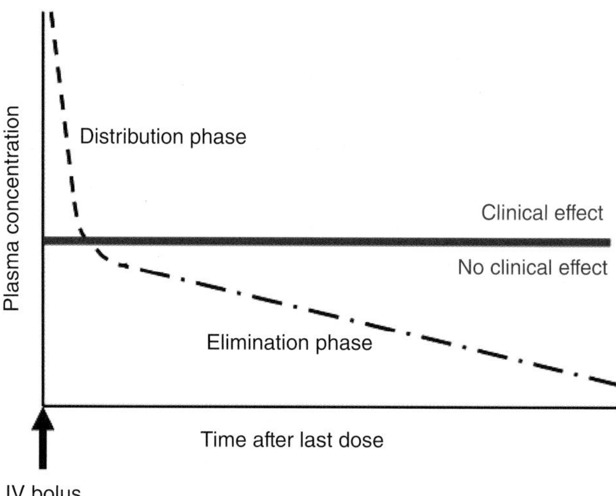

Figure 17.4 Graphic depiction of the redistribution and elimination of a rapid-acting intravenously administered drug.

The principal barrier to diffusion of compounds is the lipid bilayer. The diffusion of anesthetic agents through the BBB is largely affected by the pKa, which represents the pH at which 50% of a drug exists in its ionized form and 50% exists in the non-ionized form. Many highly fat-soluble drugs (e.g. ketamine and remifentanil) have a pKa very close to the pH of the plasma, which enables them to pass through the BBB and exhibit a very rapid onset.

Another issue of critical importance in the distribution of anesthetic drugs is the cardiac output. With high cardiac output, the drug is rapidly transported to such vessel-rich structures as the brain, heart, liver, and kidneys. Equilibration for highly lipid-soluble drugs occurs quite quickly and leads to a rapid onset. However, a patient with a lower cardiac output, such as an elderly person, will experience a slower onset of action. Since the drug is mixed with a smaller volume of blood during injection in the older person with a low cardiac output, the peak concentration is greater. Thus, a smaller induction dose must be considered in the elderly. On the other hand, because of their high cardiac output pediatric patients often require a relatively larger dose on a milligrams per kilogram basis.

Cardiac output has a somewhat different effect on the uptake of inhalation agents. As cardiac output increases, a greater volume of blood passes through the lungs, which removes more anesthetic from the alveoli. Since the partial pressure of the agent in the central nervous system cannot be greater than that in the blood, the lower level of the agent in the alveoli leads to a lower anesthetic partial pressure in the brain and therefore a delayed onset.

Tissues other than the brain may also have a high affinity for the drug. However, since these tissues receive a lower proportion of the cardiac output, there is a lower concentration of the drug in these tissues. As the concentration in the blood falls and the bonds between the drug and the receptor sites in the CNS are released, the drug leaves the brain and is redistributed to other tissues. It is this rapid redistribution that is predominantly responsible for the short duration of such drugs as propofol and remifentanil.

In the office setting, short-acting drugs are selected to rapidly achieve the desired levels of sedation, while facilitating safe discharge home in a time-efficient manner. Drug effect terminates when the drug diffuses or redistributes away from its receptor, measured as a redistribution or T1/2 α half-life. It is important to realize that variable amounts of drug will persist and slowly diffuse out from other compartments prior to metabolism, accounting for the typical postanesthetic "hangover." This is measured as the elimination or T1/2β half-life (see figure 17.4).

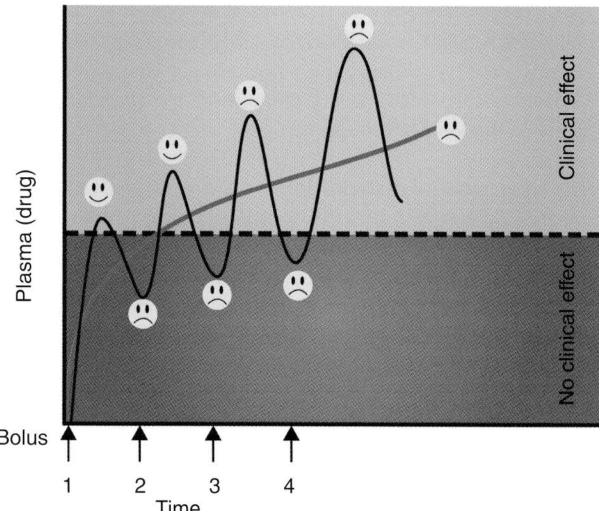

Figure 17.5 Drug accumulation of repeated dosing of drugs that are not short acting.

A common approach to office-based anesthesia includes the use of a narcotic and a benzodiazepine, and intermittent small boluses of a short-acting sedative and hypnotic agent, either methohexital or propofol. This "bump and run" approach, although utilitarian, has limitations and shortcomings, especially when any but the shortest acting drugs (propofol) are administered more than once. As seen in Figure 17.5, repeat bolus dosing of drugs whose clinical effect has dissipated, but still remains in muscle and fat tissue compartments, can lead to repeated instances of overdose and underdose, with an increasing average plasma drug concentration that is maximal at the end of the case. This situation leads to repeated underdosing leading to recall, pain, movement, and poor surgical conditions, as well as repeated overdosing, leading to loss of airway tone, apnea, adverse cardiovascular changes, and prolonged recovery. At the end of this scenario, when the patient is expected to wake up and go home, drug concentrations in the body are at their highest level.

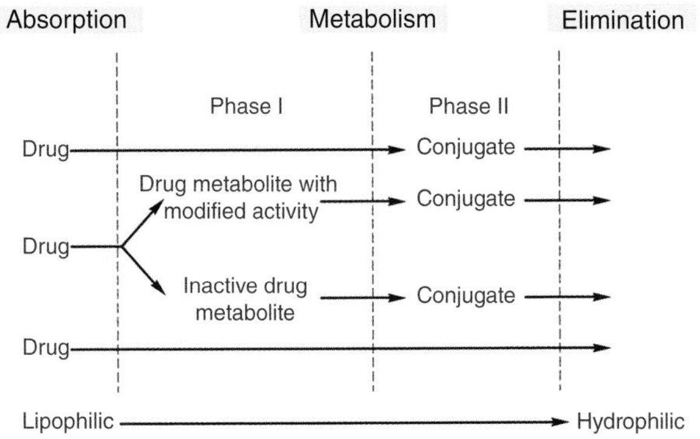

Figure 17.6 Common pathway for metabolism and elimination of drugs.

Biotransformation and elimination

For those anesthetic drugs that are highly lipid soluble, excretion through the kidneys requires a transformation of the drug into a polar water-soluble form. For the majority of agents this transformation takes place in the liver in two phases. In *Phase I* reactions, a functional group such as -OH, $-NH_2$, or -SH is either added or unmasked by the activity of enzymes termed the *cytochrome P450 isoenzymes*. Some Phase I metabolites are sufficiently polar that they can be excreted without further transformation. However, those that are not undergo a second reaction termed a *Phase II* reaction. This reaction involves a combination of the Phase I metabolite with an endogenous substance such as glucuronic acid, an amino acid, or an acid such as sulfuric or acidic acid (see Figure 17.6).

The rate at which biotransformation takes place affects the rapidity of drug elimination, and therefore recovery. Various anesthetic drugs exhibit a wide range in the rate at which they are biotransformed and eliminated. A pertinent example is the very rapid biotransformation of propofol, which is ten times that of the ultra-short-acting barbiturates. Although much of the elimination of propofol is through the traditional pathways with biotransformation in the liver and excretion through the kidneys, there is also elimination involving other tissues, including the lungs. In recent years pharmacologic research has led to the development of anesthetic agents that do not require biotransformation in the liver. One such agent is remifentanil which is biotransformed through the action of esterases that are found throughout the body. Because of the widespread presence of these esterases, the biotransformation of remifentanil is far faster than that of any of the other currently available opioids (Coda, 2009).

References

Angel, A. Thalamus. In: Antognini, J. F., et al. (eds.) *Neural Mechanisms of Anesthesia*, New Jersey: Humana Press Inc., 2003.

Antognini, J. F. and Carstens, E. Anesthetic effects on the reticular formation, brainstem and central nervous system arousal. *In:* Antognini, J. F., et al. (eds.) *Neural Mechanisms of Anesthesia*. Totowa, New Jersey: Humana Press Inc., 2003.

Becker D.E. Pharmacodynamic considerations for moderate and deep sedation. *Anesth Prog* **59**: 28–42, 2012.

Coda, B. Opioids. In: Barash, P. G. (ed.) *Clinical Anesthesia*, 6th edn Philadelphia: Wolters Kluwer/Lippincott Williams & Wilkins, 2009.

Rang, H. P., et al. *How Drugs Act: General Principles*. Rang & Dale's pharmacology, 7th edn, Churchill Livingstone, 2011.

Roberts, F., and Freshwater-Turner, D. Pharmacokinetics and anesthesia. *Br J Anaesth* **7**: 25–29, 2007.

Schnider, T. W. and Minto, C. F.. Analgesics: Receptor ligands α2 adrenergic receptor agonists. *In:* Evers, A. S., Maze, M. (eds.) *Anesthetic pharmacology: Physiologic principles and clinical practice: A companion to miller's anesthesia*. New York: Churchill Livingstone, 2004.

18 Local anesthetic pharmacology

Roy L. Stevens[1] **and Robert C. Bosack**[2]
[1]Private Practice General Dentistry for Patients with Special Health Care Needs, Oklahoma City, OK
[2]University of Illinois, College of Dentistry, Chicago, IL, USA

The safe and effective worldwide use of local instills a false sense of security, which can limit the ability to anticipate, avoid, identify, accept, or manage complications with the use of these drugs. A complete understanding of the pharmacology of local anesthetics will reward the clinician with the ability to improve their safe and effective use on their patients.

Mechanism of action

Local anesthetic drugs reversibly block sodium (Na^+) channels, which inhibit depolarization by preventing the influx of Na^+, ultimately denying impulse propagation. They are not specific to the trigeminal nerve and can act at Na^+ channels throughout the body, including both the heart and the brain, and will exert clinically noticeable effects in those organs if sufficient concentrations are reached. The clinician is able to control the total anesthetic dose, anesthetic concentration, and inclusion and type of vasoconstrictor. The precise location of injection cannot be visualized and is approximated by the use of anatomic landmarks to instill the anesthetic volume close to but not in the intended nerves. Once the solution is injected into the tissues, it diffuses radially outward along concentration gradients, hindered by bone, muscle, fat, fibrous tissue, or ligaments. Immediately after injection, the volume begins to be cleared from the injection site via local vasculature, bringing the drug into central circulation and to the brain, heart, and liver (the site of amide metabolism). Vasoconstrictors prolong the duration by slowing the rate at which the anesthetic is carried away from the intended site. Only a very small percentage of the injected volume ever reaches the intended nerve.

Local anesthetics must be both water and lipid soluble to exert their action. All local anesthetic molecules contain three moieties, each conferring a different property: a lipophilic (neutral) benzene ring and a hydrophilic (ionized) tertiary amine, which are linked together by an intermediate ester or amide (see Figure 18.1). Local anesthetics are weak bases, where ionized and unionized forms exist in equilibrium. The tertiary amine allows the drug to be in solution in the cartridge and prevents precipitation when injected into the interstitial fluid. The aromatic ring allows the drug to penetrate anatomic structures and the nerve sheath, in order to gain access to sodium channels. Once inside the axoplasm, it is the ionized moiety that facilitates protein binding to sodium channels to block sodium influx. A sufficient concentration of the anesthetic must be present to block a sufficient (critical) length of the neuron to prevent nerve transmission. The intermediate linkage determines the route of elimination: esters are hydrolyzed in the blood stream by plasma esterases to the notoriously allergenic para-aminobenzoic acid (PABA), while amides are metabolized by hepatic microsomal enzymes (CYP 450 isoenzymes).

Although drug properties do not sort independently, onset of anesthetic action and potency tend to increase with the lipid solubility of the anesthetic molecule and the amount of unionized moiety at tissue pH. In this context, each local anesthetic can be further characterized by pK_a, which is the pH where [ionized fraction] = [unionized fraction]. Drugs with relatively higher pK_as or, conversely, tissues with low pH (<7.4, as seen with inflammation) will favor the water soluble, hydrophilic moiety and inhibit drug penetration into the nerve. Duration of action can be correlated with the degree of protein binding, which is thought to facilitate binding at the Na^+ channel. (see Table 18.1).

Vasoconstrictors

Vasoconstrictors are used in combination with local anesthetics to constrict arterioles (α-adrenergic stimulation) in order to maintain higher drug concentrations at the target site by delaying vascular absorption (Brown and Rhodus, 2005). Duration and profundity of anesthesia are often increased, while systemic toxicity is reduced as the anesthetic drug enters the circulation more slowly, and in closer pace with redistribution and metabolism. Epinephrine can be added in various dilutions (see Table 18.2). Direct α1 stimulation constricts mucosal arterioles, while direct β stimulation increases heart rate and contractility and dilates skeletal muscle vasculature, if or when a sufficient amount reaches those sites. Epinephrine, with equal α and β properties, can trigger tachycardia, while maintaining a stable mean arterial pressure. Levonordefrin favors α stimulation over β stimulation, which predicts less frequent or severe tachycardia, while triggering an increase in mean arterial pressure (Malamed, 2013). These drugs interfere with their own absorption at the site of injection, but once they enter the blood stream, both are rapidly (5–10 minutes) deactivated by catechol-O-methyl transferase (COMT). Therefore, while vasoconstrictors prolong local anesthetic action, their side effects, fortunately, are short-lived. Vasoconstrictor additives lower the pH of the anesthetic solution and require the addition of a sulfite antioxidant. As such, onset of action is prolonged as the ionized moiety is favored.

Summary

Most concepts in anesthesia are difficult to confirm because of the inability to perform randomized, prospective trials changing only one variable, due in large part to patient variability and medical research ethics. That having been said, it is logical to presume that

Anesthesia Complications in the Dental Office, First Edition. Edited by Robert C. Bosack and Stuart Lieblich.

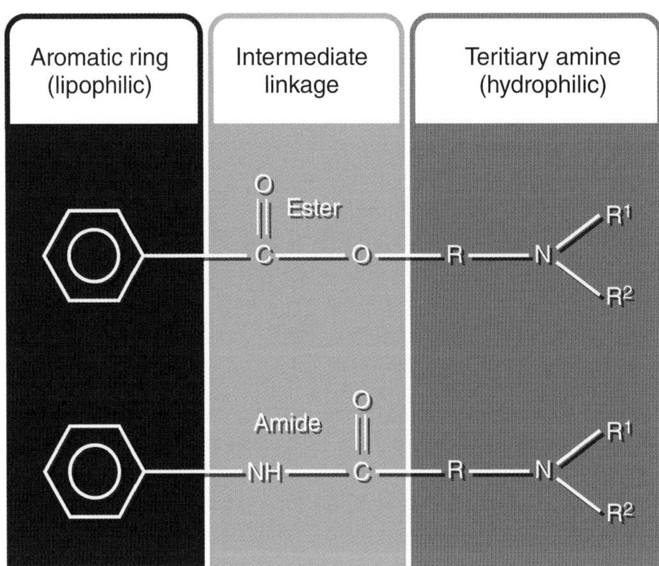

Figure 18.1 Basic chemical structure of the Ester and Amide local anesthetics

Table 18.1 Local anesthetic drug properties.

Local anesthetic	Vasodilating ability	pK_a	Onset	% ionized at pH 7.4	% protein binding	Duration	Lipid solubility	Potency
Bupivacaine	Most	8.1	Slowest	83	95	Longest	Great	Most
Lidocaine	Intermediate	7.9	Fast	76	64	Moderate	Low	Moderate
Mepivacaine	Least	7.6	Faster	61	77	Moderate	Lowest	Least
Prilocaine	Intermediate	7.9	Faster	76	55	Moderate	Lowest	Moderate
Articaine	Intermediate	7.8	Fastest	70	95	Shortest	Greatest	Moderate

Adapted from Moore and Hersh, 2010 and Yagiela, 2011.

attaining and maintaining a sufficient concentration of an anesthetic drug at the intended nerve site will enhance clinical effect. Clinically, this translates into the following statements.

1 Increasing the dose (# of cartridges, drug concentration) can hasten onset, enhance profundity, and prolong duration of anesthesia.

Table 18.2 Quantity of epinephrine in a 1.8cc cartridge.

Dilution	Concentration (mg/ml)	mg in 1.8 cc cartridge
1:1,000	1.0	x
1:10,000	0.1	x
1:50,000	0.02	0.036
1:100,000	0.01	0.018
1:200,000	0.005	0.009

Table 18.3 Quantity of local anesthetic in a 1.8cc cartridge.

Units	Formula	Example (2% lidocaine with 1:100,000 epi)
mg/ml	% × 10	20 mg/ml
mg/cartridge	% × 18	38 mg/1.8cc cartridge

2 Improving the accuracy of injection hastens onset, and enhances the duration and profundity of anesthesia.

3 Rapid injection of large volumes tends to distend or dissect connective tissue barriers, enlarging the field of anesthesia, but often causing post-injection inflammation and discomfort.

4 Increasing the amount of lipophilic free base improves drug passage through tissue planes and into the nerve, hastening the onset and profundity of anesthesia.

5 Faster onset and more profound anesthesia is more likely in nerves positioned peripherally in nerve trunks, as compared to a more central, anatomically protected location.

The concept of a "safe" or "maximum allowable dosage" appears often and with sometimes significant variation in the literature, leaving clinicians confused. The dose numbers are usually based on lean body weight and assume an extravascular injection during an interval shorter than the time it takes the body to redistribute and metabolize the drug (1 – 2 hours). For obvious reasons, maximum ceiling doses should be respected regardless of patient size. Patients with obesity are not necessarily able to tolerate a larger dose, as adipose tissue is hypovascular and less metabolically active. Dose recommendations vary in a tight range among authors and are also subject to individual variation. Doses become cumulative when two different amide drugs are used together (see Tables 18.3 and 18.4). There is variance of opinion regarding whether the addition of a vasoconstrictor increases the maximum recommended dose.

Table 18.4 Maximum allowable doses.

Drug	Max dosage (mg/lb)	Max adult dose (mg)	mg/cartridge	Max cartridges adult	Max cartridges 50lb child	Max cartridges 40lb child	Max cartridges 30lb child
2% lidocaine with 1:100,000 epi	3.3	500	36	13	4.5	3.6	2.7
4% articaine with 1:100,000 epi	3.3	500	72	7	2.3	1.8	1.4
3% mepivacaine	2.6	400	54	7	2.4	1.9	1.4
2% mepivacaine with 1:20,000 levonordefrin	2.6	400	36	11	3.6	2.8	2.1
4% prilocaine	4	600	72	8	2.7	2.2	1.6
0.5% bupivacaine with 1:200,000 epi	0.6	90	9	10	3.3	2.6	2

Adapted from Moore and Hersh, 2010 and Yagiela, 2011.

References

Brown, R. S. and Rhodus, N. L. Epinephrine and local anesthesia revisited. *Oral Surg Oral Med Oral Pathol Oral Radiol Endod* **100**: 410–418, 2005.

Malamed, S. F. *Handbook of Local Anesthesia*, 6th edn. St. Louis: Elsevier Mosby, 2013.

Moore, P. A. and Hersh, E. V. Local anesthetics: pharmacology and toxicity. *Dent Clin N Am* **54**: 587–599, 2010.

Yagiela, J. A. Local Anesthetics, *in* Yagiela, J. A., et al. (eds): *Pharmacology and therapeutics for dentistry*. St. Louis: Mosby Elsevier, 2011.

19 Enteral sedation agents

Richard C. Robert
University of California at San Francisco, Department of Oral and Maxillofacial Surgery, San Francisco, CA, USA

The medications utilized for enteral sedation were originally developed for insomnia. The oldest and most widely used of these is the benzodiazepine triazolam (Halcion®), which has both a rapid onset of action and a short duration of action. Similarly to the other benzodiazepines discussed earlier in this chapter, this hypnotic agent acts at the benzodiazepine receptor $GABA_A$. In addition to triazolam, other longer acting benzodiazepines have been utilized. These include lorazepam (Ativan®) and alprazolam (Xanax®).

In recent years, pharmacologic research has led to the development of novel non-benzodiazepine hypnotics that also act on $GABA_A$ receptors, but in a slightly different manner. Two of these agents that have found a place in enteral sedation in dentistry include zolpidem and zaleplon. The $GABA_A$ receptor may contain a wide variety of subunits. The more recently developed hypnotics zolpidem and zaleplon act at the newly defined benzodiazepine ω-1 receptor subtype (Dionne, 1998).

Triazolam

Triazolam has been used for enteral sedation in dentistry due to several desirable attributes. Its onset is rapid and peak blood levels are reached in approximately 1 hour. It is also eliminated rapidly in comparison to other benzodiazepines with an elimination half-life of 2–3 hours. Its short elimination half-life and lack of long-acting metabolites render it relatively free of residual daytime effects. Although triazolam has been found to be quite effective for shorter procedures, its duration of action is not adequate for longer procedures. Consequently, many dentists now utilize it in incremental doses as described below.

The recommended dosage of triazolam is 0.25–0.5 mg for adults with a dose of 0.125 mg for geriatric patients. Triazolam is rapidly absorbed with a mean absorption half-life of approximately 22 minutes and a mean minimal absorption efficiency of approximately 85%. Triazolam exhibits the full range of benzodiazepine actions including sedation, anxiolysis, amnesia, and relaxation (Pakes, 1981). Studies have shown oral administration of triazolam to reduce the levels of anxiety and even resting heart rate when a preoperative dose is given for third molar extractions (Lieblich).

Zolpidem

Zolpidem (Ambien®) is a non-benzodiazepine hypnotic that was developed as an alternative to triazolam due to its specificity to the ω-1 benzodiazepine receptor. As such, it has weaker anxiolytic, anticonvulsant, and milder relaxant effects than do benzodiazepines. Zolpidem has a rapid onset of action, which is usually 20–30 minutes and a bioavailability of approximately 70%. In patients with normal hepatic flow and function, the plasma half-life is approximately 2 hours. However, clearance is markedly reduced in the elderly and in patients with chronic hepatic insufficiency. Like triazolam, zolpidem comes in two strengths for adults, 5 and 10 mg. The 10 mg dose is usually considered to be equivalent to 0.25mg of triazolam. In the elderly a dose of 5 mg of zolpidem is considered to be equivalent to 0.125mg of triazolam. Zolpidem can be administered and it reaches peak effect within a half-hour (Holm, 2000.)

Zaleplon

A second non-benzodiazepine with affinity to the omega-1 benzodiazepine receptor is zaleplon (Sonata®). As in the case of zolpidem, its chemical structure is unrelated to the benzodiazepines and it shares the characteristics of the omega-1 benzodiazepine agonists. Its onset is quite rapid with effects apparent in 15–30 minutes and a peak plasma concentration in 1 hour. There is extensive first-pass elimination and an oral bioavailability of approximately 30%. As an omega-1 benzodiazepine receptor antagonist, zaleplon does not impair psychomotor function or memory. Similarly to zolpidem, zaleplon exhibits minimal anxiolytic potential, less amnesia, and minimal antiseizure activity. It lacks some of the effects of the benzodiazepines, and this results in minimal next-day residual effects and no significant impairment of driving ability on the morning after administration. The usual recommended hypnotic dose of zaleplon in adults is 10mg. For oral sedation and dentistry, zaleplon has been found to be most practical for short appointments of less than 1 hour and whenever rapid recovery is important (Heydorn, 2000).

The sublingual incremental dose triazolam technique

The use of sublingual administration was adopted to circumvent the rather erratic absorption of triazolam via the oral route. There can be a 2–3 fold range in plasma concentrations after PO administration of triazolam. Sublingual administration provides both more efficient and less variable bioavailability. With the conventional oral route, following absorption across the gut wall, the portal blood system delivers the drug to the liver before it enters the systemic circulation. The drug can be metabolized within the gut wall itself or in the portal blood, but most commonly in the liver. These diminutions in bioavailability have been termed "first-pass elimination." However, when drugs are absorbed through the mucosa, they pass via the

Anesthesia Complications in the Dental Office, First Edition. Edited by Robert C. Bosack and Stuart Lieblich.

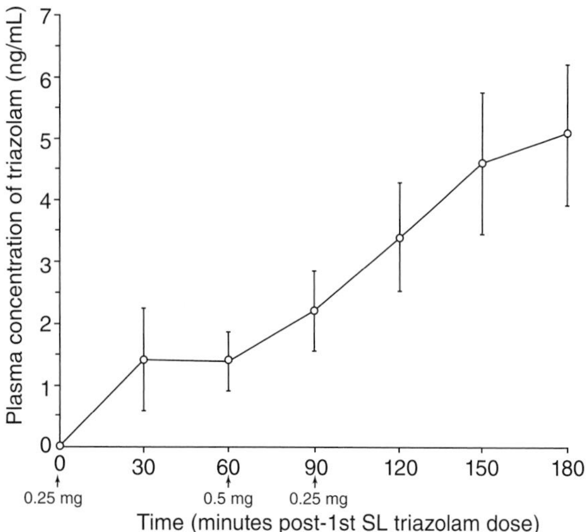

Figure 19.1 Plasma concentrations of triazolam after incremental sublingual administration, Source: Jackson et al, 2006. Reproduced with permission of Lippencott Williams & Wilkins.

venous drainage to the superior vena cava which provides protection from first-pass metabolism. The sublingual approach has been found to provide greater anxiolytic activity, but is not accompanied by greater incidence of side effects such as psychomotor impairment. The bioavailability of triazolam administered by the sublingual route is on average 28% greater than that given by the oral route. The sublingual route has also been found to be efficacious for the administration of premedication for intravenous anesthesia for oral and maxillofacial surgery (Dionne, 2006).

Summary

There are many variables that confound the ability to accurately predict the pharmacokinetic and pharmacodynamic behavior of drugs when administered via the oral route. These include variable firs-pass hepatic metabolism, presence of food in the stomach, digestive efficiency, and the distribution to *and redistribution* from plasma proteins, fat, and muscle compartments. This is evidenced by variability of clinical effect, onset, peak, duration, and offset of drug action. It is challenging at best to predict a point in time when redosing is appropriate and safe, based on clinical parameters only. Jackson (2006) has demonstrated the possibility of deep sedation or general anesthesia with bispectral index scores (BIS) consistent with general anesthesia with incremental sublingual dosing of triazolam (see Figure 19.1).

Reversal of enteral sedation

Whenever sedation or anesthesia is administered, there is always concern regarding the termination of effects or rescue from levels deeper than planned, including ventilatory depression and upper airway obstruction. The benzodiazepine antagonist flumazenil was developed for intravenous reversal of the effects of benzodiazepines. When enteral sedation is provided by dentists who do not have expertise in venipuncture and intravenous therapy, reversal becomes more problematic. Although sublingual and submucosal administration of flumazenil has been studied in animal models, the single clinical study assessing the efficacy of sublingual flumazenil concluded, "a single intra-oral injection of flumazenil at 0.2 mg cannot be used to immediately rescue over-sedation with triazolam." (Hosaka, 2009) Furthermore, it has been suggested that additional dosages of up to 0.6 – 1.0 mg would entail a volume too large to safely inject sublingually. Thus, at this time it does not appear that there is an efficacious approach by the oral route for reversal of patients who have undergone enteral sedation with benzodiazepines. It is doubtful that the non-intravenous administration of flumazenil would be sufficient in dose or time of onset to successfully rescue a patient from ventilatory inadequacy (Weaver, 2011).

References

Dionne, R. A., et al. Assessing the need for anesthesia and sedation in the general population. *JADA* **129**: 167 – 173, 1998.

Dionne, R. A., et al. Balancing efficacy and safety in the use of oral sedation in dental outpatients. *JADA* **137**: 502 – 513, 2006.

Heydorn, W. E. Zaleplon – a review of a novel sedative hypnotic used in the treatment of insomnia. *Expert Opin Investig Drugs* **9**: 841 – 858, 2000.

Holm, K. J. and Goa, K. L. Zolpidem: an update of its pharmacology, therapeutic efficacy and tolerability in the treatment of insomnia. *Drugs* **59**: 865 – 889, 2000.

Hosaka, K., et al. Flumazenil reversal of sublingual triazolam: a randomized controlled clinical trial. *JADA* **140**: 559 – 566, 2009.

Jackson, D. L., et al. Pharmacokinetics and clinical effects of multidose sublingual triazolam in healthy volunteers. *J Clin Psychopharmacol* **26**: 4 – 8, 2006.

Lieblich SE, Horswell BH: Attenuation of anxiety in ambulatory oral surgery patients with oral triazolam. *J Oral Maxillofac Surg* **49**(8):792 – 796, 1991.

Pakes, G. E., et al. Triazolam: a review of its pharmacological properties and therapeutic efficacy in patients with insomnia. *Drugs* **22**: 81 – 110, 1981.

Weaver, J. The fallacy of a lifesaving sublingual injection of flumazenil. *Anesth Prog* **58**: 1 – 2, 2011.

20 Parenteral anesthetic agents

Richard C. Robert
University of California at San Francisco, Department of Oral and Maxillofacial Surgery, San Francisco, CA, USA

Barbiturates

Methohexital and thiopental (ultra-short acting barbiturates) are weak acids that are poorly soluble in water at a neutral pH. The agents are formulated as water-soluble sodium salts with sodium carbonate added to maintain an alkaline pH of 10–11. The alkalinity produces several problems, primary of which is the potential for extensive tissue damage in the case of extravasation or an intra-arterial injection. In addition, the barbiturates that are weak acids can induce precipitation of drugs that are weak bases, including opioids, lidocaine, rocuronium, and labetalol. The high pH has been shown to prevent bacterial growth following reconstitution.

The ultra-short-acting barbiturates fall into two principal classifications, thiobarbiturates and oxy-barbiturates. Thiopental has a sulfur atom that increases its lipophilicity. This results in an increase in potency, a more rapid onset, and a shorter duration of action. Lipophilicity is also increased by alkylation at $N-1$, as in the case of methohexital, which is actually a methylated oxybarbiturate. The alkylation is responsible for some of the agent's excitatory side effects (Hemmings, 2010).

Pharmacodynamics

Barbiturates induce loss of consciousness through their interaction with the gamma-aminobutyric acid (GABA) neurotransmitter system in the areas of the brain that control consciousness. Barbiturates also directly activate opening of the chloride channel of the receptor as well as decrease the rate of dissociation of GABA from its receptor, which increases the duration of the GABA-activated opening of the channel. Although the contribution of $GABA_A$ channels is predominant, recent studies indicate that NMDA receptors also play a role.

Pharmacokinetics

The small barbiturate molecules are highly lipophilic. The rapid crossing of the blood–brain barrier leads in turn to a rapid loss of consciousness, which usually takes place within approximately 20 seconds or one arm-to-brain circulation. The effect dissipates as the drugs become redistributed to the other components of the vessel-rich group as well as muscle, skin, fat, and other tissues. Thus, the pharmacokinetic profile of the barbiturates is the typical three-compartment model that is commonly seen with other lipophilic anesthetic agents as illustrated in Figure 20.1. Thiopental has a relatively long elimination half-life of approximately 11 hours, nearly three times as great as that of methohexital, which has an elimination half-life of approximately 4 hours (Reves, 2010). In the 1960s this characteristic of methohexital was one of the primary considerations in its replacing thiopental as the preferred agent for office-based anesthesia for oral and maxillofacial surgery. Barbiturates are highly protein bound.

Both thiopental and methohexital are metabolized in the liver to largely inactive hydroxyl derivatives. However, at large doses thiopental undergoes a desulfurization resulting in the production of pentobarbital, which can have long-lasting CNS effects. As noted above, methohexital is cleared 3–4 times more rapidly than thiopental, which results in a much shorter elimination half-life.

Effect on organ systems

Both thiopental and methohexital lower peripheral vascular resistance and cardiac output. Hypotension is less likely with methohexital due to a compensatory tachycardia. Since a part of the hypotensive response is due to direct myocardial depression, these agents must be used in caution in patients with myocardial disease.

Similarly to most drugs used for general anesthesia, the ultra-short-acting barbiturates cause a dose-dependent respiratory depression. This is due in large part to a blunted medullary ventilatory response, primarily hypercapnia, and to a lesser extent, hypoxia. In contrast to propofol, laryngeal and tracheal reflexes are not depressed and may be heightened to some extent, which leads to a higher incidence of laryngospasm than is seen with propofol.

Adverse effects

Paradoxical excitement can occur with the use of methohexital when administered in subanesthetic doses. This has been described as a central disinhibitory effect, or hyperalgesia, which is often triggered by pain and notably, any stimulation, for example, inflation of a blood pressure cuff. Attendant signs include tachycardia, hypertension, tearing, sweating, and tachypnea. A decrease in GABA receptor sensitivity or an increase in receptor number is the suggested cause. The development of acute tolerance to intravenous methohexital has also been postulated but never proved (Barratt et al., 1985). Management can include the use of other agents for aborting the case.

In general, barbiturates, including thiopental, have potent anticonvulsive properties. However, methohexital has increased central excitatory side effects. It can trigger epileptogenic activity as well as elicit involuntary muscle movements, such as tremor, twitching,

Anesthesia Complications in the Dental Office, First Edition. Edited by Robert C. Bosack and Stuart Lieblich.

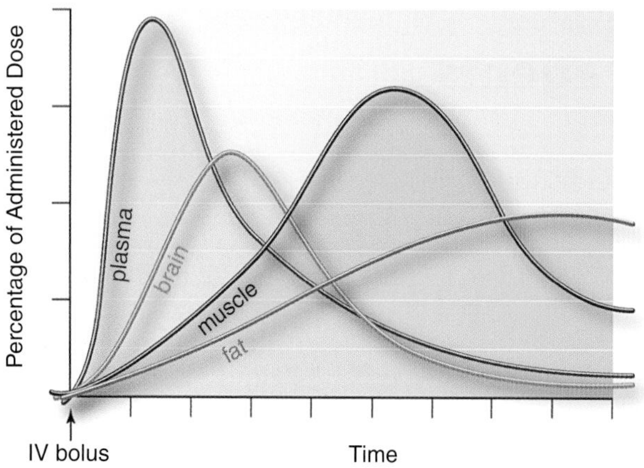

Figure 20.1 The distribution of lipophilic drugs to the VRG (vessel-rich group), the MG (muscle group), and the FG (fat group), consistent with a three-compartment model.

and hiccups. Rockoff and Goudsouzian (1981) has suggested that alternative agents to methohexital be considered in patients with psychomotor, temporal, or complex seizure disorders.

Prolonged hangover is also possible in situations where methohexital has been repeatedly administered as this lipophilic drug will accumulate in fat compartments and leach out slowly. These cases are often called "stormy" – the patient never quite falls asleep, remains combative throughout the procedure, and takes a long time to recover.

A rare complication that can be encountered with barbiturate anesthetics is their ability to induce acute intermittent porphyria. In porphyria, there is a partial deficiency in the enzymes that are involved in heme synthesis. In the absence of the enzymes there is an overproduction and buildup of porphyrin-containing heme precursors. Clinically, this gives rise to acute attacks of gastrointestinal, neurological, and behavioral disturbances. Barbiturate anesthetics induce hepatic enzyme production, which has been shown to trigger the syndrome. Barbiturates are contraindicated in patients with porphyria (Martone et al., 1991).

Non-barbiturate intravenous anesthetics

Propofol

Propofol is a unique intravenous sedative and hypnotic agent, supplied as 1% oil in a white emulsion of soybean oil, glycerol, and purified egg lecithin. This emulsion provides a favorable medium for bacterial growth, which requires the addition of a bacteriostatic agent to retard bacterial growth (ethylenediamenetetraacetic acid, EDTA, sodium metabisulfite, or benzyl alchohol). Strict aseptic handling of this drug includes single-patient use (1 patient – 1 vial – 1 syringe) within 6 hours of needle contamination.

A sulfite-containing formulation has been found to be associated with allergic reactions (Marik, 2004); however, there is only sparse data (You et al., 2012) to support the avoidance of propofol in egg-allergic or soy-allergic patients (Murphy et al., 2011; Dewachter et al., 2011, Tashkandi, 2010). Egg allergy is typically triggered by proteins in the egg white (lecithin is derived from yellow yolk), and the soy in propofol is devoid of allergenic components during the refining process. In addition, egg allergies that become apparent in childhood are rarely lifelong. Approximately, 2/3 of infants who are allergic to eggs "outgrow" their egg allergy by age 7. Hypersensitivity reactions with propofol anesthesia are significantly less frequent than reactions due to methohexital or penicillin. The following language persists in the product insert for propofol: "Propofol Injectable Emulsion is contraindicated in patients with allergies to eggs, egg products, soybeans and soy products" (AAP, 2010).

Pharmacodynamics

Propofol exerts its action at the $GABA_A$ receptors in the reticular activating system to achieve dose-dependent anxiolysis, sedation, amnesia, and general anesthesia. Unlike the barbiturates, however, there appear to be two $GABA_A$ receptor channels that are sensitive to propofol. The first, which contains a B_3 subunit, is directly activated, resulting in rapid chloride channel opening (Bali and Akabas, 2004). This site is different from the benzodiazepine receptor site and has a profound and immediate effect on the opening of the chloride channel, inducing general anesthesia. However, when propofol is given at lower doses and used as a sedative agent, it binds to a second receptor, which contains B_1 and B_2 subunits but does not contain the B_3 subunit. In this setting, propofol exerts its effect by facilitating the action of GABA to promote chloride conductance in a manner slightly similar to benzodiazepines, rather than directly opening the channel.

Additional actions include immobility, which accompanies loss of consciousness (Trapani et al., 2000), a post-anesthetic sense of well-being, and antiemetic activity, which improve patient comfort and satisfaction.

Pharmacokinetics

Distribution of propofol, similar to that of most highly lipid-soluble agents, tends to follow a three-compartment distribution model based on vascularity. In this setting, it has a distribution half-life of 1–8 minutes. There is extensive binding to erythrocytes and plasma proteins, leaving only approximately 2% of the administered dose capable of crossing the blood–brain barrier (Mazoit and Samil, 1999).

Since redistribution is dependent in large part on vascularity, patient factors have a profound effect on the response of a given patient to the agent. Primary patient factors include age, gender, and body weight. The pediatric patient in an age range of approximately 4 to 5 up to 11 or 12, exhibits very rapid redistribution and requires as much as a 50% increase in dose on a milligram per kilogram basis. If an adequate induction dose is not given, the child will often react violently to the painful stimulation of local anesthetic needles and this visceral response is often accompanied by an increase in salivation, which can precipitate a laryngospasm.

In those of advanced age with diminished circulatory capacity and a lower cardiac output relative to body mass, redistribution takes place more slowly. It is prudent to reduce dosages by 25–30% in patients older than 60 and by an additional 15–20% per decade in each of the decades thereafter. This results in doses that are in the realm of sedative rather than anesthetic levels for propofol.

Redistribution is more rapid in women (Hoymork and Raeder, 2005), which can result in the need for a 10–15% greater dose on a milligrams per kilogram basis in females as compared to males. Those with obesity and obstructive sleep apnea pose special challenges, even for such a relatively safe drug as propofol. The distribution pattern in these patients is such that dosages based on body weight are far too great and can lead to a relative "overdose." Consequently, in this setting the induction dosage should be based on lean body mass rather than on total body weight.

Although much of the dissipation of the effect of propofol is due to redistribution, the agent is also rapidly removed from the body by metabolism, predominantly in the liver. Metabolic clearance exceeds hepatic blood flow, suggesting metabolism at extrahepatic sites (Fechner et al., 2003). Its rate is approximately 10 times that of thiopental and some of the biotransformation appears to take place in the lungs and the kidneys. Metabolites conjugated in the liver are very rapidly excreted with only 1% appearing unchanged in the urine. Interestingly, renal insufficiency or even chronic renal failure tends to have little effect on the clearance of the parent drug.

Effects on organ systems

Propofol can reduce arterial blood pressure due to impairment of sympathetic vasoconstriction and possibly via a direct effect of nitric oxide on the vascular endothelium. Although in younger patients much of the hypotensive effect is countered by stimulation such as local anesthetic injections, special caution must be observed in the elderly, where a blunting of baroreceptors can be exaggerated, which hampers a compensatory increase in heart rate. Factors other than patient age that can influence the hypotensive effect of propofol include the size of the induction bolus and the rate at which it is administered. The dose can be reduced by administration of small doses of pre-induction medications including midazolam and opioids.

Similarly to barbiturate intravenous anesthetics, propofol causes respiratory depression, in large part due to a blunting of the chemoreceptor response to hypercapnia. It is most pronounced following bolus administration and can be accompanied by a period of apnea. However, as in the case of post-induction hypotension, the respiratory depression can be countered to a significant extent by the painful stimulation of local anesthetic injections. Since the latter are performed in virtually all oral and maxillofacial surgery and dental procedures, the period of apnea rarely becomes problematic in propofol anesthesia in dentistry.

As compared to barbiturates, propofol does have some positive influences on the respiratory system. It has a mild bronchodilating effect, although not nearly as great as that which is seen with ketamine. In addition, it tends to diminish upper airway sensitivity and reflexes. Consequently, it is usually possible to suction the hypopharynx for removal of secretions with little potential for laryngospasm. There is no histamine release with the use of propofol.

In addition to inducing hypnosis, propofol has several other effects in the central nervous system. These include the postanesthetic euphoria and antiemetic effect mentioned previously, as well as anticonvulsive properties. Interestingly, there have been a few case reports of long-term postanesthetic seizures associated with patients who received propofol. However, neither an unequivocal causal relationship nor a mechanism has been proved (Sinner and Graf, 2008).

When compared to methohexital, in many cases propofol can cause more profound apnea, more hypotension, less tachycardia, more pain at the injection site, greater depression of laryngeal reflexes, less myoclonus, more sedation, less nausea and vomiting, less hangover, and a smoother recovery.

Adverse effects

Pain on injection is the most notable adverse effect of propofol administration. This is most frequently encountered during the administration of the initial bolus rather than during maintenance of anesthesia. It can usually be overcome by the slow injection with “barbotage” of 1cc of lidocaine 1% without epinephrine immediately prior to administration of the bolus of propofol. In this technique, the syringe plunger is moved back and forth during the administration of the lidocaine to keep the lidocaine solution in contact with the endothelial surface of the vein. Ketamine can be successfully utilized in the same manner. Then, when the bolus is administered, the IV rate can be increased maximally to “wash in” the propofol rapidly rather than leaving it in contact with the vessel wall at the venipuncture site.

Contraindications include patients with lipid metabolism disorders or patients with sulfite allergy (with preparations containing metabisulfite). Caution is prudent in patients who have demonstrated anaphylaxis to eggs.

Ketamine

Ketamine is a rapidly acting general anesthetic agent that produces dose-dependent unconsciousness, amnesia, and profound analgesia. Ketamine depresses neuronal function between the thalamus (which relays sensory information from the reticular activating system to the cortex) and the limbic cortex (awareness of sensation), while simultaneously stimulating parts of the limbic system. This “dissociative anesthesia” puts the patient in a detached, cataleptic-like state, unaffected by sensory input. Some reflexes remain unaffected, including the corneal and light reflex, and pharyngeal and laryngeal reflexes of cough, sneeze, and swallow; however, these should never be assumed to be protective. Excessive lacrimation, salivation, and increased skeletal muscle tone can be noted, often occurring with purposeless but coordinated movement. In addition to dissociation, ketamine has a number of other interesting anesthetic effects including analgesia, sympathetic stimulation (which often tends to cause hypertension), and profound bronchodilation (Kohrs and Durieux, 1998).

Pharmacodynamics

Ketamine noncompetitively antagonizes the action of glutamate at the N-methyl-D-aspartate (NMDA) receptor, by binding at an allosteric site on the receptor, effectively blocking pain perception. The NMDA receptor is also involved with memory formation, which can explain ketamine’s amnestic properties. The intense analgesia produced by ketamine approaches that which can be obtained with therapeutic opioid levels, and this analgesia is present in subanesthetic doses, which persists after anesthetic effects have dissipated. Ketamine is also active at μ and κ opioid receptor sites. The psychotomimetic effects it exhibits may be due in part to its activity at the κ opioids sites. Ketamine has an inhibitory effect on muscarinic acetylcholine receptors, which is the most likely explanation for the bronchodilation and increase in secretion that accompanies ketamine administration (Sinner and Graf, 2008).

Pharmacokinetics

Similarly to propofol, ketamine is highly lipid soluble, and it crosses the blood–brain barrier rapidly. Its effects can be noted within seconds of intravenous administration and peak within approximately 1 minute. Redistribution is rapid with a redistribution half-life of approximately 10–15 minutes. The duration of ketamine anesthesia is directly proportional to the administered dose and is prolonged in the presence of other anesthetic agents. Protein binding is much less than that with other anesthetic agents, which also contributes to a shorter duration of action, especially at lower doses.

Ketamine undergoes *N*-demethylation and hydroxylation in the liver. The metabolites are conjugated and excreted in the urine with only approximately 4% of the parent compound excreted unchanged. Its elimination half-life is approximately 2 to 3 hours, and in children elimination is approximately twice as rapid as that seen in adults.

Effects on organ systems

The cardiovascular effects of ketamine differ from virtually all other anesthetics in that it causes an increase in blood pressure, heart rate, and cardiac output (White et al., 1982). These effects are often countered by prior administration of a benzodiazepine, especially midazolam. When ketamine is administered along with propofol, the hypertensive effect of the ketamine "balances" the hypotensive effect of propofol, such that the patient's blood pressure during induction tends to be more stable than when either drug is administered independently. The cardiovascular stimulation is due to enhanced sympathetic nervous system activity.

Unlike barbiturates and propofol, ketamine exhibits a minimal response to hypercapnia and has little effect on central respiratory drive. Consequently, it is associated with far less respiratory depression than virtually all other anesthetic agents, and in contrast to the other agents it preserves functional residual capacity (FRC) in children. Central sympathetic stimulation, which increases blood pressure and heart rate, is also responsible for the potent bronchodilation properties of ketamine. This can be particularly helpful in the treatment of asthmatic patients and has been another reason that ketamine currently so often finds a place alongside propofol in the balanced anesthetic used in OMS and dental offices. On the negative side, ketamine increases oral and pharyngeal secretions that can lead to laryngospasm. This can be largely overcome by premedication with an antimuscarinic. Overall ketamine is a very safe anesthetic agent with a high therapeutic index (Reich and Silvay, 1989).

The role of ketamine in office-based anesthesia

Ketamine can be used as a primary anesthetic as well as in combination with propofol. The complementary effects of low-dose ketamine in a propofol-based anesthetic truly provide balance to the technique. In that balance, ketamine provides dissociation to augment hypnosis and sympathetically mediated cardiovascular stimulation to counter the hypotensive effects of propofol. It adds analgesia while propofol provides none. It also possesses significant bronchodilation, which helps to counterbalance the respiratory depression that is inherent in the anesthesia provided by most other agents. The combination of ketamine with propofol reduces the dose of propofol required. These attributes have generated considerable interest in the agent within the last decade, and it is likely that it will continue to play a significant role in office-based anesthesia.

Adverse effects

The most notable adverse effect associated with the use of ketamine is the occurrence of adverse emergence phenomena, including vivid dreaming, agitation, fear, excitement, combativeness, and visual auditory, proprioceptive, and confusional hallucinations. Frequency is dependent on a number of factors, and is averaged from multiple reports to be approximately 30%. The onset of these reactions usually occurs with the first verbal contact, and may result from a misinterpretation of external stimuli with the patient. Risk factors include higher doses, an age range from 10 to 15 yrs, female gender, and patients with frequent vivid dreams, and personality and psychiatric problems. Pretreatment with benzodiazepines was found to significantly decrease the incidence of these reactions (Kothary and Zsigmond, 1977). Resolution is spontaneous and is facilitated by minimizing tactile, verbal, and visual stimulation by recovery in a dimly lit, quiet room. Continual monitoring is mandatory.

Other adverse effects include excess lacrimation, sympathetic stimulation, and slight increase in the frequency of nausea and vomiting. Like propofol, there is no reversal agent for ketamine.

Benzodiazepines

Midazolam and diazepam are the two intravenous benzodiazepines used most frequently in the dental office. Midazolam has several advantages over diazepam including water solubility, more rapid onset and offset, and less pain on injection.

Diazepam is highly lipophilic; as such it is combined with propylene glycol to exist as a solution for injection, which accounts for the pain on intravenous injection and greater risk of thrombophlebitis. Midazolam is water soluble and exists with an open imidazole ring in solution. This ring closes at physiologic pH, allowing the molecule to become highly lipid soluble.

Pharmacodynamics

Benzodiazepines are thought to enhance the binding of GABA to the $GABA_A$ receptor and/or potentiate chloride conductance into the cell, increasing the threshold for action potential, which inhibits nerve transmission. This binding accounts for the dose-dependent anxiolytic, amnesic, hypnotic, anticonvulsant and muscle relaxant effects of benzodiazepines. The enhancement of GABA rather than direct stimulation of the $GABA_A$ receptor is thought to account for a possible "ceiling effect," which can limit the degree of CNS depression with the isolated use of benzodiazepines.

Pharmacokinetics

Midazolam is approximately 3–6 times more potent than diazepam and has a more rapid onset.

The benzodiazepines undergo biotransformation in the liver involving both Phase I and Phase II pathways, but there are significant differences in the two agents. Midazolam is rapidly oxidizes in Phase I, which leads to greater hepatic clearance. The oxidative pathways can be impaired by patient characteristics such as advanced age or systemic compromise such as cirrhosis. Certain drugs such as cimetidine can compete with cytochrome P450 enzyme function, which is particularly impaired in the case of diazepam. In addition, patients who have a high level of alcohol consumption have an increased clearance of midazolam that may be due to microsomal enzyme induction.

Although both diazepam and midazolam have active metabolites, those of diazepam, including oxazepam and desmethyldiazepam, are more long-lasting and prolong the drug's effects. Profound sedation may be seen in patients with renal impairment. Overall, the clearance rate of midazolam is much greater than that of diazepam.

Effects on organ systems

The initial popularity of benzodiazepines for sedation and intravenous anesthesia has usually been attributed to their relatively minimal hemodynamic and respiratory effects. There is a slight decrease in systemic vascular resistance, and the baroreflex may be marginally impaired; but overall there are relatively minimal adverse hemodynamic effects.

Benzodiazepines do produce dose-related central respiratory depression, which is more pronounced with midazolam. Depression becomes manifest 3 minutes following midazolam injection and may become apparent more quickly when the initial bolus is delivered rapidly. When significant depression occurs, it may remain for 60–120 minutes. The benzodiazepines and opioids produce additive (synergistic) effects, and the depression may lead to apnea, which must be monitored closely and managed appropriately (Nordt and Clark, 1997).

Benzodiazepines are effective anticonvulsants. Both diazepam and midazolam increase the threshold for seizure initiation and can be utilized for treatment of seizures, including those that are due to excessive doses of local anesthetics. A mild muscle relaxant effect can also occur.

Adverse effects

An interesting central nervous system effect of the benzodiazepines is the phenomenon of paradoxical disinhibition, when anticipated anxiolysis and sedation is replaced with restlessness and agitation. These episodes can continue for an extended period of time and occur more frequently when higher doses of benzodiazepines are used. They are encountered more often in children and teens as opposed to adults.

Overall, the benzodiazepines used for intravenous anesthesia have been relatively safe. However, recovery of psychomotor and cognitive function can be lengthy, especially in patients of advanced age.

As indicated above, thrombophlebitis can occur after intravenous injections of diazepam because of the addition of propylene glycol.

Alpha-2 Agonists and Dexmedetomidine

In the 1970s, clonidine was noted to have potent sympatholytic properties, and cardiologists adopted it for the treatment of hypertension. However, it became apparent that the drug had sedative properties that ultimately led to clonidine's use for premedication and as an ancillary drug in general anesthesia. This became the first use of an α_2 adrenergic receptor agonist for anesthesia. Ultimately a second α_2 agonist, dexmedetomidine was isolated for use in humans.

Pharmacodynamics

Both clonidine and dexmedetomidine are α_2 agonists; however, dexmedetomidine has an eightfold greater affinity for the alpha 2 receptor. The sedative action of α_2 agonist is through normal sleep-inducing pathways and is consequently similar to natural sleep.

Pharmacokinetics

Dexmedetomidine has a distribution half-life of approximately 6 minutes. Its elimination half-life is 2–3 hours and it has a pharmacokinetic profile consistent with a 3-compartment model that is unaltered by age, weight, or renal failure. It undergoes extensive biotransformation in the liver, and its pharmacokinetics is markedly affected by hepatic insufficiency (Schnider and Minto, 2004).

Effects on organ systems

The most important hemodynamic effects of dexmedetomidine are bradycardia and decreased systemic vascular resistance. Following bolus injection, there is an initial increase in blood pressure with a decrease in heart rate. The initial increase in blood pressure is due to the peripheral α_2 effects leading to vasoconstriction. As the initial decrease in heart rate dissipates, blood pressure begins to fall. Within the dose ranges required for significant sedation there are relatively minor effects on respiratory function. In an animal model, dexmedetomidine appears to block histamine-induced bronchoconstriction.

Although dexmedetomidine has not found a place in the armamentarium of agents for office-based anesthesia, its alpha-2 agonist congener clonidine has been used quite successfully as anesthetic premedication, especially in pediatric patients. It provides anxiolysis, sedation, enhancement of postoperative analgesia, and reduced postoperative nausea and vomiting (PONV). There is a considerable body of literature on its use in Europe, and the agent is now receiving attention for this application in the United States.

Adverse effects

Although the natural sleep-like hypnosis of dexmedetomidine is desirable, it is challenging to capitalize on this attribute clinically. Because of its hemodynamic actions, especially its tendency to cause bradycardia, it is difficult to give either rapid or large boluses of dexmedetomidine to achieve the desired level of sedation. Loading doses must be relatively small and delivered quite slowly, usually over a 15–20 minute time frame, and following discontinuation there is a prolonged period of recovery. These attributes are not conducive to its being utilized as a primary anesthetic agent in dentistry.

Opioids

Opioids most commonly used in the dental office are fentanyl and meperidine, as well as pentazocine and nalbuphine, which are mixed agonist–antagonists.

Pharmacodynamics

Opioids exert their effect by interaction with various opioid receptors, primarily the mu receptor. The analgesic effects of opioids are due to two factors: direct inhibition of the ascending transmission of nociceptive transmission from the dorsal horn of the spinal cord and activation of descending inhibitory circuits sent from the midbrain to the dorsal horn of the spinal cord (Sessle, 1999). Other intended dose-dependent effects of opioids include cognitive impairment, mood alteration, sedation, and blunting of airway reflexes. The euphoria and tranquilization produced by opioids is thought to involve dopaminergic pathways. The opioids do not have any significant effect on the areas of the brain involved in memory. These findings would be consistent with experience with opioid-based "balanced anesthetics," which have fallen out of favor. Even with high-dose opioid levels, patients complain of having been aware of their procedures and have recall of intraoperative events.

Pharmacokinetics

Fentanyl and meperidine have a rapid onset within minutes of intravenous injection (meperidine has a slower onset and delayed offset) with rapid redistribution to fat and muscle compartments. In addition, there is a relatively high uptake of opioids by the lungs. Peak activity requires more time, making both drugs difficult to titrate. Clinical duration is 2–4 hours.

Both drugs are metabolized in the liver and excreted by the kidneys. Norfentanyl is clinically inactive; however normeperidine is 1/2 as potent as meperidine as an analgesic, but 2–3 times as potent as a central nervous system stimulation. As such, it has pro-convulsant properties. Since it has a far longer elimination half-life than the parent compound, these effects can be particularly severe in patients with renal disease. In addition, meperidine has strong anticholinergic properties, which can lead to disruption of cholinergic transmission in the CNS that in turn lead to agitation, confusion, delirium, and possible memory deficits. Finally, meperidine has been implicated in mood state alteration resulting in fear, anger, and anxiety.

Effects on organ systems

The most significant cardiovascular effect of the opioids is their tendency to cause vagally mediated bradycardia (meperidine can cause tachycardia) and vasodilation from a sympatholytic effect. Overall, inclusion of opioids as a part of balanced intravenous anesthetic tends to impart hemodynamic stability (Fukada, 2010).

Perhaps the most profound adverse systemic effect of opioids is the respiratory compromise due to a blunted hypercapnic response, which causes a slowed respiratory rate and protracted expiratory time. The very young and the very old are more sensitive to these respiratory depressant effects of opioids. This respiratory depressive effect is magnified when opioids are used with benzodiazepines and hypnotics.

Opioid agonist/antagonists

In the early 1970s, a true opioid antagonist naloxone was introduced on the market. Over the next decade, agents that exhibited both agonistic and antagonistic activity were developed in an attempt to find an effective analgesic agent that had little abuse potential. Two of the primary agents in this category include pentazocine and nalbuphine. Nalbuphine is competitive at μ receptor sites but acts as an agonist at κ receptors. Pentazocine is a weaker μ receptor antagonist but maintains κ agonistic activity.

Similarly to other opioids the agonist/antagonists provide analgesia and sedation but cause limited respiratory depression. Both pentazocine and nalbuphine exhibit a "ceiling effect" for respiratory depression i.e., mild respiratory depression is seen at low doses but there is not a proportionate increase in respiratory depression with higher doses. This characteristic is more pronounced with nalbuphine. Additional effects of pentazocine include elevation of blood pressure and cardiac work and dysphoric reactions. Nalbuphine does not usually produce undesirable cardiovascular effects and elicits dysphoric reactions only in exceedingly high doses. Pentazocine has a plasma half-life of 4–5 hours and nalbuphine 3 hours.

The clinical use of the agonist/antagonist has been limited by their undesirable side effects, their limited analgesic effects, and their relatively long plasma half-lives (Yaksh and Wallace, 2010).

Adverse effects

In addition to respiratory depression, bradycardia, and hypotension, there are other adverse side effects and drug interactions associated with the use of opioids. These include pruritis (itching), particularly on the nose the upper lip, which is often triggered by the presence of a nasal cannula, hypothermia and shivering, and nausea and vomiting. Shivering consumes oxygen, which can be problematic in patients with coronary artery disease or respiratory disease. Nausea is due to stimulation of the chemoreceptor trigger zone in the medulla. Once this occurs, CTZ may exhibit a lower threshold for stimulation by other emetogenic events, e.g. premature ambulation. The incidence of opioid-induced nausea and vomiting can be markedly reduced when it is administered concomitantly with propofol as a part of a balanced anesthetic. However, additional antiemetics can be considered, and a combination of ondansetron and dexamethasone has been found to be particular effective.

Another respiratory concern in the administration of opioids is chest rigidity, which has been occasionally reported with fentanyl. Chest wall rigidity is addressed in Chapter 35.

Interaction between meperidine and monoamine oxidase inhibitors can trigger the serotonin system. This is addressed in Chapter 36 (Table 20.1).

Table 20.1 Cardiovascular effects of frequently used parenteral anesthetic agents.

Drug	Heart rate	Blood pressure	Ventilation	Bronchodilation
Methohexital	↑	↓	↓	–
Propofol	–	↓	↓	↑(mild)
Ketamine	↑	↑	↓ (mild)	↑
Midazolam	–	–	↓ (mild)	–
Fentanyl	↓	↓	↓	–

References

Bali, M. and Akabas, M. H. Defining the propofol binding site location on the gabaa receptor. *Mol Pharmacol* **65**: 68–76, 2004.

Barratt, R., et al. In influence of sampling site in the distrubution phase kinetics of thiopentone. *Anaesth Intensiv Care* **56**: 1385–91, 1985.

Dewachter, P., et al. Anesthesia in the patient with multiple drug allergies: are all allergies the same? *Curr Opin Anesthersiol* **24**: 320–325, 2011.

Hemmings, H. C. Jr., The pharmacology of intravenous anesthetic induction agents: a primer. *Anesthesiology News [Online]*, **36**: 10, 2010.

Fechner, J., et al. Pharmacokineticss and clinical pharmacodynamics of the new propofol prodrug GPI 15715 in volunteers. *Anesthesiol* **99**: 303–313, 2003.

Fukada, K. Opioids In: Miller, R. D., ed. *Miller's Anesthetsia* 7th edn Philadelphia: Churchill Livingstone/Elsevier, 2010.

Hoymork, S. C. and Raeder, J. 2005. Why do women wake up faster than men from propofol anaesthesia? *Br J Anaesth* **95**: 627–633, 2005.

Kohrs, R. and Durieux, M. E. Ketamine: Teaching an old drug new tricks. *Anesth Analg* **87**, 1186–93, 1998.

Kothary, S. P. and Zsigmond, E. K. A double blind study of the effective anti-hallucinatory doses of diazepam prior to ketamine anesthesia. *Clin Pharmacol Ther* **21**: 108–109, 1977.

Marik, P. E. 2004. Propofol: Therapeutic indications and side-effects. *Curr Pharm Des* **10**: 3639–3649, 2004.

Martone, C. H., et al. Methohexital: a practical review for outpatient dental anesthesia. *Anesth Prog* **38**: 195–199, 1991.

Mazoit, J. X. and Samil, K. Binding of propofol to blood components: Implications for pharmacokinetics and for pharmacodynamics. *Br J Clin Pharmacol* **47**:35–42, 1999.

Murphy, A., et al. Allergic reactions to propofol in egg-allergic children. *Anesth Analg* **113**: 140–144, 2011.

Nordt, S. P. and Clark, R. F. Midazolam: a review of therapeutic uses and toxicity. *J Emerg Med* **15**: 357–365, 1997.

Propofol Product Insert. AAP Pharmaceuticals, Schaumburg, IL 2010.

Reich, D. L. and Silvay, G. 1989. Ketamine: An update on the first twenty-five years of clinical experience. *Can J Anaesth* **36**: 186–197, 1989.

Reves, J. Intravenous anesthetics. In: Miller, R. D. (ed.) *Miller's Anesthesia*. 7th edn, Philadelphia: Churchill Livingstone/Elsevier, 2010.

Rockoff, M. and Goudsouzian, N. G. Seizures induced by methohexital. *Anesthesiol* **54**: 333–335, 1981.

Schnider, T. W. and Minto, C. F. 2004. Analgesics: Receptor ligands α2 adrenergic receptor agonists. In: Evers, A. S. and Maze, M. (eds.) Anesthetic pharmacology : Physiologic principles and clinical practice : a companion to miller's anesthesia. New York: Churchill Livingstone, 2004.

Sessle, B. J. Neural mechanisms and pathways in craniofacial pain. *Can J Neurol Sci* **26**: S7–S11, 1999.

Sinner, B. and Graf, B. M. Ketamine. *Handbook Exp Pharmacol* **182**: 313–333, 2008.

Tashkandi, J. My patient is allergic to eggs, can I use propofol? A case report and review. *Saudi J anaesth* **4**: 207–208, 2010.

Trapani, G., et al. Propofol in anesthesia. Mechanism of action, structure-activity relationships, and drug delivery. *Curr Med Chem* **7**: 249–271, 2000.

White, P.F., et al. Ketamine – its pharmacology and therapeutic uses. *Anesthesiol* **56**: 119–136, 1982.

Yaksh, T. L. and Wallace, M. S. 2010. Opioids, analgesia, and pain management. In: Brunton, L. L., et al. (eds.) *Goodman and Gilman's The Pharmacological Basis Of Therapeutics.* 12th edn, McGraw-Hill Professional, 2010.

You, B., et al. A Case of Propofol-Induced Oropharyngeal Angioedema and bronchospasm. *Allergy Asthma Immunol Res* **1**: 46–48, 2012.

21 Inhalational anesthetic agents

Charles Kates[1], Douglas Anderson[2], Richard Shamo[3], and Robert Bosack[4]

[1] University of Miami Miller School of Medicine, Departments of Anesthesiology and Surgery and Section of Oral/Maxillofacial Surgery, Department of Surgery, Jackson Memorial Hospital Miami, FL, USA

[2] Oregon Health Sciences University, Department of Anesthesiology and Peri Operative Medicine, Portland, OR, USA

[3] Memorial Hospital of Sweetwater County, Rock Springs, WY, USA

[4] University of Illinois, College of Dentistry, Chicago, IL, USA

The term "anesthetic" refers to a class of chemical moieties that produce three effects: analgesia (absence of pain), amnesia (absence of recall), and sleep (loss of consciousness). In the absence of local anesthesia, all three effects are essential for a patient to tolerate a painful surgical procedure. Although nitrous oxide is often categorized as an anesthetic agent, it cannot be predictably used for this purpose, in the absence of other agents.

Nitrous oxide pharmacology

Physical properties

Nitrous oxide (N_2O) (Figure 21.1) is the most widely used of all inhalational anesthetics. Better known by the name "laughing gas" because of the euphoria often experienced when inhaled, it is a colorless, non-halogenated, ultra-short-acting anesthetic gas. It has been described as odorless, or having a slightly sweet or fruity odor. It is the only inorganic agent of the inhalational anesthetics; in contrast to the other more potent agents, nitrous oxide exists as a gas at room temperature. It is typically stored in pressurized metal cylinders where its gas and liquid phases exist in a state of equilibrium, resulting in a constant pressure of 750 psi until nearly all of the nitrous oxide has been depleted. Similarly to oxygen, N_2O will support combustion, but it is not explosive. Although it is considered a weak anesthetic, its relatively safe pharmacologic profile and ease of titration have led to its frequent use as an agent to lower the MAC of other volatile and intravenous agents in patients undergoing general anesthesia. These properties, along with its noninvasive means of delivery and anxiolytic effects, contribute to its almost universal use in both the dental setting and the surgical operating room.

Pharmacodynamics

N_2O is a weak anesthetic gas, with analgesic and anxiolytic properties at subanesthetic concentrations. While the comprehensive mechanism of action for N_2O has not been fully elucidated, it is known that the analgesic properties of N_2O are related to both spinal and supraspinal release of endogenous opioids (Emmanouli and Quock, 2007). As this pathway is not fully developed in early childhood, N_2O may not be as effective in this group of patients. The role of opioid receptors is clearly demonstrated by the fact that administration of naloxone, an opioid antagonist, reverses the analgesic effects of N_2O (Gillman et al., 1980).

There is also evidence that N_2O stimulates $GABA_A$ receptors that in turn trigger an anxiolytic signaling pathway; however, the exact mechanism remains to be elucidated. Further evidence of the GABA receptor pathway involvement in the anxiolytic effects elicited by N_2O is the fact that this agent can be blocked by the administration of flumazenil, a GABA receptor antagonist. Studies on rats suggest that the NMDA (N-methyl-D-aspartate) receptor plays a role in the anesthetic property. It is believed that N_2O blocks the excitatory influence of the NMDA glutamate receptors, thus reducing its excitatory effects on the nervous system (Jevtovic-Todorovic et al., 1998). It is also possible that the anesthetic property could be mediated partially through the GABA receptor.

Although it is considered relatively weak among modern anesthetics, anesthesia was, in fact, one of the first uses of N_2O. As the minimum alveolar concentration of N2O is 104% in adults and 109% (Murray et al., 1991) in children, general anesthesia is unlikely, but still possible when N_2O is used at atmospheric pressure as the sole agent. When delivered in its highest concentrations in the operating room, N_2O demonstrates an amnestic quality, which is believed to be due to inhibition of nicotinic acetylcholine receptors (Avidan et al., 2008).

Pharmacokinetics

The partial pressure (tension) that is exerted by a gas is proportional to its concentration in air. Room air contains 20% oxygen; therefore, at 1 atmosphere (760 mmHg), the pressure exerted by oxygen is 152 mmHg (760 mmHg $\times$ 0.2, ignoring the effect of moisture.). When gas is in contact with blood, it dissolves in blood proportional to its partial pressure. The amount of gas that dissolves in blood is determined by its solubility. The more soluble the agent, the greater the amount dissolved in blood, which is pharmacokinetically inactive, as dissolved gas does not exert pressure or tension. Pressure (tension) gradients drive gas movement in the body, from inspired gas to alveoli, to blood and to tissues and in the reverse, when inspired gas is turned off. Gases with low blood solubility exist mostly in the gaseous state (therefore in limited quantity), exerting a tension that drives its diffusion in or out of the plasma. Gases

Anesthesia Complications in the Dental Office, First Edition. Edited by Robert C. Bosack and Stuart Lieblich.

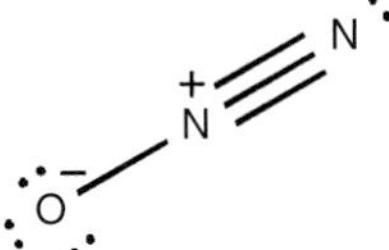

Figure 21.1 chemical structure of nitrous oxide. Note the lack of any organic components. The oxygen molecule is bound to nitrogen, preventing its use for respiration.

Table 21.1 Partition coefficients of volatile anesthetics at 37°C.

Agent	Blood/gas	Brain/blood	Muscle/blood	Fat/blood
Isoflurane	1.4	2.6	4.0	45
Desflurane	0.42	1.3	2.0	27
Sevoflurane	0.65	1.7	3.1	48

Table 21.2 Select factors that determine pressure gradients and movement of inhalational agents.

- P_I – inspired partial pressure (concentration) of inspired gas
- P_A – alveolar partial pressure
- P_a – partial pressure in arterial blood
- P_{br} – partial pressure in the brain
- CO – cardiac output
- Blood/gas partition coefficient

with high solubility (which permits it to be carried in the blood in substantial quantities) need time to reach equilibrium and exert a tension, which tends to slow down the rate of diffusion in or out of the plasma. The blood : gas partition coefficient quantifies the equilibrium concentrations of the gas in air and dissolved in blood, with small numbers indicating low solubility (see Table 21.1).

Nitrous oxide is relatively insoluble in blood: it is held in less quantity and diffuses faster than the more soluble oxygen or volatile gases (see Table 21.2). However, nitrous oxide is approximately 30 times more soluble than nitrogen. Closed spaces in the body contain 80% nitrogen, whose even lower solubility limits its rapid removal by the blood. Entrance of N_2O, whose relatively greater solubility permits it to be carried by blood in substantial quantities (compared to nitrogen), is not countered by an equal loss of nitrogen. This results in an increase in volume and expansion of a complaint space (bowel, pulmonary bullae) or an increase in pressure in a noncompliant space (eye, middle ear, obstructed sinus.) Having the patient to breath 100% oxygen for several minutes prior to administering N_2O "washes out" nitrogen, which permits the N_2O to achieve a higher concentration, and hence quicker onset.

The partial pressure of any gas rapidly achieves equilibrium in the alveoli, blood, and tissue (brain.). Increasing the partial pressure of any gas in the alveoli, by increasing the delivered concentration (partial pressure), will hasten its onset. Nitrous oxide is often used in combination with other gases to hasten induction. When inhaled with other volatile gases, the insoluble N_2O leaves the alveoli more rapidly, augmenting diffusion gradients to increase the movement of N_2O into the alveoli. The rapidly moving N_2O increases the tracheal inflow of other gases. N_2O initially expands the alveoli, which then contracts as N_2O leaves the alveoli and enters the blood, shrinking the alveolar volume, which subsequently increases the concentration of the second gas.

When gases are turned off, the opposite situation occurs, as N_2O is thought to enhance the rate of emergence from anesthesia with volatile gases. Nitrous oxide leaves the blood and rapidly enters the alveoli, diluting the concentration of oxygen. This "diffusion hypoxia" is not clinically significant; however, it is still prudent to allow the patient to breath 100% oxygen at the end of the case to scavenge the remaining N_2O (Brodsky et al., 1998, Becker, 2008).

N_2O does not accumulate within the body and leaves unchanged from the bloodstream into the lungs (Yagiela et al., 2004) where it is exhaled. There are no active metabolites.

Physiologic effects

Nitrous oxide has long been regarded for its relative safety and neutral physiologic impact. As mentioned previously, it is frequently combined to lower the MAC of other general anesthetics in order to achieve the desired level of anesthesia while decreasing the required dose of each anesthetic. Its rapid onset and offset enhance the ability to accurately titrate doses to the desired effect. Another major benefit of adding N_2O to a balanced technique is the ability to reduce the dose of other agents while maintaining clinical effect, which hopefully decreases the frequency and severity of adverse side effects.

In adults, nitrous oxide possesses mild sympathomimetic properties (Hohner and Reiz, 1994), leading to release of catecholamines and a mild increase in peripheral vascular resistance. However, it also acts as a mild direct myocardial depressant, masking much of the sympathetic effects and yielding a mild stimulatory effect on the cardiovascular system. In contrast, children tend to experience overall mild cardiovascular depression.

While N_2O has been demonstrated to increase respiratory rate, it also decreases tidal volume, leaving minute ventilation essentially unchanged in healthy patients. Slightly unique among inhalational anesthetics is the fact that N_2O is nonirritating to the airway; thus, it is well suited to pediatric and asthmatic patients. It has, however, been reported to induce gagging in patients with hyperactive gag reflexes and thus could conceivably present a possible risk for aspiration.

The most significant reported impact of nitrous oxide upon the respiratory system is its ability to cause depression of the hypoxemic drive. Even amounts as small as 0.1 MAC can cause significant depression of the normal response to hypoxia. Given the diffusion hypoxia phenomenon described above, this can cause a potentially serious situation in which hypoxia is not recognized and hypoxic end organ injury can occur.

Adverse effects

When used intermittently (<6 continuous hours) and with effective scavenging, nitrous oxide has a high degree of safety with only very rare morbidity involving patients with significant medical conditions. There are, however, some important risks and potential complications that must be considered prior to its administration. These include depression of hypoxic pulmonary drive in patients with COPD (theoretical), accumulation of N_2O in closed air spaces in the body, blood dyscrasias, and myeloneuropathic changes (tingling, weakness, memory impairment, and incoordination, among others).

Patients with COPD can be at elevated, albeit theoretical, risk from the administration of nitrous oxide, because of the supplemental oxygen that is co-administered with N_2O. Ventilatory drive in these patients is dependent upon arterial oxygen saturation rather than on

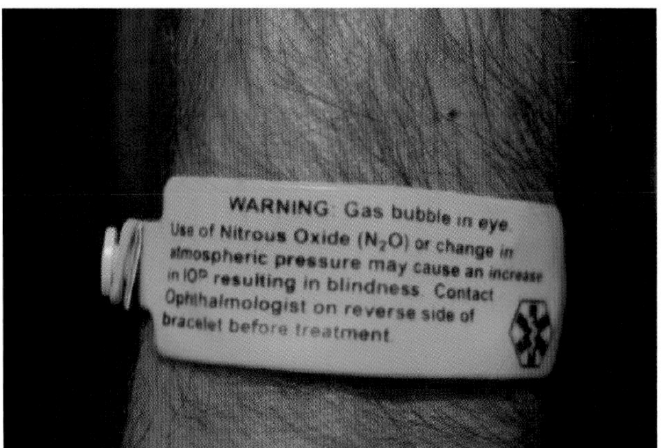

Figure 21.2 A patient arm band advising against the use of N_2O because of recent eye surgery.

the levels of carbon dioxide. The administration of oxygen at high flow rates during sedation with nitrous oxide prevents hypoxia, and can decrease respiratory rate. The resultant increased CO_2 retention can worsen respiratory acidosis, which, in many COPD patients, is likely to already exist.

N_2O can increase the volume or pressure of closed air spaces in the body, as N_2O enters closed spaces more rapidly than nitrogen can escape. This phenomenon can lead to rupture of emphysematous pulmonary bullae due to volume expansion. In situations where volume expansion is limited due to lack of compliance, pressure will increase, leading to further damage and even loss of vision in patients with retinal detachment or recent eye surgery in which an intraocular bubble may remain postoperatively (Fu et al., 2002; Vote et al., 1992) (see Figure 21.2). Other situations in which N_2O administration could be problematic include middle ear infections with blocked eustachian tubes, which can lead to tympanic membrane injury or pain in obstructed sinuses.

N_2O irreversibly oxidizes the cobalt atom in Vitamin $B_{12,}$ thereby reducing the activity of B_{12}- dependent enzymes (methionine synthase) (Deacon et al., 1978).

Methionine synthase plays a role in transforming folate into its active form, which is important for DNA synthesis as well as red and white blood cell formation (Koblin et al., 1982). This suggests a potential for serious hematologic consequences, which are rare when nitrous oxide is used intermittently in the dental office. Nitrous oxide should be avoided in patients with Vitamin B_{12} or folate deficiencies.

Inhibition of the methionine synthase enzyme can also result in low levels of methionine with chronic, low dose, or long-term abuse of N_2O. These patients classically present with Lhermitte's sign (shooting sensations on flexion of the neck; Layzer et al., 1978) as well as tingling, weakness, memory impairment, and incoordination. This deficiency is believed to be related to degenerative neurologic changes resulting from inhibition of the transmethylation process necessary to maintain the myelin sheath (Flippo and Holder, 1993). Methionine has been used with some success in the treatment of nitrous-oxide-induced neuropathy (Stacy et al., 1992).

In patients with the rare autosomal disease, type III homocystinuria, the tetrahydrofolate reductase enzyme is defective. Administration of N_2O in such patients can lead to thromboembolic events and thus should be avoided (Yamade and Hamada, 2005).

Another potential reaction involves patients taking bleomycin chemotherapy within the last 12 months. These patients are more vulnerable to pulmonary fibrosis if exposed to high concentrations of O_2. As at least 30% oxygen must necessarily accompany nitrous oxide administration, N_2O should be avoided in these patients (Fleming et al., 1988).

There are some patients in whom N_2O administration may cause postoperative nausea and vomiting. In such patients, including propofol and dexamethasone in the sedation protocol can help prevent this complication.

Data do not support the notion that exposure to trace amounts of N_2O is associated with impaired fertility, spontaneous abortion, or increased cancer risk (Weimann, 2003); however, some concerns linger (Rowland et al., 1992). Owing to fears of possible association of N_2O use with spontaneous abortion and potential birth defects, NIOSH has arbitrarily selected a time-weighted average of <25 ppm as the maximum allowable concentration for the duration of exposure (McClothin et al., 1994).

Clinical use

Recent data from the American Dental Association indicates that over 70% of dental practitioners use nitrous oxide (ADA, 2007). This is largely due to public acceptability of the drug and its relatively safe profile as an anesthetic. Most states within the United States do not require special permits to administer N_2O in the dental office. For reasons discussed above, it serves as an ideal agent for relatively minor dental procedures or as an adjunct to intravenous sedation in more complicated procedures. In order to maintain public approval of nitrous oxide as well as the privilege to administer nitrous oxide in private dental practice, several safety precautions have been employed to avoid potentially life-threatening mistakes that could occur.

Nitrous oxide use should be avoided in patients with

- vitamin B_{12} deficiency,
- COPD or pulmonary bullae
- upper respiratory infections with nasal congestion
- recent middle ear infections
- eye surgery within the last 3 months
- bleomycin chemotherapy within the past 1 year
- children with type III homocystinuria.

Safety measures

The widespread use of nitrous oxide in both the dental and operating room settings requires the employment of a number of safety precautions and strict attention during use in order to ensure safety and perpetuate the favorable reputation of nitrous oxide.

In an effort to prevent incorrect connections between nitrogen and oxygen tanks to the delivery system, a Pin Index Safety System exists, which prevents nitrous oxide tanks from being plugged in to oxygen hoses and vice versa. After many years of use, however, these pins could fail and be lost, allowing indiscriminate connection to either gas. For this purpose, the Diameter Index Safety System was developed such that the diameter of the hoses and connectors as well as the thread pattern for each gas connection is different, making improper hose connections nearly impossible. In addition, the hoses are color coded so that blue nitrous tanks are plugged into blue nitrous supply hoses, and green oxygen tanks are plugged into green oxygen supply hoses. Nitrous delivery units for use in dental operatories also have built-in regulators to limit the percentage of nitrous to oxygen ratio to no more than 70% nitrous, ensuring that a patient never receives less than 30% oxygen. In fact, if oxygen delivery fails or the tank is empty, modern delivery systems contain a safety valve that stops administration of all gases and allows ambient air to enter the mask.

Another inherent safety feature with nitrous oxide as given in the dental operatory is that the delivery and respiratory components for nitrous administration are not a closed circuit; thus even at the highest delivery concentration of 70% nitrous, the patient is not limited to the 30% oxygen delivery through the system because mouth breathing is almost always possible. Even with these "fail-safe" measures, however, equipment and fail-safe mechanisms still require frequent inspection and maintenance, and these safeguards do not protect against errors in plumbing that could occur during building construction.

As mentioned previously, the use of scavengers is mandated to reduce levels of nitrous oxide in ambient air. The inability to maintain a perfect nasal hood seal and the presence of an open mouth limit the efficacy of the scavenging systems. For this reason, it is a good idea to have ventilation ducts at low levels in the operatory because nitrous oxide is heavier than O_2 and will accumulate on the floor. In addition, ventilation systems should remove air from inside to outside the building. Infection control is also a potential safety issue and should be addressed by ensuring that masks and tubes are sterilized or changed after each use.

In cases where the patient is slow to wake up from anesthesia or appears to be deepening in level of anesthesia despite decreasing the level of N_2O, it is possible that there may be a mechanical failure or installation error. If the practitioner suspects that there may be failure of safety features, removal of the patient's mask or replacement with oxygen flowing from a separate system is the recommended course of management.

Technique of N_2O administration in the dental office:

1. Inspect equipment, all connections, and scavenger systems for obvious signs of failure in safety mechanisms or leaks.
2. Always have an assistant in the room with any type of sedation.
3. Baseline vital signs should be obtained and recorded.
4. Continuous visual monitoring should be done during the delivery of N_2O.
5. An appropriately sized mask (comfortable but sealed) should be selected for the patient and fitted appropriately.
6. Start with 100% O_2 at 6L per minute initially and assess patient for effect for 1–2 minutes.
7. Titrate N_2O in 5-10% increments every 3–5 minutes until the desired effect is achieved.
8. Discourage talking and encourage nasal breathing.
9. Limit total exposure duration to <6 hours.
10. When finished, turn off N_2O and administer 100% O_2 for 3–5 minutes.
11. Check vital signs at the end of the case to ensure they are within 20% of baseline prior to discharging the patient.

End point of proper sedation

Effective N_2O sedation/analgesia should induce positive mood changes: happy, pleasant, relaxed, sense of well-being, modest euphoria, and warmth. The patient should remain cooperative. While protective reflexes should remain intact, gag reflex may be diminished. Patients also may report a diminished sense of the passage of time while under nitrous oxide sedation. They may be less alert and less concerned with surroundings. Extremities may feel tingly or heavy, with a mild decrease in muscle tone. Speech can gain a nasal quality.

Oversedation

Signs or symptoms of oversedation include hysterical laughter in a patient who is otherwise difficult to manage. Patients may also experience a dysphoric or uncomfortable feeling, floating sensation, slurred or incoherent speech, delayed response to questions, and 'altered hearing or a humming sound. In some cases of severe oversedation, patients may become confused, agitated, unable to move or speak, or may be lose consciousness. Other signs of oversedation include nausea, vomiting, sweating, and increased heart rate and blood pressure.

Special Considerations

Modifying factors that affect the way in which patients respond to nitrous sedation must also be considered. Concomitant administration of CNS depressants as well as advanced age will increase the relative potency of nitrous oxide whereas younger age, chronic alcohol abuse, and concomitant use of sympathomimetic drugs decrease its relative potency. Thus, careful attention to titrating the level of sedation to the individual rather than a common numerical value at which most patients feel the desired effects is essential.

Potent Inhalational anesthetic agents

Pharmacodynamics

The exact mechanism of action of inhalational anesthetic agents has not been fully elucidated; however, interaction with the GABA receptor is one of many probable actions. Sevoflurane, desflurane, and isoflurane are the only halogenated anesthetic agents currently available in the United States.

Pharmacokinetics

Gases move between air, pulmonary alveoli, blood, and brain by simple diffusion, from regions of high to low partial pressure. As expected, these concentration gradients are constantly changing with the movement of gases. Some of the parameters that determine these pressure gradients are listed in Table 21.3. The letter "P" is an abbreviation for partial pressure.

The partial pressure of any gas rapidly reaches equilibrium in the alveolus, arterial blood, and brain, such that the concentration (partial pressure) of any agent in one compartment reflects the concentration in the other compartments.

$$P_A = P_a = P_{br}$$

Factors that affect the partial pressure of the anesthetic gas in any of these "compartments" include the inspired concentration of the anesthetic gas, the uptake of gas by the blood (solubility (blood/gas partition coefficient)), alveolar ventilation (respiratory rate x (tidal volume − dead space), cardiac output, cerebral blood flow,

Table 21.3 Characteristic of inhalational agents and nitrogen (Data from Martin, 2010).

Agent	MAC (potency)	Blood:Gas partition coefficient (solubility)
Nitrogen	–	0.014 (least soluble)
Desflurane	6.0	0.42
Nitrous oxide	105 (least potent)	0.47
Sevoflurane	2.0	0.65
Isoflurane	1.2	1.4 (most soluble)

and tissue uptake of inhaled gases (which depends on partition coefficients and blood flow). Clinically, induction and recovery are most rapid with agents with low blood/gas partition coefficients. Factors that lead to fast induction with a gaseous agent are listed in Table 21.4

The MAC (minimum alveolar concentration) is an indicator of anesthetic potency. It is defined as the minimum alveolar concentration of an anesthetic at 1 atomosphere that produces immobility in 50% of those patients when exposed to a noxious stimulus (Eger, 1984). Notably, the MAC necessary to tolerate laryngeal manipulation and endotracheal intubation without coughing is oftentimes greater than that needed for a surgical incision (see Table 21.2). Factors that alter MAC are shown in Table 21.5.

Termination of anesthetic effect occurs when gases are turned off and concentration gradients are reversed. Volatile agents are exhaled largely unchanged, with hepatic metabolism and urinary excretion playing only a very minor role.

Characteristics of individual gases

Isoflurane (see Table 21.6)

Isoflurane is nonflammable and in spite of a mildly pungent odor, it can be inhaled without much difficulty. It exhibits minimal cardiac depression, and cardiac output is generally maintained with occasional tachycardia, as carotid baroreflexes are largely preserved. Mild beta-adrenergic stimulation can lower arterial blood pressure and reduce systemic vascular resistance while increasing blood flow to muscles.

Table 21.4 Select factors that lead to fast induction with a gaseous agent.

1 High delivered concentration of agent (concentration effect)
2 Low blood/gas solubility
3 Patent airways, healthy and ventilated alveoli, and functional respiratory membranes
4 Hyperventilation (rate and depth)
5 Low cardiac output

Table 21.5 Select Factors that change MAC.

- Factors that increase MAC
  - Youth
  - Drugs that release catecholamines
  - Chronic alcohol abuse
- Factors that decrease MAC
  - Old age
  - Anemia
  - Hypotension
  - Acute alcohol or substance abuse
  - Local anesthetics
  - Parenteral anesthetic agents

As is true of all inhalation agents, except for nitrous oxide, even low concentrations of isoflurane will blunt normal physiological response to hypoxia and hypercapnia. There is a rapid fall in minute ventilation, and it can be slightly irritating to upper airway reflexes. Because it is an ether, it causes some bronchodilatation.

There is an increase in cerebral blood flow and intracranial pressure, with a reduction in cerebral metabolic oxygen requirements, providing some brain protection during episodes of cerebral ischemia.

Some relaxation of skeletal muscles occurs, so the addition of less muscle relaxant is required to achieve adequate surgical operating conditions as compared to a N_2O/intravenous anesthetic technique.

The drug is metabolized to trichloroacetic acid, and because of its limited metabolism, there is little, if any, risk of liver damage. There are no contraindications to the use of isoflurane, with the exception of malignant hyperthermia (MH).

Desflurane

Desflurane has a very high vapor pressure, which requires a special heated and pressurized vaporizer to produce clinically useful concentrations. It is highly insoluble in blood, and therefore it has a very rapid onset and recovery period. "Wake up" times are 50% more rapid than with isofluane. Unfortunately, desflurane is only 25% as potent as the other currently available inhalation potent anesthetics, which makes it far less efficient, that is, a MAC of 6.6% versus 1.2% for isoflurane.

The main disadvantage of desflurane is its pungency, which makes it difficult to breath as an induction agent. Desfluane is irritating to the airway, which often results in a high incidence of laryngospasm, breath-holding, coughing, and salivation. Cardiovascular effects are similar to those of isoflurane, so a rapid increase in concentration can lead to a transient elevation in heart rate, blood pressure, and catecholamine levels. However, it does not increase coronary arterial blood flow as does isoflurane. Its respiratory effects include a decrease in tidal volume, an increase in respiratory rate, an overall decrease in alveolar ventilation, and depressed respiratory response to carbon dioxide.

Desflurane causes cerebral vasodilatation, an increase in cerebral blood flow, and intracranial pressure at normal blood pressure and normal CO_2 levels. There is a decline in the cerebral metabolic rate and therefore a decrease in cerebral oxygen consumption. As with other agents of this class, there is a dose-dependent relaxation of skeletal muscles. It has no nephrotoxic effects and LFTs are unaffected with no hepatic injury. There is minimal metabolism. However, there is greater degradation of dry carbon dioxide absorbent, which can produce significant levels of carbon monoxide. Desflurane is contraindicated in patients who have severe hypovolemia, a history of MH or intracranial hypertension. As is true of other halogenated agents, it potentiates non-depolarizing muscle relaxants.

Table 21.6 Clinical pharmacology of volatile anesthetic agents.

Agent	Blood pressure	Heart rate	Tidal volume	Respiratory rate	Hepatic metabolism
Isoflurane	–	+	–	+	Minimal
Desflurane	–	+ or no change	–	+	Minimal
Sevoflurane	–	No change	–	+	2–3%

Sevoflurane

Sevoflurane is non-pungent and very easily inhaled, making it a near ideal agent for inhalation induction. It is highly insoluble, allowing for rapid induction and recovery. Sevofluane causes a mild depression of cardiac contractility and vascular resistance, but has more depression of cardiac output than either isofluane or desflurane. Its respiratory effects are similar to that of isoflurane, and it causes an increase in cerebral blood flow and intracranial pressure similar to isoflurane. It also decreases cerebral metabolic requirements, and it impairs cerebral autoregulation. As with other halogenated agents, it provides some skeletal muscle relaxation.

There is a decrease in portal vein flow and an increase in hepatic arterial blood flow. Similarly to isoflurane, it is metabolized in the liver through the P-450 system.

There is some evidence that sevoflurane can degrade soda lime producing a nephrotoxic substance called *compound A*. This is probably of no clinical significance; however, a new carbon dioxide absorbent known as Amsorb has been developed, which is not subject to this degradation (Kharasch et al., 2002).

Clinical applications

Isoflurane mask induction

Start with a concentration of 1% in oxygen or oxygen plus N_2O. Increase the concentration by 0.5% to 1% every two to three breaths, or as tolerated, until the patient loses consciousness. The maintenance concentration for isoflurane is between 0.4% to 2% with or without N_2O.

Possible complications:

1 Isoflurane is not the drug of choice for obese patients unless it is supplemented with intravenous agents.
2 It frequently causes tachycardia when it is employed without basal narcosis.
3 Isoflurane is pungent, and therefore can cause laryngospasm during mask induction.
4 It is easy to overdose patients, but it reverses as readily as it overdoses.
5 It works well with intubated patients as an adjunct to narcotic anesthesia.
6 Recovery is rapid, but there is a fairly high incidence of laryngospasm.

Desflurane

Desflurane is a very rapid-acting anesthetic and must be carefully controlled. It is important to use this agent with an agent monitor for both inspired and exhaled anesthetic concentration for safe patient delivery. As previously stated, the agent is not useful for inhalation induction and has limited value in the oral surgery setting, but has been used very successfully for longer anesthetic where it is used for maintenance of anesthesia with an endotracheal tube or LMA. It is typically delivered in concentrations of 4–11% for induction and 2.5–8.5% for maintenance.

Sevoflurane mask induction

Sevoflurane is an excellent agent for mask induction.

The traditional method:

1 Begin with an inspired concentration of 3% with or without N_2O/O_2.
2 Increase the concentration by 1% for every three breaths, or as tolerated until loss of consciousness is reached.
3 Maintenance concentrations vary between 0.5% and 3%, depending on number factors including local anesthesia or supplemental intravenous agents.

The one-breath technique:

1 Premedicate with an antimuscarinic and low dose benzodiazepine.
2 Pre-flood the breathing circuit with 8% sevoflurane plus 50% N_2O/O_2.
3 Have the patient do a forced exhalation.
4 Place the fully sealed facemask (avoid mask leak) over the patients mouth and nose and have the patient do a forced inhalation, followed by breathholding.
5 Expect loss of consciousness in 15–30 seconds.
6 Ventilate with an 8% concentration for 1–2 minutes or until induction is complete.
7 Spontaneous ventilations will resume.
8 Expect partial upper airway obstruction, easily correctible with an oral airway (sevofluane is very forgiving of upper airway stimulation), with little likelihood of laryngospasm.

Possible complications:

There are almost no caveats to the use of sevoflurane. It is a nearly ideal agent for dental anesthesia use, particularly if an inhalation induction is desired. Overdosage is rapidly reversed, and laryngeal reflexes are depressed before anesthetic levels are achieved. This is a double-edged sword since depression of laryngeal reflexes can invite silent foreign body aspiration. Sevoflurane can also be used as part of a traditional balanced anesthetic technique with intravenous induction, gas maintenance, and basal narcosis.

The Advantages of Inhalation Anesthetics:

1 It allows for the maximum control of anesthetic depth.
2 It depresses upper airway reflexes at low concentration (except desflurane) and is very useful as a primary or adjunctive anesthetic modality.
3 When patients are discharged, they are fully well, with little chance of silent airway obstruction when no longer under professional supervision.
4 When properly utilized, there is little or no nausea and vomiting associated with these drugs.
5 It is possible to utilize halogenated anesthetics as sole anesthetic drugs.

Disadvantages of Halogenated Inhalational Anesthetics:

1 They are relatively expensive compared with intravenous agents.
2 It is advisable to use a hospital-grade anesthetic apparatus to deliver these drugs.
3 All halogenated agents are malignant hyperthermia triggers, and an adequate supply of dantrolene and other appropriate medications must be readily available should an MH event occur.

Summary

A brief review of the science necessary for understanding the practical administration of halogenated inhalation anesthetics has been presented along with some practical advice on its administration. Emphasis has been directed toward the avoidance of perioperative complications with these drugs by approaching their use with a sound fundamental scientific understanding of their application in modern office-based dental and oral surgical practice.

References

American Dental Association Survey Center. 2007 *Survey of Current Issues in Dentistry: Surgical Dental Implants, Amalgam Restorations and Sedation*. Chicago: American Dental Association, **2008**, pp 11–13.

Avidan, M. S., et al. Anesthesia Awareness and the bispectral index. *N Engl J Med* **358**: 1097–1108, 2008.

Becker, D. E. and Rosenberg, M. Nitrous oxide and the inhalation anesthetics. *Anesth Prog* **55**: 124–131, 2008.

Brodsky, J. B., et al. Diffusion hypoxia: a reappraisal using pulse oximetry. *J Clin Monit* **4**: 244–248, 1998.

Deacon, R., et al. Selective inactivation of vitamin B12 in rats by nitrous oxide. *Lancet* **2**: 1023–1024, 1978.

Eger, E. I. *Anesthetic Uptake and Action*. Baltimore: Williams and Wilkins, 1984.

Emmanouli, D. E. and Quock, R. M. Advances in understanding the actions of nitrous oxide. *Anesth Prog* **54**: 9–18, 2007.

Fu, A. D., et al. Complications of general anesthesia using nitrous oxide in eyes with pre-existing gas bubbles. *Retina* **22**: 569–574, 2002.

Fleming, P., et al. Bleomycin therapy: a contraindication to the use of nitrous oxide-oxygen psychosedation in the dental office. *Pediatr Dent* **10**: 345–6, 1988.

Flippo, T. W. and Holder, W. D. Neurologic degeneration associated with nitrous oxide anesthesia in patients with vitamin B12 deficiency. *Arch Surg* **128**: 1391–95, 1993.

Gillman, M.A., et al. *Paradoxical effect of naloxone on nitrous oxide analgesia in man Eur J Pharmacol* **61**: 175–177, 1980.

Hohner, R. and Reiz, S. Nitrous oxide and the cardiovascular system. *Acta Anaesthesiol Scand* **38**: 763–766, 1994.

Kharasch, E. D., et al. Comparison of Amsorb, sodalime, and Baralyme degration of volatile anesthetics and formation of carbon monoxide and compound a in swine in vivo. *Anesthesiol* **96**: 173–82, 2002.

Koblin, D. D., et al. Nitrous oxide inactivates methionine synthetase in humer liver. *Anesth Analg* **61**: 75–78, 1982.

Jevtovic-Todorovic, V., et al. Nitrous oxide (laughing gas) is an NMDA antagonist, neuroprotectant and neurotoxin. *Nature Med* **4**:460–463, 1998.

Layzer, R. B., et al. Neuropathy following abuse of nitrous oxide. *Neurology* **28**: 504–506, 1978.

Martin, J. L. Inhaled anesthetics: metabolism and toxicity. In Miller, R. D., (ed.) *Miller's Anesthesia* 7th edn. Philadelphia: Churchill Livingstone Elsevier, p. 640, 2010.

McClothin, J., et al. Center for disease control technical report: control of nitrous oxide in dental operatories. DHHS (NIOSH) Publication No. 94–129, 1994.

Murray, D. J., et al. The additive contribution of nitrous oxide to isoflurane MAC in infants and children. *Anesthesiol* **75**: 186–190, 1991.

Rowland, A. S., et al. Reduced fertility among women employed as dental assistants exposed to high levels of nitrous oxide. *New Engl J Med* **327**: 993–997, 1992.

Stacy, C. B., et al. Methionine in the treatment of nitrous-oxide-induce neuropathy and myeloneuropathy. *J Neurol* **239**: 401–403, 1992.

Vote, G. J., et al. Visual loss after use of nitrous oxide gas with general anesthetic in patients with intraocular gas still resistant up to 30 days after vitrectomy. *Anesthesiol* **97**: 1305–1308, 1992.

Weimann, J. Toxicity of nitrous oxide. *Best Prac Res Clin Anaesth* **17**: 47–61, 2003.

Yagiela, J., et al. *Pharmacology and Therapuetics for Dentistry*. 5th edn. St. Louis: Mosby, 2004. P 287–289, 774–5.

Yamade, T. and Hamada H. General anesthesia for patient with type III homocystinuria (tetrahydrofolate reductase deficiency). *J Clin Anesth* **17**: 565–567, 2005.

22 Antimuscarinics and antihistamines

Richard C. Robert
University of California at San Francisco, Department of Oral and Maxillofacial Surgery, San Francisco, CA, USA

Antimuscarinics

Mechanism and site of action

Atropine and glycopyrrolate are used in the dental office as antisialogogues because of their inhibitory effect on salivary gland secretion. In addition, atropine is often beneficial as a first-line choice for hemodynamically significant bradycardia. These drugs are competitive antagonists of muscarinic acetylcholine receptors. They are also called *anticholinergic* or *parasympatholytic*, although these terms are less specific. Muscarinic receptor sites are shown in Table 22.1.

Pharmacodynamics and pharmacokinetics

Atropine blocks salivary and bronchiolar secretions and increases cardiac output by blocking the muscarinic slowing of the heart at the SA and AV nodes. As an antisialogogue, it is less potent, and has a more rapid onset and shorter duration when compared to glycopyrrolate (see Table 22.2). The drying of secretions together with the relaxation of the smooth muscles of the airway may help protect against laryngospasm. The use of atropine as an antisialogogue may be useful in preventing excess airway secretions sometimes seen with ketamine. It is slightly antiemetic (unlike glycopyrrolate) and may decrease PONV associated with opioids, but it reduces the opening pressure of the lower esophageal sphincter, increasing the risk of passive regurgitation. Unlike glycopyrrolate, atropine is a tertiary amine, which readily crosses the blood–brain barrier, possibly leading to CNS effects. Atropine can decrease excitation sometimes seen with the use of methohexital, due to a mild sedative effect at lower doses. Atropine is contraindicated in patients with narrow-angle glaucoma, as dilation thickens the iris peripherally, causing a narrowing of the iridocorneal angle, which blocks drainage of aqueous humor, which increases intraocular pressure. Symptoms of acute angle-closure glaucoma include severe pain in the eye, erythema, blurred vision, seeing halos around lights, and systemic complaints such as headaches and nausea and vomiting. It has been suggested that a patient who has severe eye pain, a markedly red eye, subjective loss of vision, and nausea in the immediate postoperative period should have an ophthalmologic examination to rule out acute angle-closure glaucoma (Lachkar and Bouassida, 2007). Atropine should also be avoided in cases where tachycardia may be harmful, such as severe coronary artery disease. Elderly patients may be more susceptible to the CNS effects of atropine, even at smaller doses. The adult intravenous dose is .5 mg, and can be repeated up to 3 mg.

Glycopyrrolate is a quaternary amine that is unable to cross the blood–brain barrier. Therefore, it exerts more of its effects peripherally with pronounced antisialagogue activity and less tendency to cause tachycardia. Although in general, glycopyrrolate has more desirable properties as an antimuscarinic premedication, it has downsides as well, one of which is its tendency to cause urinary retention in older male patients who suffer from benign prostatic hypertrophy. The possibility of significant urinary retention, which can occasionally require catheterization, tends to limit the use of glycopyrrolate in this patient population. Although glycopyrrolate is an excellent antisialagogue, its duration of action is somewhat longer than desired and may extend to 7–8 hours following administration. Consequently, patients should be advised of this effect, and fluid replenishment during the immediate postoperative period encouraged. The usual dose is 0.005–0.01 mg.kg or 0.2 mg IV in adults.

Another concern in the use of antimuscarinics is their use in elderly patients, especially those taking multiple medications, which may have anticholinergic effects. Diminution of acetylcholine levels in the CNS has been implicated in the development of cognitive dysfunction and is even a contributing factor in dementia. Consequently, atropine should be used with caution in this patient population.

Antihistamines (H_1 receptor antagonists)

Histamine is a member of a family of biologically active amines sometimes called "autacoids" (derived from Greek meaning "self-remedy"). Autacoids function as neurotransmitters and involve a wide variety of receptors. In addition to histamine, the family includes serotonin, prostaglandins, leukotrienes, and cytokines. Historically, those drugs which were perceived to be antagonists of the actions of histamine were termed antihistamines. However, it has become apparent that there is not a single histamine receptor, but four, which are designated as H_1, H_2, H_3, and H_4. The term "antihistamine" includes those drugs that antagonize the action of histamine at the H_1 receptor.

Anesthesia Complications in the Dental Office, First Edition. Edited by Robert C. Bosack and Stuart Lieblich.

Table 22.1 Select muscarinic receptor sites.

	Organ	Stimulation	Inhibition
Post-ganglionic sympathetic receptor	Sweat glands	Excessive sweating	Anhydrosis
Post-ganglionic parasympathetic receptor	Salivary glands	Excessive salivation	Xerostomia
	Sinoatrial node	Bradycardia	Tachycardia
	AV node	Decreased conduction velocity	Increased conduction velocity
	Bronchiolar smooth muscle	Bronchoconstriction	Bronchodilation
	Gastrointestinal smooth muscle	Increased motility	Decreased motility
	Eye	Miosis, near vision	Mydriasis, far vision

Table 22.2 Comparative pharmacology of atropine and glycopyrrolate.

	Onset, IV	Duration, IV (minutes)	CNS effect	Airway secretions	Heart rate
Atropine	1–2 minutes	15–30	Low dose sedation, then stimulate	↓	+++, may see paradoxical bradycardia initially or at low doses
Glycopyrrolate	15 minutes	120–480	None	↓	+/0

The agents

The first generation of antihistamines includes diphenhydramine, tripelennamine, chlorpheniramine, cyclizine, hydroxyzine, and promethazine. Although these agents blocked some of the undesirable actions of histamine, most tended to cause sedation and drowsiness. Pharmacologic research continued and a second generation of H_1 receptor antagonists, for example, loratadine were formulated in the 1980s. A charged side chain was added, which imparted a lower lipid solubility with commensurate inability of these agents to pass through the blood–brain barrier (Del Cuvillo et al., 2006).

Mechanism and site of action

H_1 receptor subtypes are widely distributed in the body in the smooth muscle, endothelium, and the brain. In the brain, histaminergic neurons are found in the hypothalamus and project to several major areas of the brain, notable of which are those involved in sleep, wakefulness, and processing of memory. They relax the smooth muscle, decrease vascular permeability, and decrease pruritus. However, many of the actions of drugs in this class are not due to their actions at the H_1 receptor site. A significant portion of the attributes of the antihistamines are due to the action at the receptor sites of agents with which they share a chemical similarity, such as the phenothiazines and anticholinergics.

Distribution, metabolism, and elimination

Following injection, first-generation H_1 antagonists are widely distributed, and easily pass through the blood–brain barrier due to their lipid solubility. Most undergo extensive biotransformation by CYP450 enzymes in the liver and may form active metabolites. Excretion is by the kidneys with an elimination half-time of approximately 4–8 hours for most of the agents, but can go up to several days for others. They are eliminated more rapidly in children than in adults and more slowly in patients with significant liver disease. They tend to induce hepatic microsomal enzymes, which, interestingly, may actively facilitate their own metabolism (Du Buske, 1996).

Effects on organ systems

A common characteristic of most firs-generation H_1 antagonists is their sedative properties. Part of their sedative effect may be due to their direct effects on the hypothalamus and the related areas that control wakefulness discussed above. However, some of the sedation that attends these agents is due to the similarity between their chemical structures and other drug families such as the phenothiazines, e.g., promethazine, and the piperazines, e.g., hydroxyzine. It is these sedative effects that have often prompted the use of the latter drugs in dentistry, especially for sedation in children.

Several of the first-generation H_1 receptor antagonists have been found to exhibit a relatively high level of efficacy as antiemetics. This appears due to their ability to counteract motion sickness mediated by the vestibular apparatus. Diphenhydramine, dimenhydrinate, and meclizine have been found to be particularly efficacious, but vary in their tendency to cause sedation. For instance, diphenhydramine can cause significant sedation and has been utilized as a sleep aid. Promethazine is a phenothiazine as well as an H_1 receptor antagonist and exerts part of its antiemetic activity by blocking D_2 receptors in the chemoreceptor trigger zone.

H_1 receptor antagonists also have actions consistent with activity at several other non-H_1 receptor sites. These include an antimuscarinic type effect, which leads to urinary retention; an alpha-receptor-blocking effect, which may cause hypotension; and serotonin-blocking actions as well (Skidgel et al., 2011).

A final, rather interesting attribute of one of the H_1 antagonists is the ability of diphenhydramine to function as a local anesthetic. It is injected as a 1% solution and has been utilized in a number of settings including dental anesthesia and the emergency room for patients purported to be allergic to local anesthetics. Its onset of action is usually about 5 minutes, but reports vary widely as to the duration from approximately 15 minutes to up to 3 hours. The injection itself does tend to be somewhat more uncomfortable than local anesthesia, but its effectiveness is reportedly greater than that of procaine.

The role of antihistamines in office-based anesthesia

The primary uses of antihistamines in dental anesthesia have been largely dependent upon properties unrelated to antagonism at the peripheral H_1 receptor sites. In particular, agents such as promethazine and hydroxyzine have been primarily utilized as sedatives and antiemetics. Today, their use as sedatives has been largely supplanted by the benzodiazepines, but they continue to be used in the treatment of allergic reactions and as antiemetics.

References

Del Cuvillo, A., et al. Comparative pharmacology of the h1 antihistamines. *J Investig Allergol Clin Immunol* **16**: Suppl 1, 3–12, 2006.

Du Buske, L. M. Clinical comparison of histamine h1-receptor antagonist drugs. *J Allergyt Clin Immunol* **98**: S307–S318, 1996.

Lachkar, Y. and Bouassida, W. Drug-induced acute angle closure glaucoma. *Curr Opin Ophthalmol* **18**: 129–133, 2007.

Skidgel, R., et al. Histamine, bradykinin and their antagonists. *In:* Brunton, L. L., et al. (eds.) *Goodman and Gilman's the Pharmacological Basis of Therapeutics*, 12th edn. New York: McGraw-Hill, 2011.

23 Drug interactions

Kyle Kramer[1] and Richard C. Robert[2]
[1]Indiana University, Department of Oral Surgery and Hospital Dentistry, Indianapolis, IN, USA
[2]University of California at San Francisco, Department of Oral and Maxillofacial Surgery, San Francisco, CA, USA

Introduction

Historically, drug interactions of anesthetic agents have been looked upon as troublesome, unintended side effects of the agents. However, gradually it was realized that some side effects could be balanced alongside the primary effects of the anesthetic agents utilized in the balanced anesthetic approach (Rosow, 1997). An example is the opposing effects of propofol and ketamine on systemic blood pressure. When unopposed, the blood pressure effects of either can be detrimental, i.e. patients can develop dangerously low blood pressure with the administration of propofol and dangerously high blood pressure with ketamine. However, if modest levels of the two agents are administered concomitantly, the blood pressure effects of each tend to be neutralized and the patient remains relatively normotensive.

Unintended adverse interactions occur with medications that a patient is currently taking, notwithstanding interaction of anesthetic drugs administered by the anesthesia provider. There is a direct correlation between the risk of drug interactions and the number of medications a patient is currently taking. A retrospective study from 2000 found that the risk of an adverse drug reaction occurring is 9.8 times more likely once patients concurrently take three or more medications (Mannesse et al., 2000). It must be stated that not all drug–drug interactions are clinically significant. There are factors that the dentist should be aware of that may either increase or decrease the risk of these interactions. It is crucial for clinicians to be aware of the potential for these adverse drug interactions in order to primarily prevent them from occurring, and if a patient were to present with an adverse event, to be able to identify and promptly initiate management (see Table 23.1). This chapter reviews adverse reactions and interactions for drugs commonly utilized in dentistry and dental anesthesia.

Table 23.1 Risk factors and adverse drug interactions.

Risk factors associated with *increased* incidence of adverse drug interactions	
Patient factors	Age extremes Multiple existing comorbidies: • Cardiovascular disease • Pulmonary disease • Neurological disease • Renal disease • Hepatic disease Pregnancy or nursing Unreported or illicit drug use/abuse
Pharmacologic factors	Narrow therapeutic index Chronic administration or use Hepatic microsomal enzyme inducers or inhibitors Impairers of normal renal physiology
Risk factors associated with *decreased* incidence of adverse drug interactions	
Patient factors	Most dental patients ASA I and II Elective procedures predominate
Pharmacologic factors	Short-term administration Minimal need for chronic administration or use Wide therapeutic index

Types of drug interactions

Many of the drugs commonly used in dentistry, medicine, and anesthesia interact with specific cellular receptors that naturally exist within the body. These drug–receptor relationships can be classified as agonists, antagonists, or partial agonist/antagonists. Unanticipated or abnormal responses may arise when there are other drugs present that cause a disruption to normal drug functioning. These altered responses can be classified as antagonism, potentiation, summation, synergism, and unexpected drug effects (Yagiela et al., 2004).

Antagonism

Antagonists bind to specific receptor sites, but unlike agonists, do not trigger any activation of the receptor. An antagonistic process can occur with the administration of a drug that specifically acts to counter or reverse a previously administered agonist. Antagonistic interactions can be further classified as competitive or noncompetitive. Competitive antagonists are capable of occupying the same target receptor-binding site as the agonist, thereby preventing its binding. Activity or inactivity of the receptor depends on which molecule (agonist or competitive antagonist) is able to occupy

Anesthesia Complications in the Dental Office, First Edition. Edited by Robert C. Bosack and Stuart Lieblich.

the receptor-binding site. Receptor site occupation heavily depends on the quantity of molecules (agonist versus competitive antagonist) available for binding in addition to the quantity of free binding sites. Noncompetitive antagonists bind in a different location than the agonist receptor binding site, and produce a conformational change in the protein structure that effectively inactivates or closes the agonist binding site. Alternatively, noncompetitive antagonists can also bind to the same receptor site as an agonist; however, unlike competitive antagonists, they cannot be overcome by increasing the number of available agonist molecules. A common example of competitive antagonism is the use of flumazenil to reverse the sedative effects of benzodiazepines. Flumazenil functions by competitively binding to the benzodiazepine receptor, which is located on the GABA ion channel, effectively displacing and temporarily preventing further receptor binding and activation by other benzodiazepine molecules. An example of a noncompetitive antagonist is aspirin, which irreversibly acetylates cyclooxygenase (COX), inactivating the COX enzymes (Golan, 2008). Any increase in the COX substrate, arachidonic acid, will fail to produce any products due to the aspirin-induced blockade.

Potentiation

Potentiation involves the concurrent administration of two drugs, producing a greater clinical effect of one drug than otherwise would occur if administered alone (Yagiela et al., 2004). The key component to potentiation is that the receptor sites for the involved drugs are different as are the expected clinical effects. A common example of potentiation includes the marked respiratory depression produced when opioids are administered concurrently with benzodiazepines. While opioids are able to depress the respiratory drive, this effect is much greater when administered with benzodiazepines.

Summation

Summation occurs when more than one drug is administered, all of which interact with similar receptors, producing either infra-, supra- or simply additive effects, which neither drug typically produces alone (Page, 2002; Yagiela et al., 2004). This process usually involves concurrent administration of multiple drugs within the same class. For example, a patient who received oral triazolam (Halcion) preoperatively and intravenous midazolam (Versed) intraoperatively is likely to demonstrate the summative (additive) effects of combining two benzodiazepines.

Synergism

Synergistic effects occur when drugs that have different mechanisms of action but produce similar clinical effects are administered, producing an end result that is greater than either drug could produce alone. An example of synergism would include the marked CNS depression observed when utilizing propofol in conjunction with etomidate or a barbiturate. All drugs involved are GABAergic, but activate different sites on the GABA receptor.

Unexpected drug effects

An unexpected drug effect is defined as a novel response that occurs when two drugs are concurrently administered, neither of which is capable of producing this response alone, even in excessive doses (Yagiela et al., 2004). For example, it was recently discovered that the antidepressant paroxetine (Paxil) and the cholesterol-lowering drug pravastatin (Pravachol) can unexpectedly produce hyperglycemia (Tatonetti et al., 2011). This is an effect that neither drug is known to produce alone.

Mechanisms of drug interactions

The altered drug function/response can also be classified by the mechanism of drug interaction: pharmacodynamic, pharmacokinetic, or pharmaceutical (Yagiela et al., 2004).

Pharmacodynamic interactions

Almost all drugs function by altering, either positively or negatively, naturally occurring cellular or physiologic processes. These alterations caused by the administered drugs can be defined as the pharmacodynamic response, or "what the drug does to the body." With the administration of additional drugs, interactions can occur that impact the cellular or physiologic process modifying the initial drug's clinical effect. Types of responses produced by pharmacodynamic interactions have already been discussed and include antagonism, potentiation, summation, synergism, and unexpected drug effects.

Pharmacokinetic interactions

Pharmacokinetics can be defined as what happens to the administered drug as it moves throughout the body, or "what the body does to the drug." Pharmacokinetic mechanisms include processes such as drug absorption, distribution, redistribution, metabolism, and excretion. Drug interactions that alter any of these pharmacokinetic processes can cause significant variations in clinical responses. Drugs administered by the enteral route are subject to first pass hepatic metabolism, while parenteral (including sublingual) routes of administration are not. Enteral drugs are first absorbed from the gastrointestinal tract into the blood, which then immediately goes to the liver. On its initial or first pass through the liver, the drug may be metabolized to a greater or lesser extent, depending on the individual drug involved, before traveling throughout the body to interact with its receptors. This phenomenon can lead to altered clinical effects, especially when the activity of the hepatic microsomal enzyme system that is frequently involved in metabolism of drugs is influenced by the presence of other drugs as well. Increased first pass metabolism can lead to reductions in peak plasma levels and duration for drugs inactivated by the liver. For example, a dentist may prescribe an oral analgesic (hydrocodone) for postoperative pain to a patient who is also being treated with an antiepileptic drug. The oral analgesic, if normally metabolized by the liver, may experience a shorter and/or a lower maximal analgesic response due to the increased activity (induction) of hepatic microsomal enzymes by the antiepileptic drug. Induction of the specific CYP450 enzyme of the hepatic microsomal enzyme system will affect not only the extent of first pass metabolism, but also phase I metabolism (oxidation, reduction or hydrolysis) and phase II metabolism (conjugation reactions with compounds such as glucuronic acid to enhance excretion), thus leading to reduced plasma levels and decreased clinical duration of the analgesic drug. Inhibition of the cytochrome P450 enzymes may lead to toxic levels of a drug due to impaired hepatic metabolism. For example, a patient taking the histamine H2-receptor antagonist cimetidine may become oversedated if concurrently given triazolam (Klock, 2008). Parenterally administered drugs are also susceptible to altered pharmacokinetics by alterations in distribution, redistribution, metabolism, and/or excretion.

Pharmaceutical interactions

Drug interactions of this class are relatively rare in dentistry. Pharmaceutical interactions are best defined as an incompatibility of two drugs, which may manifest, for instance, as a precipitate-producing chemical reaction, often inactivating both drugs (Yagiela et al., 2004; Klock, 2008). Drugs should be administered individually, and the intravenous line should be cleared of the previous drug before administering a different drug. Of mention, glucocorticoids should never be mixed other agents.

Interactions with drugs commonly used in dentistry

Interactions with epinephrine

Epinephrine is the most common catecholamine administered on a routine basis by dental professionals. Epinephrine has several important potential drug interactions that can impact dental patients. Most of these drug interactions fall within the pharmacokinetic category due to interacting drugs causing alterations in the normal life cycle of catecholamine molecules. Other sympathomimetics, including ephedrine and phenylephrine may also be similarly affected.

Interactions with epinephrine and TCAs, SNRIs, sNRIs, and amphetamines

Antidepressant classes that have a potential for significant drug interactions with catecholamines and select sympathomimetics are tricyclic antidepressants (TCAs) such as amitriptyline (Elavil), serotonin-norepinephrine reuptake inhibitors (SNRIs) such as venlafaxine (Effexor), desvenlafaxine (Pristiq), and duloxetine (Cymbalta) and selective norepinephrine reuptake inhibitors (sNRIs) such as atomoxetine (Strattera). These antidepressant medications exert their potentiating effects by inhibiting the presynaptic reuptake of serotonin and/or norepinephrine from the synaptic cleft. In addition to indirectly stimulating the presynaptic release of dopamine along with the other catecholamines discussed above, amphetamines also function by impairing dopamine, serotonin, and norepinephrine reuptake transporters (Tarter et al., 1998). These neurotransmitters are synthesized slowly and require their own reuptake after release to help maintain normal neuronal stores. Inhibition of the reuptake transporters initially decreases the concentration of presynaptic catecholamines available for release into the synapse. These presynaptic stores are slowly replenished over time. In addition, impairment of the reuptake transporters can lead to prolonged and increased catecholamine levels within the synaptic cleft. Potential drug interactions can manifest as a prolonged and/or heightened sympathetic response (tachycardia and/or potentially hypertension). The increase in sympathetic activity may be triggered by administration of an indirect (ephedrine) or direct (epinephrine) acting agent. It is recommended that the vital signs of patients be appropriately monitored before and after the administration of vasopressors in local anesthetic solutions. Administration of adrenergic agonists, specifically epinephrine, is not contraindicated in patients taking these classes of medications as long as care is taken to prevent accidental intravascular injection, and the patient is sufficiently monitored to prevent additional drug administration unless vital signs stay within 20% of baseline.

Interactions with epinephrine and non-selective β blockers

It is crucial that dentists be aware of the potential drug interaction between nonselective beta blockers (e.g., propranolol or sotalol) and epinephrine. As a direct-acting adrenergic agonist, epinephrine acts on α1, α2, β1, and β2 receptors. Activation of peripheral α1 receptors causes vasoconstriction; however, activation of the β2 receptors peripherally within the skeletal muscle causes vasodilation. These offsetting effects help prevent system-wide vasoconstriction and a massive increase in the systemic vascular resistance when epinephrine is administered. Administration of exogenous epinephrine to a patient taking a nonselective beta blocker can precipitate a hypertensive crisis. This interaction is a direct result of unopposed α1 vasoconstrictive activation by the epinephrine due to the nonselective beta blocker preventing vasodilatory activation of the β2 receptors within the skeletal muscle. Preventive options include elimination of the epinephrine in the local anesthetic or gingival retraction cord, reducing the concentration and total dose of epinephrine given (e.g., no more than 40 micrograms), or spreading out the injections of epinephrine-containing local anesthetic throughout the appointment rather than giving it all at once at the beginning.

Interactions with epinephrine and MAOIs

Monoamine oxidase inhibitor drugs (MAOIs) function by inhibiting monoamine oxidase, which is one of the main enzymes involved in catecholamine metabolism, specifically in the presynaptic degradation of the naturally occurring catecholamines (dopamine, norephinephrine, serotonin and epinephrine). Inhibition of this process leads to increased catecholamine concentrations primarily within the presynaptic terminal. MAOI-As, such as phenylzine (Nardil) and tranylcypromine (Parnate), are a class of medications that are used as antidepressants, although with much greater frequency in the past than today. MAOI-Bs, such as selegiline (Eldepryl), are more selective for dopamine than for catecholamines in general and are used primarily for the treatment of Parkinson's disease (Klock, 2008). Potentiation of their clinical effects is not a concern when administering exogenous direct-acting catecholamines, such as epinephrine, because a large percentage of the epinephrine injection is metabolized via catecholamine-O-methyl transferase (COMT) rather than by MAO (Yagiela et al., 2004). However, phenylephrine and dopamine are metabolized by MAO, so avoiding these drugs in patients taking MAOIs is appropriate. Administration of sympathomimetics that act indirectly, such as ephedrine, via the presynaptic terminal triggering the release of stored catecholamines, is especially prone to potentiation as there is an increased quantity of catecholamines in storage vesicles due to the inhibition of MAO. Potentially, this may cause a large "bolus" of released catecholamines, prompting severe tachycardia and hypertension. Historically, it was recommended that patients stop MAOIs 2 weeks prior to surgery. However, that was not always possible in emergent/urgent cases. In fact, current recommendations no longer include this mandatory 2-week delay (Stoelting et al., 2008). Cessation of therapy with MAOIs also increases the potential of precipitating the return of psychological symptoms (i.e., depression or a psychotic episode). Appropriate alternatives currently include avoiding the use of indirect-acting sympathomimetics and, when required, utilizing direct-acting sympathomimetic agents (Klock, 2008). Appropriate monitoring is recommended in order to identify and manage prolonged or heightened drug responses.

Interactions with benzodiazepines

Benzodiazepines are largely metabolized in the liver via the cytochrome P450 enzyme system. Specifically, benzodiazepines are rendered inactive once conjugated with glucuronide but may have pharmcologically active metabolites before being conjugated (Yagiela et al., 2004). Enzymatic metabolism within the gut also serves as an extrahepatic metabolic pathway for several benzodiazepine compounds including triazolam, a drug of special interest to dentists. Benzodiazepines are eliminated in the bile and urine, which can be problematic for patients with hepatic or renal dysfunction. In addition, benzodiazepines with clinically significant active metabolites that have very long half-lives, such as diazepam (Valium), can further complicate issues for patients with hepatic or renal impairment.

Interactions with benzodiazepines and metabolic inducers

Drug that induce microsomal enzymes may cause a decrease in the peak effect of orally administered benzodiazepines and/or the duration of sedation produced by the administered benzodiazepine. These altered clinical effects can usually be overcome when utilizing parenteral routes due to the ease of titration. Enteral routes along with parenteral routes that do not easily facilitate titration are most at risk for significant interactions.

Interactions with benzodiazepines and metabolic inhibitors

There are several drugs and drug classes that are documented as inhibitors of the various enzymes involved with benzodiazepine metabolism. (see Table 23.2). Cimetidine, an H2 antagonist, inhibits CYP 3A4 hepatic enzymes, which are primarily involved in the metabolism of clonazepam and diazepam. Metabolism of midazolam and triazolam is similarly impaired by diltiazem and verapamil in addition to cimetidine (Yagiela et al., 2004; Klock, 2008). Several antibiotics, specifically erythromycin and clarithromycin, along with ketoconazole and itraconazole, both antifungals, are known to inhibit oxidative microsomal enzymes (Yagiela et al., 2004). Patients currently on antiviral therapy are also at risk for impaired benzodiazepine metabolism due to inhibition of hepatic microsomal enzymes.

Table 23.2 Examples of cytochrome P450 inducers and inhibitors (Page, 2002; Yagiela et al., 2004; Klock, 2008).

Cytochrome P450 *inducers*	Cytochrome P450 *inhibitors*
Chronic Alcohol use (Ethanol)	Antibiotics (Macrolides)
Antiepileptics	• Erythromycin
• Phenytoin (Dilantin)	• Clarithromycin
• Carbamazepine (Tegretol)	Antifungals (-azole)
• Oxcarbazepine (Trileptal)	• Ketoconazole
Barbiturates	• Itraconazole
• Pentobarbital	• Fluconazole
• Phenobarbital	Antivirals (Protease Inhibitors)
Glucocorticoids	• Ritonavir
Thiazolidineodones (TZD's)	• Indinavir
• Pioglitazone (Actos)	• Nelfinavir
Tobacco smoke	Histamine H2 Antagonists
Tuberculocidal Antibiotics	• Cimetidine (Tagamet)
• Rifampin	• Ranitidine (Zantac)
Isoniazid	Non-dihydropyridine Calcium Channel Blockers
	• Verapamil
	• Diltiazem
	Proton Pump Inhibitors
	• Omeprazole (Prilosec)
	SSRI Antidepressants
	• Fluoxetine (Prozac)
	• Paroxetine (Paxil)
	• Sertraline (Zoloft)

Just as inducers can seriously impact the clinical effects of several benzodiazepines, inhibitors also can disrupt the "normal" response. Common responses secondary to impaired metabolism potentially include unintended oversedation, airway compromise secondary to soft tissue, or muscle relaxation and unconsciousness. Routes of administration that permit easy titration are less hazardous in that smaller doses can be given incrementally until the desired clinical endpoint is reached. Orally administered benzodiazepines are most likely to be negatively impacted by inducers.

Interactions with benzodiazepines and other CNS depressants

Concurrent administration of benzodiazepines and other CNS depressant drugs produces synergistic effects that can result in profound sedation, unconsciousness, respiratory depression, and muscle relaxation leading to obstruction of the upper airway. Depending on the clinical situation, the presence of these other CNS depressive drugs may or may not be known to the anesthesia provider. Balanced anesthetic techniques commonly utilized in dentistry may include other CNS depressant drugs, such as propofol or methohexital. Several additional anesthetic adjunctive medications, for example, diphenhydramine, hydroxyzine, and promethazine, produce CNS depression and mild sedation. Similarly to alcohol, the sedative effects can be greatly increased when administered concurrently with benzodiazepines. Clinicians should take appropriate measures to prevent and be prepared to manage any potential complications arising from unintended oversedation.

Interactions with opioid agonists

Interactions with opioid agonists and benzodiazepines

The concurrent administration of two or more benzodiazepines will produce summative (additive) effects. The same summative effects occur when combining two or more opioid agonists. Benzodiazepines and opioid agonists administered together often elicit synergistic effects and/or potentiation, producing clinical effects that quantitatively exceed what each drug would typically produce when administered alone. This well-known interaction between opioid agonists and CNS depressant drugs (benzodiazepines) is often purposely utilized when administering a balanced sedative or anesthetic technique. One of the main advantages is the reduction in sedative or anesthetic requirements caused by the synergistic effects, thereby decreasing the dosages of each individual drug required. Unfortunately, the degree of synergism is highly variable among patients, which may be problematic for clinicians inexperienced or inadequately prepared to manage or rescue an unexpectedly oversedated patient.

Special considerations with meperidine

As an opioid agonist, meperidine (Demerol) has historically been utilized in the provision of analgesia, sedation, and anesthesia. With the discovery of newer short-acting opioid agonists, such as fentanyl and remifentanil, the use of meperidine has declined. Meperidine has several qualities that differentiate it from the other opioid agonists. The molecular structure of meperidine shares some similarities with atropine, a potent anticholinergic. As such, administration of meperidine often produces mild tachycardia as a result of its parasympatholytic action. Meperidine undergoes hepatic metabolism, producing the active metabolite normeperidine, which is a proconvulsant. Meperidine and normeperidine are renally eliminated, so patients with impaired renal function have an inherently higher risk of complications from elevated levels of these compounds (Yagiela et al., 2004).

Interactions with meperidine and MAOIs, SSRIs, and SNRIs

As discussed previously, MAOIs inhibit the normal presynaptic metabolism of catecholamines, including serotonin. Selective serotonin reuptake inhibitors (SSRIs) and SNRIs both cause increased synaptic concentrations of serotonin due to impaired reuptake. One of the unique properties attributed to meperidine administration is the increase in serotonin activity (Yagiela et al., 2004). When meperidine and drugs from any of these classes are given concurrently, there is a potential for massive increases in serotonin concentrations, potentially leading to serotonin toxicity. Serotonin toxicity, or serotonin syndrome, may manifest clinically as tachycardia, hypertension, sweating, confusion, and agitation, which may become life threatening. In fact, the main impetus behind changes in regulating medical resident work hours was a patient in New York named Libby Zion, whose death in 1984 was contributed partly to serotonin toxicity stemming from drug interactions between meperidine and MAOIs (Kramer, 2010). There have been sporadic case reports regarding the serotonin toxicity for patients taking other antidepressants with serotonergic activity. However, the majority of reports have involved interactions with MAOIs. It is a contraindication to administer meperidine for patients who are taking MAOI within two weeks of meperidine for patients currently taking MAOIs.

Interactions with NSAIDs

One drug class frequently utilized in dentistry is the nonsteroidal anti-inflammatory analgesics (NSAIDs), which are commonly employed to manage postoperative pain, inflammation, and edema (Garcia Rodriguez et al., 2011). NSAIDs function by inhibiting cyclooxygenase (COX) enzymes, which play a crucial role in the metabolism of arachidonic acid, a byproduct of cell membrane breakdown. Currently, three isoforms of COX have been identified. COX-1 is a constitutive enzyme present in all cells except red blood cells. It helps regulate the production of prostaglandins involved in homeostatic "maintenance." These enzymes play important protective functions within the gastrointestinal and renal systems in addition to being involved in helping regulate hemostasis. COX-2 is an inducible enzyme, produced mainly in response to inflammation and cell damage. COX-3 has been theorized to exist within the central nervous system. In addition, it has been hypothesized to be the enzyme responsible for the clinical effects of administered acetaminophen; however, this is still rather controversial (Smith, 2009). Unlike COX-1, COX-2 does not have a gastrointestinal protective role (Page, 2002). Nonselective COX inhibitors, such as ibuprofen, inhibit both COX-1 and COX-2 and are associated with an increased risk of GI side effects, especially with prolonged use. NSAIDS, by virtue of their inhibition of COX enzymes, have the potential to impair renal blood flow due to decreased production of prostaglandins that help regulate the afferent renal arterioles (Yagiela et al., 2004). COX enzymes are also involved in the production of thromboxane A2, which is a potent vasoconstrictor and which facilitates platelet aggregation. Utilizing selective COX-2 inhibitors allows the clinician to reduce inflammation and pain without causing any gastrointestinal side effects such as gastritis and ulcers. However, selective COX-2 inhibitors are associated with an increased risk of thrombotic cardiovascular side effects, including myocardial infarction and thrombotic stroke. This is due to the decreased production of prostacyclin relative to the production of thromboxane A2. The imbalance between prostacyclin and thromboxane A2 produce a prothrombotic environment, which in patients with existing cardiovascular disease may lead to thrombotic cardiovascular events (Garcia Rodriguez et al., 2011).

Interactions with NSAIDs and warfarin (Coumadin)

Warfarin (Coumadin), an anticoagulant, is commonly used to prevent the formation of blood clots associated with a variety of conditions such as deep venous thrombosis, atrial fibrillation, and prosthetic heart valves. The anticoagulant effect of warfarin can vary depending on the amount of free drug circulating unbound to albumin in the blood. NSAIDs, which are highly protein-bound drugs, displace warfarin from the plasma protein albumin, which leads to an increase in the concentration of free warfarin. In addition to the increased anticoagulant effect resulting from the additional free warfarin, NSAIDs also inhibit thromboxane A2, which is a crucial enzyme for facilitating platelet aggregation (Yagiela et al., 2004). This may effectively cause the complete collapse of the normal hemostatic response due to inhibition of both the clotting cascade and the platelet aggregation mechanism. Finally, NSAIDs are ulcerogenic to the gastrointestinal system and frequently cause a bleeding ulcer. As a result, the use of NSAIDs is contraindicated for patients currently taking warfarin.

Interactions with NSAIDs and ACE inhibitors, ARBs

With primary hypertension becoming so prevalent in our society, it is extremely common for patients to present to the dentist while taking angiotensin-converting enzyme inhibitors (ACE inhibitors) such as lisinopril or captopril, or angiotensin receptor blockers (ARBs) such as losartan. These classes of antihypertensive drugs work within the renin–angiotensin system to prevent the normal functioning of angiotensin II (AT-II), which is a potent vasoconstrictor. Normally produced in response to hypotension, one of the areas AT-II works is within the renal system, specifically on the efferent renal arteriole. By vasoconstricting this arteriole, the pressure gradient and filtration rate within the glomerulus are maintained. ACE inhibitors and ARBs prevent either the production of AT-II or the binding of AT-II, respectively, which in turn causes a decrease in systemic blood pressure. NSAIDs impair the COX-produced enzyme PG I -2, which helps regulate vasodilation of the afferent renal arteriole (Yagiela et al., 2004). Decreased PG I- 2 production inhibits vasodilation of this arteriole, which decreases the afferent renal blood flow, leading to increased risk of renal ischemia and possibly acute renal failure (Page, 2002). Patients who take NSAIDs concurrently with ACE inhibitors or ARBs are at risk for loss of the mechanisms responsible for regulating renal blood flow.

Use of long-term NSAID therapy, for chronic pain, for example, may lead to decreased antihypertensive effectiveness as well. This antihypertension antagonistic effect reflects the decrease in renal blood flow, further activating the renin–angiotensin system in addition to increasing the sympathetic tone. This phenomenon tends to surface once NSAID therapy extends beyond 10-14 days. Patients who are likely to require prolonged NSAID therapy should be monitored for renal dysfunction periodically, typically by evaluating for changes in their blood urea nitrogen (BUN) or creatinine (Stoelting et al., 2008).

Interactions with NSAIDs and immunosuppressive drugs

Medical advances have made possible a multitude of life-saving modalities including a wide variety of organ transplants. In order to prevent the rejection of the transplanted organ and/or tissue, patients are required to take immunosuppressive drugs. These drugs function to suppress the body's immune system, preventing acute rejection of the transplanted organ or tissue and chronic graft-versus-host disease. Many commonly prescribed immunosuppressants, such as methotrexate, cyclosporine, or tacrolimus, are highly protein bound, renal toxic compounds (Page, 2002). Patients on these drugs who take NSAIDs concurrently are at an increased risk of renal toxicity leading to acute renal failure. The mechanism behind this drug interaction involves the protein (albumin) binding of the NSAIDs, which displaces the immunosuppressant drug from the circulating albumin. This general increase in the concentration of circulating free drug ultimately increases to a point where cellular damage occurs within the kidney. Current recommendations include avoidance of NSAIDs for patients on post-transplant immunosuppressant therapy (Stoelting et al., 2008).

Interactions with NSAIDs and lithium

Lithium is a cation and is used primarily as a mood stabilizer to treat a variety of psychiatric illnesses such as bipolar disorder or schizoaffective disorders. Patients on lithium are at risk of a pharmacokinetic drug interaction if NSAIDs are administered concurrently. NSAIDs can alter the sodium concentration within the kidney, leading to increased reabsorption. This directly impacts the renal excretion of lithium, leading to retained lithium cations and increased systemic concentrations (Page, 2002). Current recommendations include either avoidance of NSAIDs or reducing the lithium dosage along with monitoring for signs of lithium toxicity (Stoelting et al., 2008).

Conclusion

Drug interactions can be helpful or a hindrance to the clinician depending on the situation. Significant interactions exist with drugs that are commonly used in dentistry outside the realm of sedation or anesthesia. As such, the prudent clinician must be able to identify and avoid drug interactions that are likely to cause harm to the patient.

References

Garcia Rodriguez, L. A., et al. NSAID use selectively increases the risk of non-fatal myocardial infarction: a systematic review of randomized trials and observational studies. *Plos One* **6**: e16780, 2011.

Golan, D. E. *Principles of Pharmacology: the Pathophysiologic Basis of Drug Therapy*. Philadelphia: Wolters Kluwer Health/Lippincott Williams and Wilkins, 2008.

Mannesse, C. K. , et al. Contribution of adverse drug reactions to hospital admission of older patients. *Age Ageing* **29**: 35–39, 2000.

Klock, P. A. Drug interactions for the anesthesiologist. Annual Meeting of the American Society of Anesthesiologists, Orlando, 2008.

Kramer, M. Sleep loss in resident physicians: the cause of medical errors? *Front Neurol* **1**: 128, 2010.

Page, C. P. *Integrated pharmacology*. New York: Mosby, 2002.

Rosow, C. E. Anesthetic drug interaction: an overview. *J Clin Anesth* **9**: 27S–32S, 1997.

Smith, H. S. Potential analgesic mechanisms of acetaminophen. *Pain Physician* **12**: 269–280, 2009.

Stoelting, R. K., et al. *Stoelting's Anesthesia and Co-existing Disease*. Philadelphia: Churchill Livingstone/Elsevier, 2008.

Tarter, R. E., et al. *Handbook of Substance Abuse: Neurobehavioral Pharmacology*. New York: Plenum Press, 1998.

Tatonetti, N. P., et al. Detecting drug interactions from adverse event reports: interactions between paroxetine and pravastatin increases blood glucose levels. *Clin Pharmacol Ther* **90**: 133–142, 2011.

Yagiela, J. A., et al. *Pharmacology and Therapeutics for Dentistry*. St Louis: Elsevier Mosby, 2004.

SECTION 5

Monitoring

24 Limitations of patient monitoring during office-based anesthesia

Robert C. Bosack[1], and Ken Lee[2]
[1]University of Illinois, College of Dentistry, Chicago, IL, USA
[2]Ostrow School of Dentistry at USC, Los Angeles, CA, USA

"Vigilance" is the motto of the American Society of Anesthesiologists (Bacon, 1996). It is defined as the action or state of keeping careful and continuous watch for possible danger or difficulty. Among the many techniques and medical devices that can be used to monitor ventilation and perfusion, parameters that are *expected to change* during surgical/anesthetic intervention, none is more important than the use of the senses of sight, sound, and touch, which require physical proximity of the anesthetist to the patient during anesthesia and recovery. Monitoring loses value when the clinician is not cognizant of its inherent limitations or is unable to accept and act upon abnormal information.

The American Society of Anesthesiologists (2010) have set forth "Standards for Basic Anesthetic Monitoring" to encourage quality patient care during anesthesia. Selected standards are summarized in Table 24.1, as they pertain to open airway cases. A host of other organizations have similarly published monitoring guidelines for their members, with occasional variances to this document. It remains difficult, if not impossible to demonstrate that robust monitoring does not improve outcomes, given the fact that patients can quickly and unexpectedly move between levels of sedation with drug administration.

Ostensibly, the goals of patient monitoring are to improve situational awareness, identify levels of anesthesia (Table 24.2) and quickly and accurately diagnose episodes of deleterious changes in oxygenation, ventilation, or circulation, in order to avoid patient injury. Table 24.3 outlines methods of cardiopulmonary monitoring for office-based anesthesia. Electronic monitors are used to provide information that cannot be obtained through the senses of sight, sound, and touch. Temperature is monitored when patients are exposed to triggering agents for malignant hyperthermia, namely, volatile gases and succinylcholine.

Direct visualization

Direct visualization allows one to assess the color of the skin and blood, the movement of the chest wall, and the movement of the reservoir bag on the airway circuit. Although it is often assumed that a pulse oximeter will reveal hypoxemia prior to the onset of cyanosis (see Table 24.4) or darkening of the blood, this is not always the case (Wright, 1992).

The frequency, coordination, and rhythm of ventilation can be ascertained as well as some indication of the depth of ventilation, when baggy clothing or dental bibs do not obstruct the view. Normal ventilation is viewed as a gradual, smooth chest wall expansion that pulls the abdominal wall up, often hiding the descent of the diaphragm and protrusion of the abdomen. Inspiratory attempts during upper airway obstruction are jerky, with collapse of the chest wall, sternal retraction, and exaggerated protrusion of the abdomen – characterized as "Rocking Boat" phenomena. The clinician should remain cognizant that visually detected signs are often lagging indicators of pathologic events that have triggered the finding. Direct visualization also monitors patient movement, grimacing, or tears, which can indicate inadequate anesthesia and/or painful stimulation. Listening to a patient talk or hearing hiccups is a guarantee that ventilation is occurring. It is difficult to watch and be aware of everything, while working and focusing intraorally. It is for this reason that anesthesia assistants remain a vital part of the anesthesia team.

Pretracheal auscultation

Similar to murmurs, upper airway noise can only be heard when air is moving with sufficient velocity or through a constricted lumen, or both. The use of a pretracheal stethoscope (Figure 24.1 and 24.2) usually allows the clinician to hear movement of air or presence of secretions in the upper airway, although sounds from the impedance of airflow at any level in the airway (supraglottic snoring, glottic crowing or subglottic wheezing) can be transmitted. As such, the pretracheal stethoscope is sensitive, but not specific. This modality provides the most rapid detection of apnea.

Pretracheal auscultation optimizes, but does not duplicate ventilatory monitoring when used in conjunction with capnography (see Table 24.5). Extraneous ambient sounds (drilling, conversation, mechanical room air conditioners, suction noises) can interfere with auscultation. It is difficult to evaluate the adequacy (depth) of ventilation with a stethoscope.

Anesthesia Complications in the Dental Office, First Edition. Edited by Robert C. Bosack and Stuart Lieblich.

Table 24.1 Standards for basic anesthetic monitoring (ASA, 2010).

Standard I – Qualified anesthesia personnel shall be present in the room throughout the conduct of all general anesthetic, regional anesthetics, and monitored anesthesia care

Standard II – During all anesthetics, the patient's oxygenation, ventilation, circulation, and temperature shall be continually evaluated.

- Oxygenation
  - Objective – to ensure adequate oxygen concentration in the inspired gas and the blood during all anesthetics
    - Blood oxygenation – During all anesthetics, a quantitative method of assessing oxygenation such as pulse oximetry shall be employed. When the pulse oximeter is utilized, the variable pitch pulse tone and the low threshold alarm shall be audible to the anesthesiologist or the anesthesia care team personnel. Adequate illumination and exposure of the patient are necessary to assess color.
- Ventilation
  - Objective – to ensure adequate ventilation of the patient during all anesthetics
    - Every patient receiving general anesthesia shall have the adequacy of ventilation continually evaluated. Qualitative clinical signs such as chest excursion, observation of the reservoir breathing bag, and auscultation of breath sounds are useful. Continual monitoring for the presence of expired carbon dioxide shall be performed unless invalidated by the nature of the patient, procedure, or equipment. Quantitative monitoring of the volume of expired gas is strongly encouraged.
    - During regional anesthesia (with no sedation) or local anesthesia (with no sedation), the adequacy of ventilation shall be evaluated by continual observation of qualitative clinical signs. During moderate or deep sedation the adequacy of ventilation shall be evaluated by continual observation of qualitative clinical signs and monitoring for the presence of exhaled carbon dioxide unless precluded or invalidated by the nature of the patient, procedure, or equipment.
- Circulation
  - Objective – to ensure the adequacy of the patient's circulatory function during all anesthetics.
    - Every patient receiving anesthesia shall have the electrocardiogram continuously displayed from the beginning of anesthesia until prepared to leave the anesthetizing location.
    - Every patient receiving anesthesia shall have arterial blood pressure and heart rate determined and evaluated at least every 5 minutes.
    - Every patient receiving general anesthesia shall have, in addition to the above, circulatory function continually evaluated by at least one of the following: palpation of a pulse, auscultation of heart sounds, or pulse oximetry.

Pulse oximetry

Oxygen in the blood exists in three forms: gaseous, dissolved (gaseous and dissolved remain in equilibrium), and oxygen attached to hemoglobin. Gaseous oxygen, under tension in arterial blood, is able to diffuse across cell membranes to meet metabolic demands, and is immediately replaced by the oxygen released by hemoglobin. A pulse oximeter continuously and noninvasively measures heart rate and estimates the percentage of oxyhemoglobin/total hemoglobin in arterial blood (SpO_2). The partial pressure (tension) of oxygen in arterial blood can then be estimated with the oxyhemoglobin dissociation curve.

It is impossible for blood to transport enough gaseous oxygen or to dissolve enough oxygen to meet heightened metabolic demands. Hemoglobin in the red blood cell behaves as a temporary reservoir for large amounts of oxygen, with each molecule permissively binding four molecules of oxygen. The binding of the first molecule is difficult; however, once bound, it facilitates binding and increases the affinity of subsequent molecules until four oxygen molecules are bound. The reverse is also true: it is difficult for a fully bound hemoglobin molecule to release the first molecule of oxygen, but once it does, the release of subsequent oxygen molecules is facilitated. This biochemical phenomenon gives rise to the classic sigmoid shape of the oxyhemoglobin dissociation curve (see Figure 24.3). For this reason, the oximeter has been described as a "sentry standing on the cliff of desaturation." Observation of the curve identifies the rapid and severe change in slope that occurs at a saturation of 90%, corresponding with a PaO_2 of 60 mmHg. Subsequent decreases in saturation occur rapidly at this point.

The oximeter functions as both a spectrophotometer and a plethysomograph. The probe, usually placed on a digit, emits two different wavelengths of light: red (660 nm) and infrared (940 nm). Oxyhemoglobin absorbs more infrared and less red as compared with deoxyhemoglobin. A photodetector picks up the difference in absorption that occurs in pulsatile (arterial) blood and converts it to a percentage number using a complex algorithm. "Normal" SpO_2 is approximately 95%, inferring a PaO_2 of 80 mmHg. The terminology of the concentration of oxygen in humans is shown in Table 24.6.

In spite of its universal and effective use, there are multiple limitations with pulse oximetry.

1 *Failure to detect hypoventilation or early apnea when supplemental oxygen is administered.* Prior to and during anesthesia, patients are given supplemental oxygen to breathe, as a method to delay the onset of hypoxemia during a period of apnea. With this process, oxygen displaces nitrogen in the functional residual capacity (reservoir) of the lung and becomes a continuous supply in the absence of ventilation. Supplemental oxygen also increases (insignificantly) the amount of oxygen dissolved in the plasma as shown by the oxyhemoglobin dissociation curve. Even with PaO_2 values approaching 600 mmHg, hemoglobin saturation still may not reach 100%.
2 *Delayed detection of hypoxemia.* The oximeter has been termed a "lag monitor" providing "yesterday's news." The delay is due to signal averaging (5–8 seconds), the delay in circulation time from the lungs to the probe (20–35 seconds), exacerbated by decreased cardiac output and poor perfusion, and a delay caused by patient motion (light anesthesia, shivering, seizure), which makes venous blood somewhat pulsatile (Trivedi et al., 1997). Recent advancements in technology have overcome some of these limitations.
3 *Environmental conditions leading to erroneous saturation measurements.* Ambient light may falsely depress pulse oximeter readings. Improper probe placement can prevent both wavelengths of light form passing through the tissue to be sensed, altering the reading. Electromagnetic radiation from cell phones or electrocautery devices can also interfere with oximetry (Ralston et al., 1991).
4 *Patient conditions leading to erroneous saturation measurements.* Unfortunately, pulse oximetry can be least accurate when patients need it the most. Hypoperfusion at the site of measurement tends to yield a falsely low reading. Such instances include irregular rhythms and low pulse amplitude, secondary to hypotension, hypovolemia, vasoconstrictor usage, or cold ambient temperature. Deeply pigmented skin can falsely lower readings, as a bluish tinge often appears in the nail beds of these patients. Abnormal hemoglobins also diminish accuracy. Carboxyhemoglobin (as can occur with recent exposure to cigarette smoke) absorbs red light (660 nm) identical to oxyhemoglobin. As a result, oximeter readings can be falsely elevated by 5–10% in

Table 24.2 Continuum of depth of sedation: definitions of general anesthesia and levels of sedation/analgesia* (Adapted from Practice Guidelines for Sedation and Analgesia by Non-Anesthesiologists, 2002 (with permission)).

	Minimum sedation (Anxiolysis)	Moderate sedation/analgesia (conscious sedation)	Deep sedation/analgesia	General anesthesia
Responsiveness	Normal response to verbal stimulation	Purposeful† response to verbal or tactile stimulation	Purposeful† response after repeated or painful stimulation	Unarousable
Airway	Unaffected	No intervention required	Intervention may be required	Intervention often required
Spontaneous ventilation	Unaffected	Adequate	May be inadequate	Frequently inadequate
Cardiovascular function	Unaffected	Usually maintained	Usually maintained	May be impaired

*As sedation is a continuum, individual patient responses are variable and may not exactly follow these categorizations.
†Reflex withdrawal from a painful stimulus is not considered a purposeful response.

Table 24.3 Methods of cardiopulmonary monitoring during office-based anesthesia.

Oxygenation – amount of oxygen in the blood and tissues
- Visual inspection of the color of the blood, skin, and mucous membranes
- Pulse oximetry

Ventilation – movement of gas between environment and alveoli
- Verbal communication with the patient
- Visual inspection for chest excursion, signs of obstruction, movement of the reservoir bag
- Pretracheal auscultation
  - Upper airway noise – snoring, crowing
  - Lower airway noise – wheezing
- Capnography

Circulation
- Palpation of radial or carotid pulse
- Electrocardiography – heart rate and rhythm
- Sphygmomanometry
- Pulse oximetry – pulse rate and rhythm

Table 24.4 Cyanosis.

Cyanosis – a bluish/purple coloration seen on the skin, nail beds, and mucous membranes. It is less noticeable in patients with pigmented skin, where there is a decrease in peripheral perfusion (vasoconstriction) or in rooms with poor lighting. It is an approximate, and at times, unreliable clinical indicator that there is not enough oxygen in the blood (hypoxemia.) It occurs in several situations:
- When there is approximately 5 g/dL of reduced (deoxygenated) hemoglobin in the capillaries. Anemic patients (who have less overall hemoglobin) can be hypoxemic without reaching the 5 g/dL value needed to cause cyanosis, while a patient with polycythemia can be cyanotic without hypoxia. In a patient with normal hemoglobin concentrations, 5 g/dL corresponds to an SaO_2 of 67% (Grace, 1994).
- When there is abnormal hemoglobin. The cyanosis caused by methemoglobin (which is the oxidized form) is a more intense bluish tinge, and this becomes an unreliable indicator of the amount of reduced hemoglobin in the blood.
- With peripheral vasoconstriction. Nail beds can appear blue secondary to peripheral vasoconstriction with less than 5 g/dL reduced hemoglobin.

heavy smokers, possibly masking life-threatening desaturation. Methemoglobin has the same absorption coefficient at both red and infrared wavelengths. This 1:1 absorption ratio corresponds to a saturation of 85%, when metHgb is in sufficient concentration. Depending on the absolute percentage of oxyhemoglobin this number can be either falsely elevated or depressed.

Capnography

Capnography provides a continuous and noninvasive waveform measurement of the partial pressure of exhaled CO_2, and has become the gold standard for verification of correct endotracheal tube placement (Matevosian and Nourmand, 2004). It provides the most sensitive measurement of ventilation. In order for CO_2 to appear during exhalation, three important physiologic functions must be intact: ventilation of alveoli, a respiratory membrane that facilitates diffusion, and a functioning cardiovascular system. In the dental office, sidestream technology prevails where a sample of respiratory gases is aspirated and delivered to an infrared sensor in a monitor approximately 5 feet away from the patient. This distance causes a delay in measurement of approximately 6 seconds. The sample is usually taken from the nose, via a cannula under a nasal hood (see Figure 24.4) or integrated into a nasal cannula, which simultaneously delivers oxygen (see Figure 24.5 and 24.6). Sampling errors in open airway cases include room air or supplemental oxygen dilution of the sample or absence of CO_2 in patients who have nasal congestion or who are breathing through their mouth. In all instances, the measured end-tidal CO_2 can be 5–10 mmHg less than the normal $PaCO_2$ of ~40 mmHg.

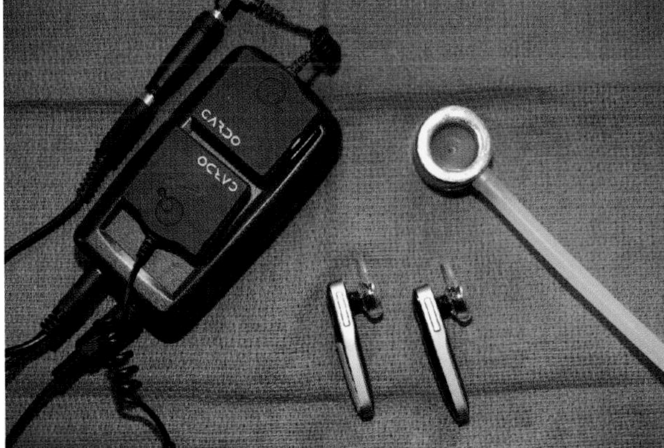
Figure 24.1 A pre-tracheal stethoscope fitted with two headsets, so that both doctor and assistant can monitor airway noise simultaneously.

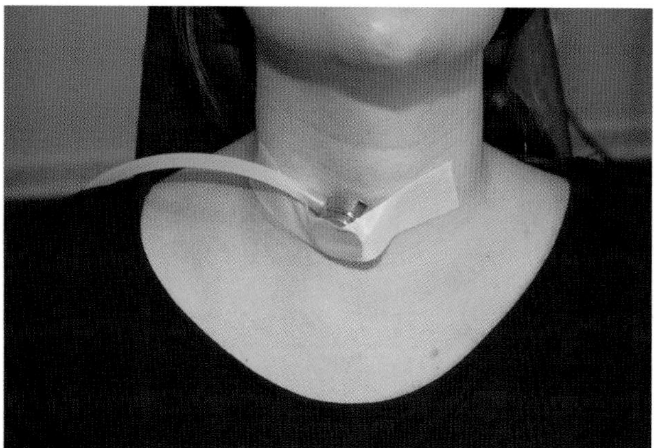

Figure 24.2 A weighted bell (see figure) is affixed to the neck with double-sided adhesive discs and further stabilized with surgical tape. Off-center placement improves tissue contact in patients with prominent larynxes.

Table 24.5 Limitations of ventilatory monitoring.

	Side stream, nasal sampling capnography	Pretracheal auscultation
Mouth breather	NO	YES
Slow, silent nasal breathing	YES	NO
Slow, silent mouth breathing	NO	NO

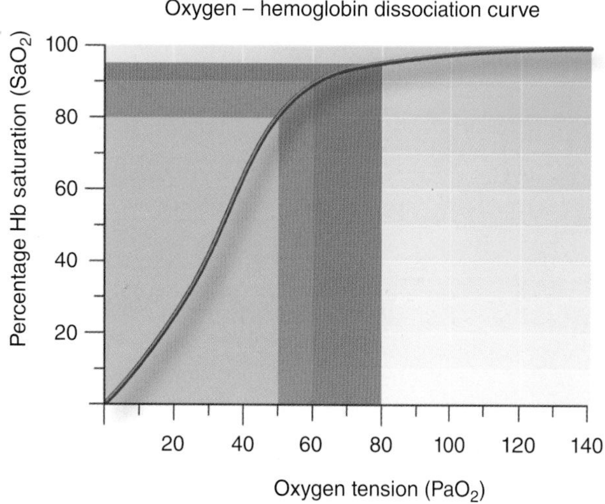

Figure 24.3 Oxygen–hemoglobin dissociation curve.

Table 24.6 terminology of the concentration of oxygen in humans.

PaO_2 – partial pressure of oxygen in the arterial blood

SaO_2 – the oxygen saturation of hemoglobin in arterial blood, as measured with blood gas, expressed as a percentage of oxyhemoglobin / total hemoglobin

SpO_2 – the oxygen saturation of hemoglobin as measured by pulse oximetry

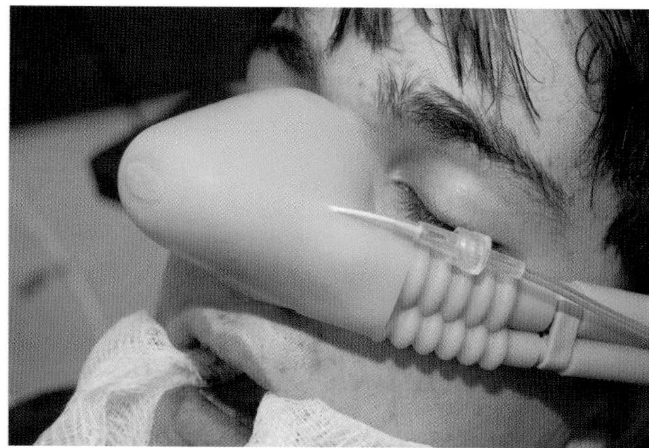

Figure 24.4 CO_2 sampling using an intravenous catheter inserted into a nasal hood.

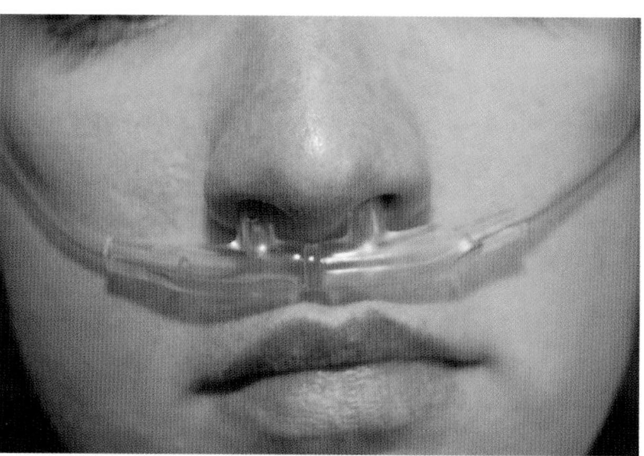

Figure 24.5 Divided nasal cannula that delivers oxygen to one prong and samples CO_2 from the other prong.

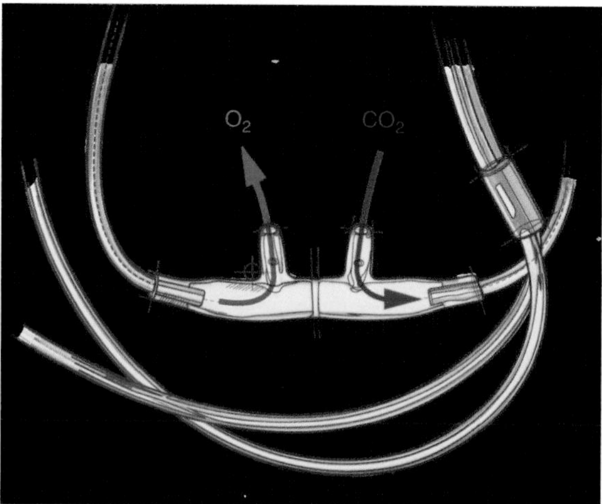

Figure 24.6 Schematic diagram of a divided cannula, which simultaneously samples CO_2 while delivering oxygen. Salter Labs, with permission.

The value of capnography lies in the visualization of a recurring waveform, which is a guarantee that CO_2 is being exhaled and ventilation is occurring through an open airway. Production

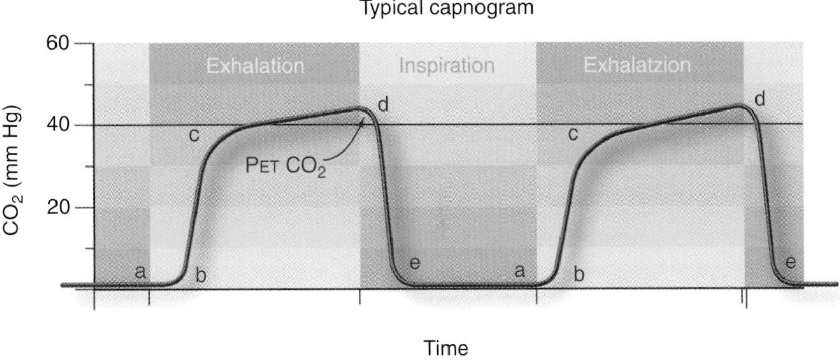

Figure 24.7 Typical capnogram.

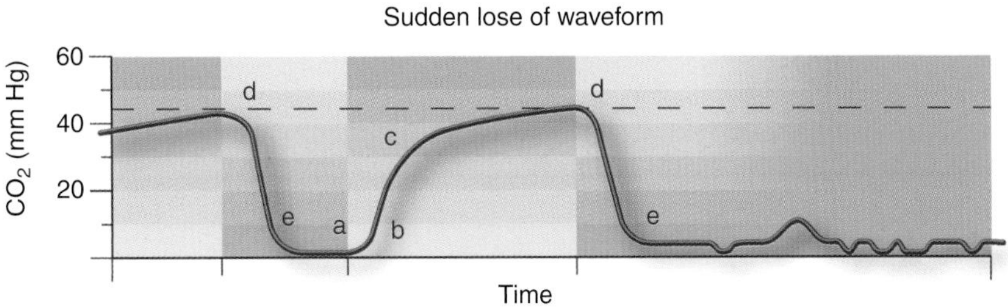

Figure 24.8 Sudden lose of waveform.

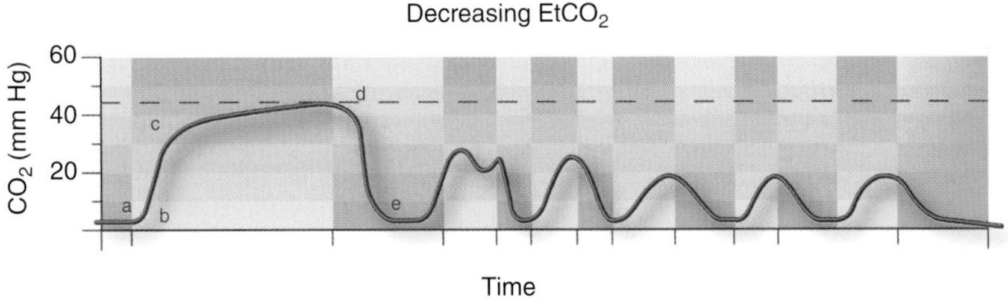

Figure 24.9 Decreasing $EtCO_2$.

and measurement of CO_2 in exhaled air implies ongoing cellular metabolism, diffusion of CO_2 to the blood stream, and circulatory transit to the lungs where it diffuses into the alveoli. In open airways, the depth and frequency of ventilations become more important than the numeric value of the $ETCO_2$.

A typical capnogram is shown in Figure 24.7.

AB – the beginning of exhalation, where air from the anatomic dead space is being exhaled.

BC – rapid rise in the concentration of exhaled CO_2, as the anatomic dead space is being filled with CO_2-rich gas from the pulmonary alveoli.

CD – alveolar plateau, where mixed alveolar gases are exhaled.

D – End – Tidal CO_2, the highest concentration of CO_2, which occurs at the end of exhalation of the tidal volume. This value provides the most accurate reflection of alveolar CO_2.

DE – inhalation starts, fresh gas rapidly replaces CO_2.

There are several possibilities of ventilatory changes that can be visually seen on the capnogram.

1 Sudden loss of waveform – apnea, laryngospasm, tube is dislodged or kinked, cardiac arrest (see Figure 24.8)
2 Decreasing height of waveform – partial obstruction to exhalation, onset of hypoventilation with sedation (see Figure 24.9)
3 Increasing height of waveform – CO_2 accumulation with prolonged hypoventilation, recovery from an obstructed airway (see Figure 24.10)
4 Increasing frequency of waveform - tachypnea
5 Decreasing frequency of waveform - bradypnea
6 Decreasing the BC slope - bronchospasm – "shark-fin" appearance (see Figure 24.11)
7 Decreasing the DC slope – slow tidal breathing

Electrocardiography (ECG)

Electrocardiography is the amplified surface recording of electrical potentials generated by depolaration of myocytes, displayed as a waveform. Myocardial contraction and pumping of blood is assumed and verified by pulse oximetry, palpation of peripheral pulses, and capnography. Electrodes are typically placed on the right arm, left arm, and left leg. Lead II (Right arm negative, Left leg positive) most closely mimics the normal orientation of the heart in the chest. Advantages of Lead II information is provided in the table 24.7. Wrist electrodes, popular in dental offices, monitor Lead I (Left arm positive and Right arm negative) and are incapable of monitoring Lead II.

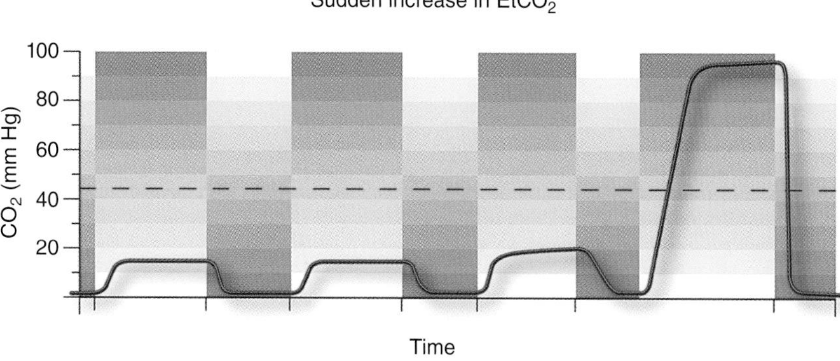

Figure 24.10 Sudden increase in $EtCO_2$.

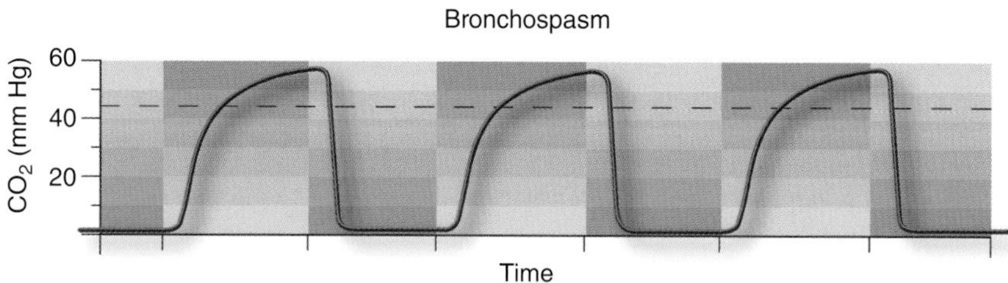

Figure 24.11 Bronchospasm.

Table 24.7 Advantages of monitoring Lead II during office-based anesthesia.

- P waves have largest amplitude and are therefore easily identified.
- P wave changes are easily noted.
- Upgoing QRS complex, identifiable T wave.
- Best detection of heart blocks.
- Best detection of dysrhythmias (R-R′ periodicity, QRS configuration).

The dynamic ECG tracing as seen on an oscilloscope provides information about heart rate and rhythm. Monitoring of ST segment changes solely with lead II is unreliable as this lead configuration "sees" only limited portions of the myocardium.

Moving the left arm lead to the fifth intercostal space, anterior left axillary line and selecting lead I will approximate a chest lead V5, and will be a more sensitive monitor for cardiac ischemia, as seen by alterations in the position of the ST segment. This is excellent didactic information, which rarely will be put to use in a dental office. It is unlikely that a patient who requires ST segment monitoring will be anesthetized in a dental office – monitoring ST segments and performing dental surgical procedures usually cannot be accomplished simultaneously by the same person. It is also likely that disorders of pulse rate and rhythm and pressure will precede ST segment alterations in negatively screened patients who unfortunately will have ischemia in the dental office.

The limitations of office ECG rhythm monitoring with limb leads:
- No leisurely analysis or comparison with preop ECG
- Inability to monitor 12 leads continuously
- Lack of specificity of ST and T wave changes
- Interference by shivering and electrocautery

Sphygmomanometry

Sphygomomanometry is the indirect measurement of blood pressure with the use of a manual or automated inflatable compressive cuff (Beevers, 2001a,b). The gold standard is the use of a stethoscope and cuff attached to a mercury column mounted at a specific height from the floor, although environmental concerns have limited their use. Usually the cuff is applied to the upper arm, approximating the level of the heart. The cuff is inflated until the radial pulse is no longer palpable and slowly deflated. When systolic pressure is reached, blood flow becomes turbulent which creates Korotkoff sounds. The onset of the sounds heralds systolic blood pressure and the offset of sounds provides an approximation of diastolic blood pressure. The width of the cuff should cover 2/3 of the length of the upper arm, or approximate 40% of the circumference of the arm.

Sources of error in blood pressure measurement (Jones, 2003):
- Blood pressure is overestimated
  - Recent tobacco exposure or ingestion of caffeine or other stimulants
  - Anxiety
  - Use of cuffs that are too small or too loose
- Blood pressure is underestimated
  - Recording when extremity is above the level of the heart
  - Cuffs that are too large or wide
  - Overly rapid cuff deflation

Oscillometric automatic blood pressure machines are routinely used in the dental office. Pressure transducers record pressures when oscillations begin and end. Inaccuracies can occur with patient movement and in patients with high sympathetic tone. Although manufactures attest their accuracy, there are studies that show a wide variation in the accuracy of some machines (Kaufmann, 1996). Cuffs placed more peripherally on forearms or wrists tend to overestimate systolic and underestimate diastolic pressure. When considering interventional medical emergency treatment for hypertension or hypotension, the value in question should always be rechecked for accuracy, preferably by auscultation.

Measurement intervals are routinely set at 5 minutes. To improve patient comfort, lengthening this interval during light sedation is frequently entertained, as significant fluctuations in pressure are rare. In contradistinction, a 5 minute interval may be too long during emergency drug therapy for hypotension or hypertension.

References

American Society of Anesthesiologists. Standards for basic anesthetic monitoring. http://www.asahq.org/For-Members/Clinical-Information/˜/media/For%2520Members/documents/Standards%2520Guidelines%2520Stmts/Basic%2520Anesthetic%2520Monitoring%25202011.ashx (Accessed September 6, 2013).

Bacon, D. R. Iconography in anesthesiology. The importance of society seals in the 1920s and 30s. *Anesthesiol* **85**: 414–419, 1996.

Beevers, G., et al. ABC of hypertension. Blood pressure measurement. Part 1 Sphygmomanometry: Factors common in all techniques. *BMJ* **322**: 981–985, 2001a.

Beevers, G., et al. ABC of hypertension. Blood pressure measurement. Part 2 conventional sphygmomanometry: technique of auscultatory blood pressure measurement. *BMJ* **322**: 1043–1047, 2001b.

Grace, R. F. Pulse Oximetry: gold standard or false sense of security? *Med J Aust* **160**: 638–644, 1994.

Guidelines for the use of sedation and general anesthesia By Dentists. American Dental Association, 2012.

Jones, D. S., et al. Measuring blood pressure accurately: new and persistent challenges. *JAMA* **289**: 1027–1030, 2003.

Kaufmann, M. A., et al. Oscillometric blood pressure measurements by different devices are not interchangeable *Anesth Analg* **82**: 377–381, 1996.

Matevosian, R. and Nourmand, H. Monitoring. In: Hines, R. L., ed. *Adult Perioperative Anesthesia*. Philadelphia: Elsevier Mosby, 2004.

Practice Guidelines for Sedation and Analgesia by Non-Anesthesiologists. *Anesthesiol* **96**: 1004–17, 2002.

Ralston, A. C., et al. Potential errors in pulse oximetry. *Anaesthesia* **46**: 202–206, 1991

Trivedi, N. S., et al. Effects of motion, ambient light, and hypoperfusion on pulse oximeter function *J Clin Anesth* **3**:179–183, 1997.

Wright, S. W. Conscious sedation in the emergency department: the value of capnography and pulse oximetry. *Ann Emer Med* **21**: 551–555, 1992.

SECTION 6

Preparation for adversity

25 Crisis resource management

Joseph Kras
Washington University in St. Louis, Department of Anesthesiology, St. Louis, MO, USA

Crisis Resource Management (CRM) is a useful and practical method of training all office personnel to mange unexpected medical emergencies in the dental office. There is no way of absolutely preventing all emergencies from occurring. Successful management of critical incidents involves more than individual knowledge and skills. Being able to work together as a team as well as manage a team are important skills that are most often neglected in traditional training.

At first glance, there would seem to be few similarities between an aircraft carrier deck, a control room in a nuclear plant, the flight deck of a jumbo jet, and a dental office. However, when looking at why unexpected critical incidents occur and how to manage them, the resemblances are striking. Critical incidents happen not just because of personal errors but also because of ways that a number of factors work together to allow errors to occur. Once an incident is triggered, the highest chances of a successful outcome occur when systems are already in place to rapidly identify critical incidents, as well as systems in place to manage them.

What is CRM?

CRM (see Table 25.1) is a type of training meant to prepare participants to manage all of the "human factors" that enter into the causation, propagation, and management of critical incidents. Although medical knowledge and skills (ACLS, intubation, etc.) are both important and necessary, these are not the things that are directly taught during a CRM focused course. Instead, members of teams are taught how to recognize and minimize the causes of errors, when and how to appropriately challenge authority, how to maintain what in aviation is termed "situational awareness," and how to recognize and manage all available resources during a crisis.

In December 1972, Eastern Air Lines flight 401 crashed into the Everglades, after crew members distracted by a malfunctioning landing gear indicator light failed to notice that the autopilot had been accidently disconnected. Almost exactly 6 years later, in December 1978, United Airlines flight 173 crashed into suburban Portland Oregon after it ran out of fuel. Although a crew member had commented on the low level of fuel prior to the crash, the crew's attention was absorbed in diagnosing a landing gear problem, and no one integrated and prioritized this information properly, until it was too late. In both of these cases, simple errors were not managed properly, which resulted in the crew being distracted from their normal duties, and ultimately ended in several people dying needlessly.

Starting in 1980, United Airlines instituted what it initially termed Cockpit Resource Management. The terminology later changed to Crew Resource Management, to reflect the fact that non-cockpit flight and ground crew would also be involved. The training rapidly spread to other North American airlines. Although the content of training programs has changed over the years, all programs have in common the goal of assisting the crew in maximizing their performance, in order to increase safety. After initial resistance amongst aviators, acceptance rapidly grew as they appreciated the training's benefits.

In medicine, the adoption of CRM methods to the education of trainees and practitioners paralleled the development of the computerized full-body simulator. Such simulators began to be developed in a few different centers in the late 1980s. Development was spurred by the introduction of powerful personal computers as well as by increasing public demand that patients should not be used as "guinea pigs." Unlike simpler Resusci-Annie™ type simulators, full-body computerized simulators are able to replicate a much more robust set of physiological responses. Investigators became interested in marrying these more advanced simulators to the concepts of CRM, and starting in 1990 Anesthesia Crisis Resource Management (ACRM) courses were taught at Stanford University (Gaba et al., 2001).

Error prevention, occurrence, and detection

Until about the 1990s, if one attended a surgical morbidity and mortality (M and M) conference, when a case with a bad outcome was presented one would have witnessed a concerted effort to find the one thing done by the one person that led to the bad outcome. But just as aviation experts had discovered in the 1980s, researchers and practitioners in medicine also came to the conclusion that there is seldom one cause for any adverse outcome. Rather, most adverse outcomes result from the interaction of multiple factors that work together to facilitate the end result.

Consider the following scenario:

> Dr. K, an oral and maxillofacial surgeon, has been a bit sleep deprived because his 6 year old had an asthma attack last night. His first procedure of the day was unexpectedly complicated, and took 30 minutes longer than the time allotted. Dr. K's office, like many others, has been subject to sporadic shortages of various drugs, and is now using thiopenthal instead of propofol for sedation. Unbeknownst to him, the pharmacy that supplies his drugs substituted a similar looking 2 ml (50 mg) vial of nitroprusside for a 2 ml (8 mg) vial of dexamethasone. Neither the pharmacy technician nor the nurse in the office stocking the drugs noticed the mix-up.

Anesthesia Complications in the Dental Office, First Edition. Edited by Robert C. Bosack and Stuart Lieblich.

Table 25.1 Elements of crisis resource management.

- Before and during the crisis
  - Anticipate and plan
  - Know your environment
  - Designate leadership
  - Establish role clarity
  - Use cognitive aids
- During the crisis
  - Call for help early
  - Mobilize all resources
  - Allocate attention wisely
  - Use all available information
  - Communicate effectively
  - Distribute the workload

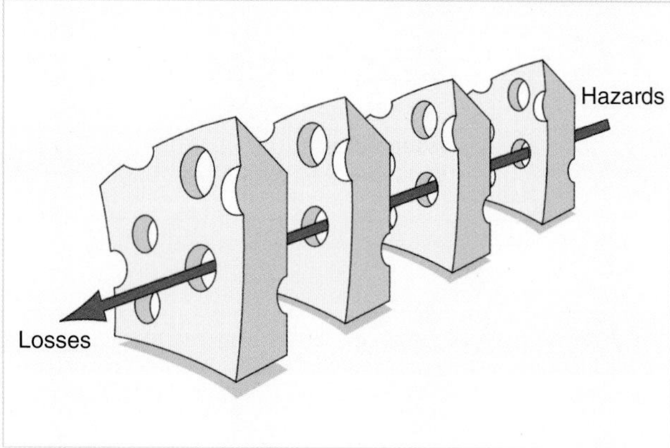

Figure 25.1 The Swiss cheese model of how defences, barriers, and safeguards may be penetrated by an accident trajectory. Source: Reason 2000. Reproduced with permission of BMJ Publishing Group Ltd.

> Dr. K's nurse draws up drugs for the following case. She follows her usual procedure of showing the vial to Dr. K right after drawing up the vial and labeling the syringe. Both are hurrying a bit, and do not notice the vial of nitroprusside/dexamethasone mix-up, while they are paying more attention to getting the thiopenthal diluted correctly. As they begin sedating their next patient, they give what they think is 8 mg of decadron, but is instead 50 mg of nitroprusside. The patient almost immediately loses consciousness. Initially thinking the patient has suffered a vasovagal reaction, the chair is repositioned to fully supine, and the airway is supported. Dr. K and his nurse also recheck the thiopenthal dilution, to ensure they have not inadvertently overdosed the patient. The patient rapidly turns blue, and full resuscitation is started. Despite a prolonged code, the patient dies.

What was the cause of the tragic outcome in this situation? Was it the doctor and nurse wrongly confirming the drug identity when it was drawn up? Was it the pharmacy technician supplying the wrong drug to the office? Can one not say that the company using a "look-alike" label, fatigue, distraction when using less familiar drugs, and production pressure played some role? Although most situations do not have quite so many readily identifiable causes, it is also true that most bad outcomes are rarely due to a single cause.

Some broad categories of sources of error include the environment (embracing both the physical environment as and the culture of the workplace), the knowledge and skill of personnel (both individually and collectively), the patient (including all of their physical and emotional makeup), and random factors (fatigue, abnormal distractors and disruptors, natural disasters, etc.).

Psychologist James Reason has put forward the "Swiss Cheese" model to explain why bad outcomes occur (Reason 2000; see Figure 25.1). In any complex environment, there will be both multiple opportunities for errors to occur and multiple efforts to prevent them from occurring. The defenses are represented by the pieces of cheese, while the opportunities for error are represented by the holes in the cheese. Mechanisms in place to prevent errors may include such things as policies (e.g., work hour restrictions), guidelines (e.g., two people should check medications when they are drawn up), or education requirements (e.g., requiring that anesthetics only be administered by qualified practitioners). Opportunities for errors may be such things as technical flaws (e.g., mechanical failure of parts), latent errors (e.g., disease states in the patient), or process violations (e.g., omitting performing a "time out" prior to starting a procedure).

Errors will always occur. The goal is to prevent as many errors from occurring as possible, catch errors once they occur as early as possible, and remediate as many errors as possible before permanent harm comes to a patient. How can this be accomplished?

First, rather than assuming that all is going well (which is what most clinicians do at "baseline"), one should be constantly proving to oneself that the patient is doing well. The human mind wants everything to be fine. Thus when abnormalities occur, a common response is to tell ourselves that "everything's OK", even when it is not. If a pulse oximeter reading falls, rather than assume that it is due to a mechanical aberration, the clinician should search for possible causes for the abnormal reading (such as airway obstruction or oversedation causing a decreased respiratory drive), while also checking for other sources of information to confirm or disprove our tentative diagnosis.

Second, the clinician needs to realize that another common flaw in human thinking occurs when the same (incorrect and unsuccessful) initial thought process is replayed over and over, with an expectation of different results (failure to abandon incorrect reasoning). Examples include failure to revise a plan when new information is obtained, failure in prioritizing problems properly, and failure to properly implement a plan once formed (Gaba et al., 2001). Once the decision is made to intervene, humans tend perseverate on completing a task, to the detriment of completing other more important tasks. Time management becomes much harder during a crisis, as perception of time is skewed by the sympathetic response, and a multitude of items competing for attention leaves little room for task prioritization.

Humans perceive their environment, process it through cognition, and then take action (St. Pierre et al., 2010). Activation of the sympathetic nervous system (fight or flight response) has the positive effect of preparing for action, by making sense organs more active and facilitating concentration on the triggering problem. When that system is overstimulated, hearing becomes less acute and tunnel vision (figuratively and literally) occurs.

The environment contains many "latent factors" (Gaba et al., 1994) that may long remain dormant, until the time comes when they contribute to an adverse outcome. Perhaps the area where the drugs are drawn up in the scenario above is somewhat poorly lit, such that it makes it harder to read the labels on the vials. Practicing scenarios with the clinical team can help to uncover some of these latent factors. A regular review of the environment should be conducted to ferret out others.

In looking at professional pilots, Jensen identified five of what he termed "hazardous attitudes," which could interfere with correct response, or even lead to counterproductive responses (Jensen, 1995). These were (1) a "macho" attitude (I'll show you), (2) an "anti-authority" attitude (rules aren't meant for me), (3) "impulsivity" (something must be done-NOW!, (4) "invulnerability" (Nothing really bad has happened to me before), and (5) "resignation" (What's the use, everything's bound to fail). If such attitudes are self-recognized, they can be corrected with internal self-talk. If not recognized, it is incumbent upon other members of the team to offer correction and redirection.

In the 1972 and 1978 crashes mentioned above, an important factor common to both was a strong captain of the plane that other crew members were loath to question. While effective leadership in a crisis is certainly important, all leaders need to be open to input from their team for information, alternative diagnoses, and therapies, as well as accepting constructive criticism during a crisis. Staying focused on doing what is best for the patient can help in keeping our own egos in check.

Decision-making during critical incidents

Making decisions under pressure is never a simple undertaking. One must be able to proceed with a constant flow of imperfect (and sometimes conflicting) information. It is crucial to quickly assimilate and process such information, weed out that which is deemed unimportant, prioritize what is left, test this information against prior medical knowledge and experience, make tentative differential diagnoses, decide on a proper course of action, manage resources effectively, constantly reevaluate the situation in light of new information, and do all this in a timely manner. Reading about how to do this can be helpful, but practicing such skills (during mock critical incidents) can be more effective in solidifying these skills.

If at all possible, whoever is leading the response (and a leader should be designated) should endeavor to not be actively engaged in carrying out tasks. In other words, when possible delegate things (such as starting IVs, giving drugs, intubating, CPR, etc.) to others. It is hard enough to lead a team during a crisis, without also having to dedicate precious time and energy to performing functions that will distract you. Of course, one does what he/she has to do, and if no one else is trained or able to perform a task, then you must do it yourself.

Decision aids may help orient us during a critical situation. One that has been used in the aerospace industry is the acronym FOR-DEC (St. Pierre et al., 2010), which stands for Facts (gathering information), Options (deciding possible courses of action), Risks (and benefits of various options), Decision (making a plan), Executing (the plan), and Check (checking to see if the plan is still valid, given new information). Another acronym that can be used is Boyd's OODA Loop (Azuma et al., 2006), which stands for Observe (take in facts), Orientation (process what the information means), Decision, and Action (execute and monitor the decision). The processing of facts is also sometimes termed "Situational Awareness."

Communication

Part and parcel of any training in CRM is incorporating practice in effective communication. Breakdowns in communication are often cited as contributing causes to crisis situations in various settings (Buyck and Lang, 2002; Reader et al., 2007). Failure to speak up because of fear of being wrong or intimidation, failure to confirm communication is received (closing the loop), and neglecting to include necessary facts are all common errors of communication during critical incidents. Communication errors also occur commonly between people of different training and status (Greenberg et al., 2007). Most CRM programs use videotaping of simulated incidents to evaluate and teach skills in communication. Reviewing one's own performance is a strong motivator to self-improvement.

A good leader not only controls the medical response to an emergency but also controls communication during an event. There can be problems of both too much, as well as too little, communication. If everyone is talking at once, then information is likely to be lost, and it is difficult to know if someone has truly received the information one was trying to convey. Good leaders seek input from those around them, address requests to specific people, and wait for a "read back" of what was just requested. Effective leaders also seek input from those around them, as they may have information or expertise that the leader does not at that time.

Clear, unambiguous language is preferable during all medical communication, and especially during critical incidents. When transferring care of a critically ill patient, the SBAR system (situation, background, assessment, response) provides a clear structure that can help ensure that information is transmitted effectively (IHI, 2011).

Who should train, and how often?

By now it should be obvious that CRM training is not just for the doctor, and should even include more than just the healthcare practitioners. All people in the environment can benefit from such training, as (1) they all have a role to play and (2) by all training together (and cross training in other people's roles) participants will both appreciate better what others are doing, as well as be more able to assist each other/substitute for others when a crisis occurs.

Training should occur on a regular basis. As with all learning, breaking it up into smaller chunks and spreading it out will provide much better retention and higher level of performance in a real emergency. Running through possible emergency scenarios for an hour or two on a quarterly basis would be more effective than 10–12 hours on a weekend every 2 years. As with BLS and ACLS, training every 2 years should be looked at as the minimum standard. Ideally, one should have someone from outside the office/clinic conduct the training, as they may see some things that are not as obvious to those that work there all the time. But if this is not possible, it is still possible to conduct sessions on a regular basis. Chapter 26 covers some specifics on what areas should be covered, as well as how to design scenarios.

References

Azuma M, Daily R, Furmanski C. A review of time critical decision making models and human cognitive processes, *Aerospace Conference*, 2006 IEEE, 2006.

Buyck D, Lang F. Teaching medical communication skills: a call for greater uniformity, *Fam Med* **34**(5):337–43, 2002.

Gaba D, Howard S, Fish K, et al., 2001. Simulation-based training in anesthesia crisis resource management (ACRM): a decade of experience. *Simul Gaming* **32**(2) 175–193, 2001.

Gaba D, Fish K, Howard S. *Crisis management in anesthesiology*. Churchill Livingstone, 1994.

Greenberg C, Regenbogen S, Studdert D, Lipsitz S, Rogers S, Zinner M, Gawande A. Patterns of communication breakdowns resulting in injury to surgical patients. *J Am Coll Surg* 2007;**204**:533–540.

Institute for Healthcare Improvement (IHI). Effective teamwork as a care strategy - SBAR and other tools for improving communication between caregivers. On demand presentation. http://www.ihi.org/IHI/Programs/AudioAndWebPrograms/Effective+Teamwork+as+a+Care+Strategy+SBAR+and+Other+Tools+for+Improving+Communication+Between+Careg.htm# (Accessed June 6, 2011).

Jensen RS. *Pilot Judgment and Crew Resource Management*. Ashgate Publishing, Vermont. 1995

Reader F, Flin R, Cuthbertson B. Communication skills and error in the intensive care unit. *Curr opin crit care* **13** (6) pp. 732–736, 2007.

Reason J. Human error: models and management. *BMJ* **320**: 768–770, 2000.

St. Pierre, M., Hofinger G., Buerschaper, C. *Crisis Management in Acute Care Settings*. Springer, 2010.

26 Simulation in dental anesthesia

Joseph Kras
Washington University in St. Louis, Department of Anesthesiology, St. Louis, MO, USA

Simulation is a technique in teaching and assessment that has grown in popularity in medicine over the last two decades. It may be task oriented, or used to train and reinforce personal responses and team interactions in complex situations. By immersing personnel in realistic situations and utilizing realistic cues, participants should be able to function to a higher level of competence during real incidents. Simulated scenarios should cover the most common incidents that occur in a particular practice setting, as well as rare but catastrophic occurrences. Designing and running simulations in your own office can be an effective way to maintain preparedness of you and your staff.

Definition and short history

Britannica's online dictionary gives the following as one definition of simulation: "… a research or teaching technique that reproduces actual events and processes under test conditions" (Britannica 2011). Simulation has probably been around (in one form or another) as long as man has inhabited the earth. Simulation is a technique used to teach, and does not refer to a specific type of equipment. The weatherman uses models to predict what the weather will be like days to months later, law students argue cases in "moot" court, and armies take part in war games. School children take part in fire drills. All are examples of simulation.

Simulation may be used to train people in specific tasks, as well as to train teams to work together more effectively. Generations of dental students have been trained to restore teeth using a typodont dental simulator. They, and millions of others, have also learned to correctly perform CPR while using a Resusci-Anne™ mannequin. Neither of these simulators are very sophisticated, but they are still very effective in training people to competency in sets of specific skills.

Although the first computerized mannequin used in medicine dates back to the late 1960's (Cooper and Taqueti, 2004), it was not until the mid 1980's that the idea of incorporating computerized simulation into medical training took off. This was facilitated both by the decreased cost and increased power of portable computers, as well as increasing demands from the public not to be used as "guinea pigs" during medical treatment.

Starting in the late 1980's researchers in the departments of anesthesiology at Stanford University and the University of Miami independently developed high fidelity full body computer controlled simulators, and developed a teaching curriculum to go with them (Cooper and Taqueti, 2004). By the mid 1990's the concept of teaching practitioners through the use of simulators was well on the way to becoming entrenched in the anesthesiology community. Virtual reality simulation has been used in training responders to critical situations, as well as surgeons to competence (Gallagher et al., 2005). As of 2011, simulation has been widely incorporated into training of doctors, nurses, and other allied health professionals.

Goals and uses of simulation

Simulation is a tool that can be used in teaching as well as evaluation. When looked at from a medical perspective, simulation can be used to teach individual tasks, allow deliberate repetitive responses to common situations, expose practitioners to uncommon but serious incidents, re-create untoward incidents so that responses can be studied, and allow group interactions to also be studied. Individual responses to crises can be evaluated, as well as group dynamics and effectiveness.

Multiple advantages to training and evaluating personnel using simulation can be had. These include being able to break complex tasks into smaller subtasks that can be mastered separately, the ability to repeat selected situations until trainees master the desired responses, and being able to expose practitioners to rare situations that they might not otherwise be exposed to during training. Because real patients are not being used, videotaping can be done so that participants' performances can be reviewed and critiqued with them by instructors.

Task trainers can be used in multiple ways in anesthesiology. There are trainers to teach intubation, starting IV's, central line trainers, cricothyrotomies, and fiberoptic intubations. Trainees can use these task trainers to sharpen or retain useful skills. Repeating tasks on a mannequin over and over again increases the ability of practitioners to perform them on real patients (Seymour et al., 2002).

Whole body computerized simulators can be utilized to train or test individual or group skills. Optimal class size is typically 4–7 participants. If the class is to be composed of more people than this, then it is recommended that the class be broken up into smaller components, with one group participating, while the other group(s) observe.

Teaching in a simulation environment can be done in "real time," with the instructor in the simulation room, or can be accomplished by debriefing the participants after the simulation is completed. Real time instruction is usually reserved for initial teaching of concepts to junior level trainees, while debriefing afterward is the more widely utilized form of teaching in simulation.

Anesthesia Complications in the Dental Office, First Edition. Edited by Robert C. Bosack and Stuart Lieblich.

Video recording of simulation sessions is often considered essential to the process. Recording sessions allows an "objective" observer to record what "actually" happened, as opposed to what participants "think" they did during a simulated crisis. Telling a person that a patient was pulseless for two and a half minutes before anyone noticed and started CPR is wholly different from showing him or her their performance on tape. In going over recorded sessions, participants can often be more critical of their own performance than the instructor is. It is also easier to demonstrate examples of both good as well as bad performance when there is videotape to refer to.

Although initially used primarily for teaching students and junior resident practitioners, simulation has shown its utility in instructing students and practitioners at all levels. Beginning students can learn and practice elementary physiology and pharmacology in a life-like environment. Junior residents can practice procedures on mannequins instead of patients, as well as learn the principles of patient rescue while working together as a team. Higher level trainees and established practitioners alike can reinforce earlier skills as well as learn new ones. Teams that work together clinically can also train together. By exposing members of the team to various scenarios in a simulated environment, participants can gain greater understanding of what other member's roles are, and mutually work to discover ways of preventing bad outcomes. Finally, simulated environments can present standardized scenarios, which can be used to evaluate competency of individuals and teams.

What to simulate

When one is setting up a simulation training program for staff, one of the first orders of business is to decide what things you want to teach or train. When looking to build a simulation "curriculum," there are three main areas that need to be covered. The first would be to cover common emergencies that happen in most offices on a somewhat frequent basis. Next would be rare occurrences that don't happen very often to anyone, but can be devastating if they are missed. Finally, including events that have actually occurred in your own office can be very helpful.

Including actual events that happened in your office makes simulation "come alive" to your personnel. They know this is not just a required exercise (as CPR training is sometimes approached as) and therefore everyone pays attention. And once they pay attention to such a scenario, they're more likely to also pay attention to the next scenario you include. Going over these scenarios through simulation may also have some other benefits. After an adverse event happens, there is a natural tendency to not talk about it, and just "move on". This is both because of a (sometimes quite real) fear of legal consequences, as well as fears of exposing personal inadequacies. By including such scenarios in your simulation program, one not only has the opportunity to explore them to find better ways to respond the next time they might happen, but also demonstrate to staff the group's commitment to patient care and quality improvement.

Next come common occurrences. Medicine is chock full of aphorisms, with a favorite in anesthesia being "It's hard to kill a breathing patient." It's no secret that the weight of the average American has been steadily increasing. Between 1960 and 2002, the average adult in the United States became approximately 24 pounds heavier. While height increased slightly over that time, BMI measurements increased from approximately 25–28, in both males and females (Ogden et al., 2004). Airway and ventilation problems are a leading cause of patients dying in any outpatient surgical facility, and need to be addressed. Being able to recognize and manage airway problems is an essential prerequisite to anyone giving anesthesia, in any setting.

Closely following airway and ventilation problems are cardiac problems. As the average age of the population rises, increasing numbers of patients with both diagnosed as well as undiagnosed cardiac problems are presenting for treatment. Coronary ischemia, MI, stroke, and arrhythmias should all be able to be handled by practitioners giving anesthesia.

Complications related to diabetic patients, including hyper as well as hypoglycemia are common, especially as both the average weight and age of patients continue to increase. If one takes care of children or young adults, then problems relating to asthma will also be quite common.

Drug related complications, including allergic reactions, improper dosing of drugs, and inadvertent drug swaps are not uncommon occurrences in a busy outpatient surgicenter. Being able to rapidly diagnose and treat such emergencies before they cause permanent damage to a patient is important.

Finally, uncommon but serious complications need to be covered. If they are not covered, they will never be considered as possibilities. Examples of such events are malignant hyperthermia, thyroid storm, severe hypothyroidism, pregnancy related problems, and seizures.

Practical tips in designing scenarios

Attending a structured review course on anesthetic problems can be a very useful exercise, but few people are willing and able to attend such a course more than once every year or two, and fewer still will be able to take their entire staff with them. Therefore it makes sense to set up regularly scheduled "in house" simulations, ideally once every month or two. Several advantages of doing so include the ability to customize the content to your office's particular needs, ease of incorporating training into the office schedule, ability to include all office members, and being able to have training sessions on a much more regular basis.

In designing and rolling out simulation scenarios, goals must be set. Is there a knowledge deficit that exists, such as new staff not knowing how to treat a person having an asthma attack in the office, or is the goal to solidify the actions of the entire team, such that everyone works together more effectively? If there is a knowledge deficit, simulation can be helpful for those who learn better by actual participation, rather than by reading about something in a book. Not everyone retains knowledge best by reading printed material, or listening to lectures. Many learn better by "walking through" the actions they would actually perform in an emergency situation. Also, new equipment (or equipment not often used, such as defibrillators) will be much more familiar if people actually simulate using it.

Practicing responding to crises slowly while everyone on the team walks through their own actions can also expose weaknesses in the response plan. For example, if the same person is expected both to draw up emergency drugs as well as communicate with first response personnel by phone, it helps to have an installed phone or a wireless extension that's been tested to actually work in every room. If cell phones are to be utilized to call 911 from certain parts of your facility, does the local EMS system automatically pull up a cell phone's location? These and many other facts can be worked through while walking through a response.

Having all of your staff train as a team has several advantages. Each person has particular strengths and weaknesses, and training with the actual people you have to depend on allows you to customize responses to those strengths, as well as identify weaknesses to be bolstered. Practicing scenarios with your own team in your own environment adds the benefit of having a workspace and equipment that is familiar to all. If there are potential problems related to equipment or environment, then these may be illuminated by practicing scenarios in the place you practice.

How long should a simulation scenario last? While some simulation centers prefer to utilize scenarios lasting about 45 minutes, which embed multiple "events" in the scenario, running such a scenario can become tedious, as well as tiring for participants. Our simulation group at the Washington University School of Medicine has found that scenarios lasting generally 5–10 minutes seem to work best. Each scenario can concentrate on one or two main points, which makes it easier when debriefing the participants afterwards.

There are many similarities between simulation and theater. One needs a script, actors, props, and a director. When organized courses are run, the director is a non-participant. For in-house training with a small group, it is unlikely that you would have extra personnel around. One may have the person directing the scenario also be one of the confederate actors who knows what problems are present in the scenario, and how the solution to those problems should proceed. In either case, the director sets the scene (making sure participants are provided written or verbal evidence of the initial conditions present), provides information to participants during the scenario as necessary (e.g., "Now the patient's rhythm on the monitor looks like this"), and debriefs participants at the end.

Written scripts for each scenario are necessary. They give you a concrete plan of what you are going to simulate, a plan for how you want the simulation to proceed, and should include lists of props that might be needed. Having scripts allows you to easily recreate simulations at a future date.

Props for simulations add to the sense of reality. They include all of the equipment and medicines necessary to handle a particular emergency, a series of normal and abnormal EKG strips for participants to evaluate during scenarios, and possibly a mannequin of some sort to perform CPR on, should it be necessary. Enough of the normal instruments that would be usually present during a procedure should also be present, in order to make the situation feel real to those involved.

A summary sheet for each simulation should include the following: the title of the simulation (e.g., MI in 48 y/o, impacted molar removal), the goals of the simulation (e.g., proper use of pressors, airway control, and activation of EMS system), list of props (e.g., extraction setup, code cart, "dummy" chart, normal EKG strip, EKG strip with PVC's and ST depression). One can keep a separate folder for each simulation scenario, containing the summary sheet, script, and paper and x-ray props. If one is using a programmable mannequin, the summary sheet would include settings for the mannequin. If one is using an "actor" to play the patient, then a "cue sheet" for the actor (detailing history, things they need to do, etc.) is also included in this folder.

Simulation is an effective technique for teaching new material, teaching or reinforcing team dynamics, or evaluating competency. Not only can it be effectively used in organized continuing education classes, but it can also be fairly easily incorporated into an in-house continuing education program.

References

Britannica academic edition. (definition of simulation). http://www.britannica.com/EBchecked/topic/545493/simulation (Accessed June 8, 2011)

Cooper J, Taqueti V. A brief history of the development of mannequin simulators for clinical education and training. *Qual Saf Health Care* **13**: i11–i18, 2004

Gallagher A, Ritter E, Champion H, Higgins G, Fried M, Moses G, Smith C, Satava R. Virtual reality simulation for the operating room: proficiency-based training as a paradigm shift in surgical skills training. *Ann Surg* **241**: 364–372, 2005.

Ogden C, Fryar C, Carroll M, Flegal K. Mean body weight, height, and body mass index, United States 1960–2002. CDC: advance data from vital and health statistics, *Num.* **347**: 1–18, 2004.

Seymour N, Gallagher A, Roman S, O'Brien M, Bansal V, Andersen D, Satava R. Virtual reality training improves operating room performance. *Ann Surg* 2002; **236** (4) 458–464.

27 Airway adjuncts

H. William Gottschalk
University of Southern California School of Dentistry, Los Angeles, CA, USA

The purpose of airway management during sedation or general anesthesia is to create a patent passage to allow adequate movement of oxygen into the alveoli of the lungs and the removal of carbon dioxide. Sedatives, narcotics, and hypnotics are titrated to achieve sedation and general anesthesia because there can be a variable and unpredictable response to these medications. If the patient response to medications compromises the patency of the airway, then the two most common maneuvers to restore the patency of that airway have been the chin tilt for minor obstructions and the jaw thrust for moderate to severe obstructions. If these maneuvers are ineffective, then airway adjuncts must be employed. Depending on the practitioner's level of training and competency, it may be necessary to lighten or deepen the level of anesthesia prior to the utilization of airway adjuncts.

Patients never just stop breathing. There is always a cascade of events that precede apnea or obstruction of the airway. It is important to monitor a patient's airway to be able to make the correct diagnosis of what is preventing the adequate exchange of gases in the lungs. *Apnea* is the cessation of breathing. During office-based sedation or anesthesia it is most often due to upper airway obstruction secondary to pharyngeal muscle relaxation, or decreased ventilatory drive, most often due to opioid medication. *Partial airway obstruction* is restriction of the patency of the airway to the point that it has compromised the patient's ability to receive adequate amounts of oxygen in the alveoli. A good example is snoring. Snoring is not a warm, happy, sleeping sound. It is a partial airway obstruction.

Complete airway obstruction is the cessation of breathing due to a complete blockage of the airway. Supraglottic, glottic, subglottic, and subdiaphragmatic are areas where obstruction can occur.

Most airway obstructions are *supraglottic* and involve relaxation of the musculature of the neck, which causes the tongue to contact the posterior wall of the pharynx, thereby reducing or blocking the patency of the airway. Other anatomic structures that can contribute to airway obstruction include a deviated nasal septum, nasal polyps, large adenoids and tonsils, and a large soft palate. Supraglottic obstruction can be overcome with positive pressure ventilation in most cases. *Glottic* obstructions are a partial or full laryngospasm. These obstructions must be treated with positive pressure ventilation with a bag-valve-mask, pressure demand valve, or a circle system and a full face mask. Partial or full laryngospasms that do not allow positive pressure ventilation must be treated with a paralyzing agent, such as succinylcholine, and mechanical ventilation until spontaneous respirations resume. *Subglottic* obstruction is a bronchospasm that can be precipitated by asthma, anaphylaxis, or emesis with aspiration.

Subdiaphragmatic obstruction is due to the weight of the abdominal contents against the diaphragm, which will reduce the excursive movement of the diaphragm and reduce the tidal volume of each respiration or ventilation. This is a problem with the obese patient. While subdiaphragmatic obstruction cannot in and of itself be treated with airway adjuncts, the obese patient usually has a concurrent airway obstruction due to a thick, fleshy neck anatomy. Subdiaphragmatic obstruction will respond to positioning the patient in a more upright and sitting position (see Figure 27.1). The most severe cases will require paralyzing the patient and utilizing mechanical positive pressure ventilation via a cuffed endotracheal tube. The worst-case scenario would be the apneic, obstructed, obese patient.

The purpose of airway adjuncts is to create a patent airway in the spontaneously ventilating patient, allow ventilation of the lungs via positive pressure ventilation, and secure the airway in an apneic patient. All of the available airway adjuncts provide the first two benefits, but only intubation with a cuffed endotrachael tube provides all three.

All of these devices should be immediately available during the administration of sedation or general anesthesia in the event that there is any airway compromise that positioning will not resolve.

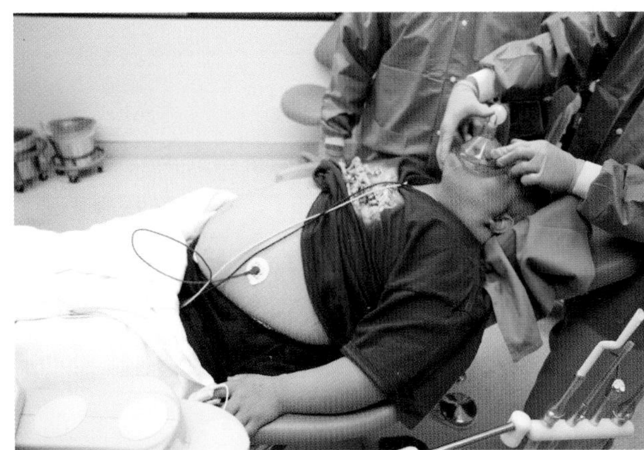

Figure 27.1 Ventilation with a full face mask in a patient with morbid obesity.

Anesthesia Complications in the Dental Office, First Edition. Edited by Robert C. Bosack and Stuart Lieblich.

Nasopharyngeal airway

Nasopharyngeal airways are flexible tubes that are inserted through the nare and extend to the hypopharynx, preventing the tongue from occluding the airway against the posterior aspect of the pharynx (Figure 27.2). These airways come in various diameters and have an increased length with an increased diameter. Their size is based on the French measuring system, with larger numbers indicating a larger diameter. The semiconscious patient tolerates these airways, but if a local anesthetic containing lubricant is utilized for their placement, they can be well tolerated into consciousness.

Oropharyngeal airway

These airways resemble a question mark and are utilized to prevent the tongue, tonsils, and pharyngeal tissue from obstructing the airway. While they can be very effective in creating a patent airway, they are also very stimulating (Figure 27.3). They have to be utilized in the unconscious patient. Improper placement of these devices will actually incorrectly position the tongue and create an obstruction of the airway. The oropharyngeal airways are also designed to allow the insertion of a suction catheter into the pharynx to remove secretions or into the stomach to remove any gastric contents. They are sized based on their linear dimension. Figure 27.4 shows a sizing technique that is helpful in preventing oversized airways from displacing the epiglottis and undersized airways from displacing the tongue posteriorly.

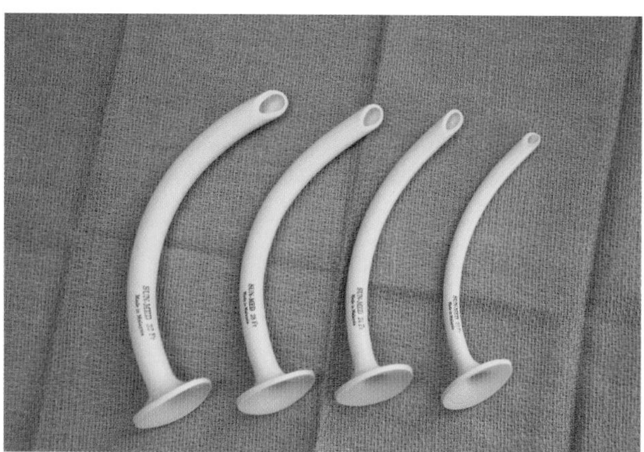

Figure 27.2 Nasopharyngeal airways.

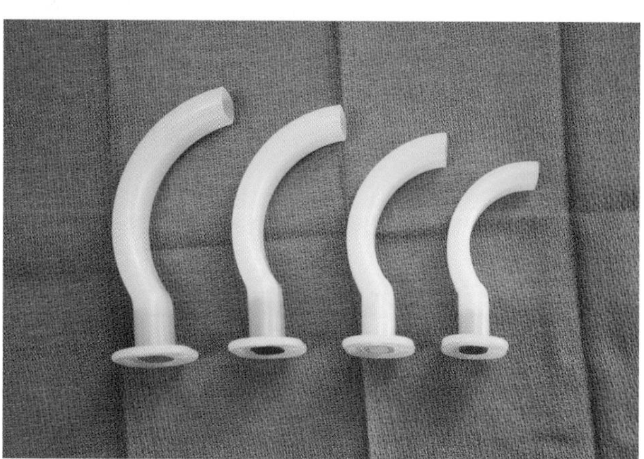

Figure 27.3 Oropharyngeal airways.

Supraglottic airways

There are several varieties of supraglottic devices that can be inserted blindly into the hypopharynx, to create a mask seal over the laryngeal inlet in order to maintain upper airway patency and facilitate ventilation. These devices include the laryngeal mask airway (Figure 27.5), which has an inflatable cuff to create a laryngeal seal, and non-inflatable devices, such as the iGel™ (Figure 27.6), designed with a soft, gel-like, non-inflatable material to create a passive laryngeal seal. The iGel™ has a gastric channel, integrated bite block, and a shape that minimizes LMA rotation. These devices tend to provide excellent protection from oral debris, but incomplete protection from aspiration of gastric contents during emesis. The King LT(S) – D™ is a disposable airway device to assist in positive pressure ventilation, by sealing inflatable balloons in the esophagus and oropharynx through a single inflation port. A separate suction port is provided (Figure 27.7).

Various levels of positive pressure ventilation are possible with these devices and depend on the patency of the larynx and bronchioles. Properly sized and appropriately positioned standard LMAs should provide a seal up to 20 cm H_2O, which should be sufficient for positive pressure ventilation in the absence of bronchospasm. It is important to note that inability to attain a laryngeal seal is rarely remediated with overinflation of the LMA cuff, which will only

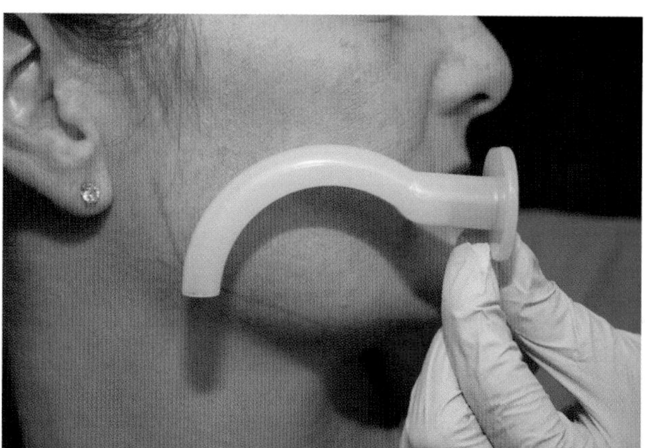

Figure 27.4 The distance from the lips to the angle of the mandible helps select an appropriately sized oropharyngeal airway.

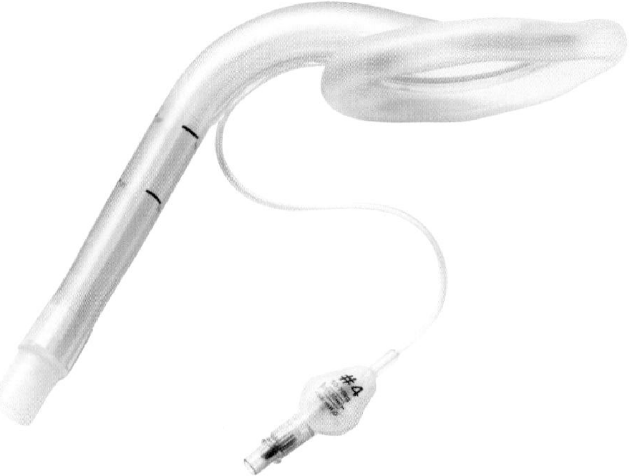

Figure 27.5 AuraOnce disposable LMA. This LMA has an anatomically correct curve for fast and easy insertion. The tip is reinforced to resist folding over during insertion, courtesy of Ambu Corp., with permission.

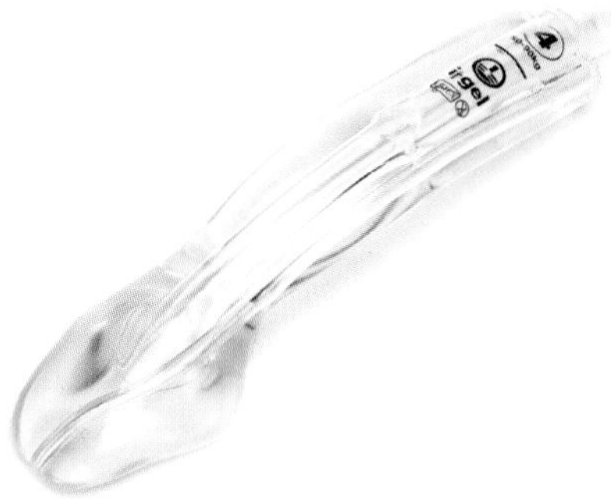

Figure 27.6 iGel™, courtesy of Intersurgical, with permission.

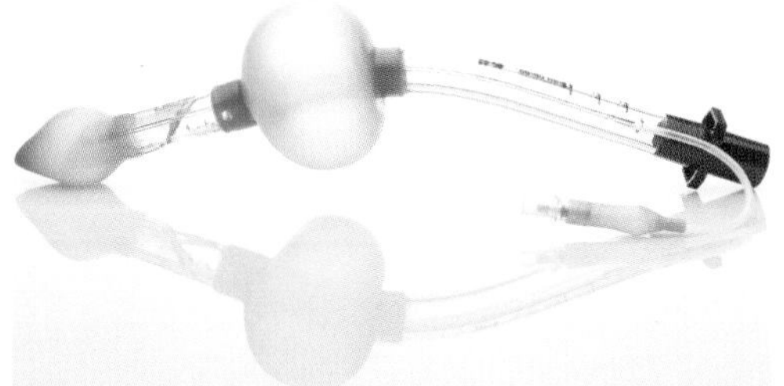

Figure 27.7 King LT (S) – D™, with permission.

decrease the compliance of laryngeal fit. Optimizing cuff position or increasing the size of the cuff can improve the seal. The suggested cuff pressure for the King LT(S) – D™ is 60dm H_2O, which may support higher ventilator pressures.

Magill forceps

Magill forceps (Figure 27.8) are grasping forceps with a scissor-like handle and blades that open in a vertical plane, similar to the jaws of an alligator. They are used to retrieve foreign bodies from the hypopharynx and to assist in the directing of an endotrachael tube through the glottic opening.

Endotracheal tube

These devices can be inserted through the oral cavity or the nasal passage (Figure 27.9). They are the gold standard of airway management because they insure a patent airway, allow for very efficient positive pressure ventilation, and protect the trachea from aspiration of oral, pharyngeal, or gastric secretions. The downside of these devices is that without routine practice in their placement, the delicate tissues of the airway and larynx can be traumatized and cause bleeding, which will make visualization of the anatomic structures of the pharynx very difficult. The airway could be further compromised, putting the patient in greater harm.

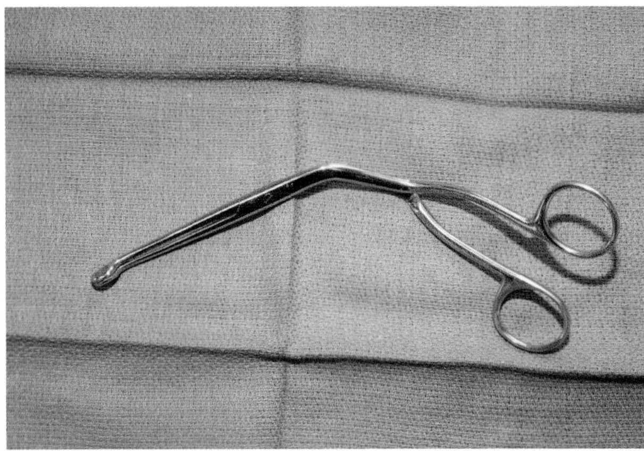

Figure 27.8 Magill forceps.

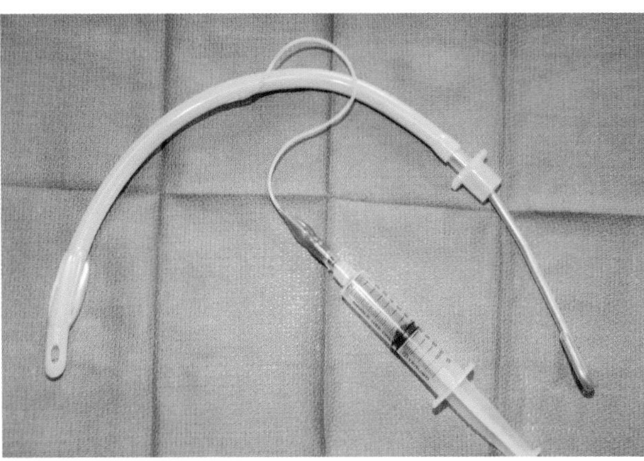

Figure 27.9 An endotracheal tube with a flexible stylet to maintain bends in the tube to facilitate placement. The tip of the stylet should never extend beyond the tip of the tube.

Endotracheal tubes are sized based on the inside diameter of the tube. The overall thickness of these tubes varies among the manufacturers. Since the opening between the vocal cords is smaller than the diameter of the trachea, these tubes have a cuff that is inflated after passing beyond the vocal cords, to seal it in the trachea.

All of the other airway adjuncts can be placed blindly. An endotrachael tube requires the use of a manual or video-enhanced laryngoscope. The video-assisted laryngoscopes have greatly improved the visualization of the trachea in even the most difficult, anterior locations of the trachea. Now, the laryngoscopy is much less traumatic than with a manual scope and there is much less postoperative discomfort and edema.

28 Intravenous fluids

Cara Riley[1], Kyle Kramer[2], and Jeffrey Bennett[2]
[1]Department of Anesthesiology, Children's Hospital Colorado, Aurora, CO, USA
[2]Indiana University, Department of Oral Surgery and Hospital Dentistry, Indianapolis, IN, USA

Introduction

The fluid status of patients undergoing surgery is altered during the perioperative period, with patients often arriving for the procedure with a significant fluid deficit. It is the responsibility of the anesthetist to restore fluid balance in order to maintain hemodynamic stability and improve the rate and quality of recovery. Isotonic crystalloid solutions, such as 0.9% normal saline and lactated Ringer's, are frequently employed for such fluid therapy in the dental office.

The significance of acquiring intravenous access for sedation or general anesthesia extends beyond the administration of pharmacological agents. Intravenous fluid (IVF) therapy is an important component of the surgical and anesthetic treatment, even for minor procedures in the ambulatory setting. Administering IVF helps correct preexisting fluid deficits, manage maintenance fluid requirements, and offset fluid losses or shifts associated with surgery. IVF also aids in counterbalancing the vasodilatory effects common to many anesthetic agents. Furthermore, optimization of fluid therapy positively influences the patient's postoperative course, reducing complications and supporting recovery (Hamilton, 2009). Adequate attention to appropriate IVF administration is therefore key to a successful procedure.

An important concept in IVF therapy is that of fluid compartments (see Figure 28.1). Water comprises about 60% of the total weight of the human body. Total body water (TBW) is distributed in two main compartments within the body: the extracellular fluid (ECF) and the intracellular fluid compartments (ICF). The ICF contains approximately two-thirds of the TBW, while the ECF holds the remaining one-third. The ECF is further distributed within the intravascular and interstitial fluid compartments, which hold 25% and 75% of the ECF respectively. A 70-kg male has approximately 42 liters of total body water, 28 liters within the ICF, and 14 liters within the ECF. The intravascular volume, which approximates 3.5 liters of water, comprises roughly 70% of the total blood volume as plasma. The volume of the interstitial space approximates 10.5 liters (Sabiston, 1991; see Figure 28.1).

Water distributes between these compartments freely, moving via osmosis toward areas with higher concentrations of ions, such as sodium and chloride. Areas of varying ion concentrations are the basis of tonicity, and the consideration of tonicity is important in choosing the optimal intravenous fluid to administer.

How does surgery affect fluid status?

Under normal circumstances, fluid is lost from these compartments in the form of urine, feces, sweat, and respiratory vapor. The oral intake of food and water is responsible for replenishing the fluid losses from these spaces. Surgery modifies this balance in several ways. Patients arrive for surgery with a preexisting fluid deficit after following *nulla per os* (NPO) guidelines (refer to Table 28.1), and discomfort and swelling may limit their oral intake postoperatively as well (Bennett et al., 1999). Surgery can directly lead to fluid loss as a result of bleeding, evaporation from open wounds, and the internal redistribution of body fluids known as "third spacing." Third spacing occurs when traumatized, inflamed, or infected tissue collects fluid within interstitial spaces or body cavities. This fluid collection cannot easily equilibrate with the other fluid compartments and is considered nonfunctional (Morgan et al., 2006). Up to 20% of an infused volume of IVF can be sequestered in this manner (Hahn, 2010). While direct surgical fluid losses such as these are usually significant only in major surgeries, even minor procedures exert indirect effects on fluid balance. The elimination of fluids from the body is altered, as surgery, stress, and anesthesia induce hormonal changes. Preoperative dehydration and vasodilation from anesthetic agents cause a release of antidiuretic hormone (Berleur et al., 2003), which signals the kidneys to reabsorb water. Renin and aldosterone levels likewise increase during surgical procedures, further promoting fluid retention (Hahn, 2010). The reduction in elimination is substantial, as only 5–15% of an infused crystalloid load is excreted in the surgical setting, in comparison to the normal 40–75% observed in an awake patient (Hahn, 2010).

How much fluid does the patient need?

The physical examination

It is the responsibility of the anesthetist to assess fluid status and replace fluid deficits. The physical examination is helpful to this end. Hypovolemia is suggested by lethargy, low skin turgor (the skin does not snap back into place after being pinched upwards for a few seconds), dry mucous membranes, weak peripheral pulses, a high resting heart rate with low blood pressure, and orthostatic changes (increased heart rate and decreased blood pressure) when

Anesthesia Complications in the Dental Office, First Edition. Edited by Robert C. Bosack and Stuart Lieblich.

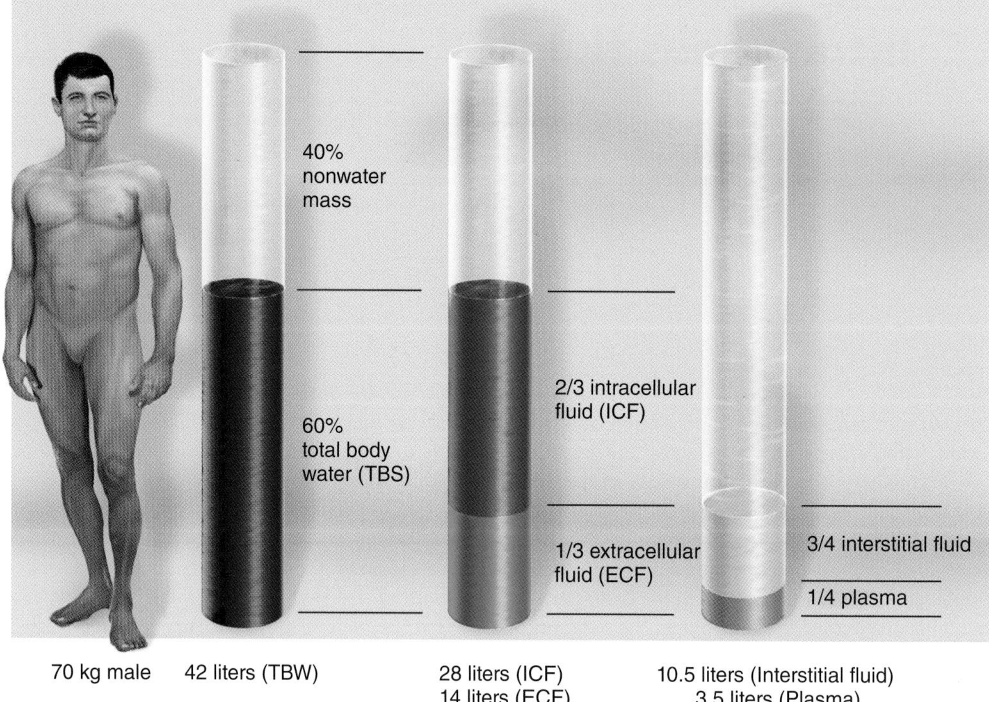

Figure 28.1 Fluid compartments in the body.

Table 28.1 Current ASA NPO guidelines (ASA, 2011).

Substance	NPO Recommendation (hours)	Examples
Clear liquids	2	Water, black, coffee, tea, juice without pulp
Breast milk	4	
Non-human milk	6	Baby formula
Light breakfast	6	Dry toast with black coffee
Fatty foods	8+	Bacon, eggs, milk, cream, butter

rapidly changing from a supine to a sitting or standing position (Morgan et al., 2006). Intraoperatively, a dehydrated patient may exhibit a more pronounced response to the hypotensive effects of anesthetic agents. A patient who is severely fluid overloaded, on the other hand, may show signs of peripheral and pulmonary edema. The latter is indicated by crackles or rales, wheezing, cyanosis, frothy pink secretions, and impaired ventilation and oxygenation. Peripheral edema can locally impair oxygen transport and worsen healing (Morgan et al., 2006). A more accurate method for assessing volume status involves the measurement of stroke volume and cardiac output, but such techniques are invasive and beyond the scope of this text (Hamilton, 2009).

The 4-2-1 rule

In determining how much intravenous fluid is to be given, it is important to keep in mind the patient's weight and hours of NPO fasting. A patient's hourly maintenance fluid requirements (for urine production, sweating, breathing, GI secretions, etc.) can be calculated following the 4-2-1 rule (Table 28.2, from ASA, 2011). This volume, multiplied by the hours without food or drink intake, estimates the patient's existing fluid deficit.

For example, a 70-kg person would have a maintenance requirement of 110 mL/hr (40 mL + 20 mL + 50 mL), which after a 10-hour fast would lead to 1,100 mL fluid deficit (110 mL × 10 hr). By convention, half of this volume is replaced in the first hour of the procedure, with the second half split equally over the next 2 hours. In addition to replacing the fluid deficit, the hourly maintenance rate is concurrently administered (110 mL/hr). Any losses from bleeding, evaporation, or third spacing can be replenished according to the extent of the surgical wound and the hemodynamic stability of the patient. The majority of oral and maxillofacial procedures are fairly noninvasive with minimal blood losses, environmental losses, or large fluid shifts, and typically do not require more than 0–2 mL/kg in additional fluid replacement. When restoring the measured blood loss, crystalloid or colloid is first administered until the risk of anemia overshadows that of transfusion, at which point red blood cells are used (Morgan et al., 2006). Crystalloid tends to be given in a 3:1 ratio to replace blood loss, and colloid in a 1:1 ratio (Morgan et al., 2006).

While administering 1 liter or more of fluid may at first seem excessive for a dentoalveolar procedure, such fluid therapy has proved beneficial to the patient in a number of studies. Receiving more than 1 liter of crystalloid during minor ambulatory surgery reduces the unpleasant symptoms of dehydration

Table 28.2 4-2-4 rule for maintenance fluid requirements (ASA, 2011).

≤10 kg	4 mL/kg/hr
11–20 kg	Add 2 mL/kg/hr
≥21 kg	Add 1 mL/kg/hr *or* Total weight in kg + 4 = mL/kg/hr

(Bungaard-Nielsen et al., 2009). Dehydration or lack of adequate rehydration can itself have adverse effects on the quality and speed of recovery from anesthesia and surgery (Bennett et al., 1999). Patients receiving more liberal fluid replacement perceived themselves to be more fully recovered with an improved sense of well-being prior to discharge, and demonstrated less residual sedation, drowsiness, fatigue, dizziness, nausea/vomiting, fewer headaches, and an overall improved outcome in the postoperative period (Bennett et al., 1999). Starting with a 1-liter bag of fluid for each adult patient is therefore good practice, as it will help optimize fluid status even if the bag remains partially unfinished at the end of the procedure. In addition, during an acute emergency, the IV will remain functional and precious time will not be wasted in changing an empty small bag. The fluid is best administered over at least 30 minutes, a goal readily achieved during average intraoperative and recovery times (Bennett et al., 1999). For longer procedures, many clinicians advocate a slow infusion rate during the majority of the surgery and increasing the infusion toward the end, provided that the vital signs remain stable. This helps prevent the discomfort of a full bladder or even intraoperative voiding, as urinary catheters are not usually placed for ambulatory dental/maxillofacial cases. In those more invasive procedures, such as orthognathic surgeries, in which a urinary catheter is utilized, the pace of IVF infusion can be more consistent, following conventional fluid replacement guidelines. Moreover, the rate of urine formation can actually be used as a tool for assessing the patient's fluid status. The production of 0.5 mL/kg/hr of urine is often used as a goal in indicating adequate hydration.

With regard to the size of catheter and the type of drip chamber to use, consideration for the age and medical condition of the patient, as well as anticipated fluid requirement, should be made. Larger bore needles can deliver higher rates of fluid infusion, but also carry an increased risk of pain on placement, failed attempts, site infection, phlebitis, and extravasation. Eighteen to 20 gauge catheters are considered all-purpose and are appropriate for the needs of most adult dental patients. Twenty-two gauge catheters are standard for pediatric patients, and can also be used in elderly patients or those with fragile veins. Sixteen gauge needles tend to be employed for blood transfusion and donation, and even larger bore catheters are placed in trauma patients for rapid fluid resuscitation. It should be noted that increasing the rate of fluid administration is possible with IV catheter of any size by using a pressure bag or rapid infuser. The type of drip chamber further influences the rate of IVF administration. Macrodrip sets generally dispense 10–15 drips per mL, whereas Microdrip sets require 60 drips per mL. A 60 drip per mL set will deliver a given amount of fluid six times more slowly than a 10 drip per mL drip chamber. It follows then that Macro-drippers are conventionally used for adult patients or when rapid infusion is anticipated. Micro-drippers allow for fine-tuning of the infusion rate and are often employed in the pediatric population. They can also be utilized when administering medications with a precise infusion rate (dopamine, e.g.) if a drug infusion pump is not available.

What kind of fluid does the patient need?

What fluid is optimal for a given patient? Patients arriving for surgery have measurable deficits of water containing small amounts of sodium, potassium, and chloride (Bennett et al., 1999); our aim is to replace such losses in kind. The available formulations of intravenous fluids differ in their composition of electrolytes and other molecules, as well as in the degree and duration of intravascular expansion they provide (Grocott & Hamilton, 2002). The two major classes of IVF are crystalloids and colloids. Blood products and special derivatives can also be administered but are not addressed in this text. Fluid therapy for dentoalveolar surgery generally involves the infusion of crystalloids such as 0.9% normal saline (NS) or lactated Ringer's (LR), with or without glucose (Morgan et al., 2006). While NS contains sodium and chloride, LR also contains calcium, potassium, and lactate (which is converted to glucose and bicarbonate in the liver) and mimics most closely the natural extracellular fluid composition (Morgan et al., 2006). LR is therefore considered the most physiological solution. It is, however, avoided in patients with liver failure in order to prevent a build-up of lactate. NS in large volumes has been associated with hyperchloremic metabolic acidosis secondary to its high concentration of sodium and chloride; this complication is of little concern in the dental office as such volumes are unlikely to be given (Grocott and Hamilton, 2002) (see Table 28.3).

Crystalloids versus colloids

After a crystalloid fluid is infused, it initially expands the intravascular plasma volume, and then equilibrates with the interstitial space. Fluid is excreted by the kidneys or lost to third spacing (Hahn, 2010). Colloids undergo less distribution to the interstitial space, and are therefore more reliable intravascular volume expanders (Hahn, 2010). Examples of colloid solutions include blood-derived products such as serum albumin, and synthetic substances such as Dextrans and hydroxyethyl starches. The key characteristic of colloids is that they contain high molecular weight substances that allow the fluid to persist intravascularly for a longer period than the crystalloids. After a 1-liter infusion of colloid, approximately 70 to 80% will remain within the intravascular space after 90 minutes. On the other hand, after a 1-liter dose of NS, only

Table 28.3 Components of common crystalloid solutions (ASA, 2011).

Solutions	Sodium (mEq/L)	Chloride (mEq/L)	Potassium (mEq/L)	Calcium (mEq/L)	Glucose (mg/dL)	Lactate (mEq/L)	Approximate pH	Osmolality (mOsm/L)
Normal saline 0.9% (NS)	154	154					5.6	308
1/2 NS	77	77					5.6	154
Lactated Ringer's (LR)	130	109	4	3		28	6.6	273
5% Dextrose in water (D_5W)					5000		4.3	253
D_5 1/4 NS	38.5	38.5			5000		4.3	329
D_5 1/2 NS	77	77			5000		4.3	406
D_5 LR	130	109	4	3	5000	28	4.9	525
Extracellular fluid	140	108	4.5	5	90–110		7.3	290

about 25% remains within the intravascular compartment (Grocott and Hamilton, 2002). Indeed, the half-life of colloid solutions is 6–12 times longer than that of the crystalloids (Grocott and Hamilton, 2002). Colloids are not without adverse effects, however. Infusion of colloid solution can lead to impairment of hemostasis, inhibition of endothelial and inflammatory cell function, and allergic reactions. They are generally used only when crystalloid resuscitation proves ineffective, prior to blood transfusion in the severely hypovolemic patient until blood products are available, or in those patients with large protein or albumin losses, such as burn victims (Morgan et al., 2006). Despite any differences, data from clinical trials fail to support the use of colloids over crystalloids in the surgical patient, as they are significantly more expensive and are not associated with improved patient outcomes (Bailey et al., 2010).

Tonicity

Crystalloids can be hypo-, iso-, or hypertonic to plasma. It is desirable to give the patient IVF with a tonicity close to that of plasma (isotonic) to allow the fluid to remain within the intravascular space for an extended period and to prevent abrupt shifts between compartments. Hypotonic solutions are rapidly redistributed from the intravascular space and do not help maintain plasma volume and blood pressure as isotonic solutions can (Bennett et al., 1999). As noted previously, isotonic crystalloids have a 25–30 minute distribution phase, such that the majority of the volume given will remain intravascularly for that time, after which equilibration with the interstitial space slowly decreases the fluid expansion to about 25% of the infused amount (Hahn, 2010). NS is isotonic to plasma, and LR is treated as isotonic in practice, although it is mildly hypotonic by the numbers. Dextrose solutions, such as D_5W, act as hypotonic solutions (Bailey et al., 2010) because the glucose they contain is rapidly metabolized after infusion and the remaining water freely distributes throughout the body. Certainly, hypotonic solutions are primarily used to replace free water losses (Morgan et al., 2006). Conversely, hypertonic solutions draw tissue fluid into the intravascular space and are reserved for use in situations such as refractory hypovolemic shock, traumatic brain injury with cerebral edema, and burn injuries (Bailey et al., 2010). Complications associated with hypertonic solutions include osmotic demyelination syndrome, rebound increases in intracranial pressure, acute renal failure, and electrolyte abnormalities (Bailey et al., 2010).

Dextrose-containing solutions

Crystalloid solutions are either sodium chloride or glucose based. The use of glucose-containing solutions is generally reserved for those patients at risk of hypoglycemia, such as young children. Hypoglycemia can alter the brain's blood flow and metabolism, and even cause neurodevelopmental impairment if it remains unrecognized (Bailey et al., 2010). The incidence of preoperative hypoglycemia in pediatric patients is between 0.5–2.5%, typically secondary to fasting and lower carbohydrate reserves (Berleur et al., 2003). Neonates and premature babies are at the highest risk. Fasting guidelines allow clear liquids up to 2 hours before surgery, but many patients fast for much longer, and fasts on the degree of 8 to 19 hours are associated with the development of hypoglycemia in children (Bailey et al., 2010). Nevertheless, blood glucose concentrations typically rise in response to surgical stress, and most pediatric patients remain normoglycemic throughout the perioperative period (Berleur et al., 2003). It follows that dextrose-containing solutions are best administered to children at the greatest risk of hypoglycemia, such as neonates, children on hyperalimentation, and those with endocrinopathies (Bailey et al., 2010). Conversely, glucose solutions can lead to hyperglycemia, which in combination with hypoxemia can cause brain cell dysfunction and death. This situation is unlikely during dental/maxillofacial procedures (Bennett et al., 1999), but hyperglycemia is also associated with an osmotic diuresis that can lead to electrolyte abnormalities and dehydration from enhanced urine production, and also increases the risk of wound infection (Berleur et al., 2003). If a dextrose-containing solution is to be used, it should be in combination with NS or ½ NS (Bennett et al., 1999) to help attenuate any alterations of electrolyte concentrations. Certainly, pediatric patients are well resuscitated with any isotonic crystalloid, such as NS or LR, which can replace both fluid and electrolyte losses.

It is clear that isotonic crystalloid solutions, like NS and LR, are well suited for IVF therapy in the dental office during procedures under sedation or general anesthesia. Special care should be given to sufficiently restoring the patient's fluid balance, which will help ensure hemodynamic stability and improve the speed and quality of recovery. Preparing a 1-liter (500 mL in children) bag for infusion, using a new bag and tubing for each case to preserve sterility, is good practice and enables the optimization of fluid status in each patient. Adequate fluid therapy will, in turn, help ensure the success of the surgical procedure as a whole.

References

Bailey, A. G., et al. Perioperative crystalloid and colloid fluid management in children: where are we and how did we get here? *Pediat Anesth* **110**: 375–390, 2010.

Bennett, J., et al. Perioperative rehydration in ambulatory anesthesia for dentoalveolar surgery. *Oral Surg Oral Med Oral Pathol* **88**: 279–284, 1999.

Berleur, M. P., et al. Perioperative infusions in paediatric patients: rationale for using Ringer-lactate solution with low dextrose concentration. *J Clin Pharm Ther.* **28**: 31–40, 2003.

Bungaard-Nielsen, M., et al. "Liberal" vs. "restrictive" perioperative fluid therapy—a critical assessment of the evidence. *Acta Anesthesiology Scandinavica.* **53**: 843–851, 2009.

Grocott, M. P. W, Hamilton, M. A. Resuscitation fluids. *Vox Sanguinis.* **82**: 1–8, 2002.

Hahn, R. Volume Kinetics for Infusion Fluids. *Anesthesiol* **113**: 470–481, 2010.

Hamilton, M. A. Perioperative fluid management: progress despite lingering controversies. *Clev Clin J Med* **76**: S28–S31, 2009.

Morgan, G. E., Jr., Mikhail, M.S., and Murray, M. J. Fluid management & transfusion. In: *Clinical Anesthesiology*. 4th edn. New York: Lange Medical Books/McGraw Hill Medical Publishing Division, 690–707, 2006.

Practice Guidelines, Preoperative fasting and the use of pharmacologic agents to reduce the risk of pulmonary aspiration: application to healthy patients undergoing elective procedures. An updated report by the American Society of Anesthesiologists Committee on standards and practice parameters. *Anesthesiol* **114**: 495–511, 2011.

Sabiston, D. C. Fluid and electrolyte management of the surgical patient. In: *Textbook of Surgery: The Biological Basis of Modern Surgical Practice*. 14th edn. 57–76. Philadelphia: Saunders, 1991.

29 Emergency drugs

Daniel A. Haas
University of Toronto, Faculty of Dentistry, Toronto, ON, Canada

Anesthesia and sedation are safe modalities for patients when administered by qualified practitioners. However, it is known that complications can still arise even for those with experience and expertise in providing sedation and anesthesia. Managing such potential adversity requires the knowledge, skills, and judgment that can be achieved with appropriate training. Part of this training requires an understanding of the drugs used for the management of such events, and it is assumed that the reader already has this knowledge base. The objective of this chapter is to review and reinforce that knowledge by summarizing their clinical pharmacology and application in adversity. The agents discussed are those commonly considered to be appropriate in an outpatient practice where anesthesia is being administered. Many of them are part of the Advanced Cardiac Life Support (ACLS) algorithms, and it is assumed that their use would follow current ACLS recommendations (Neumar et al., 2010). The discussion on each drug is organized to review the indications, mechanisms of action, pharmacokinetics, adverse effects, contraindications, dosages, and available formulations. The indications and doses for each of the drugs discussed are summarized in Table 29.1. Table 29.2 provides a synopsis of the drugs organized by the emergency for which they should be considered.

This table represents the author's suggestions for consideration. IV = intravenous. Where multiple drugs from one class are listed, such as the β-blockers or corticosteroids, it is assumed that only one of them is needed in the office. See Table 29.2 for a list of drugs that are considered essential. Vasopressin is considered optional in this context. Intraosseous injection for ACLS drugs may be utilized if intravenous access is not possible.

It is assumed that oxygen is available for all of the above events. This table represents the author's suggestions for consideration. It is not meant to be all-inclusive as additional drugs may be added. It is assumed that only one of the three β-blockers listed above would be present. The individual anesthesia provider must determine the most appropriate set of drugs for the individual practice.

Oxygen

Oxygen administration is indicated any time there is an adverse event in anesthesia. The only contraindication is anxiety-provoked hyperventilation, which is not uncommon in dentistry. In all other instances, oxygen should never be withheld. This is also true for situations where it may be considered to be relatively contraindicated, such as the patient with chronic obstructive pulmonary disease (COPD), where chronic carbon dioxide retention often results in hypoxemic respiratory drive. Short-term administration of oxygen to get patients through the emergency should not depress their drive to breathe. Previous concern regarding oxygen supplementation depressing hypoxemic drive in these patients is now known to be incorrect (Becker and Haas, 2007). For the COPD patient, one should provide oxygen to maintain oxyhemoglobin saturation above 90% (Reilly et al., 2005).

Understanding the pharmacology of oxygen resides in the knowledge of the oxyhemoglobin dissociation curve and its classic sigmoidal shape. Room air contains 20.9% oxygen, and this normally results in the oxyhemgolobin saturation approximating 98%, as read on a pulse oximeter. At this level, the curve is relatively stable. When mouth-to-mask or mouth-to-mouth ventilation is carried out as part of basic cardiopulmonary resuscitation (CPR), the exhaled carbon dioxide results in a reduction in the amount of oxygen delivered, to a level approximating 16%. Therefore, this patient is immediately at a disadvantage even when being ventilated adequately. As oxyhemoglobin saturation drops below 90%, the slope of the curve changes rapidly, resulting in decreased arterial oxygen tension. Chest compressions put the patient at a further disadvantage. Ideal chest compressions, at best, will achieve only 25-33% of the normal cardiac output (Berg et al., 2010). If cardiac arrest has been present for a period of time, lactic acidosis occurs, which will shift the oxyhemoglobin dissociation curve to the right. This results in a lower oxyhemoglobin saturation for a given partial pressure of oxygen being delivered to the lung alveoli. These facts point to the need to improve oxygen delivery whenever adversity arises.

For the patient who is spontaneously breathing, oxygen should be delivered by a full face mask, also called a non-rebreather mask, where a flow rate of 6–10 liters per minute is appropriate for most adults. This is based on the typical adult having a minute volume of 6 liters per minute. For the child, a lower flow rate may be acceptable. A nasal hood could also be used on patients who are spontaneously breathing. If the non-rebreather mask has a reservoir, a 6 liter flow rate will deliver an oxygen concentration of ~60%, and each additional L/min will increase the fraction of inspired oxygen by approximately 5%.

For the apneic patient, the fraction of inspired oxygen needs to be increased to 1.0 if possible and a positive pressure device needs to be used. The bag-valve-mask is the most common positive pressure device used. When used, the flow rate should be 10–15 liters per minute. An automated positive pressure device may be used in adults, provided that the flow rate does not exceed 35 liters per minute.

Anesthesia Complications in the Dental Office, First Edition. Edited by Robert C. Bosack and Stuart Lieblich.

Table 29.1 Drugs for management of adverse events.

Drug	Indication	Dose
Oxygen	All cases except hyperventilation	100%
Flumazenil	Benzodiazepine overdose	0.1–0.2 mg IV q2–3 min, prn
Naloxone	Opioid overdose	0.1mg IV q2–3 min, prn
Succinylcholine	Laryngospasm	0.1–0.2 mg/kg IV
Dantrolene	Malignant hyperthermia	2.5mg/kg IV, repeat prn up to 10 mg/kg
Epinephrine	Cardiac arrest	1mg IV q3-5min, prn 1:10,000, follow with 20 ml flush
	Anaphylaxis	0.01 mg/kg IV, q3–5 min, prn
	Asthma unresponsive to albuterol	0.01 mg/kg IV, q3–5 min, prn Or 0.3–0.5 mg IM (1:1,000)
Ephedrine	Hypotension	5 mg IV, q 3–5 min, prn
Phenylephrine	Hypotension with tachycardia	50–100 μg IV, q 3–5 min, prn
Vasopressin	Ventricular fibrillation, pulseless ventricular tachycardia	40 units IV push
Metoprolol	Hypertension, tachycardia	5 mg IV slow, q 3–5 min, prn (15 mg max)
Esmolol	Hypertension, tachycardia	0.5 mg/kg, IV, repeat 20 mg q3–5 min prn to max dose 100mg
Labetolol	Hypertension	20 mg IV, repeat q3–5 min, prn to max dose of 300mg
Nitroglycerin	Angina, hypertension	0.3–0.4 mg subL, repeat q5 min (3 doses max)
Amiodarone	Ventricular fibrillation, pulseless ventricular tachycardia	300 mg IV (dilute in 20ml of D5W
	Ventricular tachycardia	150 mg IV over 10 min, repeat once prn
Lidocaine	Ventricular tachycardia, (second-line drug)	1–1.5mg IV, repeat 0.5–0.75 mg/kg IV, prn
Adenosine	Paroxysmal supraventricular tachycardia	6mg IV push, follow with rapid 20 mg saline flush, repeat 12 mg after 1–2min, prn
Diltiazem		Second line drug, 15–20 mg IV, then prn 20–25 mg IV in 15 min
Verapamil		Second line drug, 2.5–5 mg IV q3–5 min, then prn 5 mg IV q15 min to a max of 30 mg
Atropine	Hemodynamically significant bradycardia	0.5 mg IV q 3–5min to a max of 3 mg
Aspirin	Angina	160–325 mg sub L
Morphine	Angina	Titrate 2 mg IV increments
Midazolam	Status epilepticus	Titrate to effect up to 5 mg
Diphenhydramine	Allergy	25–50 mg IV, PO
Albuterol	Bronchospasm	2 puffs (180μg), repeat prn
Hydrocortisone	Recurrent anaphylaxis	100 mg IV
Dexamethasone	Recurrent anaphylaxis	4–16 mg IV

Table 29.2 Drugs grouped by adverse event.

Adverse event	Essential	To be considered
Overdose	Naloxone, flumazenil	
Cardiac arrest	Epinephrine	Amiodarone, lidocaine
Tachydysrhythmia	Esmolol, labetolol, metoprolol	Amiodarone, adenosine, ditiazem/verapamil
Bradydysrhythmia	Atropine	
Anaphylaxis	Epinephrine, diphenhydramine	Hydrocortisone, dexamethasone
Bronchospasm	Albuterol, epinephrine	
Myocardial infarction	Nitroglycerin, aspirin, morphine	
Hypotension	Atropine, ephedrine	Phenylephrine
Hypertension	Esmolol, labetolol, metoprolol	
Laryngospasm	Succinylcholine	
Malignant hyperthermia	Dantrolene	
Status epilepticus	Midazolam	

There are a number of sources that can provide oxygen. A portable source should be present in every outpatient office even if there is a centrally stored supply. This portability allows for delivery of oxygen to a patient no matter where in the office the event occurs. This portable source would ideally be an "E"-size cylinder. This size has the advantage of holding more than enough oxygen to manage the event, as there are over 600 liters in a full tank, and yet is small enough to make it move easily when mounted on wheels. A full tank will show a pressure of approximately 2,200 psi. To estimate the amount of time remaining in an oxygen cylinder, one can use the following formula to get an approximation: (psi × F)/L/min = time remaining in minutes, where $F = 0.3$ for E-cylinders and 3.0 for large H-cylinders that supply central plumbing (Becker and Haas, 2007). For example, if a flow of 15 L/min is required from an E-cylinder containing 1000 psi, the time remaining would be only 20 minutes.

Reversal agents

Reversal agents are indicated to manage overdose. As benzodiazepines and opioids are routinely used in sedation and anesthesia, their reversal agents should be immediately available.

Appreciation of the pharmacology of receptor antagonists will improve the understanding of the limitations of these drugs. The binding of drugs to receptors is characterized by their affinity (attraction to and degree of binding) and efficacy (ability to trigger a response.) Drugs that bind to receptors with sufficient affinity and then cause a response are known as *agonists*. A drug can bind to a receptor and yet have zero efficacy, meaning that it causes no action.

These drugs are known as *antagonists*. Since their action is to block the effect of the relevant agonist, they are commonly referred to as *blockers*. Hence, the terms "β blockers" and "β adrenoceptor antagonists" are synonymous. Reversal agents are antagonists for specific drugs and will block, or reverse, the actions of their respective agonists.

In sedation and anesthesia, there are two specific reversal agents: flumazenil and naloxone. It is important to note that neither agent should be used to hasten discharge. Physostigmine is an older agent with limited use today, which can be used for nonspecific reversal of certain adverse events in sedation.

Flumazenil

Flumazenil (Romazicon®) is a specific antagonist to the benzodiazepine receptor and will therefore reverse all benzodiazepine actions. These actions are sedation, anxiolysis, amnesia, muscle relaxation, and anticonvulsant effect. It will reverse any benzodiazepine such as diazepam, midazolam, lorazepam, triazolam, or alprazolam. It will also reverse zolpidem (Ambien®) and zaleplon, as these drugs stimulate one of the benzodiazepine receptor subtypes. Its primary indication is the emergency reversal of benzodiazepine overdose, which has led to unconsciousness in planned moderate sedation. Secondary indications are to manage benzodiazepine-induced paradoxical reactions, postoperative drowsiness, or respiratory depression. It may also be considered as part of the management of laryngospasm where a benzodiazepine significantly contributed to the state of central nervous system depression (Heard et al., 2009).

Flumazenil is characterized by a rapid onset and short duration of action. It is more rapidly cleared and has a shorter elimination half-life as compared with any of the benzodiazepine agonists used in sedation and anesthesia. A 1 to 3 minute onset of action is expected with intravenous administration, with a peak effect in 6 to 10 minutes. The precise duration is dose dependent and therefore difficult to predict, but an estimate of 45 minutes is reasonable. The greater the level of the overdose, the greater is the likelihood that the patient will re-sedate after this period of time. It is important to note that the potential for re-sedation requires that whenever this agent is used to reverse overdose, the patient should be monitored in recovery beyond the expected duration of action of flumazenil. As an estimate, this means that monitoring should continue for at least 1 hour following its administration. This fact essentially negates its ability to "speed up recovery," if the patient is not ready for discharge at the time of administration.

There are very few contraindications to flumazenil. It should not be administered to patients having a history of dependence on benzodiazepines as it may precipitate a withdrawal reaction. It should not be given to a patient with a seizure disorder managed by a benzodiazepine, as it may trigger a seizure.

Flumazenil is formulated as a 0.1 mg/mL injectable solution in 5 and 10 mL vials. The dosage is 0.1 – 0.2 mg increments intravenously, every 2 – 3 minutes until reversal is apparent. Maximum dose is 1mg.

There is controversy over acceptable means of giving this drug (Weaver, 2011). The intended and optimal route of administration is intravenous. However, there may be instances where intravenous access is lost and cannot be immediately re-established, which triggers questions about the acceptability and efficacy of other routes of administration. Flumazenil's effectiveness when given intramuscularly has not been established. Submucosal administration has been studied in dogs (Olive et al., 2000) and humans (Hosaka et al., 2009) but failed to show adequate and safe reversal of benzodiazepine effect. Although intranasal flumazenil has been reported, there appears to be insufficient evidence to recommend this route (Heard et al., 2009; Zanette et al., 2009). Onset data in dogs show that intravenous administration had an onset of 120 seconds, sublingual had an onset of 262 seconds, and intramuscular had an onset of 310 seconds (Heniff et al., 1997). Thus, if flumazenil is indicated when the intravenous line is lost and successful venipuncture is not possible, then sublingual or intralingual administration would appear to be worth the attempt, knowing that the onset will be longer than expected compared with intravenous administration. Basic maintenance of the airway and oxygen administration should be carried out while waiting for the onset of the reversal, since there will be a relative delay. Thus, this alternate route should be considered only when there is no other choice.

Naloxone

Naloxone (Narcan®) is indicated for the emergency management of inadvertent opioid overdose. Naloxone is an antagonist for all opioid receptor subtypes, and will therefore block all of the actions of any opioid. It is indicated for emergency treatment of opioid-induced loss of consciousness when moderate sedation is intended and can be used for unintended respiratory depression, in conjunction with airway and ventilatory support.

Following intravenous administration, naloxone has an onset of action of 1 – 2 minutes and a peak effect in 5 – 15 minutes. This often makes naloxone unsuitable for the management of desaturation secondary to opioid-induced chest wall rigidity, where succinylcholine is the first choice. Similar to flumazenil, its duration of action is dependent on the extent of the overdose it is reversing, and may range from 30 – 60 minutes. Its elimination half-life is 60 minutes. Its short duration of action necessitates appropriate monitoring beyond the termination of its effect. Thus, the same considerations as with flumazenil would apply and the patient should be kept in the office for at least 1 hour after its administration for appropriate monitoring to rule out re-sedation.

Naloxone must be used very cautiously as there is the potential for significant adverse effects. Its administration may result in significant release of catecholamines and result in alterations in blood pressure, ventricular tachycardia, or ventricular fibrillation (Osterwalder, 1996). Vasoconstriction may result in a fluid shift triggering pulmonary edema. Thus, particular concern should be given to patients with cardiac disease. Seizures are possible. An additional contraindication is a current history of opioid dependence in the patient, unless the event is life-threatening and other interventions have been unsuccessful.

To minimize the likelihood of any of these adverse events, the safest technique is to titrate naloxone slowly in 0.1 mg increments to effect (Dahan et al., 2010). These may need to be repeated every 2 to 3 minutes, to a maximum of 0.8 mg. It is formulated as either a 0.4 mg/mL solution in 1 and 10 mL vials or a 1 mg/mL solution in a 2 mL vial.

Physostigmine

This drug is indicated for the treatment of central anticholinergic syndrome. Physostigmine is a centrally acting cholinesterase inhibitor, which increases acetylcholine concentration and, in turn, increases parasympathetic activity. There is no true receptor specificity as is found with flumazenil and naloxone. Central anticholinergic syndrome manifests primarily as disorientation, restlessness, confusion, and delirium. This may result from an excess of the anticholinergic drugs with central effects, namely, atropine or scopolamine, or from an excess of drugs with anticholinergic side effects such as several antihistamines, antipsychotics, meperidine, and to a lesser extent, benzodiazepines. Prior to flumazenil's release it was the only means of reversing the effects of excessive benzodiazepine. It is an indirect means of reversing this syndrome, as it is not a true receptor antagonist.

Physostigmine has an onset of action of 3 – 8 minutes and duration of action of 45 – 60 minutes. As a cholinesterase inhibitor, it often triggers cholinergic side effects such as bradycardia and hypersalivation.

Currently, its presence in the office providing anesthesia is optional as it is clearly not the drug to give for benzodiazepine overdose given the availability of flumazenil. Yet, it may offer a means to deal with anticholinergic excess or antihistamine excess. It has been reported as a means to manage post-anesthetic shivering similar to that found with meperidine and clonidine (Horn et al., 1998).

The dose is 0.5-mg by slow intravenous administration over 1 minute. It may be repeated in 10 minutes. It is formulated as 1 mg/mL solution in a 2 mL vial.

Muscle relaxants

Succinylcholine

Succinylcholine (Anectine®, Quelicin®) is a depolarizing neuromuscular blocker, indicated for the management of laryngospasm after non-pharmacologic methods have proved to be unsuccessful. These latter methods include suctioning, positive-pressure oxygen, a forceful jaw thrust, and consideration of either deepening or awakening the patient. It helps relax the vocal cords, and may proceed to cause generalized muscle paralysis, including loss of soft tissue tone of the upper airway. It is metabolized by plasma cholinesterase (pseudocholinesterase) with an elimination half-life of less than 1 minute. Its administration is associated with a number of concerns. A 1 – 2 mg/kg intravenous dose can increase plasma potassium by 0.5 mEq/L. Thus, it should not be used whenever hyperkalemia may be possible, such as in muscular dystrophy or other myotonias, and in muscle denervation or in burn patients. The subsequent increase in potassium could lead to cardiac arrest. It is a trigger for malignant hyperthermia (MH). Masseter spasm, possibly due to an inadequate dose, may be an early sign of MH; however, it is not consistently associated with MH (Littleford et al., 1991). Its use should be considered with caution in children for this latter reason. It may lead to bradycardia, particularly in pediatric patients, or if given as a second dose in adults, where asystole has been reported. These effects are attenuated with atropine pretreatment. High doses are associated with fasciculations, which can result in postoperative muscle pain. These latter side effects are not likely in doses used to manage laryngospasm.

Succinylcholine has a very rapid onset of action, the fastest of any muscle relaxant currently available. It has a short duration of action of several minutes. Rocuronium in high doses can approach the rapidity of onset of succinylcholine, but has a prolonged duration of action of muscle paralysis in those doses, limiting its value in managing laryngospasm.

When succinylcholine is used for the management of laryngospasm, a small sub-paralyzing dose of approximately 0.1 to 0.2 mg/kg IV should be administered. This is much less the full intubating dose of succinylcholine (1 – 2 mg/kg IV) used when direct tracheal intubation is planned. Intravenous access is ideal, but if the intravenous line is lost, then sublingual or intralingual administration can be used. Succinylcholine is formulated as a 20 mg/mL and as a 100 mg/mL solution in 10 mL vials. It should be stored refrigerated when it is not in the operatory for immediate availability.

Pseudocholinesterase deficiency is a rare, inherited or acquired, qualitative or quantitative condition that impairs the metabolism of succinylcholine, and can result in prolonged paralysis following its use. Acquired cases can be secondary to renal or hepatic disease, malnutrition, advanced age, and malignancy, among others. A prolonged Acholest test paper reaction or a low dibucaine inhibition number (80% is normal) are indicative of reduced pseudocholinesterase activity (Soliday et al., 2010, Leadingham, 2007, Maiorana and Roach, 2003).

Dantrolene

Dantrolene (Dantrium®) is indicated for the treatment of a malignant hyperthermia (MH) crisis. Its presence is essential in any clinic where vapor anesthetics are being used, because isoflurane, sevoflurane, and desflurane are all known triggers, as is succinylcholine. This drug interferes with calcium release from the sarcoplasmic reticulum. It decreases calcium buildup in the myoplasm and decreases hypercatabolic reactions dependent on this ion. Its elimination half-life is approximately 12 hours and its duration of action is 4 – 6 hours.

As soon as an MH crisis is identified, 2.5 mg/kg should immediately be administered intravenously, ideally through a large-bore intravenous catheter. The remainder of the MH protocol should be followed, including discontinuing administration of the volatile agent, hyperventilating with 100% oxygen at flows of at least 10 L/minute, sodium bicarbonate administration, and cooling the patient (http://medical.mhaus.org/). This dose of dantrolene may be repeated incrementally as needed, up to a total of 10 mg/kg. It is formulated as a 20-mg-per-bottle powder, which also contains mannitol. It must be prepared by injecting 60 mL sterile water into this 70 mL vial and mixing vigorously until dissolved. The administration of water into the vial may be facilitated by venting the vial with another needle; dissolution may be facilitated by using warm water. This preparation may take time and could be done by another member of the anesthetic team to allow the practitioner to attend to other aspects of patient resuscitation. The Malignant Hyperthermia Association of the United States recommends that 36 vials be kept on site if vapor anesthetics are being used, in order to stabilize the patient before transfer to hospital. This leads to the consideration of how many vials are needed for the first dose alone. A 70-kg patient (154 pounds) would require an initial bolus of nine vials (70 kg × 2.5 mg/kg / 20 mg/vial). As further examples, a 100-kg patient would require 12.5 vials, and a 30-kg child would require 4 vials for the initial dose. These possibilities and the nature of the anesthetic practice must be kept in mind for practitioners utilizing vapor anesthetics when determining the immediate availability of dantrolene.

Vasopressors

Epinephrine

Epinephrine is indicated for a number of emergencies and must be present in every dental office. There are three indications for epinephrine in this context: cardiac arrest, anaphylaxis, and albuterol-resistant asthma. Epinephrine carries the potential for a high benefit, as also a high risk if given to a patient with cardiovascular disease.

Epinephrine is an endogenous catecholamine released from the adrenal medulla, and is also found in specific neurons throughout the body. While norepinephrine is the primary postganglionic neurotransmitter of the sympathetic nervous system, endogenous epinephrine can play a role when released due to stress. It is a direct-acting agonist for all adrenoceptors, both α and β. Cardiac effects are mediated primarily due to the stimulation of β-1 receptors. This results in an increase in heart rate, force of contraction, and automaticity. The combination of increased rate and stroke volume leads to an increase in cardiac output, which, in turn, should lead to improved perfusion. During acute anaphylaxis, this increase in cardiac output will reverse the hypotension that is part of that reaction. Increased myocardial automaticity can predispose to dysrhythmias in a beating heart, but may be advantageous during cardiac arrest. Myocardial oxygen requirement increases as a result of the greater work of the heart. This can be an adverse effect, particularly in the compromised heart where an increased demand for oxygen in the presence of diminished supply may predispose to ischemia, with subsequent angina or infarction. The effects on the vasculature are primarily due to either α-1 stimulation, which induces constriction mainly in skin and mucous membranes, or β-2 effects, which include vasodilatation of the blood vessels predominantly in skeletal muscle. Increased peripheral vasoconstriction is the primary benefit of its administration during a cardiac arrest (Neumar et al., 2010).

Stimulation of β-2 receptors causes relaxation of the bronchiolar smooth muscle. This is beneficial in the emergency treatment of bronchoconstriction as found during an acute asthmatic attack when bronchodilation cannot be induced by a β-2 agonist alone. This action is also required in the management of anaphylaxis.

Intravenous administration provides a very rapid onset and a duration of action of 5–10 minutes. The dose for cardiac arrest is 1 mg intravenously, which may need to be repeated every 3–5 minutes as required (Neumar et al., 2010). Its administration follows appropriate electrical defibrillation. Each injection during cardiac arrest should be followed by a 20 mL flush with saline to improve vascular distribution during cardiac compressions.

For the management of anaphylaxis, initial doses are 0.3–0.5 mg when given intramuscularly (1:1,000) or 0.1 mg intravenously (1:10,000) (Ewan, 1998; Dym, 2001; Eisenberg and Mengert, 2001). The intravenous doses are best titrated in small increments such as 10 μg at a time. These doses should be repeated as necessary until resolution of the event. Similar doses should be considered in asthmatic bronchospasm, which is unresponsive to a β-2 agonist, such as albuterol. Intramuscular administration during cardiac arrest has not been studied, but would appear to be very unlikely to render significant effect. If intravenous access is lost or is not present, epinephrine can be administered into the endotracheal tube. If this is done, then the dose should be 2–2.5 times greater, and should be followed immediately with a 10 mL flush of saline. If intraosseous access can be achieved, then that may be used as well.

For emergency purposes, epinephrine is available in two formulations; 1:10,000 or 1:1,000. Intravenous administration should be carried out using the 1:10,000 solution (1mg/10ml), usually prepared as a prefilled syringe. Thus, for cardiac arrest, 10 mL of this 1:10,000 solution would be given. For anaphylaxis or bronchospasm unresponsive to albuterol, 0.1 mL increments of this 1:10,000 solution would be given, which is 10 μg at a time. The 1:1,000 solution (1mg/ml) is used for intramuscular or intralingual/sublingual injections. This 1:1,000 solution is prepared in an ampoule or prefilled syringe. Autoinjector systems are also present for intramuscular use, which provide a dose of 0.3 mg per injection, or the pediatric formulation, which is a dose of 0.15 mg per injection. Multiple administrations of epinephrine may be necessary for any of the above indications, and thus multiple pre-filled syringes or ampoules should be present in the office.

Vasopressin

This drug is an alternative to epinephrine in the management of ventricular fibrillation or pulseless ventricular tachycardia (Neumar et al., 2010). The dose is 40 units, to be administered as an intravenous push. Its administration follows appropriate electrical defibrillation. Given that intravenous formulations of epinephrine should be present in the outpatient anesthesia office, the need for stocking vasopressin can be considered entirely optional in this context.

Ephedrine

This drug is a vasopressor, which is indicated to manage significant hypotension. Ephedrine is a sympathomimetic, which both directly and indirectly leads to stimulation of all adrenoceptors. It has similar cardiovascular actions compared with epinephrine, except that ephedrine is less potent and has a longer duration of action, lasting from 60 to 90 minutes. The fact that both α and β receptors are stimulated is an advantage over other vasopressors such as phenylephrine, which is a selective α-1 agonist. Phenylephrine is very effective provided that an adequate volume of intravenous fluids are being coadministered. Ephedrine is preferable if hypovolemia is not addressed adequately. β-1 stimulation causes an increase in heart rate and stroke volume, thereby increasing cardiac output, which, in turn, should help maintain perfusion. The result is an improvement in both blood pressure and perfusion, thereby enhancing tissue oxygenation, one of the primary goals in the handling of any emergency. Similar precautions as noted with epinephrine administration should be considered when given to a patient with cardiovascular disease.

Ephedrine is formulated as 50 mg/mL solution. To prepare the drug to be administered, 1 mL of 50 mg should be drawn into a 10 mL syringe and diluted with 9 mL of saline or water to a total in 10 mL, resulting in a 5 mg/mL solution. It is then administered in 5 mg increments intravenously, which is 1 mL at a time, titrated to effect, until resolution of hypotension.

Phenylephrine

Phenylephrine is a specific α-1 adrenergic receptor agonist that is useful for treating hypotension, especially when tachycardia is present or when an increase in heart rate should be avoided, such as in a patient with significant ischemic heart disease. Phenylephrine produces venoconstriction, thereby improving preload and systolic pressure, and produces arterial constriction, which increases diastolic pressure. A baroreceptor-mediated reduction in heart rate may result. Its use should be accompanied by adequate fluid administration to ensure that hypovolemia is not present. Rapid administration has been associated with ventricular extrasystoles, ventricular tachycardia, and hypertension. Its duration of action is approximately 20 minutes.

Phenylephrine is typically administered by continuous intravenous infusion or in 0.1 mg intravenous increments. It is formulated as a 1% solution (10mg/ml). To prepare for intravenous administration in this context, it should be diluted twice. Initially, 1 mL of the 10 mg/mL solution should be drawn and diluted with

9 mL of saline/water to a total of 10 mL, resulting in a new 1 mg/mL solution. This should then be repeated, with 1 mL of the 1 mg/mL solution being drawn and diluted with 9 mL to a total in 10 mL, resulting in a 0.1 mg/mL solution. Most intravenous solutions, such as saline or D5W, can be used for dilution. Alternatively, one can take 1 ml of the 1% phenylephrine solution and inject into a 100-mL bag of intravenous solution to provide 0.1 mg/mL concentration. It may then be administered in 0.5 mL to 1 mL increments, meaning 50 to 100 μg at a time, titrated to effect, until resolution of hypotension. Infusion may be considered but should be done through a central line. If an infusion is used, it should be started at a dose of 100–180 μg/minute. Once the patient has stabilized, the infusion should be decreased to 40 to 60 μg/minute while titrating to response.

ANtihypertensive agents

β blockers

β blockers are widely used as oral medications for the management of a number of cardiac and non-cardiac conditions. Cardiac conditions that may be managed, at least in part, by β-blockers include hypertension, ischemic heart disease, congestive heart failure, and dysrhythmias. Non-cardiac indications include stage fright, intention tremor, and migraine headaches. For emergency purposes, they are indicated for hypertensive crises and tacharrhythmias such as paroxysmal supraventricular tachycardia, atrial fibrillation, and atrial flutter.

β-blockers, pharmacologically more correctly referred to as β-adrenergic receptor antagonists, are selective antagonists that bind to the receptor tightly with high affinity and have zero efficacy. They may bind to all of β receptors relatively equally, as does the prototype propranolol. Conversely, they may be relatively selective for one type over the other. The key is the term *relative*, as even those that are classified as selective β antagonists still have some binding to the other receptor subtype. Some may even have some intrinsic sympathetic activity by stimulating specific receptor subtypes. Examples of β-1 receptor antagonists include metoprolol, atenolol, and esmolol. There are also drugs that are mixed antagonists, blocking both α and β receptors. The prime example of this latter group is labetalol.

Sinus tachycardia may occur in patients who are not sedated deeply enough or are in pain. This is relatively easily rectified by deepening the sedation/anesthetic or achieving appropriate local anesthesia. It can also be a reflex response to hypoxia. If so, increasing the inspired concentration of oxygen should alleviate the problem. It may be a reflex response to hypotension. If so, supporting the blood pressure by administering intravenous fluids should be carried out initially. Concurrently, however, and a possible diagnostic challenge, hypotension-induced reflex tachycardia may be a result of the sedation/anesthetic being too profound. For example, propofol can lower blood pressure. If too high an infusion of propofol is the reason for the decreased blood pressure, then lowering the infusion rate will rectify the problem. This action is in the opposite direction of the light-anesthetic-induced tachycardia. The diagnosis is made by looking at the blood pressure. The patient who is too light with a tachycardia is not likely to be hypotensive at the same time. Once these other sources of the tachycardia have been addressed, and if it persists, it may then require pharmacologic intervention. There are three considerations for use in an outpatient office setting; metoprolol, esmolol, or labetalol.

Metoprolol (Lopressor®), is a β1-selective antagonist that is not expected to induce bronchospasm. Nevertheless, it should be used with caution in patients with COPD or asthma, as the blockade of β2-receptors on bronchial smooth muscle may result in bronchoconstriction. It has an elimination half-life of 3.5 hours. Its dose is 5 mg intravenously over a 2-minute period repeated up to a maximum of 15 mg. It is formulated in either 1 or 5 mg/mL concentration.

Esmolol (Brevibloc®) is another β1-selective antagonist with a very short duration of action. Its elimination half-life is 2 to 9 minutes. Its duration of action is usually under 20 minutes. Dosing recommendations list a loading dose of 0.5 mg/kg intravenously over a 30-second period initially, followed by an infusion of 0.05 mg/minute by infusion pump. An alternative approach for outpatient office use is to titrate 20 mg increments intravenously every 2 to 3 minutes until the hypertension or tachycardia resolves. The peak effects occur within 5 minutes. If there is no resolution after several 20 mg increments, one should likely discontinue this approach and consider another drug or another diagnosis. If the tachycardia does not respond to this dosage, or recurs after the effects of esmolol have waned, EMS transport should be considered. As with metoprolol, it should still be used with caution in patients with COPD or asthma. Esmolol comes in a number of formulation, both pre-mixed for infusion, or as single dose vials. It is important to note that there are two concentrations available. Both have a total of 100 mg esmolol contained within. One is a 10 mL vial at a concentration of 10 mg/mL. The other is a 5 mL vial at a concentration of 20 mg/mL. Clearly, it is crucial that the practitioner know which concentration is being used in order to prevent potential overdosing.

Labetalol (Trandate®) is a selective α1 blocker and nonselective β blocker. The ratio of α to β blockade varies depending on the route of administration. When taken orally it has a 1:3 ratio, whereas the ratio is 1:7 when given intravenously, meaning that it is 3 or 7 times, respectively, more active on the β receptors compared to α receptors. This drug does have intrinsic sympathetic activity, meaning that it has weak partial agonist effects. Although small, this means that it will not decrease resting cardiac function as much as metoprolol or esmolol, which are void of this intrinsic activity. Labetalol lowers blood pressure by blockade of the α-1 receptors in vascular smooth muscle and the β-1 receptors in the heart. Its onset of action following intravenous administration is 5–15 minutes. The elimination half-life is 5.5 hours. The duration of action is dose dependent, but ranges anywhere from 2 to as long as 18 hours. Owing to the simultaneous β-receptor blockade, the usual reflex tachycardia associated with other vasodilators does not occur. Any drug that lowers blood pressure increases a patient's risk for orthostatic hypotension. Labetalol is no exception, and patients receiving it should be assessed carefully in recovery and discharge.

For the management of an acute hypertensive episode, the initial dose of labetalol is 0.25 mg/kg over a 2-minute period followed by a repeat every 10 minutes up to a maximum dose of 300 mg. Alternatively, it can be titrated in 20 mg increments to effect. Like all non-selective β blockers, labetalol is contraindicated in patients with COPD or asthma. It is formulated at a concentration of 5 mg/mL in 4, 20, or 40 mL vials.

Nitroglycerin

This drug has two potential indications in emergency scenarios in anesthesia. It is most commonly indicated for acute angina or myocardial infarction, and is used as a sublingual formulation for this purpose. It can also be used to manage an acute hypertensive episode, where it can be administered in its intravenous formulation.

Its primary mechanism of action is through vasodilation, which results in a decrease in venous return to the heart and therefore a reduction in the work of cardiac muscle. In turn, this reduces myocardial oxygen consumption. Given that angina pectoris arises due to an imbalance in the supply and demand of oxygen in the heart, this action is beneficial. Nitroglycerin lowers blood pressure by reducing preload and subsequent cardiac output. This action may be undesirable in patients with impaired cerebral perfusion and should not be used if a cerebrovascular accident occurs.

There are contraindications for nitroglycerin. The systolic blood pressure must be at least 90 mmHg. It is contraindicated if the patient has taken erectile dysfunction agents such as sildenafil or vardenafil within 24 hours, or tadalafil within 48 hours (Kloner, 2004). It is also contraindicated if the infarction involves the inferior wall and right ventricle (Ferguson et al, 1989; Moye et al, 2005). While this diagnosis would require a 12-lead ECG analysis, successful management of these particular infarctions is dependent on improving preload, which is reduced by nitroglycerin. This emphasizes the importance of confirming that systolic blood pressure is over 90 mmHg before administering any dose of nitroglycerin.

For the management of angina or myocardial infarction, 0.3 or 0.4 mg should be administered sublingually. If necessary, this dose can be repeated twice more in 5-minute intervals provided that the systolic blood pressure remains above 90 mm Hg.

For hypertension, the tablets or spray may be used similarly to the above, or an intravenous infusion may be considered carefully by those with appropriate training. The infusion should start at 5 μg/minute intravenously and titrated every 3 to 5 minutes to effect, with close monitoring of blood pressure throughout. Increases of up to 20 μg/minute may be required.

For the management of angina or myocardial infarction it is available as 0.3, 0.4, or 0.6 mg sublingual tablets or as 0.4 mg sublingual spray. The tablets have a short shelf-life of approximately 3 months once the bottle has been opened and the tablets exposed to air or light. The spray has the advantage of having a shelf-life that corresponds to that listed on the bottle.

For hypertension, nitroglycerin is available as either an infusion solution premixed in D5W or a 10 mL ampoule at a concentration of 5 mg/mL. infusion solutions are available in 250 mL bags in the concentrations of 100 μg/mL, 200 μg/mL, or 400 μg/mL.

Anti-arrhythmic agents

Amiodarone

Amiodarone is indicated for the treatment of ventricular fibrillation or pulseless ventricular tachycardia that is refractory to defibrillation and epinephrine administration (Neumar et al., 2010). It is also indicated for stable ventricular tachycardia. It is a Class III anti-arrhythmic that works by blocking potassium channels, and to a lesser extent, sodium and calcium channels, as well as β, α, and muscarinic receptors. It decreases automaticity in the SA node. It slows conduction velocity in the AV node and increases the threshold for ventricular fibrillation. It is a negative inotrope and may cause vasodilation, thus leading to hypotension. It should not be given with other antiarrhythmics or β-blockers as it may lead to sinus arrest.

When used in the cardiac arrest algorithm for refractory ventricular fibrillation or pulseless ventricular tachycardia, it should be administered intravenously as a 300 mg bolus. To do this, it should be first diluted in 20 mL of D5W. The initial bolus may be followed by 150 mg after 3 to 5 minutes if needed. For the management of stable ventricular tachycardia, 150 mg should be given intravenously over a 10 minute period, which may be repeated if it reoccurs. Amiodarone is formulated at a concentration of 50 mg/mL in 3 mL, 9 mL, or 18 mL vials.

Lidocaine

Lidocaine has had a long history of use as an antiarrhythmic for the management of premature ventricular complexes or ventricular tachycardia. Today, it is no longer the first-line drug for these rhythm abnormalities (Neumar et al., 2010). Yet, its administration may be considered an acceptable alternative for the management of stable ventricular tachycardia when amiodarone is not available. In this context, lidocaine is classified as a Class IB antiarrhythmic, blocking sodium channels. It decreases automaticity and ventricular ectopy.

The antiarrhythmic dose is 1–1.5 mg/kg intravenously, which can be repeated at 0.5 to 0.75mg/kg intravenously if required, up to a maximum of 3 mg/kg. An infusion of 2–4 mg/minute may follow. It is available in a number of formulations, but for antiarrhythmic purposes, it is available as a 20 mg/mL solution in 5 mL premixed syringes. Premixed solutions for infusion are also available as 4 mg/mL in 250 or 500 mL bags, or 8 mg/mL in 250 or 500 mL bags.

Adenosine

Adenosine (Adenocard®) is indicated for the management of paroxysmal supraventricular tachycardias. These include stable narrow complex tachycardias, or unstable ones while waiting for cardioversion. This drug is a unique antiarrhythmic that slows conduction through the AV node. It has a rapid onset that has profound effects on the patients receiving it. Chest pain, flushing, hypotension, and bronchospasm are expected side effects of its administration. Transient sinus bradycardia or asystole may occur after its administration. It is contraindicated in asthmatics and patients taking dipyridamole or theophylline. It has a very short duration of action, making these notable side effects self-limiting. The dose is 6 mg as an intravenous push, followed by a 20 mL saline flush. If needed, this may be followed by a 12 mg intravenous push. It is formulated at a concentration of 3 mg/mL in 2 mL and 4 mL vials.

Calcium channel blockers

Calcium channel blockers are used as oral agents for the management of chronic stable angina and other cardiovascular disorders such as hypertension. For emergency purposes, they are indicated for the management of stable supraventricular tachycardias if the rhythm was not already managed by adenosine or vagal maneuvers. They are also indicated for ventricular rate control for patients with atrial fibrillation or flutter. They will also decrease blood pressure, but their emergency use is primarily as an antiarrhythmic.

These drugs are not true antagonists but they block the entry of calcium through channels in cell membranes to control the intracellular concentration of calcium. They act on the voltage-dependent calcium channels in the vascular smooth muscles as well as the cardiac muscle. Unlike fast channels that transport sodium, and are affected by drugs such as lidocaine, calcium channels are considered slow acting. These channels mediate action potentials in the SA and AV nodes of the heart. They decrease the automaticity of the SA node. They decrease conduction through the AV node and conduction velocity throughout the heart. They are vasodilators in both the systemic and coronary vasculature, and are particularly helpful for coronary vasospasm. They lead to an increase in ejection fraction and cardiac output.

Two calcium channel blockers can be considered for inclusion in an emergency drug setup for an outpatient anesthesia office: verapamil (Isoptin®) or diltiazem (Cardizem®). They both have a rapid onset of action when given intravenously, and an elimination half-life of several hours. Diltiazem dilates coronary vessels more than systemic vessels. Compared to verapamil, it is less potent with lower hemodynamic action and less of an inotropic effect. There is little effect on the cardiac output. Verapamil administration may lead to hypotension.

As an antiarrhythmic, diltiazem is given in an initial dose of 15–20 mg intravenously over 2 minutes, with an additional dose of 20–25 mg in 15 minutes if needed. Verapamil is given in a dose of 2.5–5 mg intravenously over 2 minutes, and then 5 mg may be repeated every 15 minutes up to a maximum dose of 30 mg.

Diltiazem is formulated as a 5 mg/mL solution in single dose vials of 5 mL, 10 mL, and 25 mL. Verapamil is formulated as a 2 mg/mL solution in single dose vials of 2 mL or 4 mL total.

Atropine

This antimuscarinic anticholinergic drug is indicated for the management of hemodynamically significant bradycardia. Atropine increases heart rate by blocking cardiac muscarinic receptors. Hypotension should normally be accompanied by a reflex rise in heart rate. If hypotension is accompanied by a slow heart rate, correction of this bradycardia may resolve the low blood pressure. Conversely, one should be concerned about too great an increase in heart rate in patients with ischemic heart disease. Similarly, there should be concern about any patient in whom anticholinergic effects may be problematic, such as those with acute narrow-angle glaucoma, prostatic hypertrophy, or urinary retention. It has a rapid onset and short duration of action.

For management of symptomatic bradycardia, the recommended dose is 0.5 mg initially, followed by increments as necessary until one reaches a maximum of 3 mg. Paradoxically, doses of less than 0.4 mg have been associated with induction of bradycardia, likely due to atropine's actions on the central nervous system. Atropine is available in numerous strengths, ranging from 50 μg per mL to 1 mg per mL. A concentration approximating 0.5 mg per mL would be suitable for emergency purposes.

Aspirin

Aspirin is indicated as part of the management of an acute coronary syndrome. It is well established that it reduces overall mortality from acute myocardial infarction (ISIS, 1988). Aspirin blocks the cyclooxygenase enzymes, leading to a reduction in prostaglandins, prostacyclins, and thromboxanes. Thromboxanes potently constrict arteries and promote platelet aggregation. Aspirin's role in a myocardial infarction is derived through this inhibition of thromboxane A2, as it inhibits platelet aggregation.

The purpose of its administration during an acute myocardial infarction is to prevent the progression from cardiac ischemia to injury to infarction. There is a brief period early on during a myocardial infarction when aspirin can show this benefit. For emergency use there are relatively few contraindications. These would include known hypersensitivity to aspirin or active gastric bleeding.

For this purpose, the recommended dose is 160–325 mg. Aspirin is available in multiple strengths, including 81 or 325 mg. The enteric formulations must not be used. Chewable tablets are preferred as the absorption is more rapid, but tablets that are swallowed are still acceptable. The patient should receive 2–4 chewable 81 mg tablets or one 325 mg tablet to be swallowed.

Morphine

Morphine is indicated for the management of severe pain that occurs with a myocardial infarction. It has the beneficial effects of being an excellent analgesic as well as having mood-altering properties to help manage the stress that accompanies this event. This reduction in pain and stress should minimize endogenous epinephrine release. Morphine increases venous capacitance and thereby decreases systemic vascular resistance, which will reduce preload, a beneficial effect during a myocardial infarction as it reduces the work of the heart. In turn, less oxygen is needed. It can be used if systolic blood pressure is over 90 and the patient is not hypovolemic.

The dose involves titration in approximately 2 mg increments intravenously until pain relief is accomplished. This should be guided by a decrease in blood pressure and respiratory depression. Extreme caution should be used in the elderly. It is available in numerous concentrations, including any one of 1, 2, 4, 5, 8, 10, 15, 25, or 50 mg/mL. The practitioner needs to confirm which formulation is present in order to dose safely.

If morphine is not available, then either fentanyl or nalbuphine may be considered as a second alternative (Becker and Haas, 2007).

Anticonvulsants

A seizure is normally managed by protection of the patient, while allowing the event to run its course as it is most often transient. An anticonvulsant is indicated for seizures that are prolonged or recurrent, also known as *status epilepticus*. This may require administration of a benzodiazepine, a drug group well known to all practitioners of anesthesia. All benzodiazepines share the effects of anxiolysis, sedation, anterograde amnesia, skeletal muscle relaxation, and an anticonvulsant action. It is this latter action that makes benzodiazepines valuable drugs for this emergency. In the past, diazepam was often listed as the drug of choice for *status epilepticus*. This is still acceptable provided that the intravenous line is intact, as the onset of action following intramuscular administration is very unpredictable. The presence of a water-soluble agent such as midazolam or lorazepam allows the option of using the intramuscular route in the event that the line is lost during a tonic–clonic convulsion. Lorazepam has been reported as the drug of choice for *status epilepticus* (Alldredge et al., 2001). Midazolam, however, is most likely to be present in the outpatient dental office that provides sedation and anesthesia, and could be considered as an acceptable alternative.

Any benzodiazepine should be titrated until termination of the seizure, but expected doses would be 4 mg for lorazepam, 5 mg for midazolam, or 10 mg for diazepam. Exacerbation of post-ictal depression should be expected.

Antihistamines

An antihistamine is indicated for the management of an allergic reaction. While mild non-life-threatening allergic reactions may be managed by oral administration, life-threatening reactions do require parenteral administration. They may be administered along with epinephrine and a corticosteroid as part of the management of anaphylaxis. Alternatively, they may be given alone for the sole management of less severe allergic reactions, particularly those with primarily dermatologic signs and symptoms such as urticaria.

Antihistamines may be classified as those that block either H1 or H2 histamine receptors. While some have suggested the use of both classes of drugs (Zeitler, 2001), the H1 antagonist is most commonly considered the first-line antihistamine (Ewan, 1998). These drugs block the action of histamine at the H1 receptor. They do not inhibit the release of histamine.

Diphenhydramine (Benadryl®) is the prototype of H1 antagonists. The recommended dose for adults is 25 to 50 mg, or approximately 1 mg/kg for a child. Parenteral diphenhydramine is available as a 50 mg per mL solution in 1 or 10 mL vials.

Bronchodilators

Albuterol

A selective β-2 agonist is the drug of first choice for the management of bronchospasm. If bronchospasm cannot be managed by a selective β-2 agonist, then epinephrine must be considered. The most common β-2 agonist used for this purpose is albuterol (Ventolin®), although metaproterenol (Alupent®) or terbutaline (Brethaire®, Bricanyl®) can also be considered. Albuterol stimulates the β-2 receptors on the bronchioles, leading to smooth muscle relaxation and subsequent dilation. Inhaled albuterol may stimulate β-2 cardiac receptors (when present) resulting in a transient tachycardia, but rarely have any effect of β-2 receptors on skeletal muscle vasculature. The onset of inhaled albuterol is rapid (minutes) and the peak effect occurs in 30–60 minutes, with a duration of effect of 4–6 hours. Other inhaled selective β-2 agonists could also be considered for emergency management of an acute asthmatic attack, including metaproterenol (Alupent®) or terbutaline (Brethaire®, Bricanyl®).

Albuterol is available as an aerosol for a metered dose inhaler (MDI) that provides 90 μg of drug per administration. It is also available in different solutions for use in nebulizers. The adult dose is 180 μg, which is two sprays, to be repeated as necessary. The pediatric dose is 90 μg, or 1 spray, repeated as necessary. For patients who are under anesthesia, administration may be carried out by connecting the MDI to the inspiratory limb of the anesthesia circuit and adding a spacer device. The MDI can be inserted into a large syringe, such as of 60 mL size, and then connected to the inspiratory tube (Dunteman and Despotis, 1992). Depressing the plunger of the syringe will cause the canister to release its contents of 90 μg albuterol, which will then be carried to the patient when positive pressure is applied to the oxygen flow. Multiple administrations would be needed as only a portion of the albuterol will make it to the bronchioles (Taylor and Lerman, 1991).

Corticosteroids

A corticosteroid may be indicated for the prevention of recurrent anaphylaxis or as part of the management of an adrenal crisis. Corticosteroids provide membrane-stabilizing effects, reduce leukotriene formation, and reduce histamine release from mast cells. These actions are therefore beneficial in allergic reactions. Management of an adrenal crisis involves correcting the hypotension and administering a corticosteroid. The notable drawback in their use in emergencies is their relatively slow onset of action, which approaches 1 hour even when administered intravenously. There is low likelihood of adverse responses with one dose.

A number of corticosteroids may be considered for this purpose. Hydrocortisone (Solu-Cortef®) or dexamethasone is used most commonly. The prototype for this group is hydrocortisone, which may be administered in a dose of 100 mg as part of the management of these emergencies. It is available as a powder in concentrations of 100, 250, 500, or 1,000 mg that must be reconstituted in water immediately prior to use. This can be available in vials that contain the powder and liquid separately until they are mixed together when needed.

Dexamethasone is an alternative where a dose of 4 or 5 mg would be appropriate. It is available as either a 4 mg/mL formulation in any one of 1, 5, or 30 mL vials, or as a 10 mg/mL solution in 10 mL vials.

Conclusion

The anesthesia provider should be cognizant of the drugs discussed in this chapter, yet they are not the only ones to potentially play a role in an emergency event. As only one example, if hyperkalemia is diagnosed, then insulin, calcium gluconate, and sodium bicarbonate should be considered. The final decision regarding which drugs are appropriate is at the discretion of the individual practitioner. Nevertheless, knowledge of the indications and appropriate use of the drugs described herein provides a sound basis for the management of adversity that may arise during sedation or anesthesia in an outpatient office.

References

Alldredge B.K., et al. A comparison of lorazepam, diazepam, and placebo for the treatment of out-of-hospital status epilepticus. *New Engl J Med* **345**: 631–637, 2001.

Becker, D. E. and Haas, D. A. Management of complications during moderate and deep sedation: respiratory and cardiovascular considerations. *Anesthesia Progress* **54**: 59–69, 2007.

Berg, R.A., et al. Part 5: Adult basic life support: 2010 American Heart Association Guidelines for cardiopulmonary resuscitation and emergency cardiovascular care. *Circulation* **122**: S685–S705, 2010.

Dahan, A., et al. Incidence, reversal, and prevention of opioid-induced respiratory depression. *Anesthesiol* **112**: 226–238, 2010.

Dunteman, E. and Despotis, G. A simple method of MDI administration in the intubated patient. *Anesth Analg* **75**: 304–305, 1992.

Dym H. Stocking the oral surgery office emergency cart. *Oral and Maxillofacial Surgery Clin North America* **13**: 103–118, 2001.

Eisenberg, M. S. and Mengert, T. J. Cardiac Resuscitation. *New Engl J Med* **344**: 1304–1313, 2001.

Ewan P. W.. ABC of allergies. Anaphlylaxis. *Brit Med J* **316**: 1442–1445, 1998.

Ferguson, J. J., et al. Significance of nitroglycerin-induced hypotension with inferior wall acute myocardial infarction. *Am J Cardiol.* **64**: 311–314, 1989.

Heard, C., et al. Intranasal flumazenil and naloxone to reverse over-sedation in a child undergoing dental restorations. *Ped Anesth* **19**: 795–799, 2009.

Heniff, M. S., et al. Comparison of routes of flumazenil administration to reverse midazolam-induced respiratory depression in a canine model. *Acad Emerg Med* **4**: 1115–1118, 1997.

Horn, E.P., et al. Physostigmine prevents postanesthetic shivering as does meperidine or clonidine. *Anesthesiol* **88**: 108–113, 1998.

Hosaka, K., et al. Flumazenil reversal of sublingual triazolam. A randomized controlled clinical trial. *J Am Dent Assoc* **140**: 559–566, 2009. http://medical.mhaus.org/ (Accessed June 29, 2011).

ISIS (Second International Study of Infarct Survival) Collaborative group. Randomized trial of intravenous streptokinase, oral aspirin, both, or neither among 17,187 cases of suspected acute myocardial infarction: ISIS-2. *Lancet* **2**: 349–360, 1988.

Kloner, R.A. Cardiovascular effects of the 3 phosphodiesterase-5 inhibitors approved for the treatment of erectile dysfunction. *Circulations* **110**: 3149–3155, 2004.

Leadingham, C. L. A Case of Pseudocholinesterase Deficiency in the PACU. *J Perianesth Nurs* **22**: 265–74, 2007.

Littleford, J. A., et al. Masseter muscle spasm in children: Implications of continuing the triggering anesthetic. *Anesth Analg* **72**: 151–160, 1991.

Maiorana, A. and Roach, R. B. Heterozygous pseudocholinesterase deficiency: a case report and review of the literature. *J Oral Maxillofac Surg* **61**: 845–847, 2003.

Moye, S., et al. The electrocardiogram in right ventricular myocardial infarction. *Am J Emerg Med.* **23**: 793–739, 2005.

Neumar, T. W., et al. Part 8: Adult advanced cardiovascular life support: 2010 American Heart Association Guidelines for cardiopulmonary resuscitation and emergency cardiovascular care. *Circulation* **122**: S729–S767, 2010.

Olive, F. M., et. al. Comparative pharmacokinetics of submucosal vs intravenous flumazenil (Romazicon®) in an animal model. *Ped Dent* **22**: 489–493, 2000.

Osterwalder J. J.. Naloxone - for intoxications with intravenous heroin and heroin mixtures - harmless or hazardous? A prospective clinical study. *J Clin Tox* **34**: 409, 1996.

Reilly, J. J., et al. Chronic obstructive pulmonary disease. In: Kasper D. L., Braunwald E., Fauci A. S., et al Eds. *Harrison's Principles of Internal Medicine.* 16th edn. New York: McGraw Hill , 2005. p 1547–1554.

Soliday, R. K., et al. Pseudocholinesterase deficiency: a comprehensive review of genetic, acquired, and drug influences. *AANA* **78**: 313–320, 2010.

Taylor, R. H. and Lerman, J. High-efficiency delivery of salbutamol with a metered-dose inhaler in narrow tracheal tubes and catheters. *Anesthesiology* **74**: 360–363, 1991.

Weaver, J.M. The fallacy of a lifesaving sublingual injection of flumazenil. Editorial. *Anes Prog* **58**: 1–2, 2011.

Zanette, G., et al. Intranasal flumazenil and naloxone to reverse over-sedation in a child undergoing dental restorations: comment. Letter to the editor. *Ped Anesth* **20**: 109, 2009.

Zeitler, D.L. Drugs for treating allergic reactions. *Oral and Maxillofacial Surgery Clin North America.* **13**: 43–47, 2001.

SECTION 7

Anesthetic adversity

30 Failed sedation

Roy L. Stevens[1], and Kenneth L. Reed[2]

[1]Private Practice, General Dentistry for Patients with Special Health Care Needs Oklahoma City, OK, USA

[2]Lutheran Medical Center, Dental Anesthesiology, Brooklyn, NY, USA

The goals of sedation as administered in the dental office are summarized in Table 30.1. Medications to provide analgesia, amnesia, anxiolysis, behavior control, and local anesthesia are administered enterally or parenterally to achieve these goals, which, fortunately, are frequently achieved. Unfortunately, there are isolated circumstances when sedation fails.

A precise definition of sedation failure remains elusive, which is one reason why the literature is largely silent on the issue. These situations are dependent on both patient selection and preparation, and limitations of anesthetic technique. *Underdosing* leads to unanticipated pain (if local anesthesia is inadequate), patient dissatisfaction, recall of intraoperative awareness, or inability to complete the intended procedure due to agitation or combativeness ("stormy anesthetic") (Senel et al., 2002). Underdosing often occurs because of inability or unwillingness to administer additional medication, especially when confronted with airway, ventilatory, and/or cardiovascular compromise. *Overdosing* includes prolonged sedation, patient injury, loss of airway, and adverse cardiovascular and ventilatory changes (see Table 30.2).

Typical dose response phenomena fall within 2 standard deviations of the mean response, such that "recommended" doses cause anticipated responses in approximately 95% of the patients (2 standard deviations), meaning that 1 out of every 20 patients will not respond as anticipated, due to variability in receptor number or sensitivity, bioavailability, and metabolism (see Figure 30.1).

Appropriate patient selection for office-based sedation is based on several factors, much of which is the essence of this text. Resilience, reserve, BMI, ASA physical status, and Mallampati score should all be considered. Patients with high levels of anxiety and/or poor impulse control and chronic drug abusers (alcohol included) may require medication doses higher than the practitioner is willing or licensed to administer. Yacavone et al. (2001) and Delegge (2008) report that younger age, higher income, higher education, female sex and psychological distress predispose to procedural dissatisfaction.

Patient preparation also influences sedation outcomes. Prior adverse sedation experiences often predispose negative expectations, which can be a self-fulfilling prophesy. Pain perception is uniform; pain tolerance is not. Most patients expect a certain degree of procedural discomfort; appropriate communication often changes the manner in which patients accept it. Anesthetic patient management involves much more than drug selection and administration, and includes both case refusal and potentially depth of anesthesia limit setting.

Table 30.1 Goals of office-based sedation.

- Permit, facilitate and expedite painful/threatening procedures by blocking pain and decreasing or eliminating perception
- Mitigate physical and emotional reactions to painful stimuli
- Improve patient satisfaction

Limitations of oral sedation

There is perhaps no management technique for apprehensive patients within dentistry that has received more attention in the last decade than oral (enteral) sedation. Although not a new technique, the use of oral sedatives alone or in combination with N_2O for apprehensive dental patients became popular in the late 1990s when continuing education courses began, teaching "cookbook" techniques to dentists who had no previous anesthesia or sedation training. Many still view the oral route as being safe without fear of overdose or adverse effects. Limits to these techniques are pressed with repeat oral dosing during one appointment and/or when the drugs are crushed and delivered sublingually (given per mouth, but not an oral (digestive) route) bypassing first-pass hepatic metabolism and increasing bioavailability. The use of "oral titration," multiple or "stacked" dosing has been shown to induce bispectral index scores and Observer's Assessment of Alertness/Sedation scores consistent with general anesthesia in some patients (Jackson et al., 2006), which can occur when administered by clinicians with all levels of training, but can be disastrous for clinicians with little to no formal training.

Agents typically used for oral sedation include benzodiazepines, with depth of sedation being titrated by the addition of N_2O. Triazolam [Halcion®] is commonly used (albeit "off-label") although other benzodiazepines such as alprazolam (Xanax®), diazepam (Valium®), and midazolam (Versed®) and lorazepam (Ativan®) can also be administered. Non-benzodiazepine hypnotics, including zolpidem (Ambien®), eszopiclone (Lunesta®), and zaleplon (Sonata®); and anti-histamines, including diphenhydramine (Benadryl®), hydroxyzine (Vistaril®), and promethazine (Phenergan®) have also been used.

Anesthesia Complications in the Dental Office, First Edition. Edited by Robert C. Bosack and Stuart Lieblich.

Table 30.2 Continuum of depth of sedation: definition of general anesthesia and levels of sedation/analgesia* (Adapted from Practice Guidelines for Sedation and Analgesia by Non-Anesthesiologists, 2002 (with permission).

	Minimum sedation (Anxiolysis)	Moderate sedation/analgesia (conscious sedation)	Deep sedation/analgesia	General anesthesia
Responsiveness	Normal response to verbal stimulation	Purposeful† response to verbal or tactile stimulation	Purposeful† response after repeated or painful stimulation	Unarousable
Airway	Unaffected	No intervention required	Intervention may be required	Intervention often required
Spontaneous ventilation	Unaffected	Adequate	May be inadequate	Frequently inadequate
Cardiovascular function	Unaffected	Usually maintained	Usually maintained	May be impaired

*As sedation is a continuum, individual patient responses are variable and may not exactly follow these categorizations.
†Reflex withdrawal from a painful stimulus is not considered a purposeful response.

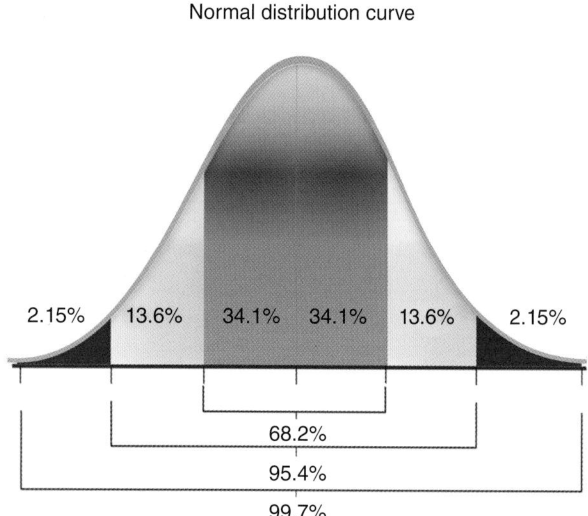

Figure 30.1 The normal distribution curve.

Oral sedation remains one of the most commonly used sedative techniques for apprehensive dental patients and if practiced using conservative drug dosages has a commendable record of safety. Yet, despite its popularity, the technique has limitations.

Latency Period

The latency period of a drug is that time between administration of a drug and the onset of clinical effects. For oral benzodiazepines latency ranges from 15 to 90 minutes, based primarily on the lipid solubility of the drug. As opposed to intravenous drugs, whose latency period is measured in seconds to minutes, the extended latency period of orally administered drugs makes titration of these drugs impossible and potentially hazardous as different patients will absorb and distribute the same drug at different rates based on a variety of factors. These factors include the volume and type of food in the stomach or small intestine, along with other enzymatic absorption factors that may be unknown to the practitioner. Patient anxiety, the presence of certain drugs including opioid analgesics, obesity, diabetes, and other considerations may each or all contribute to a delay in gastric emptying and therefore a delay in both the time of onset and peak plasma concentration of these orally administered sedative agents. The prudent practitioner must understand that the onset time described in the package insert is a best-case scenario and not necessarily applicable for their specific patient.

Oral drugs must be administered to the patient ahead of the appointment time, allowing enough time for absorption, distribution, and appearance of clinical effects before the dental procedure can begin. For this reason, some practitioners have the patient take the sedative drug at home before having an escort with a vested interest in the patient's safety drive them to the practitioner's office. Doing so, however, adds another level of risk for this type of sedation. As sedative drugs have their clinical effects along a normal distribution dose response curve, hyper-responders could become overly sedated outside the dental office without professional supervision or monitoring. In addition, should the escort become delayed getting the patient to the dental office for reasons of mechanical problems, traffic, or other reasons beyond the control of the escort, the patient could become overly sedated and develop serious airway or other compromises that could endanger his/her safety.

Empiric dosages

It is challenging to determine the ideal dose that will provide enough sedation and prevent adverse side effect. Ideal dosages of orally administered sedative drugs are often empiric and will vary among patients and even within the same patient on different days, due to variation in pharmacokinetics and pharmacodynamics. Manufacturers establish maximum recommended therapeutic dosages (MRTD) for each drug they manufacture and publish those dosages in the package insert of the particular drug (see Table 30.3). The prudent practitioner must realize that the dosages published by the manufacturer are for the approved indications of the drug. They are also the only dosages that have been demonstrated to be both safe and efficacious. Some dentists choose to administer sedative dosages in excess of the package insert recommended doses despite a paucity of evidence of safety and efficacy, especially when trying to salvage a case that should have been terminated. The dosages necessary to manage the patient's anxiety during the stimulation of a dental procedure may leave the patient oversedated once the procedure is completed and the stimulation ends.

The difficulty in proper dosing of oral sedatives makes the addition of nitrous oxide and oxygen a tremendously useful adjunct. By choosing to titrate nitrous oxide to effect after the administration of an oral sedative, the dentist is not tempted to give a large dose of the oral drug. Patients will have "baseline" sedation from the benzodiazepine and the addition of nitrous oxide and oxygen will make this technique more predictable. The patient can then be returned to

Table 30.3 Clinical characteristics of benzodiazepines.

	Midazolam	Triazolam	Diazepam	Alprazolam	Lorazepam
Oral onset (min)	15–30	30–60	60–90	45–60	90–120
Clinical duration of action (hours)	0.5–0.75	1–2	2–4	4–6	3–6
MRTD* (mg)	20	0.25	10	0.5	4

*Manufacturers maximum recommended therapeutic doses.

a lighter baseline sedation level at the completion of the procedure once N_2O is discontinued, which will improve discharge readiness. The addition of nitrous oxide and oxygen to a single oral sedative dose makes this a "titratable" technique, and increases patient safety.

Residual effects

Most agents administered orally for sedation during dental procedures have a longer postoperative effective period than drugs given intravenously. This requires careful selection of the sedative agent to match the likely time frame of the planned dental procedure (see Table 30.2). This is particularly important when patients are sent home with prescriptions for postoperative opioid analgesics, which may dangerously deepen the level of sedation once they are home when there is minimal stimulation and little to no monitoring. Deaths and injuries after discharge from professional supervision after the administration of oral sedative agents in a dental office are increasing and now represent a greater threat than do adverse occurrences arising while still in the dental office (Cote et al., 2000). Should the dental procedure be completed prior to the anticipated time, the patient must be required to remain in the dental office until they meet discharge criteria to safely leave with minimal need of follow-up monitoring. The use of lower doses of sedative drugs with supplemental nitrous oxide and oxygen lessens this risk as the nitrous oxide can be rapidly eliminated prior to discharge and the patient returned to a lighter level of impairment for escort home.

Difficult patients

Oral sedatives are very effective for milder levels of apprehension toward dental procedures. However, many patients with more severe forms of anxiety, developmental disabilities, or patients taking other psychoactive medications are poor candidates for oral sedation. The failure rate of oral sedation for these patient populations is exceedingly high. The level of sedation necessary to manage a severely phobic patient is often beyond the limitations of oral medications (and the training level of the practitioner), even with the addition of nitrous oxide and oxygen. This deeper level of sedation may require doses of agents that go beyond the manufacturer's recommended dose and place the patient into a higher risk of airway compromise that may or may not be recognized and treated by the practitioner with minimal anesthesia training. Patients with developmental disabilities oftentimes are poor candidates for oral sedation due to their total inability to cooperate during the procedure. Many times the sedative effects only confuse them more and make their cooperation less predictable. Many patients with developmental disabilities also have abnormal or difficult airway anatomy that can become problematic should high doses of sedative drug produce airway compromise. Many patients on psychoactive medications have required considerable time for their physician to balance their medication to a level that their psychological problems are managed. Addition of another psychoactive medication in the form of sedative hypnotic agents can upset this balance and cause the patient to be less than cooperative.

Limitations of parenteral moderate sedation

Compared to oral sedation, parenteral moderate sedation enjoys a much higher success rate. Drugs administered via the intravenous, intramuscular, or subcutaneous routes share many advantages over the same drugs administered orally including faster onset, greater bioavailability, ability to safely achieve deeper levels of sedation, and for intravenous administration, the ability to titrate medications to the desired level of sedation. However, as with any technique, there are limitations to this method of sedation.

Intravenous administration

The intravenous route of administration is the most frequently used technique for parenteral moderate sedation in adult patients within dentistry. This method delivers the sedative medication directly into the blood stream of the patient, bypassing "first-pass" hepatic metabolism and achieving greater bioavailability. Clinical effects are observed seconds to minutes after administration of the drug. For this reason, the sedative effects of the drugs can be quickly and effectively titrated to the desired clinical endpoint. This provides a level of safety unmatched with other methods of parenteral sedation.

Unfortunately, for all its advantages, intravenous moderate sedation does have limitations. The primary limitation involves the need for venous access. This can be problematic for pediatric, elderly, obese, or needle-phobic patients, as well as for patients with developmental disabilities or neuromuscular disorders who cannot hold still for venipuncture. For needle-phobic patients, premedication with an oral benzodiazepine or administration of nitrous oxide and oxygen sedation or both can lessen the trauma associated with the venipuncture. Application of a Eutectic Mixture of Local Anesthetics (EMLA®) cream to the area of planned needle insertion 1 hour or more prior to the procedure will lessen venipuncture discomfort. Patients with neuromuscular diseases who cannot remain still during the venipuncture might be seen at a time when uncontrolled movements are usually at their least noticeable levels. Arm boards or other stabilization devices can also be used to limit the patient's uncontrollable movements. Patients with developmental disabilities, many times, are not good candidates for intravenous moderate sedation if their lack of understanding precludes their ability to remain still during venous access. For these patients, induction of general anesthesia by inhalation or intramuscular means may be necessary in order to gain access to the vascular system. Patients with poor venous access may also present challenges for intravenous sedation. This would include obese patients, along with non-obese patients with heavy subcutaneous fat in the chosen venipuncture site that obscures visualization of the venous structures. Many elderly patients present with small caliber fragile veins that easily collapse or infiltrate because of loss of elasticity, which can cause hematomas or subcutaneous accumulation of IV fluids and medications. Previous or current intravenous drug abuse may have scarred all of the usual sites for venipuncture such that they are no longer accessible. Dehydration, due to prolonged NPO status or poor nutrition, can also make venipuncture more difficult. Anxiety causes some degree of vasoconstriction, as does the presence of low environmental temperature.

Careful tourniquet placement and palpation after dependant positioning, manual stimulation by rubbing or tapping on the vein, and warm compresses can sometimes allow the venipuncture to be successful. Use of a trans-illuminating device made specifically for locating venous structures can be as useful as tangential lighting to provide a "shadowing" effect. Some have even administered nitroglycerin paste on the skin immediately overlying the planned site of venipuncture to induce vasodilation. A dose of 0.2 mg of clonidine [Catapres®], a direct-acting alpha two adrenergic agonist, administered orally has been shown to increase forearm temperature and cause peripheral vasodilation (Hall et al., 2006). In addition to its vasodilating properties, clonidine also has mild sedative properties, making it a reasonable choice for premedication prior to venipuncture. Nontraditional intravenous sites can also be evaluated in the legs and feet if veins cannot be visualized or palpated in the hands or arms.

Intramuscular and subcutaneous administration

Intramuscular and subcutaneous sedation are parenteral techniques most frequently used in pediatric patients or for patients in whom intravenous access is not easily or readily obtainable. These techniques involve the injection of the sedative medication directly into a muscle mass or under the skin that is then absorbed through the blood vessels found in the muscle or subcutaneous structures. The vastus lateralis, the superior lateral aspect of the gluteus maximus, and the deltoid muscles are those most often used for intramuscular injections. The most common subcutaneous site is in the maxillary or mandibular buccal or alveolar mucosa. Like the intravenous route, intramuscular and subcutaneous injections require a needle stick, but unlike the intravenous route, total patient cooperation is not required. The moving patient can simply be stabilized for the few seconds required to provide the injection.

The primary limitation with intramuscular and subcutaneous sedation is the inability to establish a safe yet effective dose and the inability to titrate the sedative effects to that level. Latency to onset, although shorter than the oral route, can be much longer than the intravenous route. This slow onset is also responsible for another limitation of intramuscular sedation – that being a potentially longer duration of action due to the gradual absorption from the muscle tissue. For this reason, intramuscular and subcutaneous sedation will have a longer time to discharge than when the same drugs are administered in similar therapeutic doses intravenously.

Pediatric patients who have not developed the ability to reason are often poor candidates for moderate sedation and often require general anesthesia to achieve the goals stated above. Practitioners trained to the level of moderate sedation can be tempted to deepen the sedation to finish the intended procedure, exposing the patient to airway, ventilatory, and cardiovascular risk that the practitioner may be unable to manage.

Limitations of deep sedation

Deep sedation is generally thought be that plane on the continuum of sedation where the patient is unconscious, but may still react to pain (see Table 30.2). A common technique consists of midazolam and fentanyl, supplemented with intermittent boluses of propofol. Since the ADA Guidelines (2012) require the practitioner to be able to rescue a patient from one level deeper than the intended level of sedation, all deep sedation providers must be prepared to manage (rescue) adverse situations arising during general anesthesia, including apnea, upper airway obstruction and adverse cardiovascular changes.

Since deep sedation is not general anesthesia, profound local anesthesia is a requirement. Patients who have difficult achieving local anesthesia may fail deep sedation and may require general anesthesia for procedure completion. Deep sedation procedures may also fail in instances where the airway cannot be maintained and the practitioner is unwilling to progress to general anesthesia or place an advanced airway.

Stage II excitation, paradoxical reactions to benzodiazepines or ketamine delirium during deep sedation can result in agitation, uncontrolled patient movement, laryngospasm and/or tachycardia which may interfere with procedure completion. Prior to the introduction of propofol, methohexital was commonly used which was often excitatory in sub-anesthetic doses.

If progression to general anesthesia is not possible or desired, these adverse situations may best be managed by stopping administration of or reversing anesthetic mediations, bring the patient back to a lighter level of sedation where protective reflexes are intact, and some degree of patient cooperation may be possible. If the patient was not informed of this possibility, dissatisfaction can result. Patient safety must remain a top priority during the administration of any level of sedation / anesthesia in the dental office.

Limitations of open airway general anesthesia

It is generally thought that when minimal, moderate or deep sedation fails, the case can always be "salvaged" by deepening the level of sedation or inducing general anesthesia. With appropriate training and licensure, progressing to general anesthesia can be successful in many cases; however, there are instances where ventilatory insufficiency (due to airway loss and/or apnea) or adverse cardiovascular changes may preclude successful patient management. These instances can include medically "fragile" patients or patients with difficult airways, among others as discussed in chapter 45. Fortunately, most dental procedures can be stopped and completed on another day with a different anesthetic technique or different location of care.

References

Cote, C. J., et al. Adverse sedation events in pediatrics: analysis of medications used for sedation. *Pediatr* **106**: 633–644, 2000.

Delegge, M. H. The difficult-to-sedate patient in the endoscopy suite. Gastrointest Endoscopy. *Clin N Am* **18**: 679–693, 2008.

Hall, D. L., et. al. Oral Clondine Pretreatment Prior to Venous Cannulation. *Anesth Prog* **53**: 34–42, 2006.

Jackson, D. L., et. al. Pharmacokinetics and clinical effects of multidose sublingual triazolam in healthy volunteers. *J Clin Psychopharmacol* **26**: 4–8, 2006.

Practice Guidelines for Sedation and Analgesia by Non-Anesthesiologists. Anesthesiol **96**: 1004–17, 2002.

Senel, F. C., et al. Evaluation of sedation failure in the outpatient oral and maxillofacial surgery clinic. *J Oral Maxillofac Surg* **65**: 645–650, 2007.

Yacavone, R. F., et al. Factors influencing patient satisfaction with GI endoscopy. *Gastroinest Endosc* **53**: 703–710, 2001.

31 Complications with the use of local anesthetics

M. Anthony Pogrel[1], Roy L. Stevens[2], Robert C. Bosack[3], and Timothy Orr[4]
[1]University of California, Department of Oral and Maxillofacial Surgery, San Francisco, CA, USA
[2]Private Practice, Oklahoma City, OK, USA
[3]University of Illinois, College of Dentistry, Chicago, IL, USA
[4]Private Practice, Austin, TX, USA

Systemic complications

Psychogenic reactions

Psychogenic reactions are the most common adverse events that can occur before, during, or after local anesthetic injections in the oral cavity. Apprehension and fear are potent mental stressors that can trigger inappropriate and unrestrained behavior, hyperventilation, the "fight or flight" sympathetic response, or syncope. Attendant physiologic changes often alter heart rate, respiratory rate, and blood pressure. Occasionally, patients may demonstrate a blush (cutaneous flush) over the lower face, anterior neck, and chest (other regions possible, but not readily visible in the dental office). This emotionally triggered transient erythema is thought to result from vasodilation of cutaneous vessels in the region (see Figure 31.1). Although the etiology of flushing triggered by emotion remains obscure and the differential diagnosis burdensome, it should be differentiated from cutaneous manifestations of allergy, which usually include elevated hives and are often accompanied by an itch.

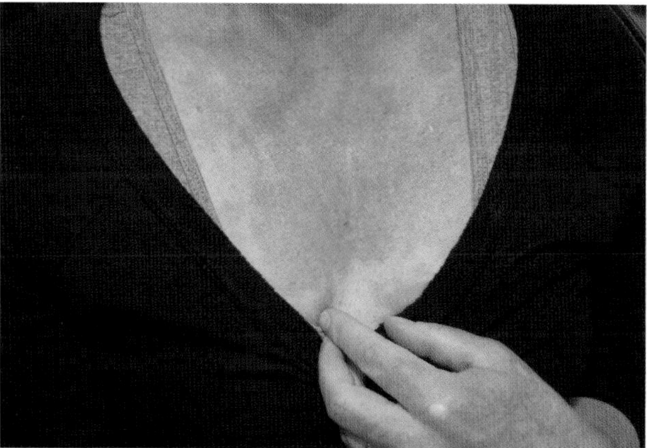
Figure 31.1 Nonallergic, emotionally triggered cutaneous flush over the anterior neck and right chest wall in a 43-year-old female.

In some cases, prevention can be accomplished with empathy and patient rapport, while medical behavioral control may be necessary in more difficult situations. Management of syncope and hyperventilation are addressed in Chapter 32.

Local anesthetic systemic toxicity

Signs and symptoms of local anesthetic overdose occur when a sufficient (toxic) concentration of anesthetic drug reaches the brain or heart, where it exerts its effect. In most cases, toxicity first manifests in the central nervous system, followed by cardiovascular involvement at much higher plasma levels. Although a typical progressive dose–response relationship remains attractive (see Figure 31.2), it may not always be clinically apparent. Signs of central nervous system toxicity include tremors, agitation, and twitching, often followed by dizziness, drowsiness, sedation, and unsteady gait. Respiratory depression, seizures, and ultimate cardiovascular collapse including bradydsyrhythmias and hypotension ensue, but are highly unlikely in doses used in the dental office (DiGregorio et al., 2010). Notably, bupivacaine demonstrates a propensity to affect cardiac tissues at "lower" toxic levels (Butterworth, 2010).

Given the generous allowance for maximal anesthetic doses for dental anesthesia, it seems likely that most cases of toxicity will involve accidental or iatrogenic overdose in lighter (smaller) or debilitated patients, or inadvertent intravascular injection. Toxicity may be more likely to occur in select clinical situations (Table 31.1). Prevention is accomplished with meticulous injection technique and compliance with maximum recommended doses. Adherence to the "rule of 25" allows for 1 cartridge of any marketed local anesthetic per 25 pounds of body weight, up to a maximum of 6 cartridges (Moore and Hersh, 2010).

Treatment in the dental office is supportive and includes airway support, oxygenation, supine positioning, and protection from injury in the event of seizure activity. The decision to "wait it out" vs. transfer to an emergency facility is based on practitioner training and experience as well as the clinical severity or progression of symptoms. Infusion of a 1.5ml/kg 20% lipid emulsion bolus has been shown to be beneficial in cases of severe toxicity, which is thought to function as a lipid sink, sequestering the local anesthetic away from the brain or heart (Weinberg, 2010). It is doubtful that dental offices would keep this drug in stock. Vital signs should be closely monitored, as hypotension and dysrhythmias can also occur with local anesthetic overdose.

Anesthesia Complications in the Dental Office, First Edition. Edited by Robert C. Bosack and Stuart Lieblich.

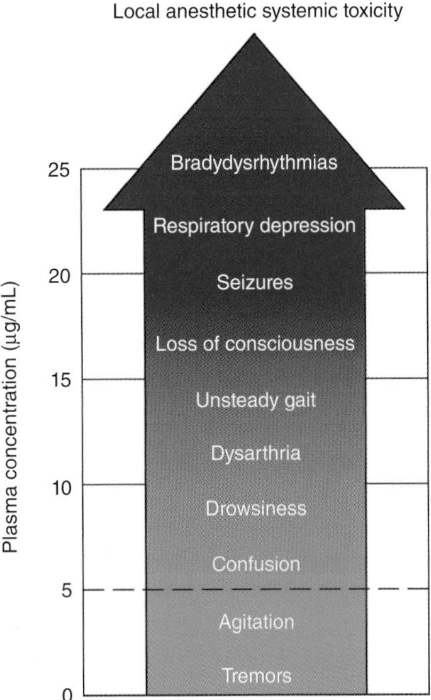

Figure 31.2 Local anesthetic systemic toxicity.

Table 31.1 Clinical situations predisposing to local anesthetic toxicity.

- Very young patients, with disproportionately larger heads
- Very old patients
- Patients with ↓ body mass or ↓ plasma proteins
  - Anorexia
  - Cachexia
- Injection into hypervascular or inflamed tissue
- Use of 3% and 4% local anesthetics without vasoconstrictors
- Repeated, rapid or intravascular injections

Acquired methemoglobinemia

Methemoglobinemia is a rare, but potentially serious complication of the administration of many drugs, most commonly due to excess accumulated metabolites of certain local anesthetics, notably, overdoses of prilocaine (ortho-toluidine) and benzocaine, which account for 90% of the reported cases (Weinberg, 2009). These metabolites oxidize the normal Fe^{2+} hemoglobin to the Fe^{3+} state. The resultant methemoglobin (Fe^{3+}) molecule displays an increased affinity for bound oxygen and a decreased affinity for both unbound oxygen and carbon dioxide. Tissue hypoxia ensues, because oxygen is not being delivered to the tissues. As methemoglobin concentration increases, SpO_2 stabilizes in the mid 80% range, regardless of the administration of supplemental oxygen. As such, the severity of the disease will not correspond to the pulse oximeter value.

The hallmark of methemoglobinemia is cyanosis (see Box 31.1), unresponsive to adequate ventilation and oxygenation, in the absence of cardiac or pulmonary disorders (Hegedus and Herb, 2005). Clinical symptoms of this disorder vary with blood levels of methemoglobin. In the awake patient, symptoms include dizziness, lightheadedness, headache, and shortness of breath. Signs include cyanosis of the lips, nail beds, and perioral regions and tachycardia. The appearance of brown blood in open surgical fields is a late finding.

Prevention includes compliance with the maximum recommended doses. Of special note, benzocaine, an ester anesthetic commonly found in topical anesthetics for dental use, has been shown to be a likely causative agent for methemoglobinemia, prompting an FDA warning in 2011 (FDA Public Health Advisory, 2001). Cetacaine™ spray (14% benzocaine) and Hurricaine™ spray (20% benzocaine) will quickly lead to overdose when sprayed for more than 1 second, or on damaged mucosa, or in dehydrated or pediatric patients. In some cases, the development of methemoglobinemia after benzocaine exposure did not correlate with the dose administered.

Mild elevations in methemoglobin are reduced by natural enzyme systems, whereas more severe and symptomatic cases overwhelm this capacity and may require treatment with 1 – 2 mg/kg of slowly administered (5 minutes) intravenous 1% methylene blue every hour up to a 7 mg/kg maximum, via a complex mechanism (Trapp and Will, 2010). Methylene blue also interferes with pulse oximetry. Regardless of its questionable efficacy, supplemental oxygen should be administered. It is doubtful that dental offices will stock methylene blue for this purpose, making early emergency transfer mandatory.

Allergy

Although true allergic reactions to amide local anesthetics and additives are extremely rare, some cases have been verified (Batinac et al., 2013). Unfortunately a small, yet significant percentage of patients will present with this history, who might have been incorrectly diagnosed by a worried clinician in the face of an adverse reaction to local anesthesia. Allergy to ester-type anesthetics (benzocaine) is possible as these drugs are metabolized to the notoriously allergenic PABA. Although this compound is also a metabolite of methylparaben, a preservative that was added to local anesthetics, it was removed from the market in 1984.

Allergy is defined as a hypersensitive immunologic state, acquired by exposure to a particular antigen; subsequent re-exposure to even much smaller doses produces a heightened capacity to react. Clinical manifestations range from mild and delayed onset to

Box 31.1

Cyanosis – a bluish/purple coloration seen on the skin, nail beds, and mucous membranes. It is less noticeable in patients with pigmented skin or in rooms with poor lighting. It is an approximate, and at times, unreliable clinical indicator that there is not enough oxygen in the blood (hypoxemia.). It occurs in several situations:

- When there is approximately 5 g/dL of reduced (deoxygenated) hemoglobin in the capillaries. Anemic patients (who have less overall hemoglobin) can be hypoxemic without reaching the 5 g/dL value needed to cause cyanosis, while a patient with polycythemia can be cyanotic without clinically significant hypoxia.
- When there is abnormal hemoglobin. The cyanosis caused by methemoglobin (which is the oxidized form) is a more intense bluish tinge, and this becomes an unreliable indicator of the amount of reduced hemoglobin in the blood.
- When there is peripheral vasoconstriction. Nail beds can appear blue secondary to peripheral vasoconstriction with less than 5g/dL reduced hemoglobin.

Table 31.2 Signs and symptoms of type I immediate-onset hypersensitivity reactions.

System	Symptom/signs
Cutaneous	• Urticaria (hive) • Pruritis (itching) • Erythema (rash) • Warm, red skin (cutaneous vasodilation) • Angioedema (asymmetrical swelling in loose tissue)
Exocrine	• Watery eyes • Running nose
Gastrointestinal	• Cramping • Nausea and vomiting
Respiratory	• Difficulty in breathing • Cough • Wheezing • Bronchospasm • Laryngeal edema
Cardiovascular	• Palpitations • Tachycardia • Hypotension

severe, acute onset and possibly a threat to life. The severity, onset, and clinical progression are quite variable and depend on the degree of antigenicity, route of exposure, dose of antigen, and anatomic clustering of reactive cells. Allergic reactions to local anesthetics have been classified as either Type I or Type IV. Type I immediate-onset (5-30 minutes) hypersensitivity reaction results from the release of mediators (histamine and SRS-A, among others) from a plethora of IgE-sensitized cells, notably mast cells and basophils. These mediators cause vasodilation, increased capillary permeability, and smooth muscle contraction, leading to hypotension, edema, and airway obstruction (bronchospasm), giving rise to the signs and symptoms in Table 31.2. It is tempting to assume an orderly progression of these findings related to the degree of allergy, but this is not always the case. Furthermore, it is impossible to predict the timing or clinical course of events. Type IV delayed onset (8–12 hours), cell-mediated reactions result from the release of mediators from sensitized T cells, which causes a more localized superficial mucosal inflammatory response.

Sulfites that are added to vasoconstrictor-containing solutions to prevent their oxidation, in theory, can act as allergens in susceptible patients. True anaphylactic reactions to sulfites are extremely uncommon, especially in the small doses contained in local anesthetic cartridges. However, it is prudent to avoid vasoconstrictor-containing local anesthetics in sulfite-allergic asthmatic patients who are intolerant to sulfite-containing foods. There is no cross-reactivity with sulfa or sulfonamides.

Prevention of allergy is easily accomplished by avoiding exposure to the known allergen. When allergy is reported or suspected, careful accrual of the past history may still be insufficient to differentiate transient facial blushing, hematoma, stress-induced asthmatic wheezing, tachycardia from intravascular or endogenous epinephrine, syncope, or idiosyncratic reaction from the signs and symptoms of true allergy. Usually, but not always, allergy to ester-type drugs will not predict allergy to amide-type drugs; however, cross-allergenicity within the amide class has been documented (Speca et al., 2010).

Referral to an allergist is appropriate if true allergy cannot be ruled out. Provocative challenge testing can be performed whereby various dilutions of the suspected allergen are sequentially introduced to various depths in the skin and waiting for a possible reaction. Drug-provocative testing, which is considered to be more reliable, uses small incremental dose escalations of the commercial preparation of the drug in the intended area of use under close medical surveillance.

A graduated treatment protocol of allergic reactions depends on the severity and urgency of symptoms. In all cases, further administration of the suspected allergen should be stopped. Close monitoring is mandatory as it is impossible to predict the clinical course of the reaction and progression of disease beyond the treatment window. Localized and limited skin reactions are managed with intervallic oral antihistamines, such as diphenhydramine 25-50 mg. Intramuscular or intravenous administration can be entertained, as predicated by practitioner training and experience and symptom severity. It is imperative to realize that antihistamines block histamine receptors and will slow down or prevent progression of symptoms, but will not reverse bronchospasm or hypotension. The onset of respiratory or cardiovascular symptoms should prompt immediate emergency medical referral. Inhaled albuterol is more effective when administered early in the clinical course of allergy and should be accompanied by supplemental oxygen. Supine positioning, intravenous isotonic crystalloids, and 0.3mg of intramuscular epinephrine (1:1,000; 1 mg/cc) are contemplated as the need arises. Allergy is also covered in Chapter 34.

Complications with the use of vasoconstrictor additives

Vasopressors contained in local anesthetic solutions will change cardiovascular parameters when sufficient concentrations are reached at β_1 receptor sites on the heart and α_1 and β_2 receptor sites on the vasculature. Concern revolves around the magnitude and duration of these changes and the ability of the patient to tolerate them. Signs and symptoms of these changes include tremor, headache, restlessness, anxiety, dizziness, palpitations, tachycardia, and hypertension. They are thought to be due to rapid systemic uptake or exaggerated effect of vasoconstrictors due to iatrogenic overdosage, intravascular injection, drug interaction, or increased patient sensitivity.

Adrenergic effects include α_1 vasoconstriction, β_1 increase in heart rate and contractility, and β_2 skeletal muscle vasodilation. Similar to other administered anesthetic agents, a clear dose–response curve for vasopressor additives does not exist, which promotes continual debate regarding what constitutes a "safe" submucosal dose, which can be an unsafe (inadvertent) intravascular dose. The issue is further confounded by the patient's ability to withstand an unanticipated drug-induced cardiovascular stimulation. Pertinent literature is limited and unable to document significant hemodynamic effects associated with the use of epinephrine-containing solutions in patients with cardiovascular disease (Brown and Rhodus, 2005; Bader et al., 2002; Niwa et al., 2001).

Regardless of origin or nature, the degree of any physiologic challenge is assessed by duration, magnitude, and ability of the patient to withstand the insult. In the case of inadvertent intravascular injection of a small dose of vasopressor, duration is usually short; the half-life of vasopressors in the central circulation is brief (minutes), as they are rapidly metabolized by catechol-O-methyltransferase (COMT). Magnitude of effect is usually proportional to dose and route of administration, which can be put into the following perspective. One cartridge of 1:100,000 epinephrine solution contains 18 μg, which is intentionally administered in submucosal or other connective tissues for infiltration or block anesthesia; versus 0.3cc of 1:1,000 solution (300 μg) administered IM to treat severe bronchospasm (a 16-fold increase); versus 10cc of a 1:10,000 solution (1000 μg) administered IV to manage ventricular fibrillation (a 55-fold increase).

The decision to use or limit the amount of vasoconstrictor is based on a risk versus benefit assessment. The benefits are increased duration and profundity of anesthesia, while reducing the need for redosing and minimizing the chance of toxicity. Profound anesthesia is more likely when vasoconstrictors are used, which protects the patient from the pain–stress response triggered by endogenous catecholamines, but will not protect against the emotion–stress response associated with fear and anxiety. The risks of vasoconstrictor inclusion are cardiovascular stimulation in a patient who may be unable to tolerate it, especially with inadvertent intravascular injection of local anesthetic with higher concentrations of the vasoconstrictor.

Given the wide variation in circumstances, it becomes difficult to totally dismiss the anecdotal, but widespread notion that 36 μg of epinephrine (2 cartridges of 1:100,000 epinephrine, within a 3 hour period) is safe for use in medically compromised patients, with the reasoning that epinephrine avoidance might lead to inadequate anesthesia, pain, and a greater than equivalent endogenous neuroendocrine response (Perusse et al., 1992). Jastak et al. (1995) suggests that 36 μg of submucosal epinephrine is equivalent to the plasma level of endogenous epinephrine secreted during mild physical exertion. The occasional physician who, when consulted, recommends epinephrine avoidance, might have concern that the patient may be unable to tolerate an unanticipated tachycardia from inadvertent intravascular epinephrine injection. In all cases, a careful injection technique should be used – with preinjection vital signs, aspiration in multiple planes, slow injection during needle withdrawal, and the use of the minimum necessary amount of vasoconstrictor. Evolving myocardial infarction, thyroid storm, acute cocaine intoxication, and dissecting aortic aneurysm are serious, life-threatening conditions that should give pause for most dental interventions, with or without vasoconstrictors.

Potential adverse drug interactions with vasoconstrictors

Potential interactions can occur between vasoconstrictors and other drugs with adrenergic activity. These interactions affect heart rate and blood pressure, and may not be clinically evident if these parameters are not measured after the injection of the vasoconstrictor. Just because they are not otherwise clinically evident does not imply that they do not occur. These reactions may be minimal because of low doses of either drug or changes in receptor activity with chronic drug administration, which restores physiologic homeostasis (Brown and Rhodus, 2005).

1 Epinephrine and nonselective β blockers (Hersh and Giannakopoulos, 2010). Epinephrine is a nonselective α and β agonist. When epinephrine is administered to a patient who is taking a nonselective β blocker, an unopposed α effect of vasoconstriction predominates, and hypertension and reflex bradycardia (compounding the bradycardia secondary to the β blocker) can occur. This interaction will not occur in patients on β_1 selective blockers, as β_2 vasodilation will offset the α_1 vasoconstriction. Examples of nonselective β blockers are provided in Table 31.3.
2 Epinephrine and phenothiazines and α blockers. Unopposed β2 vasodilation can lower blood pressure. This vasodilating effect has been called "epinephrine reversal," which promotes bleeding and shortens anesthetic action. (see Table 31.4).
3 Epinephrine and tricyclic antidepressants (Table 31.5). Tricyclic antidepressants can significantly increase the vasopressor potencies of levonordefrin and epinephrine, especially when TCA therapy has been recently started (within 2 weeks). These drugs interfere with the neuronal reuptake of adrenergic drugs (norepinephrine and 5-hydroxytryptamine (serotonin)) allowing for increased activity of exogenously administered catecholamines. TCAs permit a higher concentration of vasoconstrictor to be present at the sympathetic neuroeffector junction; as a result, vasoconstriction and cardiac stimulation (inotropy, chronotropy and dysrhythmia formation) can be commensurately increased. Caution should still be used, however, especially with the use of levonordefrin; some sources considered TCA usage a contraindication to the use of levonordefrin (Yagiela et al.,

Table 31.3 Nonselective β blockers.

Propranolol (Inderal™)
Nadolol (Corgard™)
Timolol (Blokadren™, Timoptic™)
Pindolol (Visken™)
Sotalol (Sotacort™)
Labetolol (Trandate™, Normodyne™)
Carvedilol (Coreg™)

Table 31.4 Phenothiazines and other α blockers.

Phenothiazines
Prochlorperazine + isopropamide iodide (Combid™)
Prochlorperazine (Compazine™)
Prochlorperazine + dextroamphetamine (Eskatrol™)
Perphenazine + amitriptyline (Etrafon™)
Thioridazine (Mellaril™)
Fluphenazine (Permitil™, Prolixin™)
Piperacetazine (Quide™)
Trifluoperazine (Stelazine™)
Trimeprazine (Temaril™)
Chlorpromazine (Thorazine™)
Acetophenazine maleate (Tindal™)
Perphenazine + amitriptyline (Triavil™)
Perphenazine (Trilafon™)
Triflupromazine (Vesprin™)
Promethazine (Phenergen™)
Other alpha blockers
Risperidone (Risperdal™)
Prazosin (Minipres™)
Phenoxygenzamine (Dibenzyline™)
Doxazosin (Cardura™)
Terazosin (Hytrin™)

Table 31.5 Tricyclic antidepressants.

Amitriptyline (Elavil™, Amitril™, Endep™)
Clomipramine (Anafranil™)
Desipramine (Norpramin™, Pertofrane™)
Doxepin (Sinequan™)
Imipramine (Tofranil™)
Protriptyline (Vivactil™)
Nortriptyline (Aventyl™, Pamelor™)
Combination drugs – (Etrafon™, Triavil™, Limbitrol™)
Perphenazine + amitriptyline = Etrafon™
Chlordiazepoxide + amitriptyline = Limbitrol™
Perphenazine + amitriptyline = Triavil™

Table 31.6 Monoamine oxidase inhibitors.

Isocarboxazid (Marplan™)
Phenelzine (Nardil™)
Tranylcypromine (Parnate™)
Pargyline (Eutonyl™)
Pargyline HCl/methclothiazide (Eutron™)

1985). Abrupt discontinuance of high dose TCAs can lead to cholinergic rebound, with possible symptoms of insomnia, headache, nausea, vomiting, nightmares, increased salivation, and excessive sweating.

4 Epinephrine and monoamine oxidase inhibitors (Table 31.6). MAOIs irreversibly inhibit the metabolic degradation of tyramine, dopamine, norepinephrine, and serotonin by irreversibly blocking monoamine oxidase, causing a buildup of norepinephrine within presynaptic sympathetic nerve terminals. This will lead to an increased pressor response (hypertension) from mixed or indirect-acting sympathomimetic drugs. Since both exogenous epinephrine and levonordefrin are direct acting only, neither should pose additional threat, contrary to teachings in the past. Selegiline (Elderpryl™) is a type-B-specific MAOI that is used to treat Parkinson's disease. This drug inhibits the degradation of *catecholamines*. Unlike other MAOI medications, a heightened pressor response due to an interaction between epinephrine or levonordefrin and selegiline is possible.

Localized complications

Local anesthetic failure

There are three common clinical scenarios where local anesthetic administration fails to provide adequate anesthesia.

1 *Infiltration into inflamed tissues or near painful regions.*

Inflammation is accompanied by a decrease in pH, which favors the ionized, water-soluble form of the local anesthetic. Since the lipid-soluble form is required for entry into the nerve itself, intraneural diffusion is hampered and profound anesthesia is difficult to obtain. Reinjecting the area is usually nonproductive, as local anesthetics with vasoconstrictors are acidic solutions that further lower the already acidic tissue pH. An alternative choice when block anesthesia is not possible is the use of mepivacaine, as this drug has the lowest pKa of the amide group, which increases lipid solubility in acidic conditions.

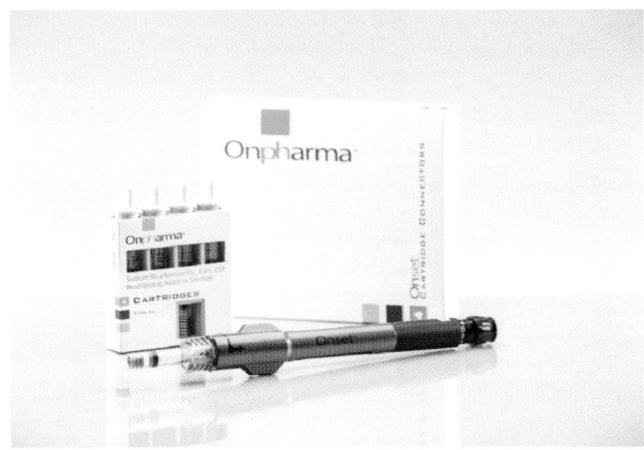

Figure 31.3 Precision buffering, courtesy of Onpharma, with permission.

2 *Inability to obtain a mandibular block*

When injection of local anesthetic solutions on the medial side of the ramus fails to produce a mandibular block (lip and chin are not anesthetized), one can assume that the anesthetic solution did not get close enough to the mandibular nerve, because of injecting too little volume OR injecting in an area not near the nerve OR injecting in a vascular area, such that the vascular supply becomes a conduit removing the anesthetic solution away from the region, faster than it can diffuse toward the target nerve. In most cases, reinjecting at a more superior and posterior position should improve the chances of obtaining a successful block for two reasons. First, "higher injections" usually cannot be too high, as gravity will help diffusion in an inferior direction in an upright patient. Second, superior injections may emulate the Gow-Gates approach, blocking the mandibular nerve superior to the mandibular foramen, often anesthetizing branches of this nerve as well. The possible disadvantage to a higher injection is that the superior locations can be more vascular, increasing the likelihood of an intravascular injection.

Proper deposition of solution near the mandibular foramen may be difficult due to a prominent medial projection of the internal oblique ridge. In these cases, entering from a more posterior approach on the contralateral side may help in proper needle positioning. In recalcitrant cases, a panoramic radiograph will help identify a possible variant position of the mandibular foramen (see Figure 31.4).

The use of articaine can be entertained to supplement an unsuccessful mandibular block, as its chemical structure increases its lipid solubility, which may enhance anesthetic diffusion. Increasing the pH of the local anesthetic immediately prior to the injection will significantly increase the concentration of the lipid soluble moiety, which theoretically will improve anesthetic concentration near the mandibular nerve. Onset of anesthesia is hastened and the burning discomfort when acidic solutions are injected is eliminated. Onpharma™ has patented a system for local anesthetic buffering, which improves consistency and ease of use (see Figure 31.3).

3 *Lip is numb, but tooth is not.*

Multiple factors can lead to this most frustrating scenario, whose etiology remains obscure. The central core theory proposes that the more central location of nerves that supply the incisors and bicuspids interferes with anesthetic diffusion (Nusstein et al., 2010). Nonmyelinated c fibers (which convey pain signals) can be more difficult to anesthetize for reasons not

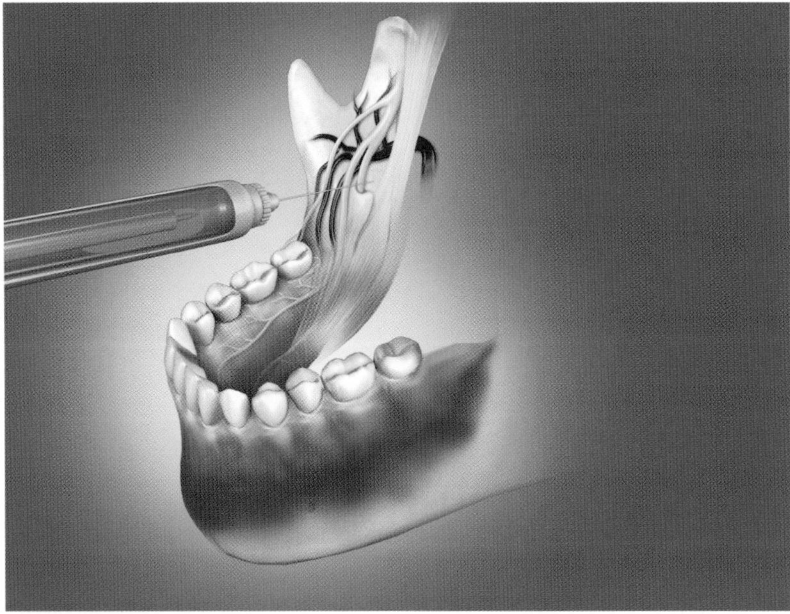

Figure 31.4 Pertinent anatomy near the mandibular foramen.

currently understood. The possibility of accessory mylohyoid or buccal nerve fibers may invite lingual or buccal anesthetic infiltration. An upregulation of Na^+ channels may occur with inflammation and pain, with or without the existence of anesthetic-resistant Na^+ channels. Finally, excess pain mediators may reduce thresholds of excitability, making complete anesthesia more difficult to attain.

Management of this situation is equally frustrating. Reinjecting with an acidic epinephrine-containing solution is usually futile in situations where the lip and chin have been successfully anesthetized. Reinjection with a buffered solution as indicated above can be of some help, as might infiltration with a more lipid-soluble agent, such as articaine (Brandt et al., 2011; Meechan, 2010). Periodontal ligament injections and intraosseus injections can be attempted as well, and appear to be of some help in these cases. It should be noted that intraosseus targets are usually quite vascular, which can rapidly increase plasma concentrations of both local anesthetics and vasoconstrictors.

Injection pain and transient facial blanching

Complaints of excessive pain during an injection can be due to several reasons, including decreased pain tolerance, rapid injection of cold or acidic solution, distending or tearing submucosal tissues, inadvertent intravascular injection, or needle tip proximity to the nerve bundle. With a careful and slow injection technique in a patient with "normal" pain tolerance, needle tip proximity to a vessel or nerve can be assumed, but never proved. In these cases, the needle should be withdrawn slightly and the injection continued. If excessive pain persists, the needle should be removed completely, and the injection should be attempted a second time, with a slightly different positioning. As will be covered later, excessive pain or feeling "electric" phenomena during an injection can be a sign that the tip of the needle is near or in the nerve bundle, a possibility leading to prolonged post-injection sensory disturbances. This occurrence should be clearly documented.

Injection pain can usually be lessened by the use of preinjection topical anesthetic, using room temperature solutions and a slow injection technique to minimize tissue distension and trauma. Counter stimulation with lip wiggling or very firm pressure can mask the discomfort of the injection. Needle gauge does not seem to influence the perception of pain (Reed et al., 2012).

Inadvertent intravascular injection, especially arteriolar, may lead to vascular spasm, blanching, and pain along the distribution of the vessel. In these instances, the location of the area of blanching follows vascular pathways with the least resistance (Figure 31.5), and can occur on both sides of the midline. It is also possible for the tip of the anesthetizing needle to irritate a small sympathetic nerve, prior to injection of anesthesia, resulting in a well-circumscribed and unilateral field of blanching, reflecting unilateral nerve distribution (Figure 31.6). Both cases are transient and should resolve in 5 to 10 minutes. Differentiation between these two scenarios is academic and does not affect clinical outcomes.

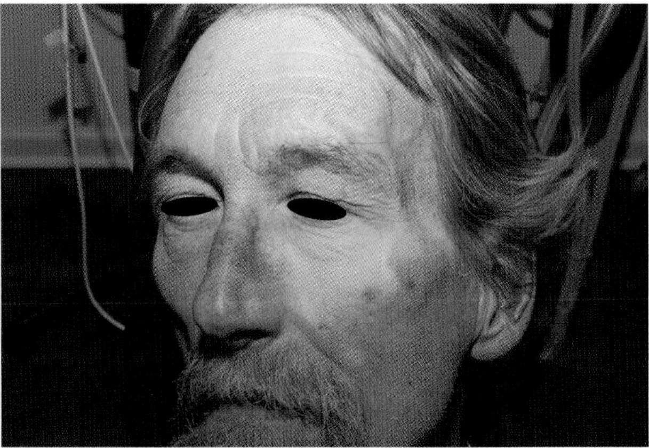

Figure 31.5 Note blanching of tissues in the left infraorbital region, after administration of a left mandibular block, associated with increased pain during the injection. The most likely explanation is inadvertent injection of local anesthetic into the maxillary artery, which carried the vasoconstrictive drug to the blanched area. Spontaneous resolution occurred within minutes.

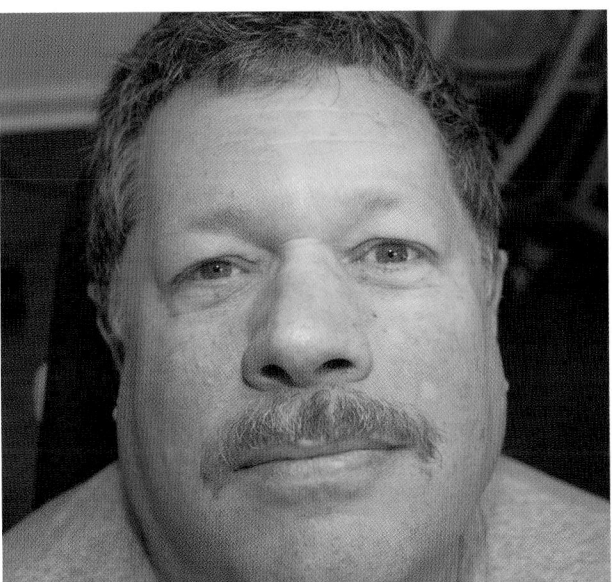

Figure 31.6 Note unilateral, instantaneous, cutaneous blanching of the distribution of the opthalmic and maxillary branches of the trigeminal nerve after mandibular block. This could be secondary to inadvertent stimulation of a sympathetic nerve that distributes to those regions. Immediate diplopia also occurred in this patient, which resolved within minutes.

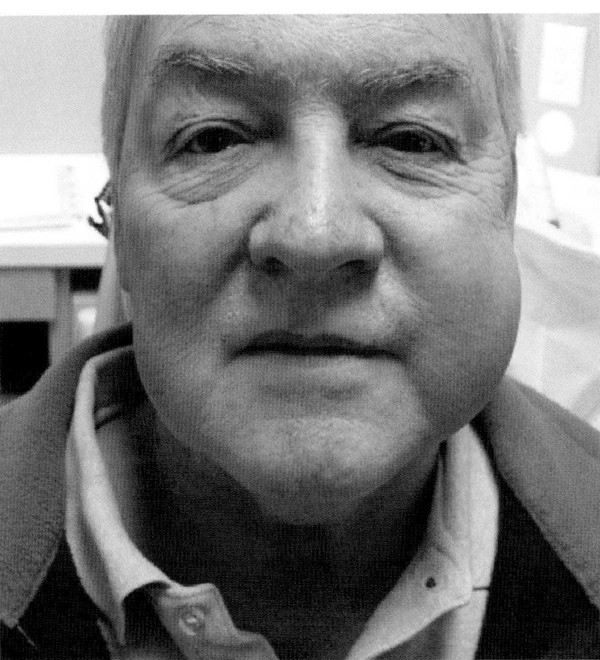

Figure 31.7 Infratemporal hematoma secondary to inadvertent arterial nicking. Notice tissue distension extraorally.

Vascular injury

Proper injection technique includes aspiration in two different planes to minimize the possibility of inadvertent intravascular injection. However, aspiration only reports the contents at the tip of the needle at the time of aspiration. A false negative aspirate is possible when the tip of the needle is just inside the lumen wall or when the negative pressure at the tip of the needle causes the vessel wall to occlude the opening before blood can enter. Intra-arterial injection carries the drug away from the heart, leading to cutaneous blanching or early signs of CNS toxicity, while intravenous injection carries the blood toward the heart, leading to cardiac stimulation if a vasoconstrictor was used. It is also quite possible for the tip of the anesthetizing needle to inadvertently puncture and disrupt the wall of a blood vessel leading to hemorrhage, which will continue until clot formation or when the pressure outside of the vessel becomes greater than the pressure inside the vessel. An arterial nick will bleed longer than a venous nick, which will result in a larger hematoma. The infratemporal fossa is a frequent site of involvement (Figures 31.7, 31.8 and 31.9).

Treatment consists of cold compresses and manual pressure for several minutes to minimize the volume of the bleed and a course of prophylactic antibiotics to prevent clot infection.

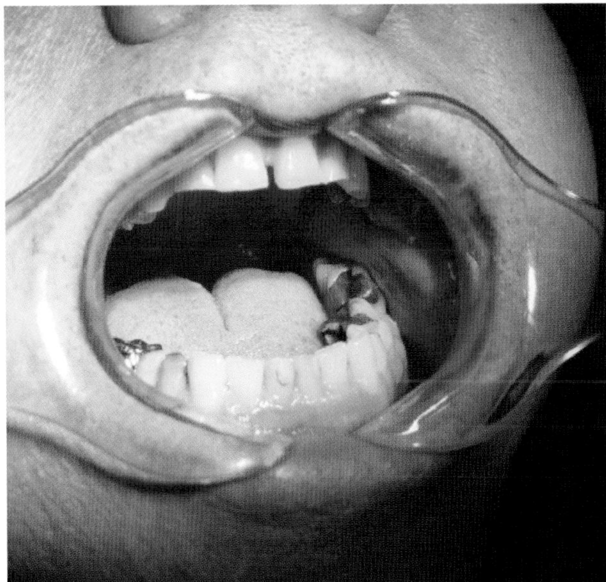

Figure 31.8 Infratemporal hematoma secondary to inadvertent arterial nicking. Notice tissue distension intraorally. This is the same patient as in Figure 31.7.

Unintended nerve involvement

In rare instances, sensory or motor nerves may inadvertently become anesthetized, leading to paralysis or anesthesia of nonsurgical regions. This may be due to increased lipid solubility of the anesthetic drug, facilitating diffusion to non-intended regions, overt misdirection of needle placement, improper depth of needle penetration, or accidental and unavoidable intravascular (arterial or venous) injection.

Acute onset of a peripheral facial nerve weakness (seventh cranial nerve) can occasionally occur after a mandibular block, especially in cases where the anterior–posterior dimension of the ramus is small. In this instance, "normal" depth of needle placement brings the anesthetic close to or into the capsule of the parotid gland as it bends medially around the posterior border of the ramus. The seventh cranial nerve is anesthetized, heralding the onset of Bell's palsy. The patient is unable to furrow the forehead, raise the eyebrow, close the upper eyelid, retract the commissure of the lips to smile, and turn down the lower lip – all on the affected side (see Figure 31.10). This condition is temporary, with resolution occurring when the anesthetic diffuses away from the facial nerve. Taping the affected eyelid in a closed position (and removal of any contact lenses) in cases of Bell's palsy caused by longer acting anesthetics (bupivacaine) is

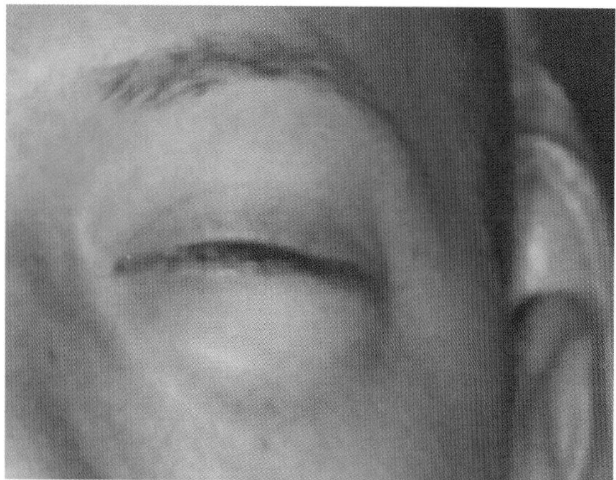

Figure 31.9 Immediate periorbital hematoma following a left posterior superior alveolar block.

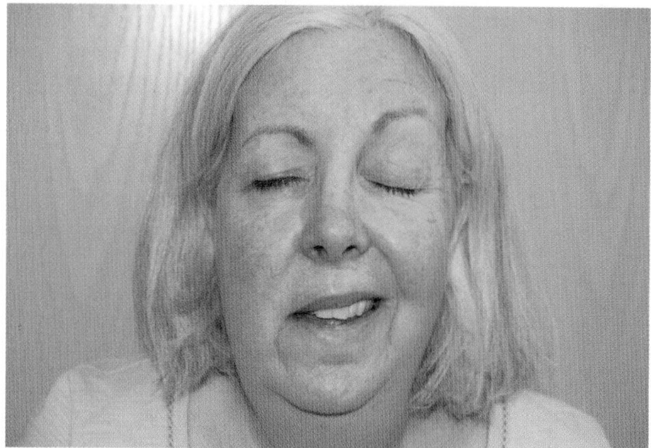

Figure 31.10 Right-sided Bell's palsy after inadvertent local anesthetic injection into the parotid capsule. Notice the inability to tightly close the right eye, inability to furrow the right forehead and raise the right eyebrow, and the inability to smile on the right side.

recommended to prevent corneal abrasion or drying. Buccal infiltration near bicuspid teeth will occasionally cause isolated weakness of the buccal or mandibular branches of the facial nerve, leading to inability to elevate or depress the lateral lip (Figure 31.11).

Acute onset of Bell's palsy after an injection of local anesthetic can also invite a diagnosis of stoke or transient ischemic attack. In most, but not all cases, a cerebrovascular event or tumor affecting the seventh cranial nerve centrally will give rise to a partial facial paralysis, preserving the ability to raise the eyebrow on the affected side (due to a central cross-over of some motor fibers), while Bell's palsy secondary to the local anesthetic solution finding its way into the capsule of the parotid gland will be a peripheral blockade of the facial nerve, affecting all muscles of facial expression on the involved side, including inability to raise the ipsilateral eyebrow. IN THE EVENT THAT YOUR PATIENT DEVELOPS A FACIAL NERVE WEAKNESS, BUT RETAINS THE ABILITY TO RAISE THE EYEBROW AND FURROW THE FOREHEAD ON THE AFFECTED SIDE, YOU SHOULD ASSUME THIS TO BE A CENTRALLY OCCURING PROCESS UNTIL PROVED OTHERWISE. IMMEDIATE TRANSPORT TO AN EMERGENCY ROOM IS NECESSARY.

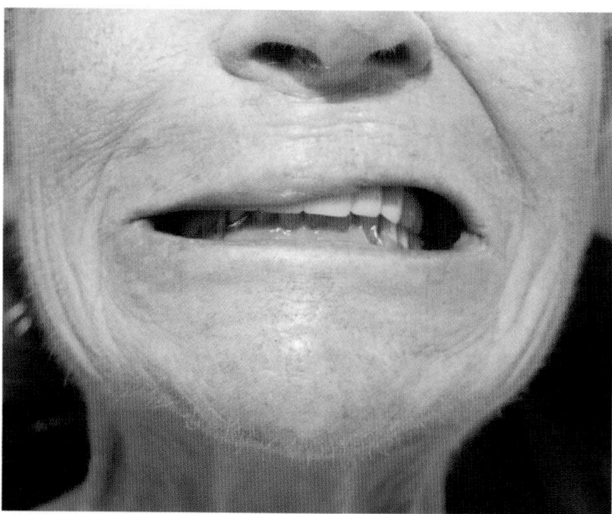

Figure 31.11 Inability to elevate the right lip after infiltration with articaine, affecting the buccal branch of the facial nerve.

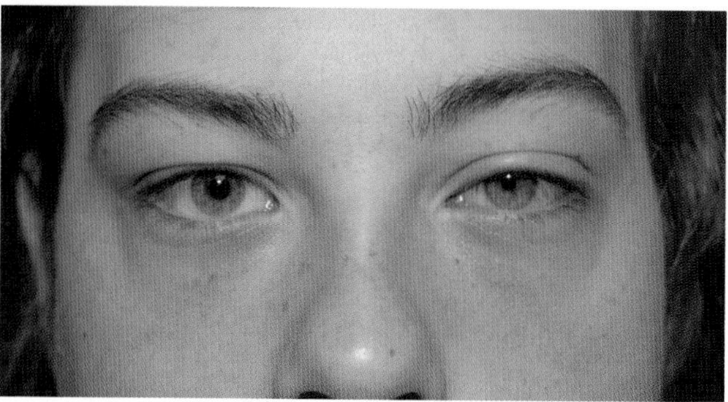

Figure 31.12 Left oculosympathetic palsy following a left mandibular block with articaine.

In extremely rare instances, the anesthetic can reach the carotid sheath, affecting cranial nerves 9-12. Anticipated signs and symptoms include hoarseness, inability to swallow, asymmetric soft palate, ipsilateral tongue deviation on protrusion, and ipsilateral sternocleidomastoid weakness – limits head turning and shoulder shrugging and tachycardia.

Sympathetic blockade (Figure 31.12) is possible following a mandibular block, especially with highly lipid-soluble anesthetics, such as articaine (Campbell et al., 1979). In this instance, five transient signs may be clinically evident:

1 Ptosis – drooping of the upper lid, as superior tarsal muscle loses sympathetic tone
2 "Upside-down" ptosis – slight elevation of the lower lid
3 Miosis
4 Enopthalmos - impression that the globe is sunk back
5 Injected (bloodshot) conjunctiva.

Opthalmologic complications

The most common problem affecting the eyes after injection of local anesthesia is paralysis of the lateral rectus muscle (Penarrocha-Diago et al., 2000). In this instance, the patient becomes unable to move the affected globe laterally, which will cause double vision in all ipsilateral fields of gaze (Figure 31.13). In all cases, the abducens nerve (sixth cranial nerve) becomes

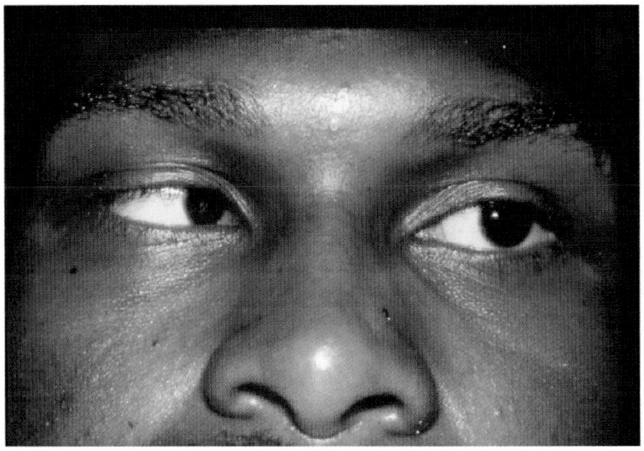

Figure 31.13 Paresis of the lateral rectus muscle on the patient's left side. He was instructed to gaze to his left; however, his left globe is unable to move in that direction.

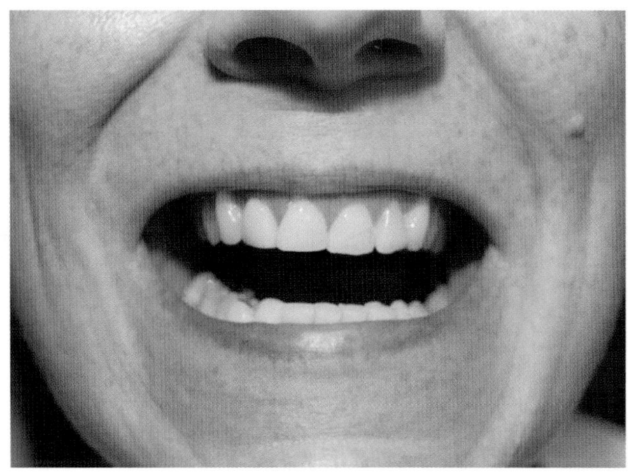

Figure 31.14 Trismus 3 days after a mandibular block injection.

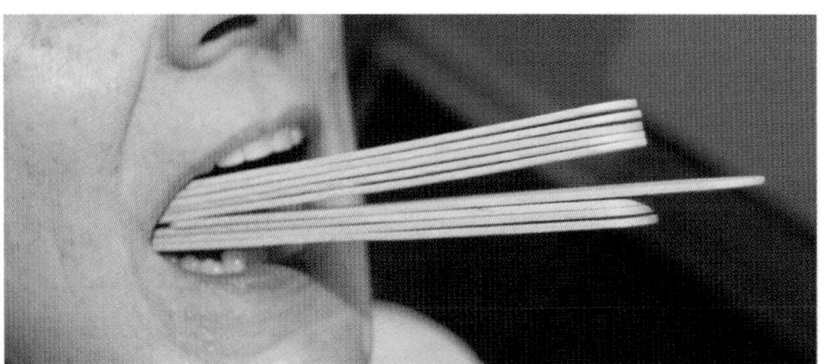

Figure 31.15 Gradual forced opening with tongue blade therapy post-injection was required to resolve post-mandibular block trismus.

anesthetized – how the anesthetic reaches that nerve is subject to debate (Magliocca et al., 2006; Boynes, 2010; Steenen et al., 2012). The posterior lateral portion of the maxilla becomes contiguous with the inferior orbital fissure. Anesthetic solutions finding their way to this region, by enhanced diffusability, deep needle positioning ("high" posterior-superior alveolar blocks), or intravascular injection will anesthetize the abducens nerve. This condition should resolve without complication. The patient must not be allowed to perform any task requiring vision, such as driving, until full resolution.

In extremely rare instances, unilateral blindness has occurred following administration of local anesthetics in the posterior maxilla, presumably because they diffuse into the area of the optic nerve. This clinical situation mandates emergent referral to an ophthalmologist. Permanent blindness, which has been reported after mandibular block, is extremely rare, but apparently possible (Tomazzoli-Gerosa et al., 1988).

Diplopia without gaze deficit has also been encountered (Figure 31.6). Autonomic interference is a proposed mechanism (Kronman et al., 1984).

Localized tissue injury

Injection of local anesthetic solutions can cause both physical and/or chemical injury (Nouette-Gaulain et al., 2012). Pressure necrosis and ischemic or chemical injury can lead to ulcerations, especially when large volumes of local anesthetics with vasoconstrictors are instilled in the tightly attached mucosa on the palate. Treatment is palliative and lesions resolve uneventfully.

Post-injection trismus is thought to result from chemical injury to the medial pterygoid muscle during attempted mandibular block injections (see Figure 31.14). It is heralded by the gradual onset of (usually) painless limitation of mandibular opening. Some cases will resolve spontaneously, while others may require gradual forced opening (brisement force), accomplished with tongue blade therapy. As shown in Figure 31.15, a stack of tongue blades is inserted between the molar teeth and held in place for several minutes, two or three times per day. An additional tongue blade is wedged in the middle of the stack to promote wider opening.

On occasion, an outbreak of viral lesions near the area of injection or following the course of the blocked nerve will occur after local anesthetic injection. It is postulated that this represents reactivation of herpes viruses that can lay dormant in the Gasserian ganglion for extended periods of time, only to recur with physical or emotional stress. Treatment is symptomatic and can involve the use of antiviral agents as clinically indicated.

Iatrogenic injury, notably lip biting (Figure 31.16,), lip sucking (see Figure 31.17), or tongue biting (Figure 31.18) during mandibular block anesthesia can occur with children, special needs patients, or patients with Alzheimer's disease. Shorter acting local anesthetics should be used, and close monitoring is necessary until the anesthesia wears off. A nonspecific α adrenergic blocker, phentolamine mesylate (OraVerse™), has been introduced to reverse unwanted, lingering soft tissue anesthesia after dental procedures have been done (Hersh et al., 2008). It is administered 1:1 by volume up to a 2 cartridge maximum in patients older than 6 years and heavier than 30 kg, and is expected to halve the recovery time. As expected, hypotension with reflex tachycardia can be a worrisome side effect.

Needle breakage

Needle breakage is a rare occurrence (Figures 31.19 and 31.20). Most reported cases involve the 30-guage needle (Malamed et al., 2010). Regardless of gauge, needles will tolerate *no more than* three bends prior to breakage; thus each time the needle is bent, one can anticipate *at least* a 33% decrease in the resistance to breakage. Breakage tends to occur with sudden and unexpected patient movement, hand grabbing, or poor technique. Adequate patient assessment with respect to his/her ability to tolerate the injection should always be performed; however, it will not be possible to anticipate adverse patient reaction and movement in spite of advance warning. The practitioner should inspect each

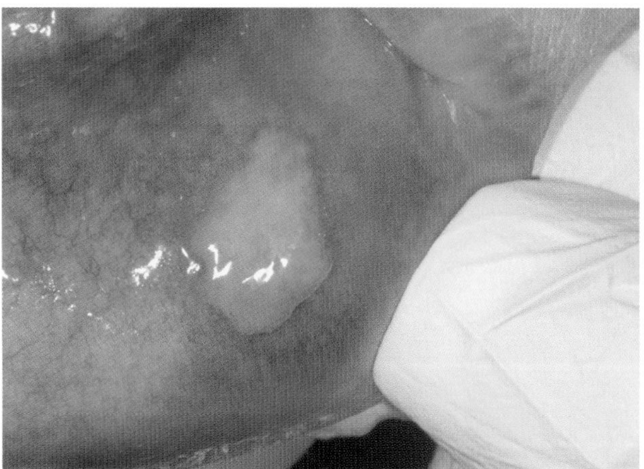

Figure 31.16 Lip biting – Note early healing of inadvertent lip biting during mandibular block anesthesia.

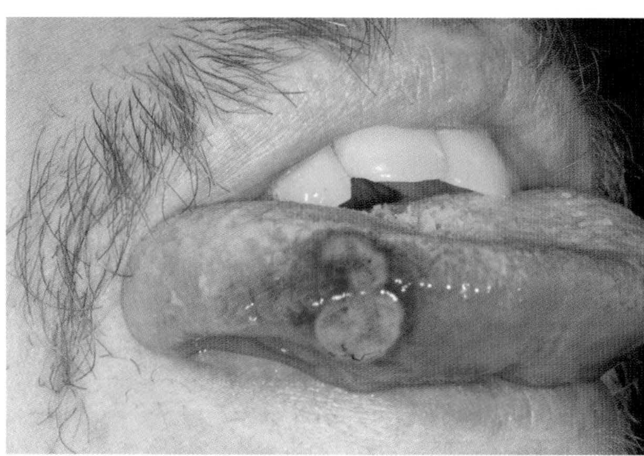

Figure 31.18 Three days status post inadvertent tongue biting after a mandibular block anesthesia.

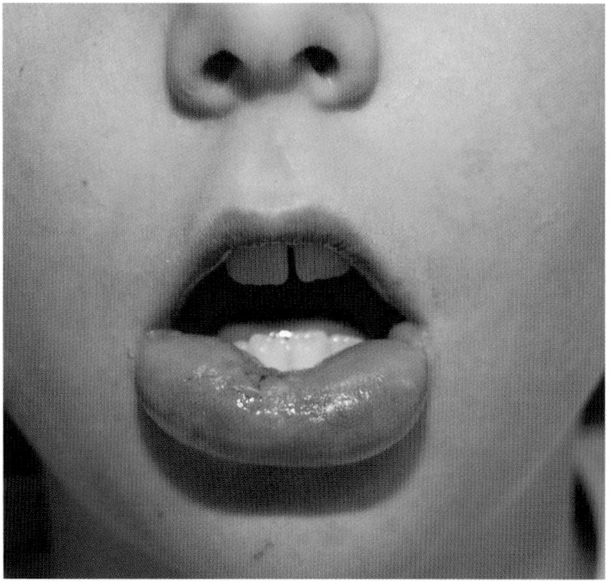

Figure 31.17 Lip sucking – this is the appearance of the lower lip of a 10-year-old male after bilateral mental nerve blocks for orthodontic bicuspid removal. Patient admitted to prolonged sucking of lip after the procedure while the lip was still anesthetized.

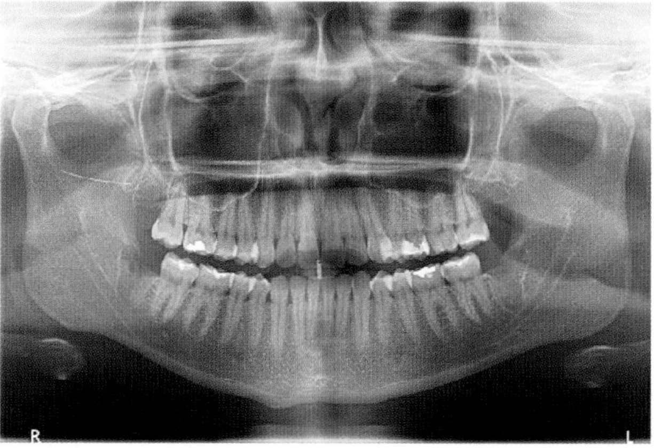

Figure 31.19 A broken 30-gauge needle is noted in the medial pterygoid space on this reconstructed CT image, courtesy of Dr. Anthony Spina, with permission.

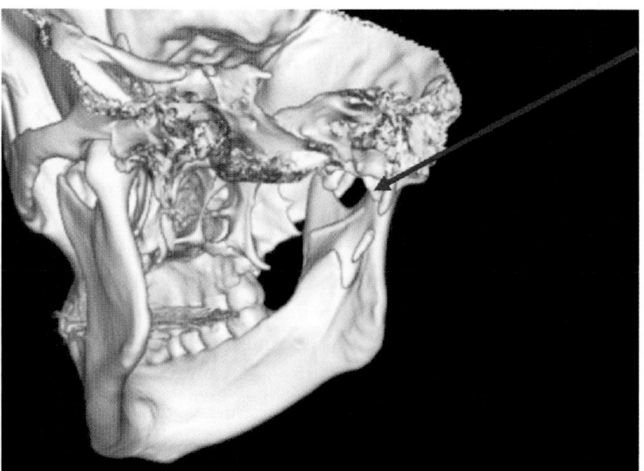

Figure 31.20 Three-dimensional reconstruction of the image in Figure 31.19, showing the precise location of the broken needle, courtesy of Dr. Anthony Spina, with permission.

needle for defects prior to usage and should minimize the number of repeated injections with the same needle. Straight line puncture and withdrawal techniques along the long axis of the needle and avoidance of full penetration to the hub can minimize breakage and improve retrieval efforts. In this manner, the clinician never loses sight of the needle. Best chances of retrieval are early, where the patient is held motionless, and the tip of the needle, IF VISIBLE, is grasped with a hemostat. If this is impossible, surgical retrieval will be necessary and appropriate referral should be made if required.

Nerve injury following local anesthetic injection

It is known that on rare occasions a local anesthetic injection, given for the purpose of anesthetizing an area of the oral cavity in order to carry out dental treatment, can cause temporary or even permanent nerve involvement, which can take the form of anesthesia, paresthesia, dysesthesia, hyperesthesia, or any combination (Pogrel et al.,

1995; Hillerup, 2008). Most cases occur as a result of an inferior alveolar nerve block but occasionally it occurs with other types of injection including even an upper anterior infiltration. Most reports are anecdotal or very small case series of a handful of cases, but there is a very small number of larger studies (Pogrel and Thamby, 2000; Harn and Durhan, 1990). These studies do seem to show that the lingual nerve is affected about twice as often as the inferior alveolar nerve, which in some ways is counterintuitive since most of the local anesthetic is deposited around the inferior alveolar nerve. However, one study has shown that in about 30% of patients, the lingual nerve may be unifascicular in the area where the needle passes for the inferior alveolar nerve block, and this might give a partial explanation in that if the patient only has one fascicle and it is affected by the local anesthetic, then there will be no alternative nerve pathways (Pogrel et al., 2003). When one takes the history from patients who have permanent nerve involvement as a result of a local anesthetic injection, it does appear that in slightly over 50% of the cases the injection was painful or different in some way from the usual injection, although in slightly under 50% of cases, patients reported that it felt just like any other injection and was no different (Pogrel and Thamby, 2000).

Studies have looked at different local anesthetic agents and of the five agents available in dental cartridge form in the United States (lidocaine, prilocaine, mepivicaine, bupivacaine, and articaine), cases have been seen with each of these local anesthetics so it appears that they all have the ability to cause this complication[6]. There have been suggestions that there may be increased incidence with prilocaine and articaine, but other studies have not substantiated this (Haas and Lennon, 1995a,b; Meechan, 2003; Pedlar, 2003a,b; van Eeden and Patel, 2002; Hillerup and Jensen, 2006; Yagiela, 2004; Pogrel, 2007).

The pattern of nerve involvement is often different from that seen from surgical causes (where the nerve has been directly damaged by a surgical procedure) and it is not uncommon for the effect to spread to involve other nerves and for there to be a patchy distribution, and in some ways this is reminiscent of the type of nerve involvement one sees with a demyelinating disease (Pogrel and Thamby, 2000).

The incidence of permanent nerve involvement from a local anesthetic injection is unknown, but estimates have varied from around 1 in 25,000 injections to around 1 per 1,000,000 injections, so by any standards it is a rare event (Pogrel and Thamby, 2000; Ehrenfeld et al., 1992). Temporary nerve involvement probably occurs 5–6 more frequently than permanent (i.e., 80–85% of cases recover spontaneously) (Pogrel and Thamby, 2000). If a nerve is going to recover it normally does so within 10–12 weeks. Late recoveries are rare (Pogrel et al., 1995).

The exact mechanism by which a nerve is permanently damaged following local anesthetic injection is unknown. The simplistic idea that this is direct needle trauma to the nerve is probably not valid since in cadaver experiments it has been proved virtually impossible to damage a nerve with a single pass of a needle (Pogrel et al., 1995). It has been suggested that if the needle hits a bone hard it will develop a barb and then while pulling back the needle the barb can damage the nerve (Stacy and Hajjar, 1994). Although this is theoretically correct, in practice most patients who suffer this damage and have an electric shock-type sensation say that they feel this as the needle goes in and not as it is being removed. Histology also shows fairly minimal nerve damage from a local anesthetic needle since it normally just separates the fascicles rather than damaging them.

An alternative theory is that the local anesthetic needle may enter the nerve and damage blood vessels that run alongside the fascicles and that it is a hematological damage to the nerve. It is known that blood around nerve fascicles is neurotoxic, and this does remain a possible mechanism (Pogrel et al., 1995).

A third theory would be that this is a neurotoxic reaction as a direct result of the chemical constituents of the local anesthetic. It is known that all local anesthetics have the potential to be neurotoxic, but generally only in much higher doses than are ever used in dental treatment (Kalichman et al., 1993; Hillerup, 2011a,b). It is also interesting that all patients seen by the author of this chapter (over 300 patients) with permanent nerve involvement from a local anesthetic injection have had previous local anesthetics with no problems whatsoever. If the patients were extremely sensitive to the possible neurotoxic effects of the local anesthetic, one would have expected it to have occurred with other local anesthetic injections.

Treatment of this condition is unsatisfactory. Many patients are given tapering steroids protocols, but there is no evidence that they confer any benefit in the long term. Similarly, vitamins, including vitamin B in all its forms, have not been shown to be helpful. Patients often take other types of supplements as well as alternative therapies such as acupuncture, but there is no evidence of any long-term benefit from them. Unfortunately, the incidence of dysesthesias is high and occurs in around 35% of patients with nerve damage as a result of local anesthetic injections (as opposed to about 10% of patients with nerve damage from wisdom tooth removal) (Pogrel and Thamby, 2000). Most of these patients must be managed medically and are often seen by a neurologist or at a pain clinic. They often receive a combination of an antiseizure medication (generally carbemazapine, gabapentin, or pregabalin) plus a low dose tricyclic-type medication and an analgesic. Surgical exploration and possible repair has not had success since the nerve involved (usually the lingual or inferior alveolar nerve) appears macroscopically, and under magnification, essentially normal. Also, if any type of corrective surgery were contemplated, it would be high up under the medial pterygoid muscle, at the site of the presumed injury, but at a site where any type of microneurosurgery would be very difficult. Nerve avulsion is a possible treatment if dysesthesia is disabling, but permanent anesthesia will result, which some patients find just as disturbing. Additionally, neuroma formation and centralized pain are possible complications of nerve avulsion.

A recent long-term study on patients with permanent nerve involvement as a result of dental treatment from all causes including local anesthetic injections shows that over time most patients do learn to cope with this problem and lead a normal life (Pogrel et al., 2011). Males appear to cope a little better than females, and the pain levels generally subside a little.

Questions arising regarding future dental treatment, as these patients are often reluctant to have an inferior alveolar block in any form, and alternative therapies need to be explored. It is possible to use intraosseous injections, or carry out dentistry under general anesthesia, or use articaine by infiltration, which has been shown to have greater penetrating power and can penetrate the buccal plate of the mandible directly and anesthetize mandibular teeth by infiltration in about 85% of cases (Currie et al., 2013).

In many cases, possible complications from local anesthesia can be added to the consent form for the dental treatment itself, so that patients realize that local anesthesia has separate risks and complications, independent of the actual dental treatment.

References

Bader, J. D., et al. A systematic review of cardiovascular effects of epinephrine on hypertensive dental patients. *Oral Surg Oral Med Oral Pathol Oral Radiol Endod* **93**: 647–653, 2002.

Batinac, T., et al. Adverse reactions and alleged allergy to local anesthetics: analysis of 331 patients. *J Derm* **40**: 1–6, 2013.

Boynes, S. G. Ocular complications associated with local anesthesia administration in dentistry. *Dent Clin N Am* **54**:677–686, 2010.

Brandt, R. G., et al. The pulpal anesthetic efficacy of articaine versus lidocaine in dentistry. *JADA* **142**:493–504, 2011.

Brown, R. S. and Rhodus, N. L. Epinephrine and local anesthesia revisited. *Oral Surg Oral Med Oral Pathol Oral Radiol Endod* **100**: 401–408, 2005.

Butterworth, J. F. Models and mechanisms of local anesthetic cardiac toxicity. *Reg Anesth Pain Med* **35**: 167–176, 2010.

Campbell, R. L., et al. Cervical sympathetic block following intraoral local anesthesia. Oral Surg, *Oral Med Oral Pathol* **47**: 223–226, 1979.

Currie, C. C., et al. Is mandibular molar buccal infiltration a mental and incisive nerve block? A randomized controlled trial. *J Endod* **39**: 439–443, 2013.

DiGregorio, G., et al. Clinical presentation of local anesthetic systemic toxicity: a review of published cases, 1979 to 2009. *Reg Anesth Pain Med* **35**: 181–187, 2010.

Ehrenfeld, M., et al. Nerve injuries following nerve blocking in the pterygomandibular space. *Dtsch Zahnarztl Z* **47**: 36, 1992.

Harn, S. D. and Durhan, T. M. Incidence of lingual nerve trauma and postinjection complications in conventional mandibular block anesthesia. *J Am Dent Assoc* **121**: 519-23,1990.

Haas, D. A. and Lennon, D. A 21 year retrospective study of reports of paresthesia following local anesthetic administration. *J Can Dent Assoc* **61**: 319–320, 1995a.

Haas, D. A. and Lennon, D. Local anesthetic use by dentists in Ontario. *J Can Dent Assoc* **61**: 297–304, 1995b.

Hegedus, R. and Herb, K. Benzocaine-induced Methemoglobinemia. *Anesth Prog* **52**: 136–139, 2005.

Hersh E. V. and Giannakopoulos, H. Beta-adrenergic blocking agents and dental vasoconstrictors. *Den Clin N Am* **54**: 687–696, 2010.

Hersh, E. V., et al. Reversal of soft-tissue local anesthesia with phentolamine mesylate in adolescents and adults. *J Am Dent Ass* **139**: 1080–1093, 2008.

Hillerup, S. Iatrogenic injury to the inferior alveolar nerve: etiology, signs and symptoms, and observations on recovery. *Int J Oral Maxillofac Surg* **37**: 704–709, 2008.

Hillerup, S. and Jensen, R. Nerve injury caused by mandibular block analgesia. *Int J Oral Maxillofac Surg* **35**: 437–443, 2006.

Hillerup, S., et al. Trigeminal nerve injury associated with injection of local anesthetics: needle lesion or neurotoxicity? *J Am Dent Assoc* **142**: 531–539, 2011a.

Hillerup, S., et al. Concentration-dependent neurotoxicity of articaine: an electrophysiological and stereological study of the rat sciatic nerve. *Anesth Analg* **112**: 1330–1338, 2011b.

Jastak, J. T., et al. *Local anesthesia of the oral cavity*. Philadelphia: WB Saunders, 1995.

Kalichman, M. W., et al. Relative neural toxicity of local anesthetics. *J Neuropathol Exp Neurol* **52**: 234–240, 1993.

Kronman, J. H., et al. The neuronal basis for diplopia following local anesthetic injections. *Oral Surg Oral Med Oral Pathol* **58**: 533–534, 1984.

Magliocca, K. R., et al. Transient diplopia following maxillary local anesthetic injection. *Oral Surg Oral Med Oral Pathol Oral Radiol Endod* **101**: 730–733, 2006

Malamed, S. F., et al. Needle Breakage: Incidence and Prevention. *Den Clin N Am* **54**: 745–756, 2010.

Meechan, J. G. Prolonged paraesthesia following inferior alveolar nerve block using articaine. *Br J Oral Maxillofac Surg* **41**: 201–207, 2003.

Meechan, J. G. Infiltration anesthesia in the mandible. *Dent Clin N Am* **54**: 621–629, 2010.

Moore, P. A. and Hersh, E. V. Local anesthetics: pharmaacology and toxicity. *Den Clin N Am* **54**: 587–599, 2010.

Niwa, H., et al. Cardiovascular response to epinephrine-containing local anesthetsia in patients with cardiovascular disease. *Oral Surg Oral Med Oral Pathol Oral Radiol Endod* **92**: 610–616, 2001.

Nouette-Gaulain, K., et al. Local anesthetic 'in-situ' toxicity during peripheral nerve blocks: update on mechanisms and prevention. *Curr Opin Anesthesiol* **25**: 589–595, 2012.

Nusstein, J. M., et al. Local anesthesia strategies for the patient with a hot tooth. *Dent Clin N Am* **54**: 237–247, 2010.

Pedlar J: Prolonged paraesthesia. *Br Dent J* **195**: 119, 2003a.

Pedlar J, Re: Prolonged paraesthesia following inferior alveolar nerve block using articaine. *Br J Oral Maxillofac Surg* **41**: 202, 2003b.

Penarrocha-Diago, M., et al. Ophthalmologic complications after intraoral local anesthesia with articaine. *Oral Surg Oral Med Oral Pathol Oral Radiol Endod* **90**: 21–24, 2000.

Perusse, R., et al. Contraindications to vasoconstrictors in dentistry: Parts I, II and III. *Oral Surg Oral Med Oral Pathol* **74**: 679–697, 1992.)

Pogrel, M. A., et al. Nerve damage associated with inferior alveolar nerve blocks. *J Am Dent Assoc* **126**: 1150–1155, 1995.

Pogrel, M. A. and Thamby, S. Permanent nerve involvement resulting from inferior alveolar nerve blocks. *J Am Dent Assoc* **131**: 901–907, 2000.

Pogrel, M. A., et al. Lingual nerve damage due to inferior alveolar nerve blocks: a possible explanation. *J Am Dent Assoc* **134**: 195–199, 2003.

Pogrel, M. A. Permanent nerve damage from inferior alveolar nerve blocks--an update to include articaine. *J Calif Dent Assoc* **35**: 271–273, 2007.

Pogrel, M.A., et al. Long-term outcome of trigeminal nerve injuries related to dental treatment. *J Oral Maxillofac Surg* **69**: 2284–2288, 2011.

Pogrel, M. A. Permanent nerve damage from inferior alveolar nerve blocks: a current update. *J Calif Dent Assoc* **40**: 795–797, 2012.

Reed, K. L., et al. Local anesthesia Part 2: technical considerations. *Anesth PRog* **59**: 127–137, 2012.

Speca, S. J., et al. Allergic reactions to local anesthetic formulations. *Den Clin N Am* **54**: 655–664, 2010.

Stacy, G. C. and Hajjar, G. Barbed needle and inexplicable paresthesias and trismus after dental regional anesthesia. *Oral Surg Oral Med Oral Pathol* **77**: 585–588, 1994.

Steenen, S. A., et al. Ophthalmologic complications after intraoral local anesthesia: case report and review of literature. *Oral Surg Oral Med Oral Pathol Oral Radiol Endod* **113**:e1–e5, 2012.

Tomazzoli-Gerosa, L., et al. Amaurosis and atrophy of the optic nerve: an unusual complication of mandibular-nerve anesthesia. *Ann Ophthalmol* **20**: 170–171, 1988.

Trapp, L and Will, J. Acquired methemoglobinemia revisited. *Dent Clin N Am* **54**: 665–675, 2010.

US FDA Public Health Advisory. Benzocaine topical products: sprays, gels and liquids - risk of methemoglobinemia. http://www.fda.gov/safety/medwatch/safetyinformation/safetyalertsforhumanmedicalproducts/ucm250264.htm (Accessed on June7, 2013).

van Eeden, S. P. and Patel, M.F. Re: prolonged paraesthesia following inferior alveolar nerve block using articaine. *Br J Oral Maxillofac Surg* **40**: 519–520, 2002.

Weinberg, G. L. Treatment of local anesthetic systemic toxicity (LAST). *Reg Anesth Pain Med* **35**: 188–193, 2010.

Weinberg, G. Banning benzocaine: of bananas, bureaucrats, and blue men. *Anesth Analg* **108**; 699–701, 2009.

Yagiela, J. A., et al. Drug interactions and vasoconstrictors used in local anesthetic solutions. *Oal Surg Oral Med Oral Pathol.* **59**: 565–571, 1985.

Yagiela, J. A. Recent developments in local anesthesia and oral sedation. *Compend Contin Educ Dent* **25**: 697–706, 2004.

32 Anesthetic adversity – cardiovascular problems

Robert C. Bosack[1] and Edward C. Adlesic[2]
[1]University of Illinois, College of Dentistry, Chicago, IL, USA
[2]University of Pittsburgh School of Dental Medicine,Department of Oral and Maxillofacial Surgery, Pittsburgh, PA, USA

Introduction

Numerous complications that can occur during the administration of office-based, open airway anesthesia can affect the cardiovascular parameters, either directly or indirectly. Most patients receiving this care present with a 4 MET functioning level, mean arterial pressures between 60 and 120mmHg (see Figure 32.1), and a sinus rhythm between 45 and 120 bpm (normal is 60 – 100 bpm), which allow them to function at "normal capacity" without symptoms of chest pain, dizziness, shortness of breath, or orthostatic hypotension. Therefore, cardiovascular problems requiring treatment during office-based anesthesia will most often represent deterioration from a normal condition, rather than an exacerbation or expression of some preoperative abnormality. Herein lies the art of patient selection. Usually, there is a cause for deterioration, which is why "remediation" of possible causes remains prominent in all algorithms. The primary goal of any resuscitative effort focuses on the maintenance of adequate perfusion of vital organs - the brain and heart (and kidney). Treatment protocols will vary with the training and experience of the provider, presence or absence of vascular access, and intended depth sedation/anesthesia. Algorithm choices are provided in this section, as well as concepts that will aid in the decisions regarding if, when, and how to treat the possible morbidities.

A schematic review of the determinants of blood pressure (Figure 32.2) emphasizes that many factors are involved with the maintenance of perfusion pressure. A clear understanding of these processes will inform treatment decisions. When a *deficiency* in one or more parameters is of sufficient severity and duration, hypotension will result. When *hypotension* is of sufficient severity and duration, treatment and/or entry into the EMS are necessary. Fortunately, the cardiovascular system has robust compensatory mechanisms to maintain adequate perfusion pressure. Intervention is contemplated when normal compensatory changes fail to maintain homeostasis.

1. When preload (venous return) is inadequate, stroke volume, cardiac output, and blood pressure will drop, in the absence of compensation by an increase in contractility, rate, and/or vascular resistance. Inadequate venous return occurs in cases of hypovolemia due to prolonged fasting, or functional hypovolemia when a significant portion of blood volume is sequestered in dilated vessels by the position of the patient and the force of gravity. Preload can be augmented by Trendelenburg positioning (legs above head), isotonic fluid boluses (Ringer's lactate or 0.9 normal saline), or vasopressors, such as ephedrine or phenylephrine.
2. Increased afterload (systemic hypertension, aortic stenosis) and/or decreased contractility (myocardial ischemia) can decrease stroke volume and cardiac output. These situations, especially when symptomatic, should be avoided in the dental office. When necessary, blood pressure can be medically lowered with β blockers or other agents.
3. Heart rates that are too fast or too slow can decrease cardiac output and blood pressure. Tachycardias decrease diastolic fill time causing decreased preload, while bradycardias decrease blood pressure when compensatory increases in vascular resistance become inadequate. Frequent premature ventricular contractions will also decrease cardiac output, because of decreased fill time and uncoordinated, inefficient contraction. Pathologic heart rates and resultant hypotension can trigger symptoms such as dizziness, palpitations, chest pain, etc. Propofol, opioids (except meperidine), and benzodiazepines tend to decrease the heart rate. Ketamine, atropine, and barbiturates tend to increase heart rate. β blockers lower pressure by decreasing the heart rate and contractility.
4. Decreased systemic vascular resistance lowers blood pressure, when compensatory increases in heart rate are insufficient. A drop in resistance occurs with syncope, propofol, barbiturates, opioids, and benzodiazepines.

General treatment protocols

Effort should consistently be directed toward the prevention of perianesthetic cardiovascular adversity, which often eliminates the requirement for any treatment. Training and experience guide the nature/extent of medical management of cardiovascular adversity, when it occurs. It is unlikely and perhaps inappropriate for any dentist to administer intravenous rescue medication during local anesthetic or oral sedation cases, where prior intravenous access

Anesthesia Complications in the Dental Office, First Edition. Edited by Robert C. Bosack and Stuart Lieblich.

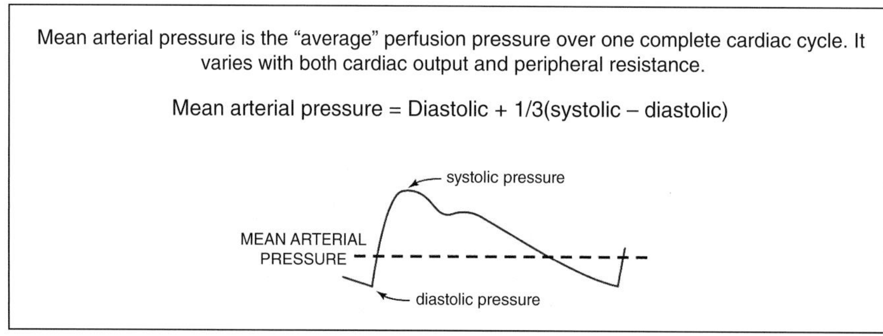

Figure 32.1 Mean arterial pressure.

has not been established, except when life-saving ACLS protocols are instituted. The use of intravenous vasoactive or cardioactive medications may also be outside the training or comfort level of the clinician administering moderate intravenous sedation. Various licensing agencies may impose other limitations. In all cases, a "start low and go slow" approach when the decision to treat cardiovascular problems is prudent.

In spite of the diverse clinical presentations of perianesthetic cardiovascular adversity, most conditions result from similar inciting events and share identical early treatment protocols. Typical triggers, which should be recognized, accepted, and remediated prior to the use of vaso/cardioactive rescue medication include hypoxemia (airway, breathing), hypotension (circulation), pain, anxiety, inadvertent intravascular epinephrine injection or levels of anesthesia that are too light or too deep.

It is prudent to be continually mindful of the fact that the abnormal parameter may be a compensatory attempt to normalize other abnormalities. For example, an increase in heart rate is a physiologic attempt to maintain perfusion during a hypotensive episode, while reflex bradycardia may occur to compensate hypertension. Treating the abnormal heart rate with adrenergic agonists or β blockers would be inappropriate in both instances.

In the dental office, the preferred order of primary assessment is airway, breathing, circulation (heart rate and blood pressure), and oxygenation (A – B – C – O), as loss of ventilation (airway obstruction or decreased ventilatory drive) is the most frequent trigger of cardiovascular emergencies. This is in contradistinction to the current American Heart Association recommendations (Travers et al., 2010), which have shifted to C – A – B, during the initial management of an unconscious patient. Final caveats include ruling out false measurement by rechecking abnormal values: retake blood pressure, check ECG leads, reposition pulse oximeter probe, and check location and patency of the side-stream capnography inlet. There is no substitute for confirmatory physical assessment of the patient (treat the patient, not the number) by noting skin color (pallor, cyanosis), chest wall movement, and breath sounds. In cases where communication can be established, the patient can be asked how they feel.

After identified triggers have been remediated, the decision to administer rescue mediation to alter blood pressure, heart rate, and/or contractility is informed by the severity and duration of the insult as well as the resilience and reserve of the patient. The spectrum of resilience and reserve (see Tables 32.1 and 32.2) ranges from the young, healthy triathlete to the obese sleep apnea patient with hypertension, systolic and diastolic heart failure with coronary atherosclerosis, and taking β blockers. As examples of each, consider the patient with patent coronary vessels better able to tolerate tachycardia vs. the patient with coronary artery disease (resilience)' or the heavily narcotized patient unable to increase rate or depth of ventilation (reserve).

Prior to treatment, the clinician should anticipate outcomes and triage options once the rescue medications wear off, which in some

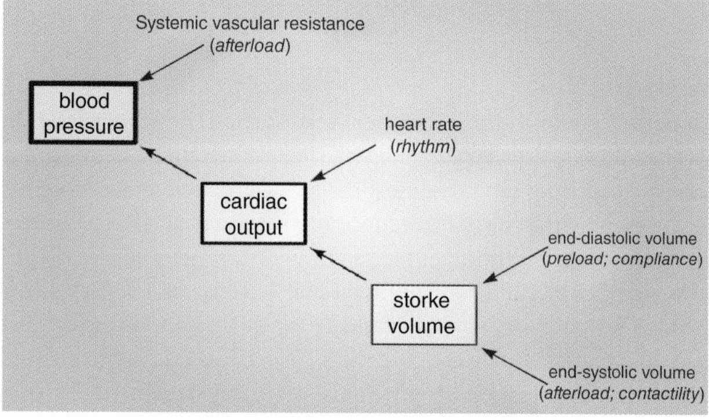

Figure 32.2 Determinants of blood pressure.

Table 32.1 Patient resilience.

Ability to tolerate insult prior to "decompensation"
- Apnea/inability to ventilate
  - Extent of pre-oxygenation
  - Size of functional residual capacity
- Hypotension, arrhythmia
  - Volume status
  - Electrolyte status, esp. [K^+]
  - Adequacy of diastolic fill
    - Patient positioning
- Hypertension, tachycardia
  - Patency of coronary vessels

Table 32.2 Patient reserve.

Ability to compensate for an increase in functional demands
- Ability to compensate for hypoxemia
  - Ability to increase rate and depth of ventilation
  - Upper airway patency
- Ability to compensate for hypotension
  - Opioids or B blockers can diminish
    - Ability to increase heart rate/contractility
    - Ability to vasoconstrict
  - Outflow obstruction (stenotic heart valves)

Table 32.3 Select drugs to manage clinically significant variances in cardiovascular parameters.

Indication	Drug/ concentration	Action	Unit Dose	Onset	Duration	Warning
Bradycardia with hypotension	Atropine, 0.4mg/ml	vagolytic	IV/IM 0.5mg q5min to a maximum of 3mg in adult	1–2 min	30–60 minutes	Low dose paradoxical bradycardia
Bradycardia and/or hypotension	Ephedrine, 50mg/ml	α and β agonist, direct and indirect	IV dilute 1 ml in 9cc = 5mg/cc	1–2 minutes	60 minutes	Avoid with MAOI; tremors, tachycardia possible
Hypotension	Phenylephrine, 10mg/ml	α agonist, direct	IV 10mg/ml, dilute 1 ml in 9cc, redilute 1ml in 9cc = 0.1mg/cc	1 minute	25 minutes	Watch for reflex bradycardia
Hypertension or angina	Nitroglycerin, 0.4mg tablet	Venous > arteriolar dilator, coronary vasodilator	0.4mg tablet, spray sublingual	1 minute	10–15 minutes	Paradoxical bradycardia, hypotension with sildenafil or tadalafil
Hypertension, PSVT, PVCs	Esmolol, 10mg/ml	β1 selective antagonist, antiarrhythmic	IV 10mg/ml, titrate up to 1mg/kg	1 minute	10–20 minutes	Avoid with CCB, greater than 1st degree heart block
Hypertension, tachycardia	Labetolol, 5mg/ml	α1 and non-selective β antagonist	IV 5mg/ml	2–5 min	2–4 hours	Caution with COPD, care with CCB
PSVT	Adenosine, 6mg/2ml	Antiarrhythmic, vago-"mimetic"	IV 6mg following by rapid 20cc saline flush	Immediate	<1 minute	Transient asystole, bronchospasm
Ventricular fibrillation or tachycardia	Amiodarone, 150 mg/3ml	antiarrhythmic	IV 150–300 mg	Minutes		Rapid administration can cause hypotension
Ventricular tachycardia	Lidocaine, 100mg/5ml	antiarrhythmic	IV 1–1.5 mg/kg	Minutes		Second line drug

cases may be sooner than the instigating trigger and resulting recurrence of the parameter that required treatment in the first place. Immediate entry into the EMS should be entertained when the clinician is faced with situations beyond the "comfort zone."

All clinicians should be familiar with a select group of medications to manage rate and/or pressure disorders, chosen on the basis of training, experience and anticipated depth of anesthesia, prior to their use. Similarly to all anesthetic agents, these drugs should be titrated to effect as one cannot accurately predict dose–response relationships. Most drugs will affect both rate and pressure and should be titrated accordingly.

Table 32.3 summarizes the pharmacology and clinical use of selected drugs that can be used to manage clinically significant variances in cardiovascular parameters. It is intended to be used as a guideline; drug choices and routes of administration are dictated by training and experience. With the exception of nitroglycerin, these medications are administered intravenously. Although some can be administered intramuscularly, indications to do so are limited.

Table 32.4 Etiology of syncope adapted from Benditt and Adkisson, 2013.

<table>
<tr><td rowspan="3">60%</td><td colspan="2" rowspan="3">Neural reflex</td><td>Vasovagal syncope</td></tr>
<tr><td>Carotid sinus syncope</td></tr>
<tr><td>Situational (cough, hysteria)</td></tr>
<tr><td rowspan="3">15%</td><td colspan="2" rowspan="3">Orthostatic Hypotension</td><td>Drug induced</td></tr>
<tr><td>Hypovolemia</td></tr>
<tr><td>Autonomic dysfunction</td></tr>
<tr><td rowspan="2">10%</td><td rowspan="4">CV cause</td><td rowspan="2">Arrhythmia (electrical defect)</td><td>Bradycardia (AV blocks)</td></tr>
<tr><td>Tachycardia (ventricular, supraventricular)</td></tr>
<tr><td rowspan="2">5%</td><td rowspan="2">Structural heart defects obstructing outflow</td><td>Aortic stenosis</td></tr>
<tr><td>Hypertrophic cardiomyopathy</td></tr>
<tr><td>10%</td><td colspan="3">Cause unknown</td></tr>
</table>

Syncope

Syncope is an abrupt, transient loss of consciousness and postural tone secondary to inadequate cerebral oxygenation. By some estimates, one in every three individuals will experience a syncopal episode during their lifetime. Incidence of syncope increases with age, with a sharp rise starting in the seventh decade (Lipsitz, 1983). The significance of syncope is quite variable, ranging from the most benign episode of vasovagal syncope progressing to an expression of underlying cardiovascular pathology: circulatory obstruction, arrhythmia, or cardiac arrest. Diagnosis and identification of underlying pathophysiology can be confounded by infrequency and the paroxysmal nature of the syncopal event. The clinical spectrum of this entity includes hypotension, dizziness, pallor, sweating, cold, moist skin with near-syncope, and loss of consciousness with syncope. An overview of the underlying pathologies, relative frequency of presentation, and clinical examples is noted in Table 32.4 (Benditt and Adkisson, 2013).

Vasovagal (neurocardiogenic) syncope is the most frequent cause of unconsciousness in the dental office, and is usually triggered by pain, sight of blood, etc., in susceptible patients. The term vasovagal describes two pathophysiologic processes that often occur simultaneously. "Vaso" refers to vasodepressor - a decrease in vascular tone and blood pressure; "vagal" refers to a heightened cardioinhibitory vagal response causing a decrease in heart rate. In spite of medical advances, there remains much to be understood about the pathophysiology of syncope – why some patients pass out and others do not.

Classic vasovagal syncope (see Table 32.5) occurs in susceptible patients in the following manner. Prolonged upright posture (kneeling, standing still) or a perceived threat – sight of blood, needle, anticipation of discomfort, etc., triggers a fight or flight sympathetic response where the heart rate is increased and blood is diverted to the larger muscle groups (legs) in anticipation of activity (β_2 vasodilator effect). Patients may complain of nausea and abdominal cramps (vagal) and may be sweating inappropriately (Figure 32.4). Diminished hearing and blurred or tunnel vision may follow. Venous return to the heart is further diminished in patients in the beach chair position without lower extremity movement. The event culminates with a compensatory tachycardia with no blood to pump. Cardiac output falls, leading to diminished blood flow to the brain. In susceptible patients, a heightened vagal response (Bezold–Jarisch response) and sympathetic withdrawal cause the heart to slow excessively, further decreasing cardiac output. When the brain is deprived of enough oxygen, the patient will lose consciousness and control of their airway. Recovery should be spontaneous, rapid, and complete in patients without underlying cardiovascular or neurologic pathology. Occasionally, a short salvo of clonic (flexion–extension) seizure activity occurs; oftentimes, this vigorous muscular activity augments venous return sufficiently to restore cerebral perfusion consciousness (see rhythm strip). ECG monitoring at the time of syncope can be frightful, as bradycardia progresses to several seconds of asystole – usually referred to as a sinus pause (see Figure 32.3). A rhythm strip recorded during a syncopal attack is seen in Figure 32.5.

Table 32.5 Characteristics of "classic" vasovagal syncope in otherwise healthy patients.

- Provoking factors indentified
  - Fear, anxiety, sight of blood, venipuncture
  - Prolonged upright posture, legs immobile
- Young, otherwise healthy patients
  - Absence of heart disease
  - Absence of hypovolemia, electrolyte disturbance
- Prodrome of nausea, warmth, anxiousness, pallor (not cyanosis), lightheadedness and/or diaphoresis
- Initial tachycardia, deteriorating to bradycardia and transient asystole
- Not preceded by shortness of breath or angina
- Loss of consciousness usually complete
- Loss of postural tone
- Incontinence is rare
- Clonic seizures (when they occur) are brief without post-ictal depression
- Rapid (not sudden) onset, short duration and complete recovery to presyncopal status

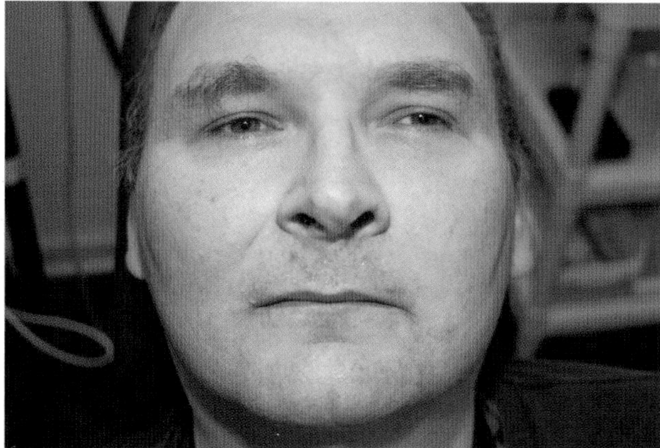

Figure 32.4 Anxious 46 y/o male presents with pre-syncopal signs of pallor, sweating and pilorection (not seen). Together with tachycardia, tachypnea and pupillary dilation, these signs are part of the "flight or fight" sympathetic response.

When "passing out" is more serious than "vasovagal syncope"

Deviation from any of the "classic" features of vasovagal syncope should invite suspicion of more serious etiology, such as orthostatic hypotension, metabolic derangement, arrhythmia, structural heart disease, stroke, or neurologic seizures (see Table 32.6; Khoo et al., 2013).

Orthostatic hypotension is defined as a 20mmHg or more decrease in systolic pressure and a 10mmHg or more decrease in diastolic pressure immediately after assuming an upright posture, or during prolonged standing or kneeling. It can be due to advanced age, antihypertensive medication, autonomic dysfunction, or hypovolemia, among others.

Metabolic derangements that can lead to syncope include hyperventilation (hypocarbia triggers cerebral vasoconstriction) or hypoglycemia, which presents with a more gradual onset and delayed recovery.

Cardiovascular causes include sudden onset tachycardias (PSVT) when palpitations immediately precede or trigger near syncope or

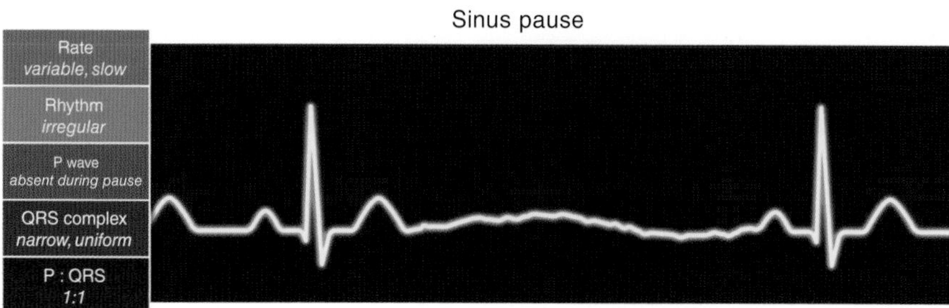

Figure 32.3 Sinus pause.

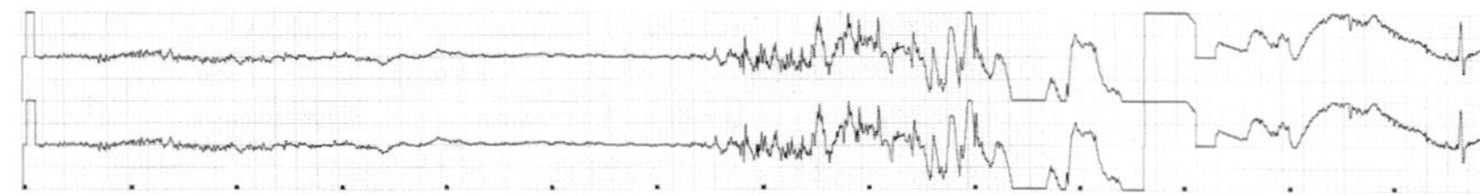

Figure 32.5 Rhythm strip. Actual rhythm strip of an otherwise healthy patient who has "passed out" after venipuncture. At the bottom of the strip, each dot represents 1 second. The patient was in asystole prior the start of this strip. Notice seizure activity at the 7 second mark, and the resumption of a normal QRS complex at the 14 second mark. In this case, the heart stopped beating for approximately 20 seconds. The decision to complete or cancel the case rests with the treating clinician.

Table 32.6 Syncope warning signs.

- Syncope + any cardiac disease/abnormal ECG/structural cardiac defect
- Age >45 years
- Prodromal chest pain, palpitations or SOB
- Syncope in the supine position
- Exertional syncope - outflow tract obstruction
- Very sudden drops or falls (no prodrome or warning)
- Incontinence of bladder, but especially bowel
- Prolonged seizure activity and/or prolonged recovery
- any loss of consciousness with cyanosis (blue coloration)

syncope, or structural heart defects leading to outflow obstructions (aortic stenosis or hypertrophic cardiomyopathy), which trigger cerebral hypoperfusion during exertion.

The patient experiencing vasovagal syncope will turn pale, but not cyanotic (blue), which might be an indication of serious cardiac or pulmonary compromise

When syncope leads to seizure activity, one must entertain a diagnosis of neurologic seizures. The seizure activity associated with syncope is of short duration, rarely involves injury, is usually not accompanied by incontinence, and ends with a quick return to normalcy. A seizure of neurologic origin usually occurs without warning, prior to loss of consciousness, is of longer duration, can involve injury and incontinence, and is followed by significant post-ictal depression, confusion, and disorientation.

Treatment protocol for syncope

1. Maintain airway, supplemental oxygen.
2. Terminate procedure, remove loose objects from mouth.
3. Prevent injury if convulsing.
4. Trendelenburg positioning – patient supine with legs higher than the heart. If semiconscious, encourage repetitive leg movement to augment venous return.
5. Crush an ammonia vaporole under the nose.
6. Apply cool packs to the forehead.
7. Contemplate etiology.

If there is no improvement with this protocol, EMS should be activated and other possibilities, such as primary seizure disorder, stroke, allergy, hypoglycemia, or myocardial infarction should be entertained.

Perianesthetic pressure disorders

Hypotension

Perianesthetic hypotension is a decrease in arterial blood pressure, referenced from a baseline value. Diminished pressure jeopardizes organ perfusion, inviting ischemia and infarct. It should be recognized that blood pressure measurements immediately prior to venipuncture or other threatening procedures may be falsely elevated, and thus not be representative of a true baseline. In general, a 20 – 30% drop in mean arterial pressure is significant and should warrant further investigation. Hypotension is more worrisome in patients with preexisting (and poorly controlled) hypertension, where organ hypoperfusion can occur at pressures considered "normal" for other patients. In otherwise normotensive patients, MAP should be maintained at or above 60–65mmHg for patients sitting in the "beach chair" position. Perfusion pressure decreases by approximately 1mmHg per centimeter above the heart. Successful autoregulation (maintenance) of cerebral perfusion is thought to occur between mean arterial pressures of 50 to 150mmHg. (see Figure 5.2) Common causes of acute decreases in blood pressure are listed in Table 32.7. To reiterate, treatment varies with the severity, duration, and estimated ability of the patient to tolerate hypotension.

Management of significant drops in blood pressure starts with cessation and stabilization of the procedure and consideration to stop the administration of (and consider reversal of) anesthetic drugs. Airway, breathing, and oxygenation should be ensured, while the pressure is rechecked. Patients who are not fully anesthetized can be stimulated. The patient can be placed in Trendelenburg position (legs above head), which can immediately increase venous return by up to 1 liter, or more depending on the size and hydration of the

Table 32.7 Contributors of acute decreases in blood pressure during office based anesthesia.

- Syncope
- Hypoxia, hypercarbia
- Volume depletion – prolonged fast, excessive sweating, diuretic usage
- Anxiety/fear/vasovagal syncope
- Pre-existing hypertension
- Anesthetic agents (expected side effect or drug overdose)
    - Propofol – vasodilation without reflex tachycardia
    - Opioids – decrease sympathetic tone
    - Inhalational agents – cardiac and vascular tone depression
- Overdose of antihypertensive medication
- Drug interaction
- Hypoglycemia
- Anaphylaxis
- Arrhythmia - frequent PVC's or infrequent QRS complexes
- Aortic stenosis
- Myocardial ischemia
- Overdose of anti-hypertensive medication
- Pulmonary embolus

patient. An isotonic intravenous fluid challenge can be simultaneously started. At this point, it is reasonable to take a "time out" and consider other possibilities as listed in Table 32.7.

There are three options for intravenous medical management of hypotension that has not responded to the above initial treatment measures. Atropine (0.5mg, titrated to 3mg) is used when hypotension is accompanied by bradycardia. Atropine increases pressure by increasing heart rate but does not alter vascular resistance. Ephedrine (5mg/cc) can be titrated to treat hypotension that is not accompanied by tachycardia. Ephedrine stimulates both α and β receptors (direct action and indirect action by stimulating the release of norepinephrine from adrenergic terminals), which will increase both heart rate and systemic vascular resistance. Onset is rapid and duration is approximately 1 hour. Tremors and tachycardia are side effects. Phenylephrine is an α agonist that increases systemic vascular resistance without increasing heart rate, and is indicated when hypotension is accompanied by tachycardia. Phenylephrine is diluted to 0.1mg/cc, which can be used as the initial dose. Onset is rapid, and offset occurs within 30 minutes. Reflex bradycardia is possible with the use of phenylephrine.

Hypertension

Perianesthetic hypertension is an increase in arterial blood pressure, referenced from a baseline value. Hypertension increases afterload and myocardial wall tension, which increases cardiac oxygen demand while decreasing oxygen supply. In these instances, ischemia often triggers tachycardia, which worsens the oxygen supply–demand balance. Theoretically, severe pressure elevation physically stresses the vasculature, inviting vessel rupture, especially in weakened regions, such as preexisting aneurysms.

Hypertensive emergencies refer to significant pressure elevations over baseline with symptoms (chest pain, headache, visual disturbance) or target organ damage (brain, kidney, eye, or heart.) Careful patient screening should make hypertensive emergencies almost nonexistent in the dental office. Hypertensive urgencies refer to pressure elevations without symptoms or evidence of target organ damage. Absolute ceiling reference values are approximated at 180/110 mmHg. In general, a 20–25% increase in systolic, diastolic, OR mean arterial pressure over baseline, validated by rechecking blood pressure, should warrant further investigation, with the realization that immediate pre-treatment pressures can be falsely elevated. Acute lowering of blood pressure in previously hypertensive patients invites hypoperfusion, as autoregulatory blood flow has been "reset" to a higher value (Immink, et al., 2004) (Figure 5.3). This emphasizes the importance of optimizing blood pressure control prior to office-based procedures and mandates a conservative approach to medical therapy in the event of elevated pressures. Blood pressure swings can be more frequent and more severe in patients with untreated hypertension (Goldman and Caldera, 1979).

Management of significant elevations in blood pressure during anesthesia starts with cessation and stabilization of the procedure. Airway, breathing, and oxygenation should be ensured, while the pressure is rechecked. Significant elevations in blood pressure in carefully screened and selected patients most often results from some type of trigger (see Table 32.8), remediation of which often leads to a lowering of the pressure.

When electing to medically treat a patient with elevated blood pressure without an identifiable cause and in the absence of end-organ damage, several factors must be considered. These include the knowledge and experience of the anesthesia provider, the age of the patient, the rapidity of pressure elevation, and any history of prior organ damage secondary to hypertension, including stroke, CAD, or renal disease. There is a lack of consensus regarding drugs or treatment thresholds (Varon and Marik, 2008). In all cases, drugs should be titrated slowly, starting with low doses, and patients should be kept in a supine position with pressures measured every 5 minutes. There is little evidence to support the practice of emergently treating elevated blood pressure in the absence of end organ damage (Shayne and Pitts, 2003)

Rapid reduction in blood pressure can be achieved with either nitroglycerin or esmolol. Nitroglycerin (0.4mg) can be sprayed or placed under the tongue of a semiconscious patient (to avoid aspiration), which will trigger a 10 – 20mmHg drop in pressure for up to 10 minutes. Nitroglycerin is more of a venous dilator than an arteriolar dilator, which decreases blood pressure by decreasing venous return, and hence the cardiac output. It is also a coronary

Table 32.8 Contributors of acute increases in blood pressure during office based anesthesia.

- Hypoxia, hypercarbia
- Neuroendocrine stress response
  - Pain/anxiety
  - Inadequate local anesthetic
  - Inadequate sedation/general anesthesia
- Intravascular injection of epinephrine
- Adverse drug interaction
- Poorly controlled pre-existing hypertension
- Rebound hypertension
  - Acute withdrawal of β blockers or α2 agonists (clonidine)
- Anesthetic drug effect
  - Ketamine
- Fluid overload
- Full bladder
- Emergence delirium
- Myocardial ischemia
- Illicit substance abuse

Table 32.9 Contributors of acute sinus tachycardia during office based anesthesia.

- Hypoxia, hypercarbia
- Hypotension
- Hypoglycemia
- Neuroendocrine stress response
  - Pain/anxiety
  - Inadequate local anesthetic
  - Inadequate sedation/general anesthesia
- Intravascular injection of epinephrine
- Drug effect
  - Ketamine
  - Atropine
  - Albuterol
  - Rebound from abrupt discontinuation of β blockers
- Full bladder
- Emergence delirium
- Myocardial ischemia
- Pulmonary embolus
- Bronchospasm
- Hyperthyroidism

vasodilator. Onset and offset are rapid (Straka et al., 1996). Esmolol (10mg/cc) is a β1 blocker at lower doses and can be safely titrated in 5 – 10mg increments to acutely lower heart rate and reduce cardiac contractility (Lowenthal et al., 1985). Onset and offset are rapid due to rapid hydrolysis by red blood cell esterases (anemia can prolong the effect of esmolol). β blockers should not be used in patients taking calcium channel blockers.

Slow reduction in blood pressure can be achieved with labetolol, which is a α1 and non-selective β blocker (Lund-Johansen, 1984). The supplied concentration is 5mg/cc, which is a reasonable starting dose to achieve onset in 2 – 5 minutes with a 2 – 4 hour duration. The β non-selectivity of this drug can trigger bronchoconstriction in susceptible patients (unlike esmolol, which blocks the β1 receptor at lower doses). Hydralazine is a peripheral arteriolar dilator, which decreases vascular resistance. Onset is slow at 5 – 15 minutes, and duration can last up to 12 hours, which makes this drug less desirable for office titrations. Precipitous falls in pressure are possible (Shepherd et al., 1980, Tietjen et al., 1996).

Sinus tachycardia

Sinus tachycardia is a sinus-originated (P wave is identified, QRS is narrow) heart rate greater than 100 beats per minute. It is commonly encountered in the dental office secondary to excess sympathetic discharge resulting from fear and anxiety, which is a prime reason for the delivery of office-based anesthesia. The sinus node receives robust autonomic innervation to enhance cardiac output to meet metabolic needs associated with increased activity. As such, some type of trigger is necessary to cause sinus tachycardia, which will manifest as a *gradual* increase in heart rate, displaying a narrow QRS complex. Fast heart rates with adequate venous return (e.g., running on a treadmill, which enhances muscular pumping to return venous blood) will increase blood pressure. As systole is an all-or-none phenomenon, even faster rates shorten diastole only, decreasing both time for ventricular filling and diastolic coronary perfusion. As expected, when heart rates increase further, venous return decreases because of less filling time, blood pressure drops, myocardial oxygen consumption increases, and oxygen supply decreases. Concomitant hypertension increases afterload, further increasing oxygen demand. Venous return is further compromised when patients sit still in a dental chair, lacking muscular pumping of lower extremity veins. Sinus tachycardias can occur with both hypotension or hypertension. Treatment is directed toward identification and remediation of the triggering factor figure 32.6.

Paroxysmal supraventricular tachycardia (PSVT)

Paroxysmal supraventricular tachycardia (see Figure 32.7) is an *abrupt* onset of a fast heart rate, originating above the bifurcation of the HIS bundle. Rates tend to be faster than simple sinus

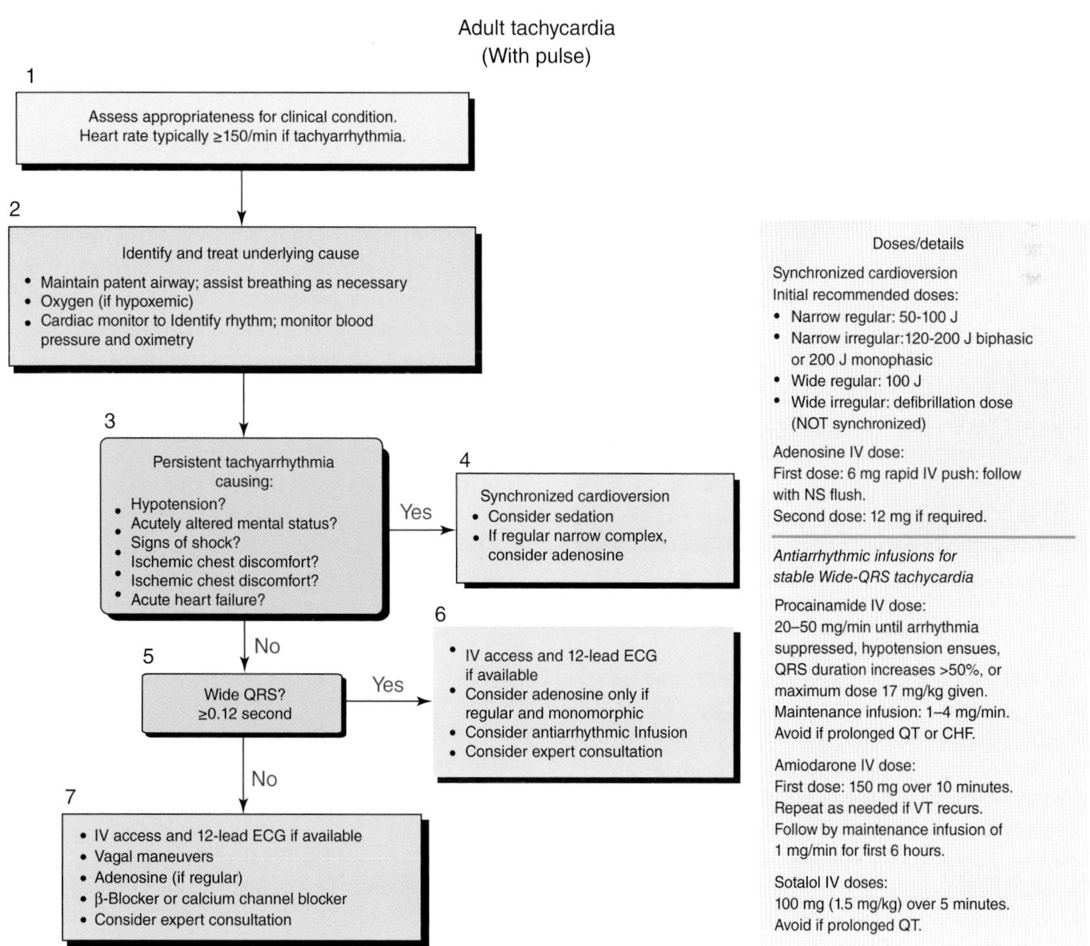

Figure 32.6 Adult tachycardia, from Neumar, 2010, with permission.

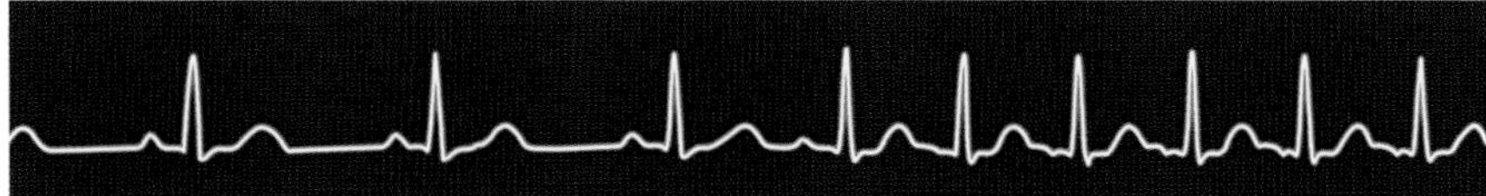

Figure 32.7 Paroxysmal supraventricular tachycardia.

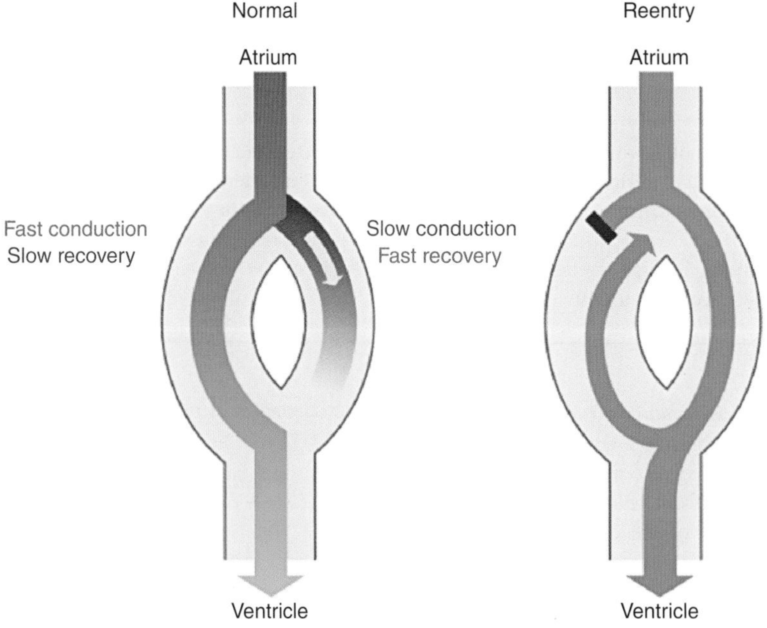

Figure 32.8 Bidirectional pathway.

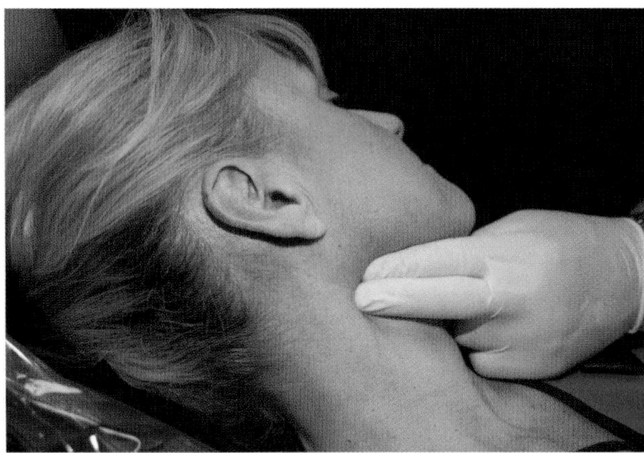

Figure 32.9 Carotid sinus massage.

tachycardia, often displaying narrow QRS complexes in the range of 170 - 180 bpm. P waves are impossible to identify as they become hidden in the previous T wave, and hence the name supraventricular. A re-entry circuit, usually within the AV node (anatomic or pathophysiologic conduction defect) must be present, which consists of two electrophysiologically dissimilar bidirectional pathways, as discussed in Chapter 5. A possible trigger for PSVT is a serendipitously timed premature atrial contraction, which momentarily stalls in the primary conduction path and is allowed to conduct down the alternate path, and then retrograde up the primary path to set up a repeated looping current or "circus movement."(see Figure 32.8).

Sudden onset of persistent tachycardia during anesthesia, in the absence of identifiable triggers, requires immediate attention. In many cases, PSVT terminates spontaneously and abruptly without treatment. If required, therapy is aimed at slowing down conduction through the AV node and increasing the refractory period or electrical interruption of the re-entry circuit during severe hemodynamic compromise. Depending on the training and confidence of the practitioner and the severity and duration of hemodynamic significance, vagal maneuvers (Valvalsa maneuver, carotid sinus massage, cold washcloth to the face), rapid infusion of adenosine, or synchronized cardioversion can be attempted (see Fig 32.6). Immediate hospital triage should be considered in recalcitrant cases and in any situation beyond the "comfort level" of the practitioner.

Carotid sinus massage, adenosine, or esmolol can be considered with a narrow complex regular PSVT supporting mean arterial pressures above 50–60 mmHg. Carotid sinus massage (see Figure 32.9) triggers a strong vagotonic reaction, slowing conduction through the AV node (one loop of the circuit) hopefully resulting in termination of this rhythm. In the absence of bruits, suggestive of carotid plaques that could be dislodged during the maneuver, the patient is placed supine with an extended neck. A steady pressure or massage is applied (similar to the force needed to indent a tennis ball) for 5 to 10 seconds, allowing 2 minutes for a response. With dysrhythmia persistence, massage on the opposite side can be attempted, while awaiting EMS entry.

Adenosine causes a transient heart block in the AV node, hopefully terminating the reciprocating dysrhythmia. Rapid (seconds) metabolism mandates fast IV administration immediately followed by a 20cc normal saline flush to get the drug to the heart prior to degradation. Dosing regimens are 6mg – 12mg – 12mg as needed at 2 minute intervals between attempts. Transient asystole is an anticipated, but sometimes worrisome, result of adenosine administration. Calcium channel blockers, esmolol, or amiodarone can be also be used. As all antiarrhythmics may be proarrhythmic, especially when used in combination, only one antiarrhythmic drug should be used per clinical scenario.

In very rare circumstances, prolonged rapid heart rates that eventually result in a mean arterial pressure <50 – 60mmHg in an otherwise normotensive patient will mandate rhythm control via electrical cardioversion or prompt entry into the EMS. Many offices have AEDs, which are not able to cardiovert at this time. Patients should be kept supine during these maneuvers, as this position improves cerebral circulation during hypotension.

The ACLS Adult Tachycardia (with pulse) is shown in Figure 32.6.

Premature ventricular complexes

In the absence of underlying cardiac disease, PVCs during anesthesia are usually triggered by sympathetic stimulation, secondary to anxiety, hypoxia, hypoxemia, pain, hypotension, or ischemia, among others. Although most PVCs are asymptomatic, responsive patients may relate symptoms of chest pain, dizziness, shortness of breath, or palpitations.

New onset of perianesthetic ventricular ectopy is an ambiguous signal. In the absence of triggers such as hypoxia or sympathetic stimulation, simple PVCs can be considered as a normal variant in patients with normal cardiac structure and ejection fractions. In contradistinction, PVCs that are increasing in number (>20% of beats), complexity, or hemodynamic significance (hypotension), especially in the absence of triggers and the presence of underlying cardiac disease, are an ominous sign that warrants immediate attention and possible emergent triage.

Treatment, when indicated, involves a search for and remediation of underlying triggers such as hypoxia, hypokalemia, sympathetic stimulation, pain, and anxiety. Anesthesia and surgery should be stopped. A defibrillator should be available in these circumstances.

β blocker therapy, such as esmolol can be considered (Cantillon, 2013). Amiodarone 50mg IV or lidocaine 0 .5-1mg/kg may also be effective. These treatments are not indicated for escape beats.

Sinus bradycardia

Sinus bradycardia is sinus-originated (P wave is identified, QRS is narrow) heart rate less than 60bpm. This is a common clinical finding, which is physiologic during sleep or in well-trained athletes with conditioned hearts having parasympathetic dominance at rest. Bradycardia is pathologic when associated with symptoms of dizziness, fatigue, weakness, angina, or shortness of breath. Triggers of acute sinus bradycardia in the office are listed in Table 32.10.

Management of sinus bradycardia during anesthesia/sedation becomes necessary when it is accompanied by a significant decrease in blood pressure. As with all other instances of hemodynamic compromise, the procedure should be stopped and stabilized, in order to devote full attention to the anesthetic situation. Airway, breathing, and oxygenation should be ensured, while the pressure is rechecked. Triggers, if present, should be identified and remediated. Medical management in the dental office, when considered necessary, includes intravenous atropine 0.5mg bolus, repeated at 3 – 5 minute intervals, up to a 3mg maximum dose. Ephedrine can be used as well. EMS triage is considered when medical treatment is unsuccessful, or at any time the practitioner is outside of the "comfort zone." Pacing can be considered per practitioner training and experience, until EMS entry.

Table 32.10 Contributors of acute decreases in heart rate during office based anesthesia.

- hypoxia, hypercarbia
- normal consequence of aging
- drug effect
  - β blocker, Calcium channel blocker, digoxin, lithium, α2 agonists
  - opioids
  - anesthetic overdose
  - repeat doses of succinylcholine
- conduction defects
  - junctional rhythm
  - heart block
- vagal stimulation
- hypothyroidism

Angina/cardiac ischemia/infarct

Myocardial oxygen demand is increased by tachycardia, hypertension, and increased contractility (among others), all of which can occur during the neuroendocrine stress response triggered by dental manipulation or inadequate anesthesia. Myocardial oxygen supply is decreased with tachycardia, diastolic blood pressure, coronary artery disease, intermittent or permanent coronary occlusion, and hypoxemia (see Table 32.11 and Chapter 5). Although variability is the rule, cardiac ischemia is often painful and can result in verbal complaints of chest pain, when patients are conversant. Depending on severity, myocardial ischemia can present with a host of other signs and symptoms, which, in some cases, progresses to myocardial infarct and possibly sudden cardiac death.

The sedated patient may be unable to communicate symptoms of acute coronary ischemia and/or acute myocardial infarction. Depending on the level of sedation the patient may display discomfort out of proportion and/or unrelated to the dental stimulus. Agitation, diaphoresis, tachycardia, hypertension, or hypotension may occur as well.

Ventricular ischemia leads to reduced compliance and contractility, thus compromising diastolic filling and forward flow. The result is a smaller stroke volume (from a stiff, poorly filled ventricle) that leads to a drop in blood pressure. Compensatory tachycardia triggered by hypotension further disrupts myocardial oxygen supply – demand balance. Atrial and/or ventricular ectopy

Table 32.11 Myocardial oxygen balance.

↓ O_2 supply	↑ O_2 demand
↓ Coronary blood flow (vessel radius)	↑ Afterload (systolic blood pressure) (valvular stenosis)
↑ Heart rate	↑ Preload (ventricular volume, filling pressure)
↓ Diastolic pressure	↑ Heart rate
↓ Oxygen delivery (O_2 saturation, [Hgb])	↑ Contractility

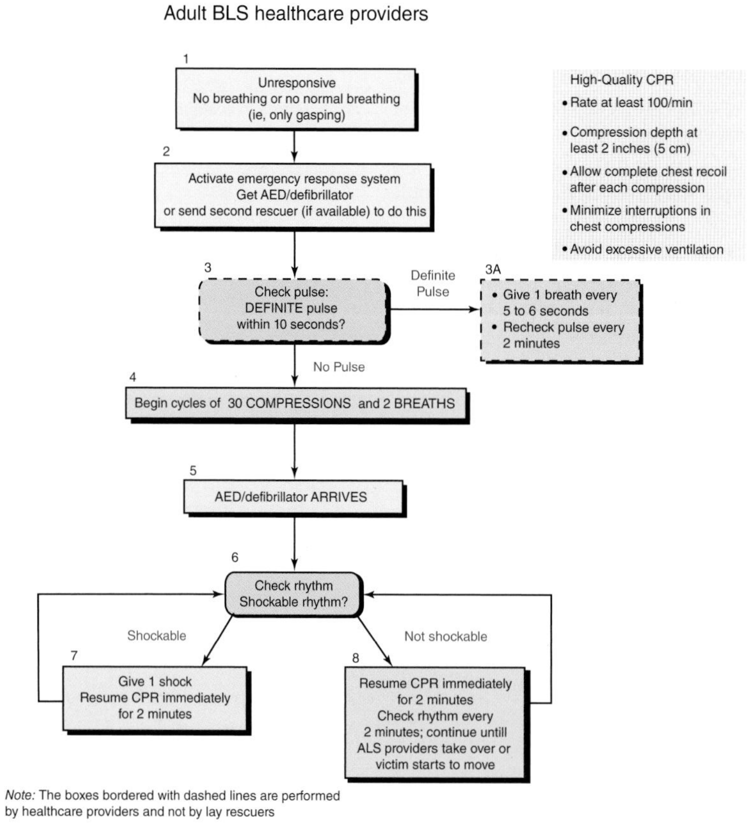

Adult BLS healthcare providers
1
Unresponsive
No breathing or no normal breathing
(ie, only gasping)
2
Activate emergency response system
Get AED/defibrillator
or send second rescuer (if available) to do this
High-Quality CPR
• Rate at least 100/min
• Compression depth at least 2 inches (5 cm)
• Allow complete chest recoil after each compression
• Minimize interruptions in chest compressions
• Avoid excessive ventilation
3
Check pulse:
DEFINITE pulse
within 10 seconds?
Definite Pulse
3A
• Give 1 breath every 5 to 6 seconds
• Recheck pulse every 2 minutes
No Pulse
4
Begin cycles of 30 COMPRESSIONS and 2 BREATHS
5
AED/defibrillator ARRIVES
6
Check rhythm
Shockable rhythm?
Shockable
Not shockable
7
Give 1 shock
Resume CPR immediately
for 2 minutes
8
Resume CPR immediately
for 2 minutes
Check rhythm every
2 minutes; continue untill
ALS providers take over or
victim starts to move
Note: The boxes bordered with dashed lines are performed
by healthcare providers and not by lay rescuers

Figure 32.10 BLS healthcare provider algorithm, Berg et al., 2010, with permission.

Adult cardiac arrest
Shout for help/activate emergency response
Start CPR
• Give oxygen
• Attach monitor/defibrilator
2 minutes
Return of Spontaneous Circulation (ROSC)
Check Rhythm
Post-Cardiac Arrest Care
If VF/VT Shock
Drug therapy
IV/IO access
Epinephrine every 3-5 minutes
Amiodarone for refractory VF/VT
Consider advanced airway
Quantitative waveform capnography
Treat reversible causes
Continuous CPR
Continuous CPR
Monitor CPR Quality
CPR quality
• Push hard (≥2 inches [5 cm]) and fast (≥100/min) and allow complete chest recoil
• Minimize interruptions in compressions
• Avoid excessive ventilation
• Rotate compressor every 2 minutes
• If no advanced airway, 30:2 compression-ventilation ratio
• Quantitative waveform capnography
- If PETCO2 <10 mm Hg, attempt to improve CPR quality
• Intra-arterial pressure
- If relaxation phase (diastolic) pressure <20 mm Hg, attempt to improve CPR quality
Return of spontaneous circulation (ROSC)
• Pulse and blood pressure
• Abrupt sustained increase in PETCO2 (typically ≥40 mm Hg)
• Spontaneous arterial pressue waves with intra-arterial monitoring
Shock energy
• Biphasic: Manufacturer recommendation (eg. Initial dose of 120-200 J): if unknown, use maximum available. Second and subsequent doses should be equivalent, and higher doses may be considered.
• monophasic: 360 J
Drug therapy
• Epinephrine IV/IO dose: 1 mg every 3-5 minutes
• Vasopressin IV/IO dose: 40 units can replace first or second dose of epinephrine
• Amiodarone IV/IO dose: First dose:300 mg bolus. Second dose: 150 mg.
Advanced airway
• Supraglottic advanced airway or endotracheal intubation
• Waveform capnography to confirm and monitor ET tube placement
• 8–10 breaths per minute with continuous chest compressions
Reversible causes
– Hypovolernia
– Hypoxia
– Hydrogen ion (acidosis)
– Hypo-/hyperkalemia
– Hypothermia
– Tension pneumothorax
– Tamponade, cardiac
– Toxins
– Thrombosis, pulmonary
– Thrombosis, coronary

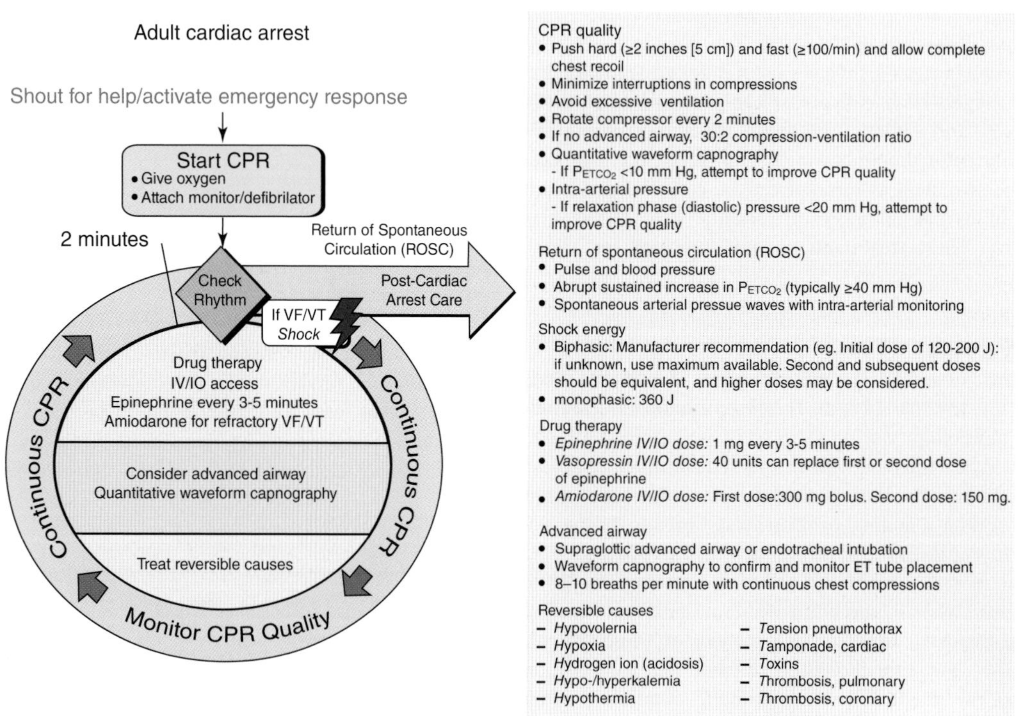

Figure 32.11 ACLS cardiac arrest circular algorithm, Neumar, 2010, with permission.

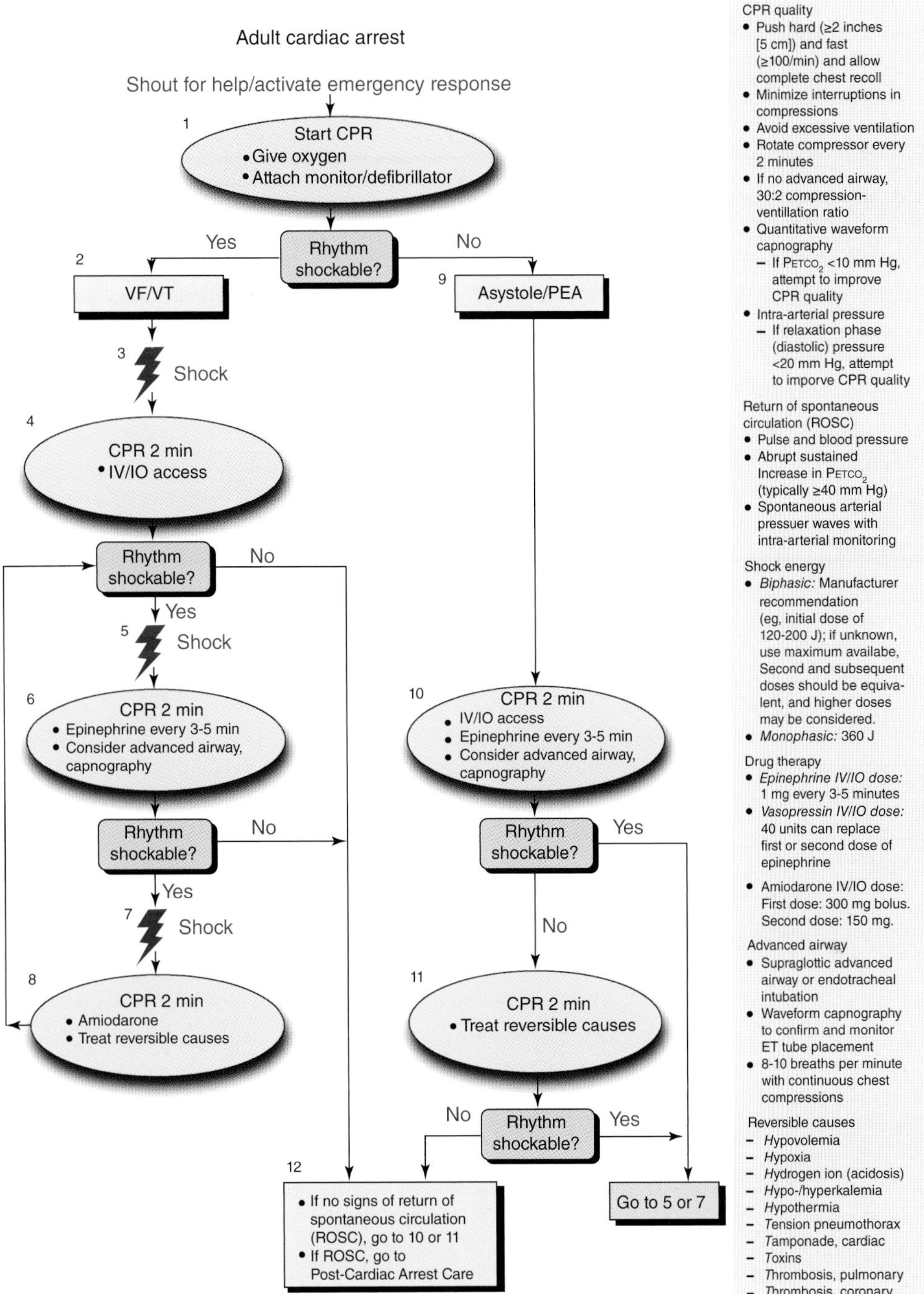

Figure 32.12 ACLS cardiac arrest algorithm, Neumar, 2010, with permission.

are common in the setting of myocardial ischemia, and can lead to more malignant dysrhythmias if not remediated in a timely manner.

Common electrocardiographic changes that may not be evident on a lead II tracing include ST segment depression or elevation more than 2mm, T wave abnormalities (flattening or inversion), or electrical abnormalities such as increasing frequency of premature ventricular complexes or the development of a new heart block.

Not all complaints of new-onset chest pain are cardiac in origin. Panic attacks, esophageal reflux, and gastritis are possibilities in the dental patient. Notwithstanding, any complaint of chest pain should be taken seriously and not prematurely dismissed as being trivial.

Management of the various presentations of this disease spectrum follow current American Heart Association protocols and depend on the clinical situation, depth of anesthesia, presence of intravenous access, practitioner training, and experience. Several AHA algorithms are included for reference. Appendix 2, Medical Emergencies in the Dental Office, includes diagnosis and management issues for those practitioners using local anesthesia and nitrous oxide analgesia only.

References

Benditt, D. G. and Adkisson, W. O. Approach to the patient with syncope. *Cardiol Clin* **31**: 9–25, 2013.

Berg, R.A., et al. Part 5: adult basic life support : 2010 American Heart Association Guidelines for cardiopulmonary resuscitation and emergency cardiovascular care. *Circulation* **122**: S685–S705, 2010.

Cantillon, D. J., Evaluation and management of premature ventricular complexes. *Cleveland Clin J Med* **80**: 377–387, 2013.

Goldman, L and Caldera, D. L. Risks of general anesthesia and elective operation in the hypertensive patients *Anesthesiology* **50**: 285–292, 1979.

Immink, R. V., et al. Impaired cerebral autoregulation in patients with malignant hypertension. *Circulations* **110**: 2241–2245, 2004.

Khoo, C., et al. Recognizing life-threatening causes of syncope. *Cardiol Clin* **31**: 51–66, 2013.

Lipsitz, L. A. Syncope in the elderly. *Ann Intern Med*, **99**: 92, 1983.

Lowenthal, D. T., et al. Clinical pharmacology, pharmacodynamics and itneractions with esmolol. *Am J Cardiol* **56**: 14F-18F, 1985.

Lund-Johansen, P. Pharmacology of combined alpha-beta-blockade II. *Haemodynamic effects of labetalol. Drugs* **28**: 35–50, 1984.

Shayne, P. H. and Pitts, S. R. Severely elevated blood pressure in the emergency department. *Ann Emerg Med* **41**: 513–529, 2003.

Shepherd, A. M., et al. Hydralazine kinetics after single and repeated oral doses. *Clin Pharmacol* **28**: 804–11, 1980.

Straka, R. J., et al. Antihypertensive agents In: Irwin, R.S., et al. (eds.) *Intesive care Medicine* 3rd edn. Boston: Little Brown, 1996.

Tang, W. Adult advanced cardiovascular life support: 2010 American Heart Association Guidelines for cardiopulmonary resuscitation and emergtency cardiovascular care. *Circulation* **122**: S729–S767, 2010.

Tietjen, C. S., et al. Treatment modalities for hypertensive patients with intracranial pathology: options and risk. *Crit Care Med* **24**: 311–22, 1996.

Travers, A. H., et al. 2010 American Heart Association Guidelines for cariopulmonary resuscitation and emergency cardiovascular care. Part 4: CPR overview. *Circulations* **122**: s676–s684, 2010.

Varon, J. and Marik, P. E. Perioperative hypertension management. *Vasc Health Risk Manage* **4**: 615–627, 2008.

33 Anesthetic adversity—respiratory problems

Charles F. Cangemi[1], Edward C. Adlesic[2], and Robert C. Bosack[3]
[1]Dental Anesthesiology, Charlotte, NC, USA
[2]University of Pittsburgh, School of Dental Medicine, Department of Oral and Maxillofacial Surgery, Pittsburgh, PA, USA
[3]University of Illinois, College of Dentistry, Chicago, IL, USA

Introduction

Airway obstruction can occur in any patient, regardless of the level of sedation or anesthesia. Proper assessment, management, and treatment of difficulties involving the upper and/or lower airway (loss of oxygenation and ventilation) are among the highest priorities of anesthetic care. In the United States, 28% of claims involving death or brain damage involved respiratory events (Cheney et al., 2006). Airway and ventilatory risk are minimized with a thorough preanesthetic assessment to guide both an anesthetic plan and an airway management plan. As the frequency of office-based surgery and anesthesia is growing exponentially, the likelihood of treating patients with compromised airways is increasing. This challenge can be met with increased scrutiny for office-based anesthesia eligibility as well as increased operator proficiency, given the limited availability of backup help should complications arise. Furthermore, even with a thorough preoperative airway assessment, the difficult airway may be difficult to predict. Langeron et al. (2000) reported that difficult mask ventilation was correctly predicted by anesthesiologists only 17% of the time. This worrisome finding should trigger frequent *office-based, in situ* airway simulation rehearsals, including the immediate availability and use of a positive pressure device (Figure 33.1) and airway tray (see Figure 33.2), stocked with emergency airway adjuncts commensurate with levels of sedation or anesthesia provided as well as the training and experience of the anesthesia provider. Having all equipment at arm's length during anesthesia prevents the diversion of attention and allows the practitioner to focus completely on the problem at hand.

Airway tray

Figure 33.2 shows an airway tray stocked with regularly maintained and appropriately sized airway devices. Trays can be customized to the level of training and practice. This tray includes the following:

1. Bag-valve-mask for positive pressure ventilation (PPV) (see Figure 33.1)
2. Oral and nasopharyngeal airways, tongue blade
3. Laryngoscope + blade selection
4. Supraglottic device and endotracheal tubes with lubricant
5. Succinylcholine and syringe
6. McGill forceps
7. Cricothyroid cannula with jet ventilation cannula
8. Suction catheter
9. Flexible stylet
10. Disposable CO_2 monitor

Respiratory problems should immediately be identified as pathophysiologic (hyperventilation, hypoventilation, apnea, chest wall rigidity) or obstructive (supraglottic, glottic, or subglottic) (see Table 33.1). Mechanical problems are also possible, such as accidental extubation, kinked tubing, disconnected tubing, or failure to properly adjust the pop-off valve in an intubated patient. Most mechanical problems are immediately obvious and rapidly corrected.

Physiologic respiratory problems

Hyperventilation

Hyperventilation is defined as an increase in the frequency (tachypnea) and/or depth or volume (hyperpnea) of respiration greater than that required for metabolic needs, resulting in a decrease in $PaCO_2$ (partial pressure of carbon dioxide in arterial blood). The etiology is variable, because of both voluntary and involuntary control of ventilation. Hysteria, anxiety, and some cases of "postanesthetic delirium" can lead to a conscious (or semi-conscious) urge to hyperventilate, while unconscious control stems from subcortical input, including hypoxemia as detected by peripheral chemoreceptors (carotid bodies) and a hypercarbia-induced increase in $[H^+]$, as detected by central chemoreceptors. The resultant tachypnea increases all lung volumes, making it more difficult for the hysterical patient to "take a deep breath and calm down." This inability to take a deep breath triggers further anxiety, exacerbating the problem. Theoretically, rapid but shallow "to and fro" air movement can lead to the reverse situation: hypoxia and hypercarbia, although this is a rare clinical situation.

The resultant respiratory alkalosis increases the affinity of oxygen to hemoglobin, resulting in an increased uptake in the lungs AND a decreased release at the tissue level. Alkalosis triggers vasoconstriction, notably in both coronary and cerebrovascular vessels. It also leads to electrolyte shifts including a decrease in potassium and a decrease in ionized calcium (due to increased binding of ionized calcium to serum albumin with alkalosis). These chemical changes lead to the clinical picture that is often associated with hyperventilation, including dizziness, confusion, visual impairment, syncope, seizure, and peripheral paresthesias (particularly lips, fingers, and

Anesthesia Complications in the Dental Office, First Edition. Edited by Robert C. Bosack and Stuart Lieblich.

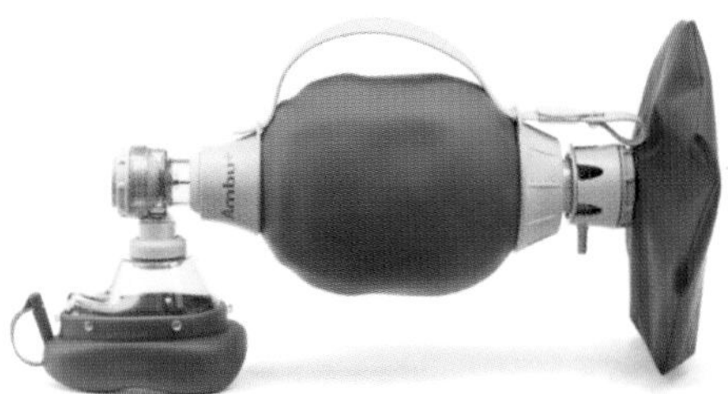

Figure 33.1 Bag-valve mask, with oxygen reservoir. Some reservoir bags supplied with nitrous oxide machines may be too elastic to permit positive pressure ventilation, courtesy of Ambu corporation.

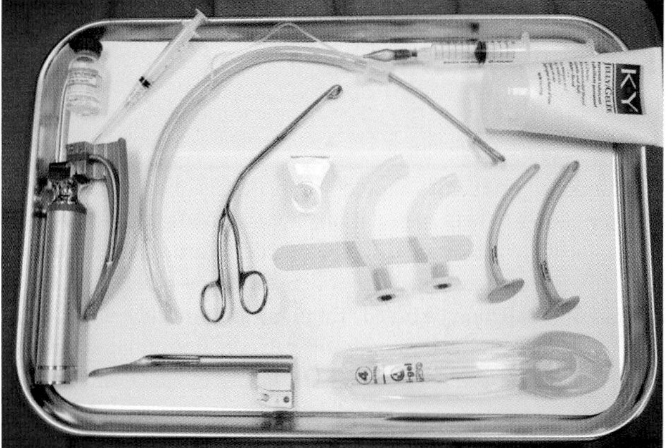

Figure 33.2 Example of airway tray.

Table 33.1 Respiratory, airway, and mechanical problems.

- Pathophysiologic
  - Hyperventilation
  - Hypoventilation
  - Drug-induced apnea
  - Chest wall rigidity
- Obstructive
  - Supraglottic – tongue falls back on posterior pharyngeal wall
  - Glottic – laryngospasm, laryngeal edema
  - Subglottic – bronchospasm, pulmonary edema, aspiration pneumonitis
  - Foreign body obstruction can occur at any level

toes), carpopedal spasm (cramping or twitching of the extremities (see Figure 33.3), tetany and muscle weakness, chest pain, and/or palpitations. These sudden onset scenarios may further upset the awake patient and aggravate the situation. Every 1 mmHg decrease in $PaCO_2$ reduces cerebral blood flow by 2%; however, this response is attenuated when $PaCO_2$ levels are less than 25 mmHg (Raichle et al., 1970).

The treatment of hyperventilation involves visual diagnosis and trigger remediation. In the acute case of conscious hysteria or panic, patience, empathy, and verbal reassurance may prove effective in some cases, while more severe situations may require anxiolytic medications. Voluntary rebreathing of expired air with a paper bag increases $PaCO_2$ in a cooperative patient, immediately reversing signs and symptoms.

Intra- or postanesthetic delirium can also trigger hyperventilation, secondary to inadequate sedation, a "stormy" anesthetic

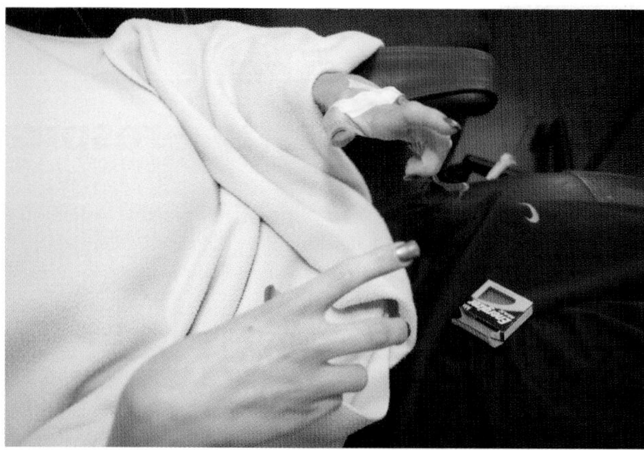

Figure 33.3 Carpopedal spasm – note involuntary flexion of the wrists and flexion-extension spasm of the finger in a hyperventilating patient.

course, or ketamine emergence delirium. While the administration of various alternate sedative, anxiolytic, or hypnotic drugs may decrease hyperventilation due to "abnormal cortical states," this course of action may be disastrous, if the "abnormal cortical state" is triggered by hypoxia from bronchospasm or pulmonary aspiration. *Agitation is always assumed to be triggered by hypoxia, until proven otherwise.*

Hypoventilation/apnea

The normal adult at rest breathes 12–15 times per minute, at a tidal (per breath) volume of 500 ml, totally 6–8 liters per minute. At rest, the body normally consumes approximately 3–4 ml O_2/kg/min and excretes 2–3 ml CO_2/kg/min. Normal $PaCO_2$ is 40 mmHg and the normal pH is 7.4.

Apnea refers to the complete absence of ventilation, while *hypoventilation* is defined as insufficient ventilation (decreased depth and/or frequency, which can lead to hypercapnia (increased $PaCO_2$) and hypoxemia (decreased PaO_2). Slow or absent ventilation is most rapidly detected by pretracheal auscultation and lack of chest wall movement, followed by capnography and finally pulse oximetry, which has the longest lag to detection. As oxygen levels decrease, cyanosis develops, as the skin color progresses from pink to white to ash and finally dark blue. Initially, hypercarbia increases anxiety; if allowed to persist and worsen, anxiety is replaced with delirium and deep sedation.

Respiratory depression is a recognized adverse side effect of narcotics, barbiturates, propofol, and benzodiazepines, especially when high doses are administered rapidly or in combination. The time to peak effect of narcotics is often delayed; subsequent impatient boluses of other drugs to quickly achieve a level of sedation can worsen respiratory depression as the effects of the narcotic reach their peak (see Table 33.2). Volatile anesthetics such as sevoflurane and isoflurane blunt the normal carotid body response to the increased H^+ concentration in hypoventilation (Stoelting and Miller, 1994). The practitioner must also be mindful of other drugs (prescribed or illicit) that the patient may be taking, such as narcotics, benzodiazepines, antihistamines, and antipsychotics, all of which can exacerbate hypoventilation.

The initial treatment of depressed ventilation depends on the intended level of sedation, the skill and practice level of the provider, the resilience of the patient, and the current SpO_2. Apnea is expected after a full induction dose of propofol prior to intubation and patients are routinely ventilated until adequate

Table 33.2 Time to peak effects of narcotics (Haas and Yagiela, 1998).

Drug	Time to peak effects (minutes)
Morphine	20
Meperidine	5–7
Fentanyl	3–5
Nalbuphine	30

levels of anesthesia are achieved. For the practitioner intending moderate sedation only, verbal, tactile, or painful stimulation can be used to encourage breathing. Drug reversal (especially opioid) can be entertained although this may take several minutes to clinical effect, and is counter-productive to the reason that the drugs were administered in the first place. Positive pressure ventilation (PPV) with a bag-valve-mask, with or without oral or nasopharygeal airways should improve the SpO_2 until the patient begins spontaneous ventilations or is connected to a ventilator.

Chest wall rigidity

Chest wall rigidity is a stiff and rigid increase in muscle tone with variable clinical presentations including glottic (Bennett et al., 1997) chest wall ("wooden chest syndrome," Coruh et al., 2013), and/or abdominal wall stiffness, often making spontaneous or PPV difficult or impossible. The mechanism is poorly understood, and for obvious reasons, this phenomenon cannot be studied, but only reported. It is usually seen soon after rapid or high doses of fentanyl, but can occur even with low doses. Vaughn and Bennett (1981) reported a case of chest wall rigidity occurring after intravenous administration of only 100 *ug* of fentanyl over 12 minutes. Ackerman et al. (1990) reported a case after two boluses of 50 *ug* fentanyl were given over 5 minutes to a 19-year-old female. Risk factors include extremes of age, dose and rapidity of opioid administration, and concomitant use of medications that alter dopamine levels (Viscomi and Bailey, 1997). Differential diagnoses include laryngospasm, bronchospasm, and complete airway obstruction.

It is often possible to maintain SpO_2 in apneic or rigid patients with an open airway, with the use of high flow 100% oxygen through a nasal cannula. Oxygen moves according to the principles of "bulk flow" (water shooting from a hose) and diffusion, the passive movement of oxygen molecules from regions of high partial pressure to low partial pressure. This technique, termed *apneic oxygenation* takes advantage of both. It is often able to maintain SpO_2 during prolonged attempts at intubation or in patients with open airway apnea (Ramachandran et al., 2010).

There are three treatment options for chest wall rigidity: narcotic reversal with naloxone, muscle relaxation with succinylcholine, or no treatment while waiting for spontaneous resolution, in instances where rigidity is triggered by short-acting opioids, such as remifentanil and where patients have been adequately preoxygenated. Attempting aggressive PPV in rigid patients will elevate intrathoracic pressure, reducing venous return leading to hypotension. The choice of reversal agent is based on the severity of the problem, the SpO_2, resilience of the patient, and the planned course of treatment. For a preoxygenated patient who is to be intubated, an intubating dose of succinylcholine (0.5 to 1.5 mg/kg) can be considered. Alternatively, the narcotic antagonist naloxone may be used, with a typical dose of 0.4 mg IV in an adult, and 10 – 100 *ug*/kg IV in children. Naloxone may be the more reasonable choice for the non-intubated patient in the outpatient setting with SpO_2 above 90%. In contrast to a neuromuscular blocker, there will be no paralysis requiring intubation or prolonged bag-mask ventilation, and if present, narcotic-induced respiratory depression will be reversed as well. Naloxone can lead to hypertension and tachycardia. In rare circumstances, cardiac arrhythmias and pulmonary edema can develop.

Obstructive airway problems

Supraglottic airway (SGA) obstruction (Figures 33.4) refers to an obstruction above the level of the vocal cords. Partial upper airway obstruction is often accompanied by audible and labored breathing, signaled by sternal retraction, flaring of nostrils, and exaggerated outward movement of the abdominal wall as the diaphragmatic descent is greater. Ventilation is often impaired, but may still be sufficient to maintain preanesthetic SpO_2, especially if the patient is breathing supplemental oxygen. With complete obstruction, ventilatory attempts (when present) can be described as a "rocking boat" movement, where jerky, exaggerated movement causes the

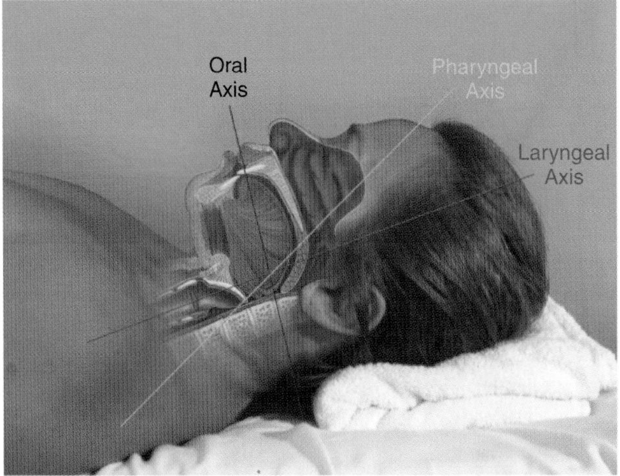

Figure 33.4 *Supraglottic airway obstruction* occurs above the level of the vocal cords. Note obstruction at the epiglottis, tongue and soft palate.

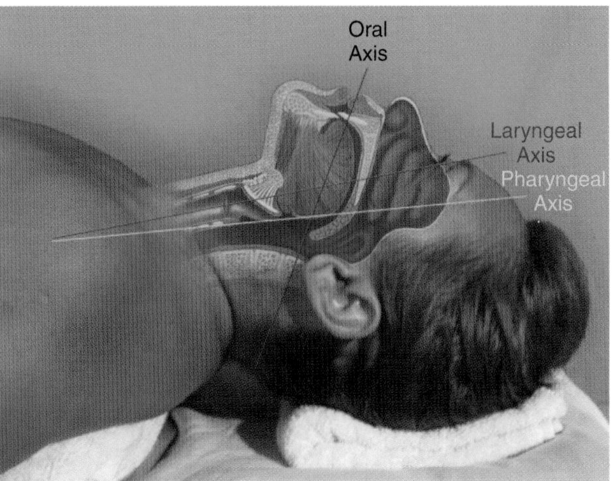

Figure 33.5 *Triple airway maneuver.* Effective opening of the airway includes flexion of the lower neck, extension of the upper neck and protrusion of the mandible to facilitate airway opening as well as direct laryngoscopy. The goal of this posturing is to optimally align the oral, pharyngeal and laryngeal axes.

chest wall to paradoxically collapse, while the abdomen protrudes (the opposite of normal, unobstructed ventilation).

The most common cause of supraglottic obstruction is relaxation of the tongue as it passively presses back to the oropharygeal wall. In these instances, a simple head tilt, chin lift, and/or jaw thrust (triple airway maneuver (see Figure 33.5) usually reopens the airway, by pulling the tongue forward and elevating the epiglottis from the posterior pharyngeal wall. When this fails, the practitioner can rotate the patient's head to the right or left approximately 30°, which can resolve the obstructions persisting after a triple airway maneuver (see Figure 33.6). Physically pulling the tongue forward with forceps, finger, or suture can also alleviate the obstruction.

Flexion of the lower neck, extension of the upper neck, and protrusion of the mandible facilitate airway opening as well as direct laryngoscopy. The goal of this posturing is to optimally align the oral, pharyngeal, and laryngeal axes (see Figure 33.5).

1. Head tilt – upper cervical extension
2. Chin lift – lower cervical flexion
3. Jaw thrust
4. Head rotation
   (a) Normal head position
   (b) Triple airway maneuver
   (c) Quadruple airway maneuver

Other adjuncts, such as placement of a nasopharyngeal airway in a conscious patient or an oropharyngeal airway (see Figure 33.7) in an unconscious patient may allow airflow past the tongue obstruction and permit adequate ventilation.

Should the presumed upper airway obstruction persist after the above maneuvers, other options will depend on the ability of the practitioner and intended level of sedation. Supraglottic devices, such as a laryngeal mask airway (LMA), iGel™, or supraglottic tube can be placed when the patient is sufficiently obtunded. Intubation can be considered as well. The possibilities of laryngospasm, bronchospasm, and foreign body obstruction should be considered.

A common reason for airway obstruction in the non-intubated, sedated patient is dental treatment on the lower arch, in which the operator is pressing down on the mandible, resulting in chin depression and tongue obstruction. Placement of the rubber dam on a posterior lower tooth can also push the tongue back and result in simple obstruction. Maneuvers described above should resolve the obstruction.

A less common reason for airway obstruction in the non-intubated patient under GA is displacement of the throat pack to the larynx or beyond. Careful attention to surgical counts and audible confirmation of pack placement and removal by the doctor with staff involvement can help prevent this occurrence. For any suspicion of a foreign object, laryngoscopy is used to inspect the hypopharynx (see Figures 33.8 and 33.9).

Glottic obstruction

Laryngospasm

Laryngospasm (see Figure 33.10) is a prolonged reflex glottic closure, maintained beyond the duration of the initiating stimulus. The duration and intensity of the spasm vary with the strength and duration of the stimulus and the depth of anesthesia. Laryngospasms are either partial (incomplete adduction of the vocal cords, associated with a high-pitched "crowing" stridor) or complete (total adduction of the vocal cords, infolding of the arytenoids and aryepiglottic folds and covered by the epiglottis, associated with total absence of air movement or airway noise) (Hagberg et al., 2008). Complete laryngospasms must be differentiated from apnea, supraglottic obstruction, chest wall rigidity, or bronchospasm.

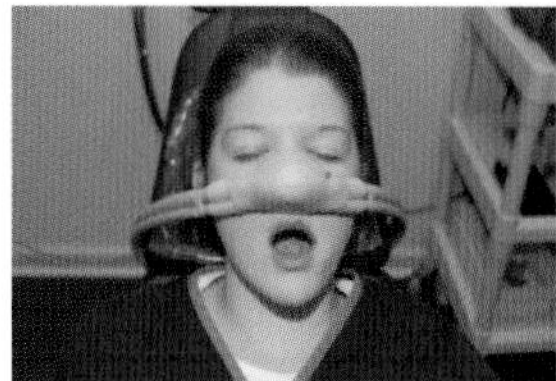
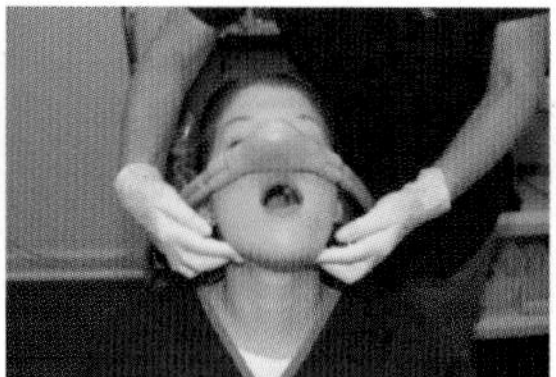
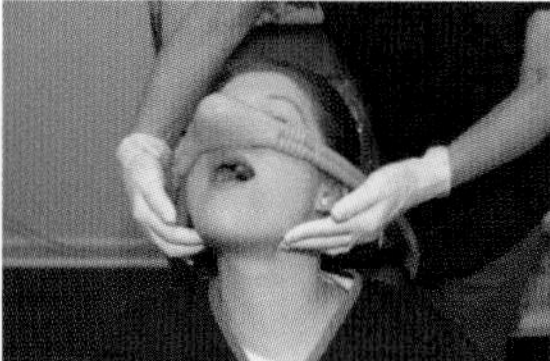

Figure 33.6 "Quadruple" airway maneuver.

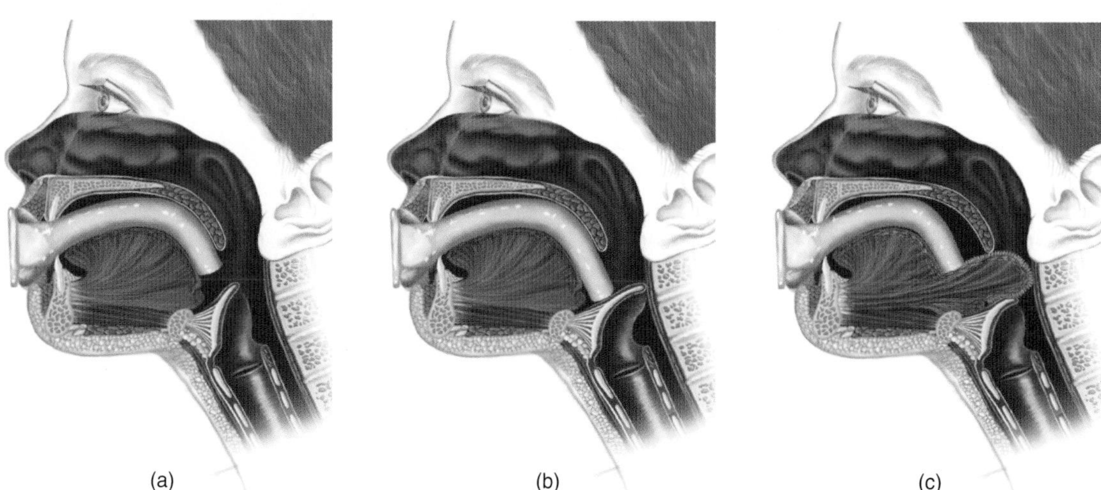

Figure 33.7 (a) Proper placement of an oropharyngeal airway. Airways that are too long (b), can obstruct the airway by pressing on the epiglottis, while airways that are too short (c) can push the tongue against the posterior pharyngeal wall, exacerbating the upper airway obstruction.

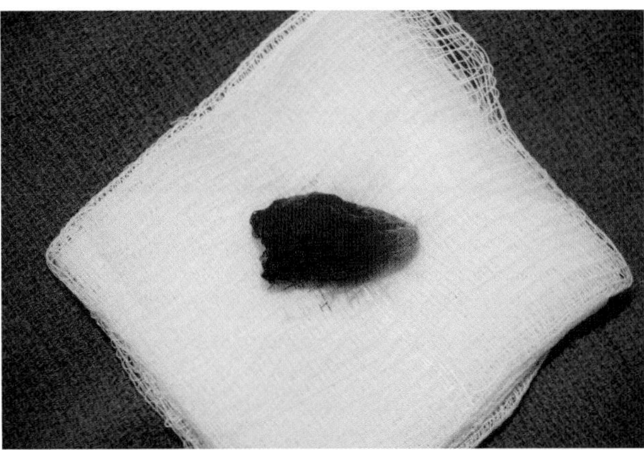

Figure 33.8 Blood soaked, untethered gauze pack, retrieved from the hypopharynx. The compressible ovoid shape can easily obstruct the airway.

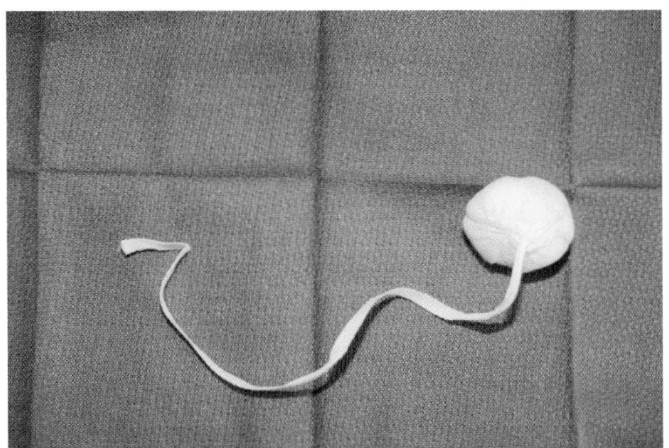

Figure 33.9 Tethered throat pack, allowing quick retrieval if displaced into the hypopharynx.

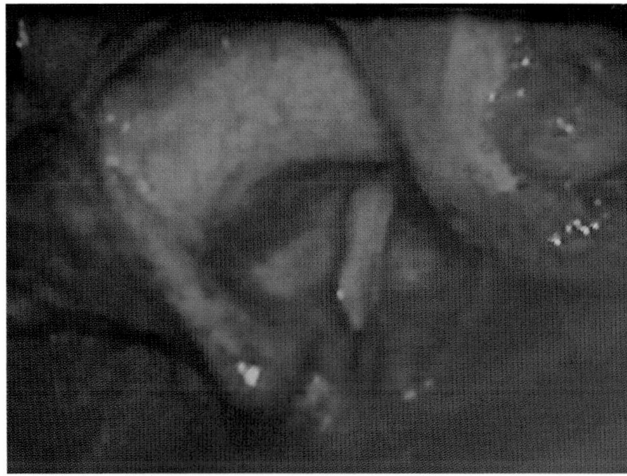

Figure 33.10 Complete laryngospasm as viewed with a videolaryngoscope. Courtesy of Dr. H. William Gottschalk.

Table 33.3 Laryngospasm risk factors.

Patient-related factors	Young age Exposure to smoke Recent URI Bronchospasm within 6 weeks (Levy et al., 1992) Upper airway anomalies
Anesthesia-related factors	Light anesthesia, painful stimuli, increased vagal tone Direct vocal cord stimulation: blood, secretions, irrigant, vomitus, LMA placement with light anesthesia Irritating anesthetic vapors – desflurane Ketamine-induced hypersecretion Barbiturates

Apnea with a patent upper airway is confirmed when a gentle push over the sternum is accompanied by the audible movement of air. Supraglottic obstruction is usually relieved with a triple or quadruple airway maneuver. Bronchospasm is often, but not always, preceded by crescendo wheezing in a patient with a history of asthma or allergy. The value of pretracheal auscultation cannot be understated in differentiating these clinical situations.

Contributory risk factors are related to both the patient and anesthesia and are shown in Table 33.3. (Al-alami et al., 2009). Avoiding these risk factors can minimize the frequency of laryngospasm. Propofol and opioids, in sufficient doses, can decrease airway responsiveness.

Consequences of laryngospasm include pulmonary aspiration, negative pressure pulmonary edema, hypoxemia, bradycardia, and cardiac arrest. Treatment should be quick and methodical. Immediate stabilization of the surgical site, followed in rapid sequence with pharyngeal suctioning, head-tilt, chin lift, jaw thrust, and head rotation often resolve the spasm. This maneuver elevates the hyoid, thereby stretching the epiglottis and aryepiglottic folds to facilitate laryngeal opening. Gentle positive pressure "flutter" ventilation distends the pharynx and can "tease" the vocal cords open. Firm inward, upward, and forward digital pressure in the depression inferior to the earlobe (laryngospasm notch) is often referenced (Larson, 1998), followed by gentle PPV with 100% oxygen via a full face mask, coordinated with inspiratory attempts if present. If open airway stage 3 anesthesia is intended and it is perceived that the patient may be too light with the resultant entry into stage 2 (the excitement plane of anesthesia), a bolus of a hypnotic such as propofol is typically given to deepen the anesthetic. If the patient is meant to be in conscious sedation and it is thought the patient has drifted too deep and into stage 2, reversal of the narcotic and possibly the benzodiazepine with naloxone and flumazenil will lighten the anesthetic depth, at which point the laryngospasm may break spontaneously. Many practitioners can be burdened with concern that deepening anesthesia might aggravate the situation, leading to a potential fatal outcome. However, the negative intrathoracic pressures generated with inspiration against a closed glottis often aggravate an upper airway obstruction and allow the persistence of unwanted airway reflexes.

If the spasm will not break, or breaks and recurs shortly thereafter, an IV dose of succinylcholine at 0.1 to 1 mg/kg (10–20mg) is administered as the definitive treatment, as per the training and experience of the provider. If a second dose is necessary, it should be increased to a full intubating dose of 1–2mg/kg. The metabolite succinylmonocholine is vagotonic, and may can trigger bradycardia in pediatric patients or with larger doses. Atropine (0.02 mg/kg IV) can be administered to attenuate this response. The short-term paralysis will relax the vocal cords and allow ventilation of the patient, although supraglottic obstruction can complicate the situation. Oftentimes, the patient will have to be manually ventilated until the effects of the succinylcholine are terminated. Alternatively, 2 ml of 1% lidocaine can be administered transtracheally or as bilateral superior laryngeal nerve blocks (Lewis, 2007). Interestingly, succinylcholine can improve facemask ventilation (Ikeda et al., 2012); however, its use can also exacerbate upper airway obstruction, especially when facemask ventilation is performed incorrectly.

Laryngospasm can occur in patients prior to intravascular access, such as during a mask induction on a child with oxygen and sevoflurane. In these instances, the use of succinylcholine or rocuronium intramuscularly can be considered. Reynolds et al. (1996) studied the intubating conditions of intramuscular rocuronium in children and determined that at a dose of 1.8 mg/kg, all children had adequate or good to excellent intubating conditions at 3 minutes. This correlates well with intramuscular succinylcholine, which at the recommended pediatric dose of 4 mg/kg produces maximal neuromuscular blocking effects at 3.5 minutes (Liu et al., 1981) although vocal cord relaxation may occur quicker. While the intramuscular route (deltoid, submental, intralingual) is not as fast as the intravenous route, it can be considered where intravenous access is difficult or impossible in the clinical time frame necessary. In patients where succinylcholine is contraindicated, such as history of malignant hyperthermia, the use of rocuronium can be considered. The onset of rocuronium 0.6 mg/kg intravenously occurs in 1–2 minutes (as compared to 30–60 seconds for succinylcholine). This is currently the fastest onset of any non-depolarizing muscle relaxant which allows its consideration in this emergency setting. It is likely that non-medical treatment will resolve partial laryngospasm, while muscle relaxants will frequently be necessary for complete laryngospasm.

Laryngeal edema

Perianesthetic laryngeal edema (see Figure 33.11) is a rare, completely unexpected expression of a severe allergic reaction, which can easily be mistaken for laryngospasm or bronchospasm, which usually accompanies it. Diagnosis is either implied by the presence of hives or angioedema or by laryngoscopy. Epinephrine is the most efficient treatment of anaphylaxis. Airway support and intubation are challenging. Laryngeal edema can also be possible after multiple traumatic intubation attempts.

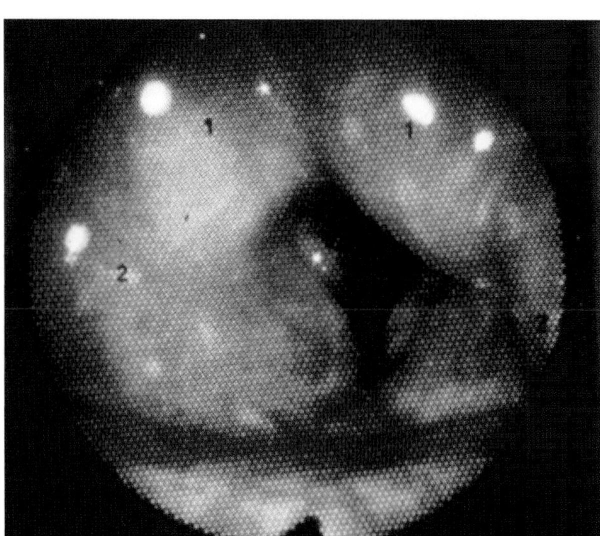

Figure 33.11 Endoscopic view of laryngeal edema.

Subglottic obstruction

Bronchospasm

Bronchospasm is a reversible constriction of the bronchiolar smooth muscle. Bronchial airway hyper-responsiveness is usually sustained by chronic inflammation, which contributes to airway obstruction (Liccardi et al., 2012). This increase in resistance leads to an increase in the work of breathing, with reduction in the ability to exhale and an increase in the time needed to do so. CO_2 retention accompanies hyperinflation of the lungs leading to tachypnea, which further interrupts exhalation. Increased intrathoracic pressures diminish venous return and obstruct right ventricular outflow, leading to hypotension. Common causes of this uncommon problem in the dental office include asthma (major risk factor), anaphylaxis, aspiration, foreign body, and physical irritation of the upper airway, including laryngospasm. A bronchospastic component is also possible with pulmonary edema. In the sedated patient with an open airway, the spectrum of signs include dropping SpO_2 (in spite of supplemental oxygen,) expiratory wheezing, unexplained tachycardia, and in severe cases, hypotension. Resistance to inspiratory airflow similar to narcotic-induced chest wall rigidity can also occur. When ventilation is still possible, although severely reduced, the capnograph will display a prolonged upstroke, indicating resistance to exhalation. The incidence of perioperative bronchospasm can occur in up to 9% of asthmatic patients (Kumeta et al., 1995).

Prevention can be maximized by a thorough history (see Table 33.4), identification of risk factors (see Table 33.5), and preanesthetic auscultation of the lungs, all of which can inform case refusal. Recent escalation of required doses of inhaled short-acting β-agonists (SABAs) may signal downregulation of the β-receptors, indicating loss of drug efficacy. In this situation, increased SABA use will exacerbate its adverse side effects – tremors, tachycardia, dysrhythmias, and hypokalemia. Importantly, there is a subset of patients with only a mild history of asthma who can experience sudden, severe bronchospasm, which can rapidly become fatal (Soubra and Guntuypalli, 2005; Rodrigo et al., 2004; Restrepo and

Table 33.4 Pulmonary history signaling increased risk of bronchospasm.

- Long history of poorly controlled asthma
- Recent drug escalation to manage symptoms, especially the addition of steroids
- Prior recent (6 weeks) hospitalizations
- Need of >2 cannisters of short-acting β-agoinst inhalers (SABA)
- Non-compliance with medication

Table 33.5 *Risk factors* for bronchospasm.

- Stress
- Obesity
- Recent exposure to triggers (smoke, weather, allergens, exercise)
- Recent URI
- Low socioeconomic status
- Gastro-esophageal reflux disease
- Physical airway stimulation – cough, laryngospasm, intubation

Peters, 2008). This presentation is thought to be more bronchospastic and less inflammatory, which will respond quicker to inhaled SABA when administered early.

Reversible components of respiratory disease should be optimized prior to anesthesia. Prophylactic pretreatment with SABAs is a common and advisable practice. Acute downregulation of β-receptors with this one-time administration is unlikely. Smoking cessation is recommended whenever possible (Shi and Warner, 2011).

The choice of anesthetic drugs and technique can influence the incidence of bronchospasm. Anesthetic drugs such as benzodiazepines and opioids are known to depress oropharyngeal muscle tone, ventilation, laryngeal reflexes, and the ability to cough. These factors can aggravate bronchospasm. With the exception of desfluane, inhaled anesthetic agents are bronchodilators and can attenuate intraoperative bronchospasm (Brown, 2000). Asthmatic patients have been shown to have a greater incidence of wheezing when exposed to barbiturates, versus propofol, which is mild bronchodilator (Pizov et al., 1995). Avoidance of drugs that cause significant histamine release, such as morphine, meperidine, and muscle relaxants is prudent. Ketamine produces a decrease in airway resistance. Adequate depth of anesthesia is imperative, as light anesthesia can also precipitate a spasm. The use of an endotracheal tube is also a risk factor, but inhaled agents coupled with propofol induction and adequate depth of anesthesia can help minimize this risk. Since the endotracheal tube is a powerful stimulus for bronchial constriction, extubation under deep anesthesia, in the absence of contraindicating factors should be considered.

Diagnosis of unanticipated bronchospasm can be challenging (see Table 33.6) When awake, patients are agitated, wheezing is often audible, and ventilation is labored, leaving only minimal time to speak in words or short phrases. Suprasternal retraction is often noted. Tachycardia, tachypnea, and dropping SpO_2 in spite of supplemental oxygenation are worrisome late findings, which can herald complete obstruction (silent chest) and cardiac arrest. "Shark-fin" capnography tracing verifies exhalation that is difficult and prolonged. Intubated cases will demonstrate increased airway pressures with prolonged expiration.

Treatment of bronchospasm during anesthesia involves prompt differential diagnosis and relaxation of bronchial smooth muscle to permit adequate ventilation. The oxygen concentration should be increased to 100% and manual bag ventilation started. During open airway cases, a variety of adapters can be used to administer SABAs with a full face mask (see Figures 33.12–33.15) Cannisters can be readily coupled to breathing circuits for intubated patients, where boluses of propofol or ketamine or increasing the concentration of volatile agent can also be entertained. If repeated SABA therapy is unsuccessful, immediate triage to emergency medical services should be contemplated. Epinephrine should be administered, either 0.15–0.3 mg deep IM or as 50 to 100 mgm intravenous boluses, as necessary. If there is associated cardiovascular collapse suggestive of IgE-mediated anaphylaxis, 0.1 mg (1cc of a 1:10,000

Table 33.6 Differential diagnosis of bronchospasm during anesthesia.

- Laryngospasm
- Chest wall rigidity
- Anaphylaxis
- Obstruction in breathing circuit with intubated patients
- Aspiration
- Pulmonary edema

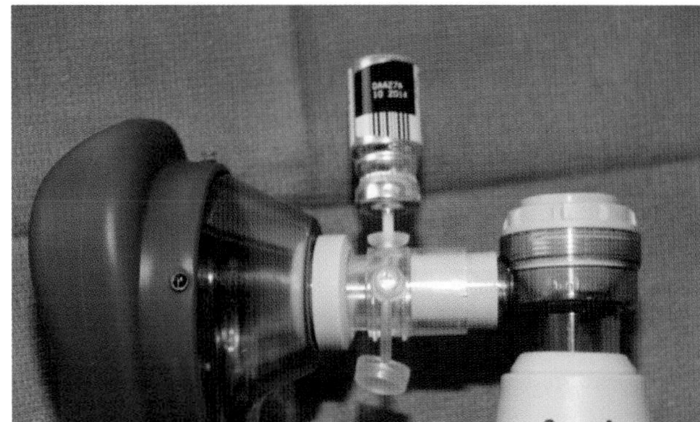

Figure 33.12 In-line delivery of inhaled SABA during facemask ventilation.

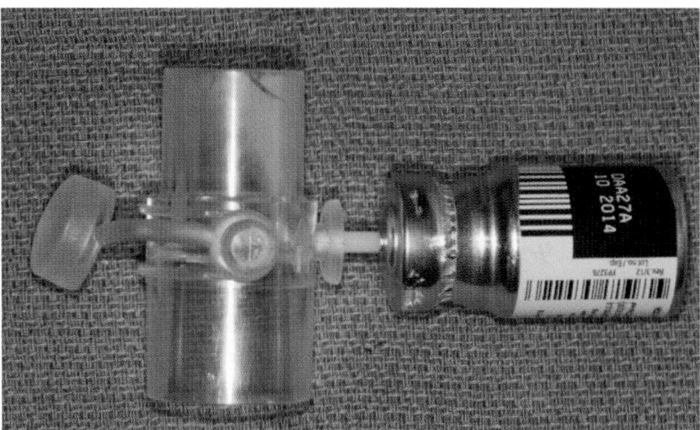

Figure 33.13 Close up view of inhaler adapter.

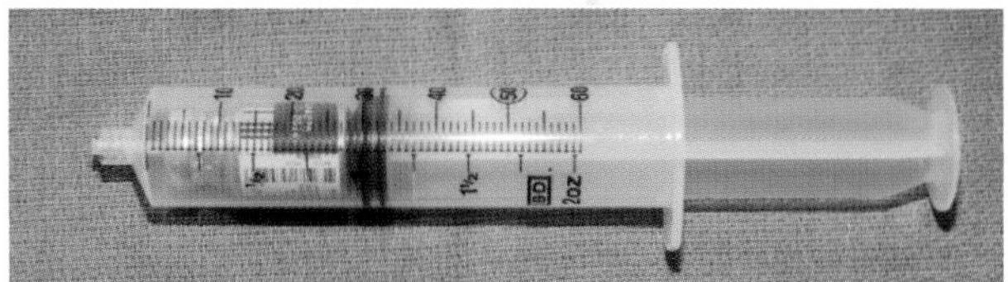

Figure 33.14 Inhaler placed in a 60cc syringe.

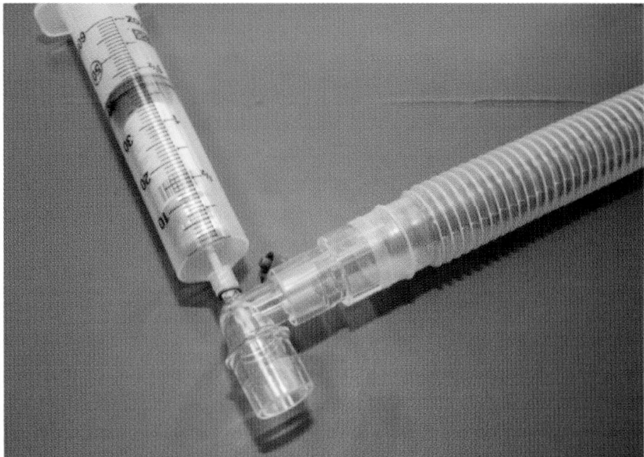

Figure 33.15 Luer Lock adapter on a 90° connector.

solution of epinephrine should be administered IV slowly over 5 minutes (Levy, 2008). Hydrocortisone 1 mg/kg IV can also be administered in spite of a delayed onset of action.

Negative pressure pulmonary edema (NPPE)

Pulmonary edema is an increased amount of fluid in interstitial spaces, which can eventually diffuse across respiratory membranes to accumulate in the pulmonary alveoli. Fluid accumulates as a result of various disease processes, which lead to increased pulmonary capillary hydrostatic pressure, increased pulmonary capillary permeability, and/or decreased alveolar pressure, among others. This presence of fluid decreases lung compliance, impairs gas diffusion, and makes lung expansion difficult. Functional residual capacity is decreased. Pathologic shunting occurs (perfusion of blood to non-ventilated portions of the lung) leading to hypoxemia.

In otherwise healthy patients presenting for dental treatment, the differential diagnosis of pulmonary edema is somewhat limited and includes iatrogenic fluid overload, anaphylaxis (bronchospasm), or severe and/or prolonged negative airway pressure. The two principle mechanisms for its development are increased hydrostatic pressure (NPPE) and increased capillary permeability (anaphylaxis and aspiration).

Negative pressure pulmonary edema (Type I, Udeshi et al., 2000) occurs as a rapid (minutes) or delayed response (hours) (Glasser and Siler, 1985) to an airway obstruction (laryngospasm, bronchospasm, aspiration, kinked endotracheal tube) where vigorous or prolonged inspiratory attempts (especially from fit and muscular patients) generate high negative intrathoracic pressure. This increases the pulmonary vascular volume and pressure, while decreasing interstitial hydrostatic pressure and alveolar pressure, such that fluid moves from the capillary beds at a rate that is greater than that which can be reclaimed by lymphatics. In severe cases, disruption of the fragile respiratory membrane can occur, as shown in animal studies (West et al., 1991; Tsukimoto et al., 1991). The ensuing hypoxia (Ciavarro and Kelly, 2002) leads to sympathetic discharge further increasing volume and pressure in the pulmonary vascular beds. Hypoxia stimulates pulmonary vascular constriction, which can increase the afterload to the right heart and decrease the preload to the left heart. The sympathetic discharge also increases systemic vascular resistance, leading to increased afterload. Cardiac output falls, oxygenation of blood is hampered, and oxygen delivery to tissues is negatively affected.

Obvious triggers include laryngospasm, prolonged snoring, inadvertent excess fluid administration (unlikely), or anaphylaxis, which typically has a rapid onset and is often accompanied by hives, angioedema, excess secretions, and hypotension. Allergy is also entertained with exposure to known or unknown allergens, such as latex, antibiotics, or muscle relaxants. Diagnosis is confirmed with the onset of rapid, shallow, labored breathing, unexplained tachycardia, and hypoxemia. Auscultation of the chest reveals wheezing and crackles. Cough can be productive with a pink, frothy sputum. The incidence is approximately 1 in 1000 patients (Krodel et al., 2010). Patients will become tachypneic, with obvious suprasternal retraction and paradoxical "rocking boat" chest and abdominal wall movement.

Treatment of pulmonary edema is based on remediation of the trigger, improving ventilation, and waiting for or facilitating reduction of interstitial pulmonary fluid. In the case of negative pressure pulmonary edema, the immediate cause, such as laryngospasm, must be corrected. Office management includes 100% oxygen delivery via a non-rebreather face mask or PPV as required to maintain oxygen saturation. The administration of SABA aerosol helps dilate bronchioles and increase the rate of fluid clearance (Mathay et al., 2000). Emergent transfer to a medical facility is considered when patients are unable to maintain $SpO_2 >$ 90%, where diuresis and continuous positive pressure ventilatory assistance can be instituted, if deemed necessary. In most cases, acute negative pressure postoperative pulmonary edema typically responds to conservative treatment. Full recovery typically occurs in 12–48 hours with early recognition and treatment.

Aspiration/foreign body ingestion

Aspiration is the soiling of the lower airways with oral, pharyngeal, or gastric contents. Requirements include the presence of sufficient volume of inoculum or particulate matter at or near the larynx along with depression or absence of the protective reflexes of coughing, swallowing, and gagging. Blood, irrigation, teeth, or tooth particles, dental materials (crowns, fillings, screws, etc.), and blood-soaked gauze can come from the oral cavity, especially in the absence of effective oropharygeal partitions (see Figure 33.16 and 33.17). Solid food or acidic gastric juice can come from the stomach, especially in patients who have not fasted sufficiently or in patients with higher gastric pressures, delayed emptying, and altered lower esophageal sphincter tone. Aspiration of solids can lead to physical obstruction in the airway and/or trigger bronchospasm in susceptible patients, while aspiration of acidic gastric juice can chemically irritate airway mucosa, leading to an asthma-like condition termed *aspiration pneumonitis* ("Mendelson's syndrome," Mendelson, 1946; Marik, 2001) with associated tachypnea, dyspnea, wheezing, tachycardia, and hypoxemia. Time of onset and severity of symptoms depends on several factors, including the type and volume of aspirate, susceptibility of the patient, and appropriateness of early treatment measures. Historically, a liquid aspirate with a $pH < 2.5$ and volume greater than 25 ml has been associated with more severe sequelae, although the validity of these cut-off numbers has been questioned. Since the dentist will not be able to measure either of these parameters, the point is moot.

The incidence of aspiration during general anesthesia ranges from 1.4 to 6.5 per 10,000 cases with a mortality rate of 5% (Ferson et al., 2008). Risk factors are listed in Table 33.7.

Prevention is best accomplished by ensuring adequate preoperative fasting (see Table 33.8), depth of anesthesia limiting setting or case refusal. The routine use of gastrointestinal stimulants, gastric acid secretion blockers, antacids, preoperative antiemetics, or preoperative anticholinergics is not recommended for patients who have no apparent increased risk for pulmonary aspiration (ASA

Table 33.7 Risk factors for aspiration.

- Morbid obesity
- Gastroesophageal reflux disease (decreased lower esophageal sphincter tone)
- Status post bariatric surgery
- Eating disorders, especially bulimia
- Difficult airways
- Diabetic gastroparesis
- opioid administration
- Young age
- Light anesthesia
- Impaired airway reflexes
- Gastric motility disorders
- Non-compliance with fasting requirements

Table 33.8 Fasting guidelines (ASA Practice Guidelines, 2011).

- Clear liquids – 2 hours
    - includes water, fruit juice without pulp, carbonated beverages, clear tea, and black coffee. Alcohol is not included
- Breast milk – 4 hours
- Infant formula – 6 hours
- Light meal and nonhuman milk – 6 hours
- Fried or fatty foods – 8 hours

Practice Guidelines, 2011). An effective oropharyngeal drape will help eliminate movement of particulate matter from the oral cavity into the hypopharynx (see Figures 33.16 and 33.17).

A common misconception is that aspiration must be witnessed to confirm diagnosis. Aspiration should be suspect with any laryngospasm, bronchospasm, or unexplained desaturation or change in vital signs. Symptoms can range from none to complete airway obstruction. In the case of lost view of a foreign body, a determination must be rapidly attempted to assess whether the object has entered the larynx or the esophagus. Signs and symptoms of aspiration can include cough, laryngospasm, wheezing, dyspnea, cyanosis, tachycardia, and hypoxemia as determined by dropping SpO_2. Esophageal displacement of foreign bodies may be void of clinical symptoms in the anesthetized patient.

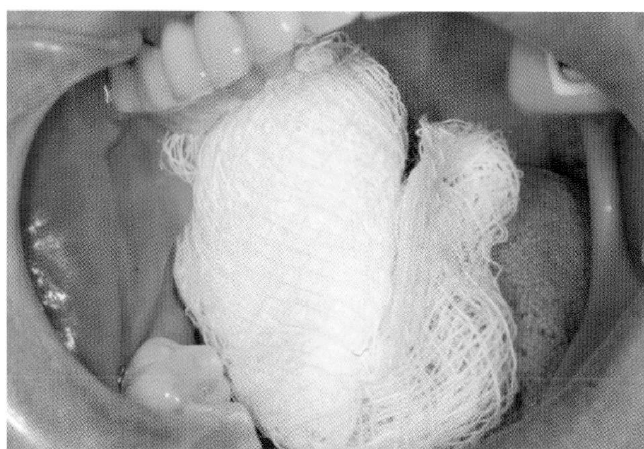

Figure 33.16 Inadequate oropharyngeal drape.

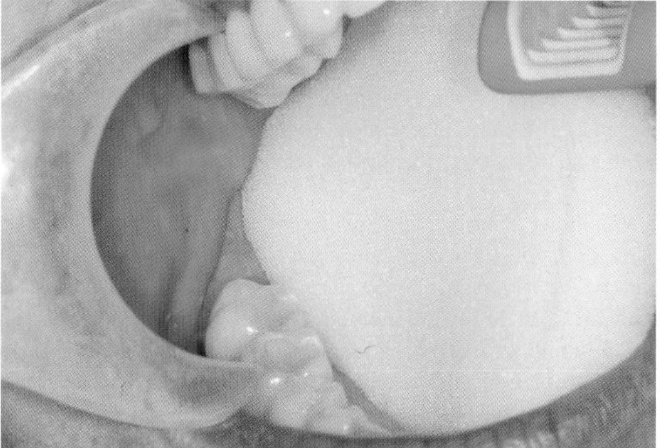

Figure 33.17 Water absorbent foam pad provides a complete oropharyngeal partition.

Acidic fluid is quite damaging to respiratory mucosa, in spite of a rapid mucosal buffering. This chemical burn is heralded by an anticipated and immediate (20 seconds) bronchospasm and an inflammatory response of vasodilation and increase in capillary permeability resulting in an exudate that can extend through the alveolar basement membrane and into the capillary endothelial cells. Compliance is negatively affected as the surfactant becomes inactivated and atelectasis and pulmonary edema ensue. Alveolar hypoxia and arterial hypoxemia are the end points and the hallmark signs of aspiration pneumonitis. Inflammatory cells appear within 1–2 hours.

Treatment of suspected or confirmed aspiration of gastric fluids/emesis focuses on the prevention of further airway involvement and management of the current clinical situation. Surgical sites are stabilized, and the patient is immediately placed in a Trendelenburg position, right side down position. The right mainstem bronchus is likely to be soiled first as it is larger and more in line with the trachea. The posture is meant to keep the aspirate on the right side and prevent it from diffusing further down the bronchiolar tree, while sparing involvement of the left mainstem bronchus. Immediate and frequent oropharygneal suction should be done. Gentle PPV with an oxygen-enriched full face mask aims to increase functional residual capacity and facilitate gas exchange. Steroids are generally not helpful (Sukumaran et al., 1980). Prophylactic antibiotics are also not indicated.

It is difficult to ascertain the true rate of aspiration during open airway anesthesia, as clinically insignificant aspiration lacks clinical signs or symptoms. Ten to thirty percent of anesthesia-related deaths are associated with cases where anesthesia-related aspiration leads to acute lung injury (Pisegna and Martindale, 2005).

When aspiration is only suspect, the dentist will be faced with a treatment decision. It is currently felt (Warner et al., 1993) that if cough or wheezing does not develop within 2 hours of the incident and if SpO_2 is within 10% of preoperative values on room air and greater than 92–93%, discharge to home can be allowed. There is no value to performing bronchoscopy or deep tracheal lavage unless there is particular matter which can be retrieved, as deep suctioning will only worsen the outcome.

Foreign body ingestion

Loss of any object to the hypopharynx, regardless of whether the final location can be determined requires immediate assessment, suction, retrieval as indicated, and stabilization of the patient. Aspiration should always be presumed, and the patient placed in a right side down, Trendelenburg position, as a likely location is the right mainstem bronchus (Figure 33.18). This position, which can make PPV more difficult, tends to "keep" the potential foreign body cephalad and on the right side (if in fact it was there in the first place), where retrieval is easier. Pulmonary assessment for sufficient ventilation and emergency treatment such as reintubation with suctioning, PPV, immediate referral, or in the case of a small swallowed object, discharge to home must occur with appropriate referral and long term follow-up.

Ingestion of a foreign body into the esophagus is often devoid of symptoms in the anesthetized patient. For objects still in the pharynx, laryngoscopy and use of Magill forceps can facilitate retrieval. Objects entering the trachea may be retrieved if a portion is still visible through the vocal cords. Mild cricoid pressure can force a tooth that has slid inferior to the vocal cords to be pushed superiorly into the pharynx for retrieval with Magills forceps. If a complete airway obstruction occurs, open the airway and visually

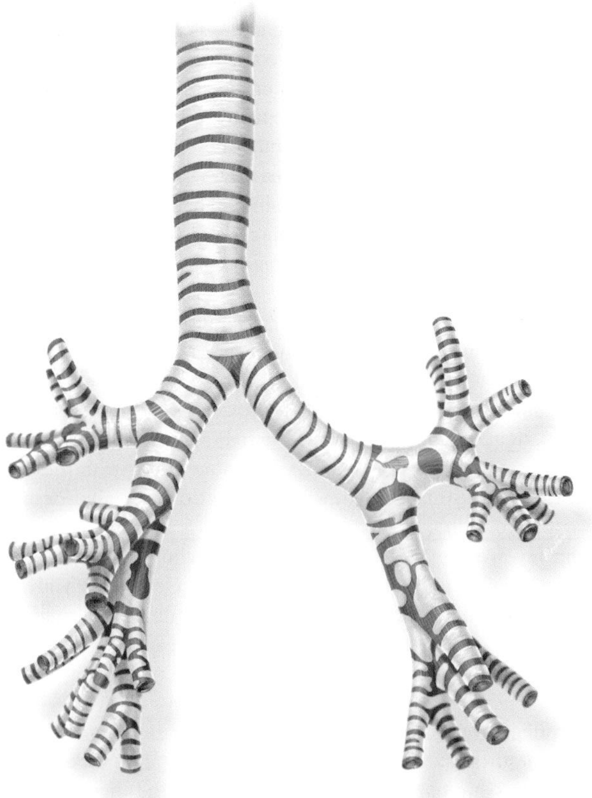

Figure 33.18 Trachea and mainstem bronchi. Note a wider right mainstem bronchus more inline with the trachea

examine the oropharynx for the presence of the suspected foreign body and remove if visible ("hook and look"). In the sedated patient, 30 chest compressions should be performed at a rate of 100 per minute, followed by 2 ventilations after checking the oral cavity for the presence of the foreign body. For objects that are not retrievable past the vocal cords, bronchoscopy will be urgently required for definitive treatment. For objects that have entered the esophagus, abdominal radiographs are indicated if the object is radiopaque, such as a tooth. Endoscopy is indicated for sharp objects, or non-radiopaque or elongated objects that pose a high risk of esophageal injury. Endoscopy is also indicated for objects that have a diameter of 2 cm, a length of 5–7 cm, and are eccentrically shaped and prone to perforation or enlodgement (Parolia et al., 2009). Symptoms of an object passing through the GI tract can include abdominal distension, discomfort, fever, vomiting, and passing of rectal blood. Small, rounded objects with a width of less than 2 cm and a length less than 6 cm can be discharged to home with strict instructions to return immediately if any symptoms of enlodgement or perforation develop. Perforation of the esophagus can cause acute mediastinitis. Symptoms include chest pain, dyspnea, and pain upon swallowing. Perforation below the esophagus will cause symptoms of acute peritonitis, and includes abdominal pain, fever, sinus tachycardia, possible diffuse abdominal rigidity, and development of ileus paralyticus (intestinal paralysis), which can cause nausea and vomiting. CT scan of the abdomen can be useful in locating the trapped object and is the image of choice if perforation and/or abscess is suspected.

Table 33.9 Difficult airway definitions.

Difficult airway: the clinical situation in which a conventionally trained anesthesiologist experiences difficulty with facemask ventilation of the upper airway, difficulty with tracheal intubation, or both.
Difficult facemask or supraglottic airway (SGA) ventilation: the clinical situation where it is not possible for the anesthesiologist to provide adequate ventilation because of one or more of the following problems: inadequate mask or SGA seal or excessive resistance to ingress or egress of gas. Signs can include absent chest wall movement, loss of breath sounds, wheezing, cyanosis, gastric distension, dropping SpO_2, inability to detect expired CO_2, hypoxia, tachycardia, and/or arrhythmia.
Difficult SGA placement: SGA placement requires multiple attempts.
Difficult laryngoscopy: It is not possible to visualize any portion of the vocal cords after multiple attempts at conventional laryngoscopy.
Difficult tracheal intubation: Tracheal intubation requires multiple attempts.
Failed intubation: Placement of the endotracheal tube fails after multiple attempts.

Adapted from ASA practice guidelines for the management of the difficult airway (2013)

Cannot ventilate, cannot intubate (CVCI)

The "cannot ventilate, cannot intubate" lost airway scenario can be terrifying for the dentist and life-threatening for the patient, demanding rapid sequence evaluation and treatment in a most stressful and time-urgent setting. Although "patient factors" and clinical circumstance play a role, the CVCI predicament is often provider dependent. This emphasizes the importance of case selection, knowledge, experience, skill, and preparation in airway management. Inability to ventilate can result from upper airway obstruction, laryngospasm, chest wall rigidity, aspiration, bronchospasm, or mechanical obstruction in the breathing circuit.

It remains elusive to assign a predictive value to any positive findings from a history and physical examination of the airway, with the possible exception of extreme deviations from normal, such as TMJ ankylosis, tracheal stenosis, rapid hemorrhagic swelling of the tongue or oropharynx, laryngeal angioedema, or compressive tumor, among others. All methods used to predict difficult airways lack both specificity and sensitivity. A conservative approach to airway evaluation can be aptly phrased: "suspicion clinches diagnosis." Case refusal, depth of sedation limit setting, or referral to another location with additional anesthesia providers are options to consider when confronted with what appears to be a patient with a difficult airway. Knowledge, preparation, experience, ability to use, and availability of advanced airway devices also inform the decision-making process. As patients can quickly and unexpectedly move between levels of sedation, practitioners should be able to rescue a lost airway for patients who slip to one level deeper than intended. Therefore, dentists planning moderate sedation should be able to rescue a patient who unintentionally falls into deep sedation.

Definitions of various difficult airway scenarios are provided in Table 33.9. The American Society of Anesthesiologists Difficult Airway Algorithm is referenced in Figure 33.19 (ASA Practice Guidelines, 2013). This document is more relevant for intubated anesthesia rather than open airway, spontaneous ventilation cases in the dental office. In the office, sedative, hypnotic, and analgesic drugs are typically titrated to preserve those parameters while providing amnesia, analgesia, anxiolysis, and behavior control. Significant changes in this document over the past 20 years are the inclusion of the LMA as a ventilatory device, followed 10 years

DIFFICULT AIRWAY ALGORITHM

1. Assess the likelihood and clinical impact of basic management problems:
   - Difficulty with patient cooperation or consent
   - Difficult mask ventilation
   - Difficult supraglottic airway placement
   - Difficult laryngoscopy
   - Difficult intubation
   - Difficult surgical airway access
2. Actively pursue opportunities to deliver supplemental oxygen throughout the process of difficult airway management
3. Consider the relative merits and feasibility of basic management choices:
   - Awake intubation vs. intubation after induction of general anesthesia
   - Non-invasive technique vs. invasive techniques for the initial approach to intubation
   - Video-assisted laryngoscopy as an initial approach to intubation
   - Preservation vs. ablation of spontaneous ventilation
4. Develop primary and alternative strategies:

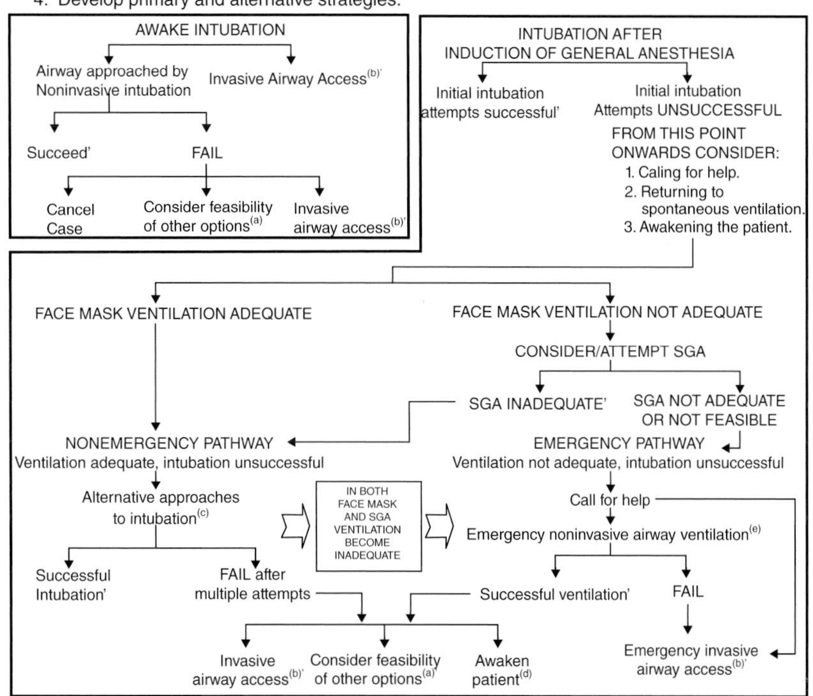

*Confirm ventilation, tracheal intubation, or SGA placement with exhaled CO_2.

a. Other options include (but are not limited to): sugery utilizing face mask or supraglottic airway (SGA) anesthesia (e.g., LMA, ILMA, Laryngeal tube), local anesthesia infiltration or regional nerve blockada. Pursuit of these options usually implies that mask ventilation will not be problematic. Therefore, these options may be of limited value if this step in the algorithm has been reached via the Emergency Pathway.

b. Invasive airway access includes surgical or percutaneous airway, jet ventilation, and retrograde intubation.

c. Alternative difficult intubation approaches include (but are not limited to): video-assisted laryngoscopy, alternative laryngoscopy blades, SGA (e.g., LMA or ILMA) as an intubation conduit (with or without fiberoptic guidance), fiberoptic intubation intubating stylet or tube changer, light wand, and blind oral or nasal intubation.

d. Consider re-preparation of the patient for awake intubation or canceling surgery.

e. Emergency non-invasive airway ventilation consists of a SGA

Fig. 1. Difficult Airway Algorithem.

Figure 33.19 American Society of Anesthesiologists: Practice Guidelines for the Management of the Difficult Airway: An updated report. Anesthesiol 118: 251-70, 2013, with permission.

later with evaluation of difficulty in placing the SGA device or ability to maintain a seal and provide adequate ventilation. Videolaryngoscopy has been introduced as an initial means of intubation and following failed intubation with direct vision rigid laryngoscopes.

Airway assessment for patients seeking office-based sedation or anesthesia

An orderly and repeatable history and examination should be performed prior to the administration of any drug capable of reducing upper airway tone or depressing ventilatory drive. Each evaluation builds on previous findings and clinical thoughts. After the patient–doctor introduction, an impression based on a brief, "arm's length" visual inspection can be readily made. Patients with obesity, audible mouth breathing (nasal obstruction,), male gender, age > 50 years, facial hair, or A–P deficient mandible are likely to present with airway risk. A history of sleep apnea, snoring, hypertension, or excessive daytime sleepiness adds credulence to this presumption.

There are six overlapping concerns that should be addressed prior to anesthesia (ASA parameters, 2013):

1. Likelihood of airway collapse with sedatives, opioids, and hypnotics
2. Likelihood of difficult mask ventilation
3. Likelihood of difficult SGA placement and ventilation
4. Likelihood of difficult direct laryngoscopy

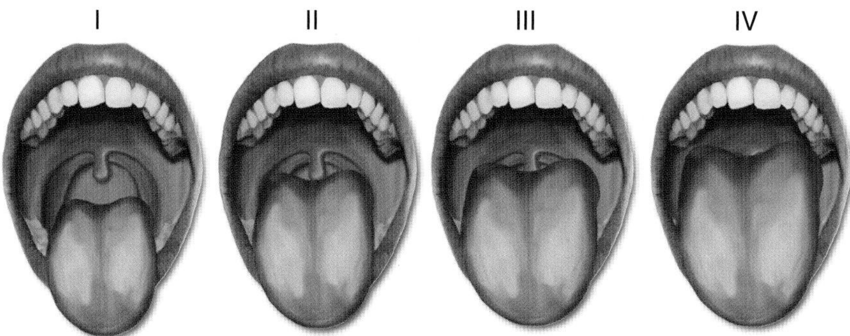

Figure 33.20 Mallampati scoring of tongue position. The size and position of the tongue are noted when the patient is asked to open wide while protruding the tongue. Class III and Class IV scores are often predictive of airway trouble, especially with other worrisome airway findings (Mallampati et al., 1985).

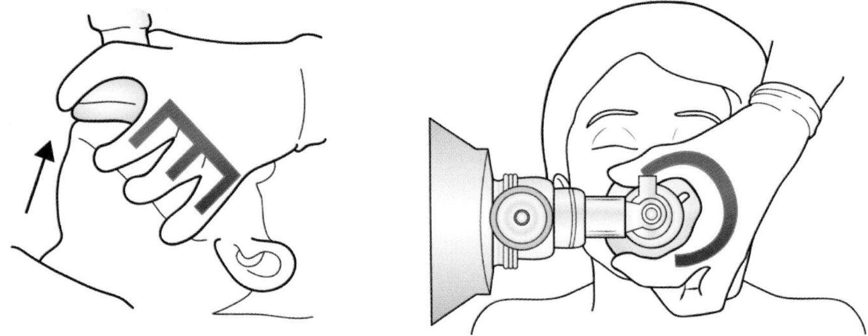

Figure 33.21 C and E positioning to maintain mask seal and head tilt, chin lift and jaw thrust.

5 Likelihood of difficult intubation
6 Likelihood of difficult surgical neck entry

Likelihood of airway collapse with sedatives, opioids or hypnotics

All muscular structures will relax to various degrees after the administration of these drugs, whether at appropriate or unintentional overdose. Airways that are already crowded in the awake state will leave little airway room after relaxation. The size and position of the tongue is characterized by the Mallampati score as shown in Figure 33.20. The tongue size is assessed as both absolute and relative to the size of the oral cavity. Narrow, constricted maxillas and retrusive, narrow mandibles with large lingual tori will make the normal-sized tongue seem large and obstructive. The depth and width of the oropharynx should also be examined, with a shallow and narrow oropharynx often having a greater tendency to obstruct (Tsai et al., 2003). The presence and size of tonsils also encroaches on airway space. Mucosal turgor may also facilitate collapse, as loose, boggy tissues are more likely pulled together during the increased negative inspiratory pressure associated with partial upper airway obstruction.

Likelihood of difficult mask ventilation

The efficacy of PPV with a full face mask is dependent on the ability to seal the mask over the mouth and nose of the patient, the size of the airway, and the resilence to lung inflation. "C" and "E" hand posturing is essential to maintaining mask seal while stabilizing the patients head in a "sniffing position." (see Figure 33.21) The seal is difficult to attain and maintain in the presence of a beard, flat nasal bridge (Oriental heritage, Trisomy 21), or with significant anterior–posterior discrepancy between the maxilla and mandible. Edentulism is accompanied by a lack of lateral cheek support and a "witch's chin" that impair mask seal. An insufficient selection of immediately available mask sizes is not helpful. Tenets of effective mask ventilation are shown in Box 33.1.

Effective mask ventilation also hinges on the ability to attain and maintain an open airway. In this instance, helpful characteristics include a flexible neck and wide range of mandibular opening and protrusion, which facilitate the triple airway maneuver that pulls the tongue forward off the posterior wall of the oropharynx.

Additional concerns relate to the size of the oral airway and patency of the larynx, trachea, and bronchi. PPV up to approximately 20 mmHg inflates the oral cavity and pushes tissues laterally. Large amounts of lateral airway adipose tissue or a strong tongue will not displace easily, necessitating pressures greater than 20 mmHg, which can inflate the stomach and encroach on lung volumes. Similarly, laryngeal obstruction, bronchospasm, pulmonary edema, rigid chest, obesity, advanced age, and pregnancy can interfere with lung inflation, especially with ineffective mask seal.

The value of simulation practice cannot be overstated. The ability to adequately perform PPV on a mannequin (see Figure 33.22) does not guarantee successful outcomes on live patients; however, the frequent, physical rehearsal of the maneuver ensures immediate availability of all equipment and facilitates a coordinated anesthesia team effort, which then allows the practitioner to focus solely on the task at hand, which is patient ventilation.

Box 33.1 Tenets of effective mask ventilation

The normal lung is very complaint and easy to distend. The normal inspiration of 500 ml requires a distending pressure of 3 cm H_2O. Similarly, the pressure required to drive gas is small, as a one liter/sec flow rate requires a pressure drop of only 2 cm H_2O (West, 2000). PPVs should be synchronized with ventilatory attempts if present. Ongoing monitoring of mask position and chest rise and fall is necessary, as one good ventilation does not guarantee efficacy of the next ventilation. Volume should be slightly less than tidal volume, but enough to observe chest rise. Overaggressive ventilation (rate and volume) leads to gastric insufflation and overinflation of the lungs, which decreases venous return, cardiac output, and blood pressure. CO_2 accumulation occurs when adequate time for passive exhalation is not permitted. Ventilatory rate should be 8–12/minute, with a cadence of 1–2 seconds per ventilation.

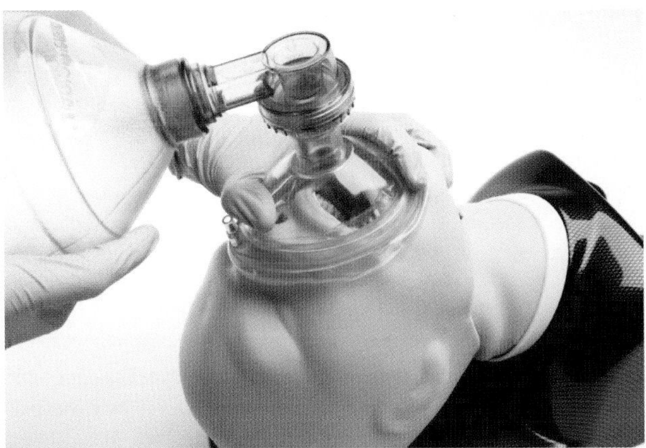

Figure 33.22 Facemask mannequin. Airsim advance, with permission, T ruCorp Ltd.

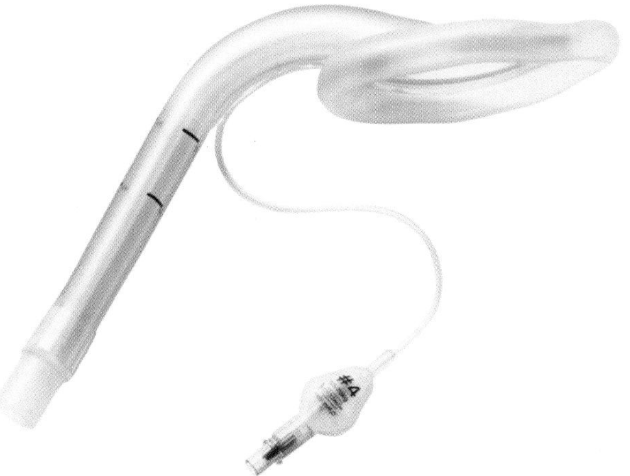

Figure 33.23 AuraOnce disposable laryngeal mask. Courtesy of Ambu corporation.

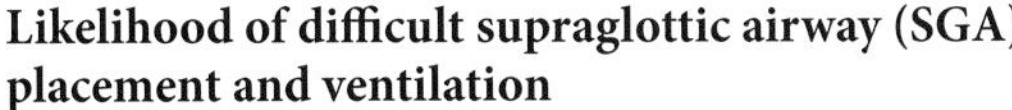

Likelihood of difficult supraglottic airway (SGA) placement and ventilation

Effective placement of an SGA with subsequent adequate ventilation requires the immediate availability of an SGA with lubrication and airway connections. The range of mandibular opening must be sufficient to pass the LMA between the incisors, approximately 20 mm. SGA ventilation will be difficult/impossible with obstruction at or below the larynx, such as due to angioedema or bronchospasm. The SGA will maintain laryngeal seal only up to approximately 20 mmHg of airway pressure, beyond which gastric inflation becomes possible. An example of a SGA is the AuraOnce® (see Figure 33.23) disposable laryngeal mask, with an angled connecting tube to facilitate placement. Problems with inflatable SGAs include shallow placement or infolding of the leading edge, both compromising an effective seal (see Figure 33.24). The iGel® SGA features a non-inflatable mask, complete with a gastric channel for suctioning and a shape that minimizes rotation (Figure 33.25). The King LT(S)-D™ is an alternate SGA, which is blindly placed into the esophagus (Figure 33.26). A single inflation port seals off both the esophagus and the oropharynx, permitting ventilation at higher pressures. A gastric suction port is also present, which aids in the decompression of inflated stomachs from prior ventilation attempts, which can promote emesis and/or interfere with descent of the diaphragm, limiting lung expansion.

Likelihood of difficult direct laryngoscopy

Direct laryngoscopy is possible when a direct line of sight to the larynx is available. This requires alignment of the oral, pharyngeal, and laryngeal axes (sniffing the morning air position), which is optimized in an anesthetized, paralyzed patient (see Figure 33.5). Attempting direct (rigid) laryngoscopy in a sedated or agitated patient can be both challenging and futile. Prominent maxillary incisors, large tongue, small mouth, and limitation of mandibular opening all interfere with this view. The laryngoscope blade is moved forward to displace the tongue laterally and anteriorly away from the line of sight. Levering the blade (Figure 33.27) displaces the larynx forward, while allowing the tongue to fall posteriorly, both of which impede the line of sight. Small tongues with ample space to accommodate displacement are ideal. A non-compliant submental space, an A–P deficient and/or small mandible and /or inability to protrude the mandible limit the potential space for tongue displacement. A high larynx also mandates exaggerated displacement of the tongue to adequately visualize the larynx. The two-fingerbreath rule estimates the thyrohyoid distance at 2 cm; shorter distances are associated with increasing difficulty of view. Direct laryngoscopy is difficult in patients who present with an anteriorly tilted larynx, as this increases the needed distance of forward tongue displacement for a straight line view (see Figure 33.28).

When a direct line of sight is difficult to attain, attention should be directed to manually moving the larynx into view. The BURP maneuver (Figure 33.29) consists of laryngeal pressure in a backward, upward, and rightward direction, which may improve the view of the glottis.

The introduction of the videolaryngoscope mitigates many issues causing difficulty with direct laryngoscopy, and renders many elements of the "traditional" airway assessment less relevant. The videolaryngoscope allows the operator to "look around corners," which facilitates laryngeal visualization as long as patients can open wide enough to allow introduction of the device into the hypopharynx. The size and position of the tongue become less important, hyperextension of the neck is not required, and there is

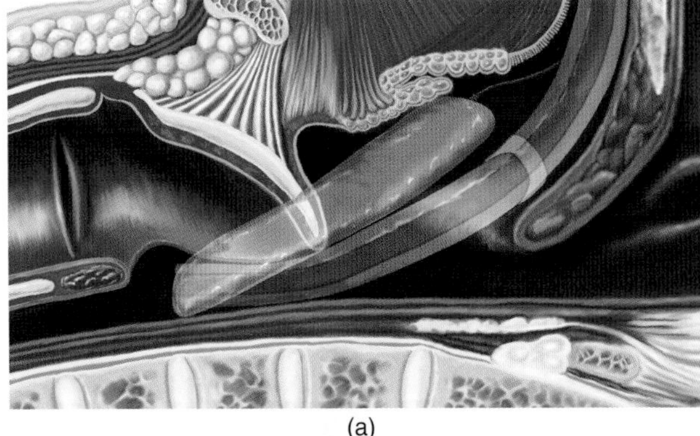

(a)

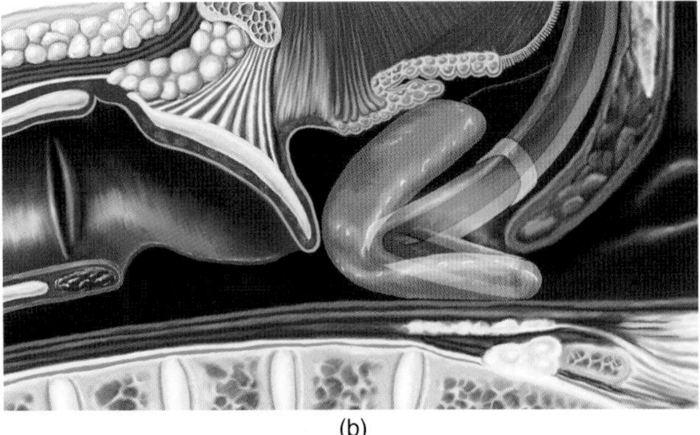

(b)

Figure 33.24 Potential problems with LMA placement. (a) Shallow placement of an LMA. (b) Infolding of the leading edge of an LMA.

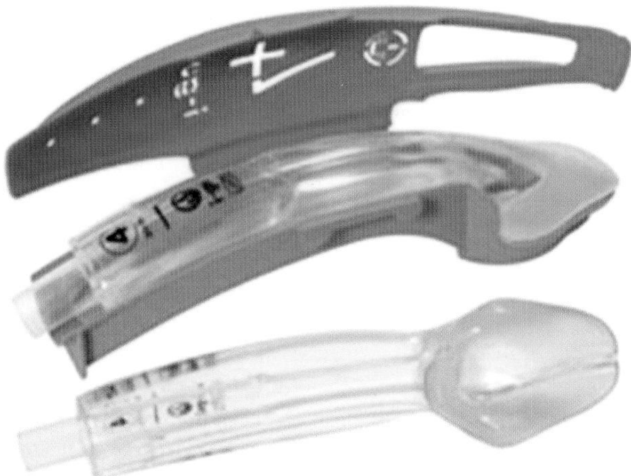

Figure 33.25 Igel, non-inflatable supraglottic airway, courtesy of Intersurgical, with permission.

less traction on the larynx, allowing videolaryngoscopy to be less stimulating and possible at lighter stages of sedation or anesthesia, commonplace with open airway anesthesia or sedation in the dental office. Although laryngeal views are improved, difficulty in passing endotracheal tubes can persist. Direct and indirect visual fields must be simultaneously monitored to prevent posterior displacement of the tongue or injury to the pharyngeal wall. The blade must be kept still to maintain view, which limits the ability to manipulate the larynx. There are numerous videoscopes currently available. The McGrath Mac® (see Figure 33.30) uses

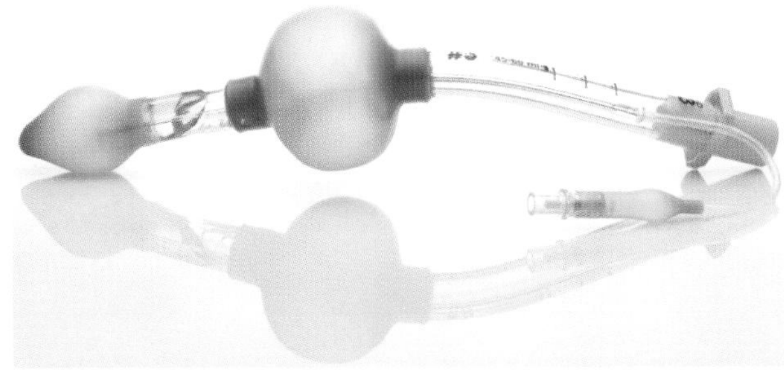

Figure 33.26 King LT airway, courtesy of Ambu corporation.

a conventional Macintosh curved blade, which can be used with either direct or indirect vision. The King Vision® videolaryngoscope (see Figure 33.31) features a gutter that guides endotracheal tube passage to the field of view. Several low cost, disposable, and multiple use videolaryngoscopes are entering the marketplace.

Likelihood of difficult intubation

Visualization of the larynx does not guarantee the ability to place the endotracheal tube through the vocal cords. Laryngeal swelling due to infection or anaphylaxis, tracheal pathology, or tracheal stenosis (congenital, or secondary to radiation or surgery) may hinder passage of an endotracheal tube past the vocal cords. In other cases, where videolaryngoscopy is used, it may be difficult to properly position the endotracheal tube for passage through the cords.

Likelihood of difficult surgical neck entry

In extremely rare instances, the clinician may be confronted with a cannot ventilate, cannot intubate situation in a patient who has received sedative, hypnotic, and/or paralytic drugs. These situations are time urgent and require immediate and decisive action on the part of the dentist, which should include a call for assistance to all staff present as well as to EMS. Extreme psychological reluctance can delay this life-saving maneuver, which aggravates time urgency. The mind is easily clouded with hopes that spontaneous improvement will somehow occur. It is in times such as these that patient resilience, reserve, and adequacy of preoxygenation play a key role and will ultimately determine the amount of time available for surgical neck entry before the onset of hypoxic brain injury. Acquisition and maintenance of skills is very difficult for the dental professional.

There are three choices for the surgical airway: the percutaneous catheter, the percutaneous cannula, and formal cricothyrotomy. Each has advantages and limitations. Practitioners who have not had training or experience in cricothyrotomy will favor the catheter or cannula approach.

Any surgical neck entry is more difficult in patients who have had a history of prior airway surgery or prior radiation, or in patients who have a tumor, pus, or blood distorting normal anatomy. Conditions that increase the distance from the skin to the cricothyroid membrane also complicate surgical airway placement. These conditions include obesity, short neck, or inability to extend the neck. Complications of surgical neck entry include inability to obtain the airway, hemorrhage, or barotrauma.

Placement of a *percutaneous catheter* for jet ventilation (high frequency, low volume) remains an attractive option for many practitioners, as it is often perceived as the least invasive approach. "Homemade" devices that adapt a large intravenous catheter to a ventilation bag (see Figure 33.33) are often ineffective, as sufficient

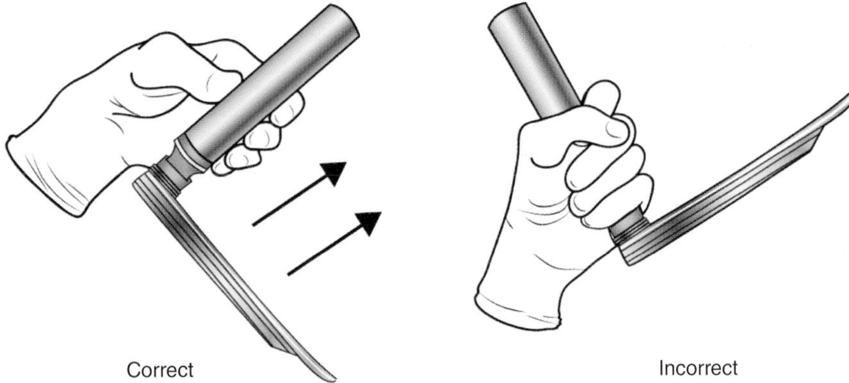

Figure 33.27 Proper laryngoscope hand position. Correct anterior-superior movement pushes the tongue out of the line of sight, while maintaining the position of the larynx. The incorrect levering of the blade displaces the larynx forward, while allowing the tongue to fall back into the line of sight.

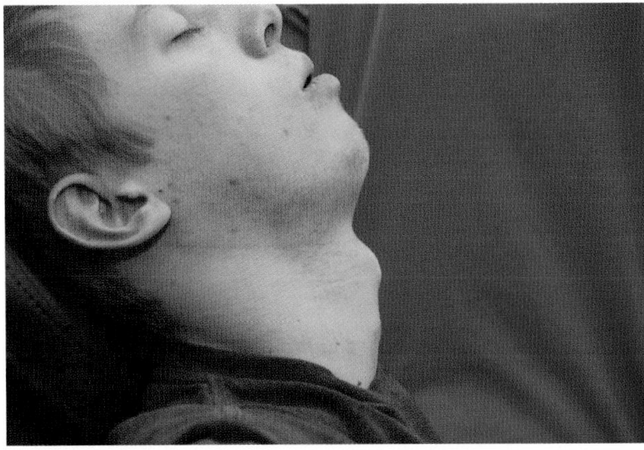

Figure 33.28 Anteriorly tilted larynx. The line of sight requires a greater anterior displacement of the mandible, which is difficult in this Mallampati II patient.

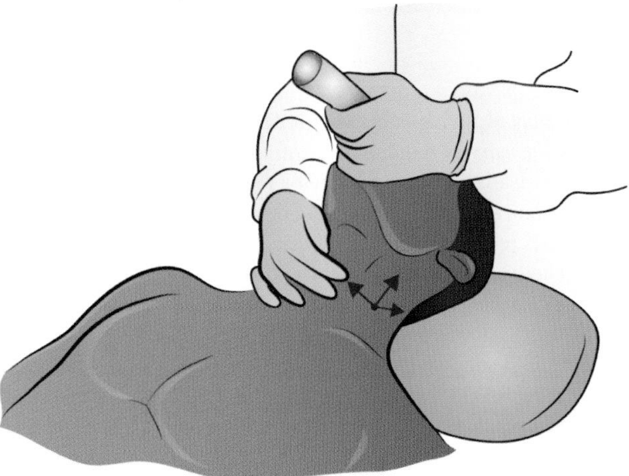

Figure 33.29 BURP maneuver – backward upward and rightward displacement of the larynx to improve the view of the glottis.

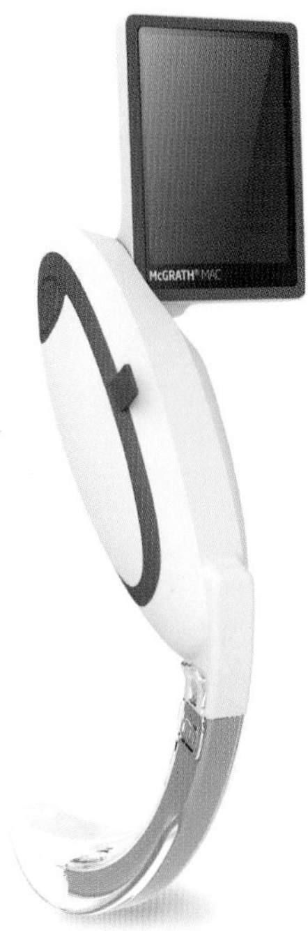

Figure 33.30 McGrath Mac® Videolaryngoscope, with permission.

movement of air through the cannula is impossible. There are several "kits" currently available, including the ENK Oxygen Flow Modulator® (Cook Medical) (see Figure 33.34). This set includes a kink-resistant 6Fr (2 mm) armored cannula over a 15 g (1.5 mm) needle that is attached to oxygen tubing via a 6 inch flexible adapter with 3 intermittently occludable holes. A 15–30L flow rate of oxygen is provided, and the holes are intermittently occluded with finger pressure at a rate of 100 times per minute. The puncture technique starts by attaching the needle to a water-filled 5cc syringe. The cricothyroid membrane is identified in the extended neck and the larynx is stabilized with the passive hand. The puncture is created, with depth verification signaled by loss of resistance and aspiration of air in the syringe. The needle must stay in the midline and must be aimed 45° caudad. The catheter must be continually held in place to prevent dislodgement. Successful use of this device depends on successful gas egress through the larynx to avoid barotrauma.

Percutaneous cannulas also require a cricoid membrane puncture, but are significantly larger than a 15 g catheter. There are several "kits" available, including the Rusch QuickTrach® (Teleflex Medical) (see Figure 33.35) which includes a 2- or 4-mm plastic cannula

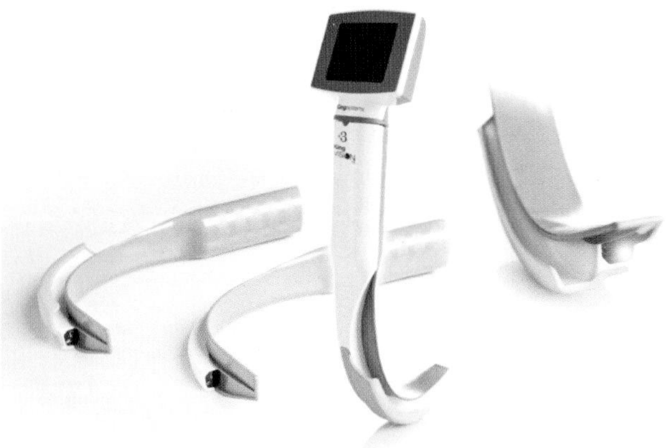

Figure 33.31 The King Vision videolaryngoscope, with permission.

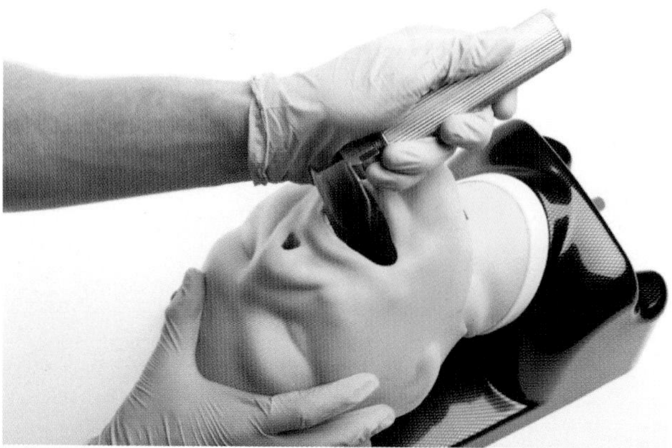

Figure 33.32 Intubation mannequin. Airsim advance, with permission, Tru-Corp Ltd.

with a safety stop and fixation flanges over the removable puncture needle with a flexible 15-mm adapter. A ventilation bag can be used with this device and exhalation can occur to some extent through the 4-mm cannula.

Cricothyrotomy is the surgical access of the airway through the cricothyroid membrane. A towel roll, tracheal hook, Trousseau dilator, Senn or Army-Navy retractors, and a 6-mm endotracheal tube or 4 or 6 Shiley tracheostomy tube must be immediately available (see Figures 33.36–33.38). The neck is hyperextended and the larynx is immobilized with the non-dominant hand, which is never released until tube placement is confirmed. The index finger of the non-dominant hand continually palpates the anatomy. The cricothyroid membrane is identified immediately inferior to the thyroid cartilage (Adam's apple). A 2- to 5-cm vertical incision (Dierks, 2008; Hart and Thompson, 2010) is made through the skin, subcutaneous tissue, and anterior fascia with a suitable scalpel blade. Blunt spreading dissection with adequate retraction facilitates identification of the membrane, which is then incised horizontally at an inferior position. The tracheal hook is placed on the superior lip of the incision and not removed until the tube is placed. The Trousseau dilator (or Kelly hemostats) dilates the stoma, while the tube is placed and secured. Ventilation is commenced and the tube is stabilized. The patient should then be transported to an emergency facility.

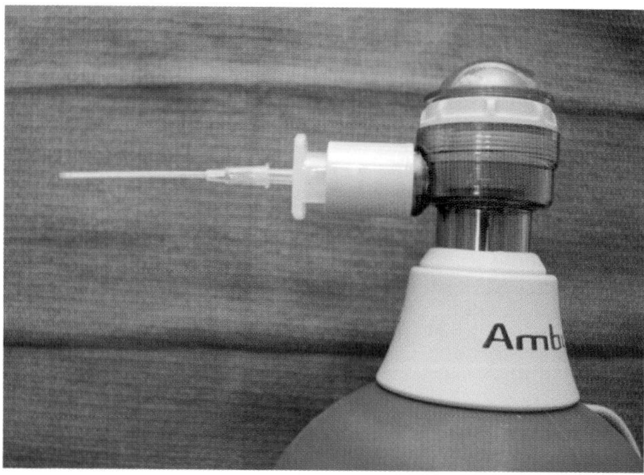

Figure 33.33 An intravenous catheter with a 15-mm adapter for ventilation bag doesnot allow effective ventilation.

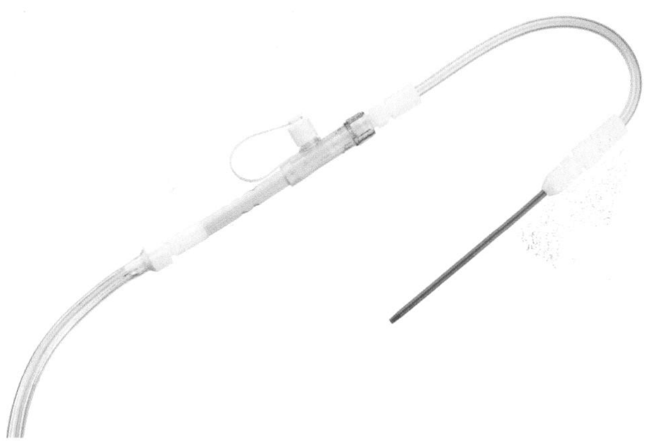

Figure 33.34 Enk oxygen flow modulator®. Permission for use granted by Cook Medical Incorportated, Bloomington, Indiana.

Lost airway algorithm for the dental professional

The loss of an airway requires an immediate assessment of the cause, coupled with advance preparation for such an event so that at least 1 back-up plan, including the use of alternate airways, blades, stylets, and tubes is readily available.

- All dental patients will present with the ability to ventilate. At some point after the administration of sedative, hypnotic, or analgesic drugs, airway sounds may cease, $ETCO_2$ tracing might disappear, and finally SpO_2 may begin to drop. Values, monitors, and probe positions should be immediately rechecked and oxygen flow and tube connections should be verified. At this point, one or more of the following will occur: 1. apnea without respiratory effort; 2. coughing, crowing, or wheezing; or 3. apnea with respiratory effort (assuming chest movement can be visualized). As it is impossible to be aware of the passage of time during high stress events, AN ANESTHESIA ASSISTANT SHOULD DOCUMENT THE TIME, AND CALL OUT TIME PASSAGE AT 30-SECOND INTERVALS, until the problem is resolved. The CALL FOR HELP is never too early; timing depends on the clinical situation, training, experience, and confidence of the practitioner.

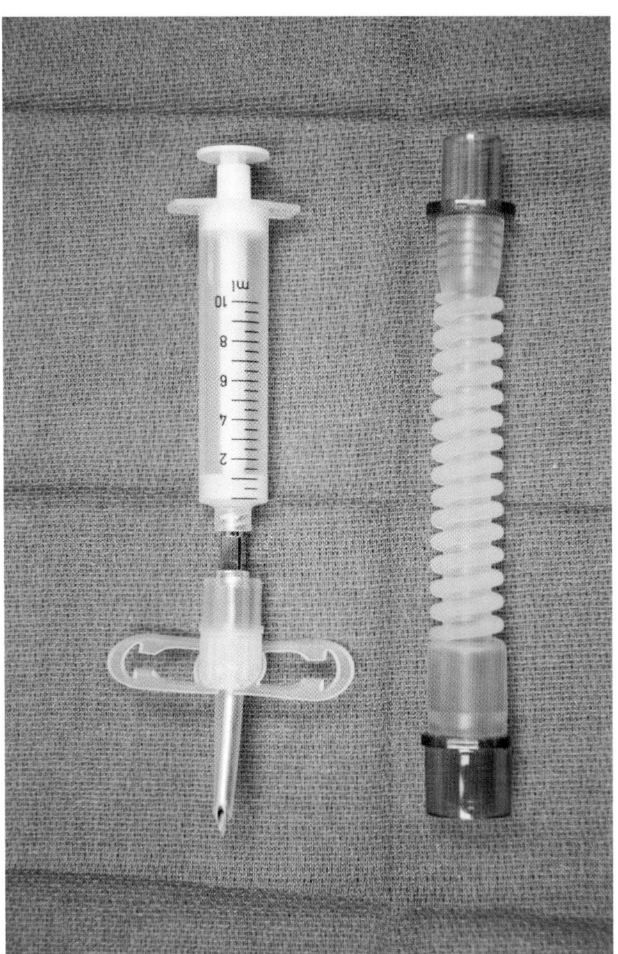

Figure 33.35 Rusch QuickTrach® TELEFLEX MEDICAL.

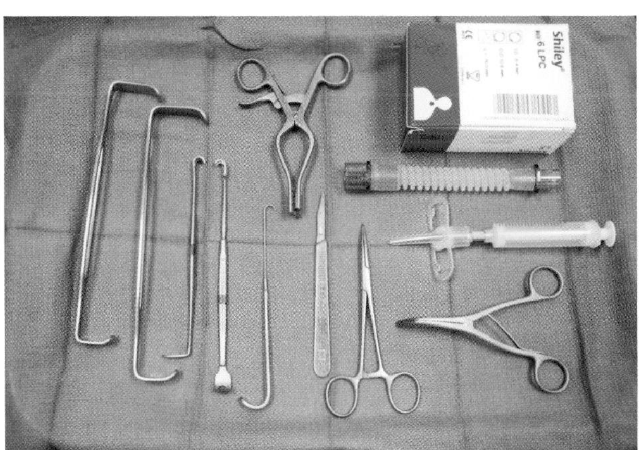

Figure 33.36 Example of a cricothyrotomy surgical tray.

All possible diagnoses should be immediately considered. This algorithm includes the full spectrum of interventions, some of which may be outside the scope or training of the sedation/anesthesia provider. The sequence of events can be modified per clinical situation. Many of these interventions are meant to be performed simultaneously.

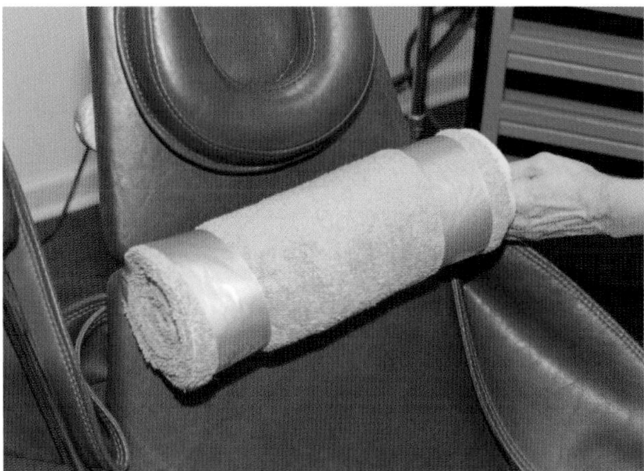

Figure 33.37 Prepared towel roll for shoulder support during neck extension prior to cricothyrotomy.

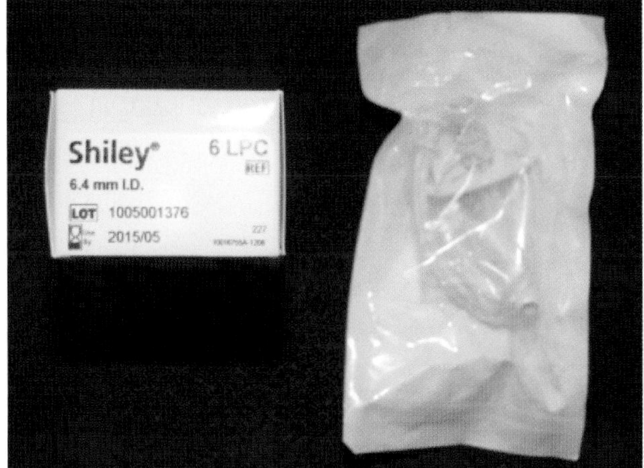

Figure 33.38 Shiley low pressure cuffed tracheostomy tube.

The dental/surgical site is packed or stabilized and untethered instruments or debris are removed. Full attention is shifted to the airway, which should be immediately reclaimed by the provider. A triple or quadruple airway maneuver is performed while the oropharynx is examined and suctioned. Lack of audible clues such as coughing, crowing, or wheezing hints toward drug-induced apnea, which is verified by a light chest compression, listening for the passage of air. If air passes, drug-induced apnea is confirmed and PPV is started, while drug reversal is entertained by practitioners not intending deep sedation or anesthesia. If no air passes, all other diagnoses again become possible. PPV should be verified by visible chest rise, which can be visualized after dental drapes are removed and loose clothing is removed or compressed in order to visually see chest movement. If PPV is impossible and the patient is unresponsive, an oral or nasopharyngeal airway is inserted to allow for air passage in the hypopharynx.

For many practitioners, thoughts of impending doom and time urgency begin to hamper thoughts and actions at this time, making drug reversal an attractive option. Variability of clinical circumstance prevents this "get out of jail card" from being 100% successful

Lost airway algorithm for the dental professional*

Loss of airway noise, $ETCO_2$ tracing and dropping SPO_2

CALL FOR HELP

VERIFY ABNORMAL VALUE, RECHECK MONITORs AND PROBES

ENSURE 100% OXYGEN DELIVERY, CHECK ALL TUBE CONNECTIONS

ASSISTANT NOTES TIME

DIFFERENTIAL DIAGNOSES (superior to inferior categorization)

- Apnea from (unintentional) drug overdose
- Upper airway obstruction – tongue falls back
- Laryngospasm
- Bronchospasm (allergy, asthma, aspiration)
- Rigid Chest
- Foreign body obstruction
- Pulmonary Edema

PACK OFF SURGICAL SITE

QUADRUPLE AIRWAY MANEUVER

Pull tongue forward as necessary

EXAMINE AND SUCTION OROPHARYNX

LIGHT CHEST COMPRESSION

Listen for air passage

YES: drug induced apnea

NO:

- Upper airway obstruction
- Laryngospasm, laryngeal edema
- Bronchospasm
- Anaphylaxis (laryngeal edema, bronchospasm
- Chest wall rigidity
- Aspiration (foreign body, emesis)

CONSIDER FULL DRUG REVERSAL OR DEEPEN ANESTHESIA

- 0.4 – 10 mg naloxone, 1 – 3 mg flumazenil

ATTEMPT POSITIVE PRESSURE VENTILATION

Consider the use of oral or nasopharyngeal airways

MUSCLE RELAXANT (succinylcholine)

SUPRAGLOTTIC AIRWAY

iGEL, LMA, King LT airway

INTUBATE

(full paralyzing dose of succinylcholine 1 – 2 mg/kg IV)

SURGICAL AIRWAY

*the sequence of these events can be modified per practitioner training, experience and confidence. This is not a checklist, but a protocol which requires regular rehearsal (Borshoff, 2011)

(Weaver, J, personal communication). In cases of unintentional drug overdose, higher doses of competitive antagonists and a longer time to clinical effect are required for clinical reversal, which increases the likelihood of pulmonary edema, dysrhythmias, and seizure. However, these adverse side effects are not significant when compared to the alternative outcome.

If laryngospasm is suspected, flutter ventilation often breaks a partial spasm, while muscle relaxants may be necessary for a complete spasm. Deepening anesthesia will often relieve laryngospasm.

If chest rigidity is suspected, muscle relaxants should be administered with low SpO_2 values, while naloxone can be considered with SpO_2 values maintained above 90%, especially for patients with "apneic oxygenation" via high flow oxygen through a nasal cannula.

If inability to ventilate persists, placement of an SGA or endotracheal tube is considered. As mentioned earlier, sedated patients can lose an airway, as easily or more so than fully anesthetized patients. Laryngoscopy is much more difficult in a sedated, combative patient versus a fully relaxed and anesthetized patient. For this reason, the less stimulating videolaryngoscope becomes an attractive option for practitioners not willing to deepen anesthesia.

If ventilation and oxygenation cannot be attained with the above methods, surgical neck entry will be necessary and life saving. A time should be established in advance when surgical neck entry will be performed, allowing 60 seconds for the procedure and assuming that irreversible hypoxic encephalopathy will commence at ~3–5 minutes without ventilation, depending on patient resilience, reserve, and degree of preoxygenation.

References

Ackerman, W. E., et al. Ineffective ventilation during conscious sedation due to chest wall rigidity after midazolam and fentanyl. *Anesth Prog* **37**: 46–48, 1990.

Al-alami, A. A., et al. Pediatric laryngospasm : prevention and treatment. *Curr Opin Anaesthesiol* **22**: 388–395, 2009.

American Society of Anesthesiologists: Practice guidelines for the management of the difficult airway: An updated report. *Anesthesiol* **118**: 251–270, 2013.

Bennett, J. A., et al. Difficult or impossible ventilation after sufentanil-induced anesthesia is caused primarily by vocal cord closure. *Anesthesiol* **87**: 1070–1074, 1997.

Borshoff, D. C. *The Anaesthetic Crisis Manual*. Cambridge: Cambridge University Press, 2011.

Brown, R. H. HRCT imaging of airway responsiveness: effects of anesthetics. *J Clin Monit Comput* **16**: 443–455, 2000.

Cheney, F. W., et al. Trends in anesthesia-related death and brain damage: A closed claims analysis. *Anesthesiol* **105**: 1081–1086, 2006.

Ciavarro, C. and Kelly, J. P. W. Postobstructive pulmonary edema in an obese child after an oral surgery procedure under general anesthesia: a case report. *J Oral Maxillfac Surg* **60**: 1503–1505, 2002.

Coruh, B., et al. Fentanuyl-induced chest wall rigidity. *Chest* **143**: 1145–46, 2013.

Dierks, E. J. Tracheotomy: elective and emergent. *Oral Maxillfacial Surg Clin N Am* **20**: 513–520, 2008.

Ferson, D., et al. Safety and hazards associated with tracheal intubation and use of supralaryngeal airways, *in* Lobato, E. B., et al. (eds): *Complications in Anesthesiology*. Philadelphia: Lippincott Williams & Wilkins, 2008, p. 119.

Glasser, S. A. and Siler, J. N. Delayed onset of laryngospasm-induced pulmonary edema in adult outpatients. *Anesthesiology* **62**: 370–371, 1985.

Haas D. A., Yagiela J. A.. Agents used in general anesthesia, deep sedation, and conscious sedation, *in* Yagiela J. A., Neidle E. A., Dowd F. J. (eds): *Pharmacology and Therapeutics for Dentistry*. New York, NY: Mosby-Year Book, 1998, p. 260.

Hagberg, C. A., et al. The difficult airway, *in* Lobato, E. B., et al., eds. *Complications in Anesthesiology*. Philadelphia: Lippincott Williams & Wilkins, 2008, p. 104.

Hart, K. L. and Thompson, S. H. Emergency cricothyrotomy. *Atlas Oral Maxillofacial Surg Clin N Am* **18**: 29–38, 2010.

Ikeda, A., et al. Effects of muscle relaxants on mask ventilation in anesthetized persons with normal upper airway anatomy. *Anesthesiol* **117**: 487–493, 2012.

Krodel, D. J., et al. Case Scenario: Acute Postoperative negative pressure pulmonary edema. *Anesthesiology* **113**:200–220, 2010.

Kumeta, Y., et al. A survey of perioperative bronchospasm in 105 patients with reactive airway disease. *Masui* **44**:396–401, 1995.

Langeron, O., et al. Prediction of difficult mask ventilation. *Anesthesiol* **92**: 1229–1236, 2000.

Larson, C. L. Laryngospasm-the best treatment. *Anesthesiolv* **89**: 1293–1294, 1998.

Levy, L., et al. Upper respiratory infections and general anesthesia in children. *Anaesthesia* **47**: 678–682, 1992.

Levy J. H., Anaphylactic and anaphylactoid reactions, *in* Lobato E. B., Gravenstein N., Kirby R. R. (eds): *Complications in Anesthesiology*. Philadelphia, PA: Lippincott Williams & Wilkins, 2008, p. 705.

Lewis, K. E. *Anaesth Intens Care* **35** : 128–131, 2007.

Liccardi, G., et al. Bronchial asthma. *Curr Opin Anesthesiol* **25**: 30–37, 2012.

Liu, L. M., et al. Dose response to intramuscular succinylcholine in children. *Anesthesiol* **55**: 599–602, 1981.

Mallampati, S. R., et al. A clinical sign to predict difficult tracheal intubation: a prospective study. *Can Anaesthetists' Soc J* **32**: 429–434, 1985.

Marik, P. E. Aspiration pneumonitis and aspriation pneumonia. *N Engl J Med* **344**: 665–671, 2001.

Mathay, M. A., et al. Alverolar epithelial barrier: role of lung fluid balance in clinical lung injury. *Clin Chest Med* **21**: 477–490, 2000.

Mendelson, C. L. The aspiration of stomach contents into the lungs during obstetric anesthesia. *Am J Obstet Gynecol* **52**: 191–205, 1946.

Parolia, A., et al. Management of foreign body aspiration or ingestion in dentistry. *Kath Univ Med J* **7**: 165–171, 2009.

Pisegna, J. R. and Martindale, R. G. Acid suppression in the perioperative period. *J Clin Gastroenterol* **39**: 10–16, 2005.

Pizov, R., et al. Wheezing during induction of general anesthesia in patients with and without asthma. *Anesthesiol* **82**: 1111–1116, 1995.

American Society of Anesthesiologists Committee on Standards and Practice Parameters, Practice guidelines for preoperative fasting and the use of pharmacologic agents to reduce the risk of pulmonary aspiration: application to healthy patients undergoing elective procedures: an updated report. *Anesthesiol* **114**: 495–511, 2011.

Ramachandran, S. K., et al. Apneic oxygenation during prolonged laryngoscopy in obese patients: a randomized, controlled trial of nasal oxygen administration. *J Clin Anesth* **22**: 164–168, 2010.

Raichle, M. E., et al. Cerebral blood flow during and after hyperventilation. *Arch Neurol* **23**: 394–403, 1970.

Restrepo, R. D. and Peters, J. Near-fatal asthma: recognition and management. *Curr Opin Pulm Med* **14**: 13–23, 2008.

Reynolds, L.M., et al. Intramuscular rocuronium in infants and children: dose-ranging and tracheal intubating conditions. *Anesthesiol* **85**: 231–239, 1996.

Rodrigo, G. J., et al. Acute asthma in adults: a review. *Chest* **125**: 1081–1102, 2004.

Shi, Y. and Warner, D. O. Brief preoperative smoking abstinence: Is there a dilemma?. *Anesth Analg* **113**: 1348–1351, 2011.

Soubra, S. H. and Guntuypalli, K. K. Acute respiratory failure in asthma. *Indian J Crit Care Med* **9**: 225–234, 2005.

Stoelting, R. K. and Miller, R. D. *Basics of Anesthesia*, 3rd edn. New York: Churchill Livingstone, 1994.

Sukumaran, M., et al. Evaluation of corticosteroid treatment in aspiration of gastric contents: a controlled clinical trial. *Mt Sinai J Med* **47**: 335, 1980.

Tsai, W. H., et al. A decision for diagnostic testing in obstructive sleep apnea. *Am J Respir Crit Care Med* **167**: 1427–1432, 2003.

Tsukimoto, K., et al. Ultrastructural appearances of pulmonary capillaries at high transmural pressures. *J Appl Physiol* **71**: 573–582, 1991.

Udeshi, A., et al. Postobstructive pulmonary edema. *J Crit Care* **25**: 508.e1–508.e5, 2000.

Vaughn, R. L. and Bennett, C. R. Fentanyl chest wall rigidity syndrome-a case report. *Anesth Prog* **28**: 50–51, 1981.

Viscomi, C. M. and Bailey, P. L.. Opioid-induced rigidity after intravenous fentanyul. *Obstet Gynecol* **89**: 822–824, 1997.

Warner, M. A., et al. Clinical significance of pulmonary aspiration during the peri-operative period. *Anesthesiol* **78**: 56–62, 1993.

West, J. B. *Respiratory Physiology: The Essentials*. 6th edn. Philadelphia: Lippincott Williams and Wilkins, 2000, p. 6.

West, J. B., et al. Stress fracture in pulmonary capillaries. *J Appl Physiol* **70**: 1731–1742, 1991.

34 Allergy and anaphylaxis

H. William Gottschalk[1] and Robert C. Bosack[2]

[1]University of Southern California School of Dentistry, Los Angeles, CA, USA

[2]University of Illinois, College of Dentistry, Chicago, IL, USA

Introduction

Allergy is a hypersensitive immunological state acquired by exposure to a particular antigen. Subsequent re-exposure to the same antigen produces a heighten capacity to react. *Anaphylaxis* (see Figure 34.1) is an acute multisystem syndrome resulting from the sudden and ongoing release of tissue mast cells and circulating basophil-derived mediators into the circulation (Sampson et al., 2006). In rare cases (1 or 2/20,000 anesthetics), immunologic or non-immunologic release of mediators can occur during anesthesia or sedation, with no predilection for age, race, or gender. Common triggers include neuromuscular blockers, latex (especially when held in prolonged contact with open surgical wounds, or in patients or healthcare providers who sustain chronic, repeated exposure to latex), and antibiotics. Less common triggers include barbiturates, opioids, and NSAIDs. Most anesthetic drugs administered perioperatively have been reported in the literature to produce anaphylaxis (Gruchalla, 2002). Succinylcholine accounted for 22.6% and rocuronium accounted for 41.3% (Mertes et al., 2003).The agents found in dental offices that are most reported to cause anaphylactic reaction are antibiotics (15.1%), latex (16.7%), and muscle relaxants (58.2%).

Risk factors include a prior history of anaphylaxis, female gender, and asthma, among others. Worrisome comorbidities, which can negatively affect outcomes of anaphylaxis, include cardiovascular and respiratory diseases and concurrent medications including β blockers or ACE inhibitors.

Pathophysiology

First-time exposure (sensitization) to an antigen triggers the clinically silent formation of antigen-specific IgE antibodies that circulate throughout the body and bind to cell membrane receptors on tissue mast cells and circulating basophils (Kemp, 2013.).

Re-exposure to the same antigen (even in minute doses) cross-bridges the membrane-bound IgE (activation), which triggers degranulation and release of preformed inflammatory mediators including histamine, tryptase, nitric oxide, and arachidonic acid metabolites, among many others. These mediators act on target tissues (see Table 34.1) and are also capable of recruiting other inflammatory cells, such as eosinophils. The recruited cells also release mediators, triggering a crescendo chain reaction.

Non-immunologic reactions occur when an antigen triggers mediator release in the absence of IgE; hence, these reactions are possible on first-time exposure. Examples include opiates and vancomycin. Clinical presentation and treatment are identical. Examples include histamine-releasing complement activation. Morphine and meperidine (and other opioids to a lesser extent, see Figure 34.2) can directly trigger histamine release from mast cells (Veien et al., 2000), which results in limited cutaneous signs (Mertes et al., 2011). ACE inhibitors can trigger isolated angioedema, possibly mediated by bradykinin.

Clinical features

Anaphylaxis is under-recognized and undertreated, especially in the absence of cutaneous signs (see Table 34.2). Onset and severity of signs and symptoms are variable and unpredictable, regardless of allergy history. As such, the appearance of a "rash" should never be dismissed as trivial. During anesthesia or sedation, patients are unable to report symptoms of itching, and patients are fully clothed, which can mask the presence of hives. Early vital sign changes associated with anaphylaxis are nonspecific and often indistinguishable from the normal range of variability during anesthesia or surgery.

Cutaneous signs include hives and angioedema. Hives (urticaria, wheal) are slightly elevated, circumscribed areas of the skin (see Figure 34.3). They are indurated, erythematous, and pruritic (itchy). Hives are due to vasodilation and transudation of fluid in superficial skin layers. Angioedema (see Figure 34.4) is a non-circumscribed, soft, asymmetrical, nonpruritic swelling in the distensible deeper soft tissues, such as the lips, tongue, uvula, or larynx. Angioedema is due to transudation of fluid in deeper tissues. Figure 34.5 is an endoscopic view of laryngeal edema, with a comparison to normal in Figure 34.6. Notably, cutaneous symptoms and signs will be masked in patients who have recently ingested antihistamines.

There are three diagnostic criteria for anaphylaxis. Anaphylaxis is likely when any one of the three criteria is met. (Sampson et al., 2006)

- Criterion I – acute onset (minutes to hours) involving skin/mucosa and either respiratory symptoms or hypotension or both.
- Criterion II – two or more of the following reactions occur rapidly after exposure to a likely antigen
  - Skin / mucosal involvement
  - Respiratory compromise
  - Hypotension

Anesthesia Complications in the Dental Office, First Edition. Edited by Robert C. Bosack and Stuart Lieblich.

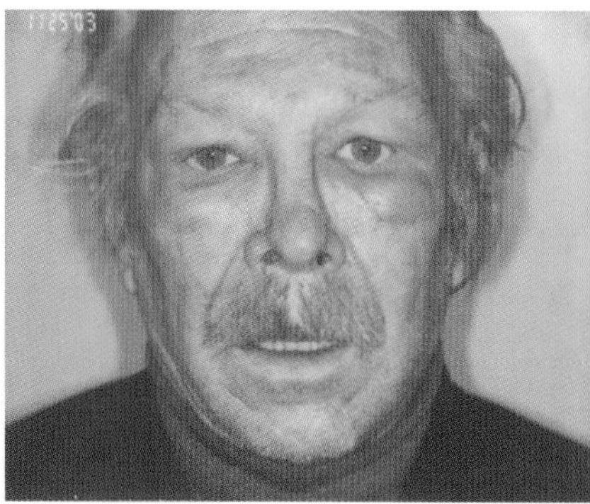
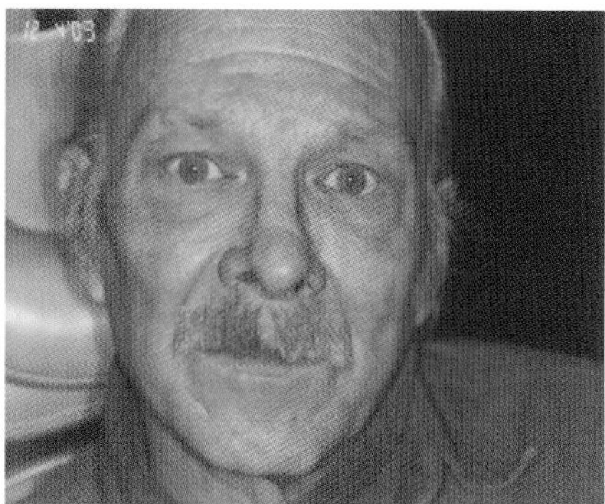

Figure 34.1 Patient on the left with classic signs of anaphylaxis: lacrimation, rhinorrhea, periobital angioedemia, shortness of breath and agitation. On the right, for comparison, is the same patient after resolution.

Table 34.1 Actions of select inflammatory mediators (Gottesman, 2011).

Mediator	Mode of action
Histamine	• Binds both H1 and H2 receptors • If released into tissue, it triggers urticaria, pruritis, flushing, and rhinorrhea. • If released into circulation, it causes dose-dependent hypotension, increased vascular permeability, and bronchoconstriction
Tryptase	• Activates complement, which triggers hypotension and angioedema
Nitric Oxide	• Vasodilation and increased vascular permeability
Arachidonic acid metabolites	• Enhances mast cell degranulation, and increases vascular permeability, vasodilation, bronchoconstriction

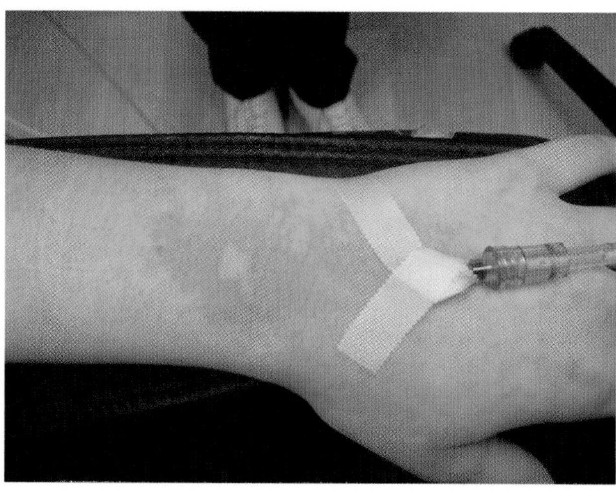

Figure 34.2 Hive located just proximal to IV site on dorsal wrist, 1 minute after injection of 50μg of fentanyl.

- Persistent gastrointestinal symptoms
- Criterion III – hypotension after exposure to a known allergen
  - <90 mmHg systolic or 30% decrease from baseline (>10 years of age)
  - <70 mmHg + [2 x age] systolic (<10 years of age)

Severity of anaphylaxis can be graded as follows (Ring and Messmer, 1977):

- Grade 1 – cutaneous – mucous signs
  - Erythema, urticaria, with or without angioedema
- Grade II – moderate multivisceral signs with cutaneous-mucous signs.
  - Hypotension, tachycardia, dyspnea, and GI symptoms possible
- Grade III – life-threatening mono or multivisceral signs
  - Cardiovascular collapse, tachycardia, or bradycardia. Dysrhythmias, bronchospasm, gastrointestinal and cutaneous/mucous signs possible.
- Grade IV – cardiac arrest.

Diagnosis

Any patient with a sudden onset of urticaria or angioedema is assumed to be having an acute anaphylactic reaction, as there are few other diagnoses for these clinical signs. However, cutaneous signs may be absent or may not be the first noted change in patient status, such as patients with unexplained tachycardia or hypotension. The severe hypotension and decrease in peripheral circulation prevent the classic signs of swelling of the tissues. In some cases, cardiac arrest is the heralding sign of severe anaphylaxis. Once epinephrine is administered and resuscitation improves circulation, cutaneous signs may develop. A majority of drug reactions occur within 10 minutes of administration.

The variability of the early clinical presentation of anaphylaxis can confound diagnosis and be mistaken for asthma, aspiration, pulmonary edema, vasovagal syncope, hypotension, and tachycardia secondary to anesthetic overdose and hypovolemia or malignant hyperthermia, among many others.

Prevention

Questions concerning allergy to frequently used drugs in the dental office should include reactions to *penicillin, codeine, iodine (surface disinfectants),* and *latex.* Many times, patients will report an allergy to medication when in fact it can be a common adverse side effect, such as nausea or itching from narcotics, or dizziness from benzodiazepines, or hypotension from propofol. Patients who have experienced syncope or epinephrine-induced tachycardia may have been erroneously informed that they are allergic to local anesthetics.

Table 34.2 Clinical features of anaphylaxis (Ledford et al., 2013).

System	Symptoms	Signs	Pathophysiology	Frequency of occurrence during anaphylaxis
Cutaneous (skin / mucosa)	Itching, burning, tingling	AIRWAY OBSTRUCTION Hives, flushing, periorbital edema, conjunctival swelling, lacrimation, angioedema (lips, tongue, uvula, larynx), change in voice quality, piloerection	Fluid extravasation Upper airway edema	80–90%
Respiratory	Dyspnea, shortness of breath, sensation of throat closure or choking, tightness of chest	BRONCHOSPASM Wheezing, stridor, cough, rhinorrhea, sneezing, nasal congestion, hypoxemia, pulmonary edema, increase in $ETCO_2$, decrease in SpO_2	Bronchoconstriction	70%
Cardiovascular	Dizziness, malaise, lightheadedness	HYPOTENSION Hypotension, syncope, incontinence, tachycardia, loss of consciousness, dysrhythmias, loss of consciousness Up to 35 % of intravascular fluid can extravasate within 10 minutes	Vasodilation and increased capillary permeability	45%
Gastrointestinal	Cramping, abdominal pain, nausea	Vomiting, diarrhea		45%
Neurologic	Anxiety, confusion, headache			15%

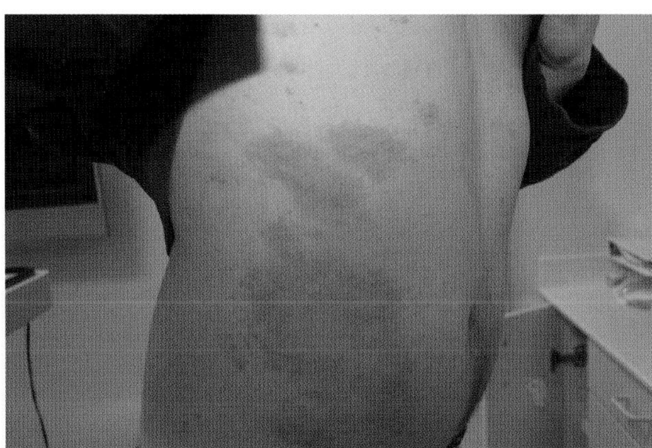

Figure 34.3 (Hives) Hives on the right thoracic wall triggered by a penicillin allergy.

The question of local anesthetic allergy occasionally surfaces. Allergic reactions to amide type anesthetics are extremely rare, while allergy to esters (such as Hurricaine™ or Cetacaine™) is more common, as these drugs are metabolized to the notoriously allergenic PABA (para-amino benzoic acid.) Direct questioning about the occurrence of rash, itching, and rhinitis helps establish the presence of allergy. If in doubt, it is unwise to challenge the patient with a "test dose," as even minute amounts of allergen can trigger full-blown anaphylaxis in susceptible patients.

There is no data in the literature that suggests that pretreatment of a patient with a history of allergy, atopy, or asthma with an antihistamine or corticosteroid will be effective in preventing true anaphylactic reactions. In fact, pretreatment can give the clinician a false sense of security, because even when large doses of corticosteroids have been administered, anaphylactic reactions have occurred (Levy et al., 1986).

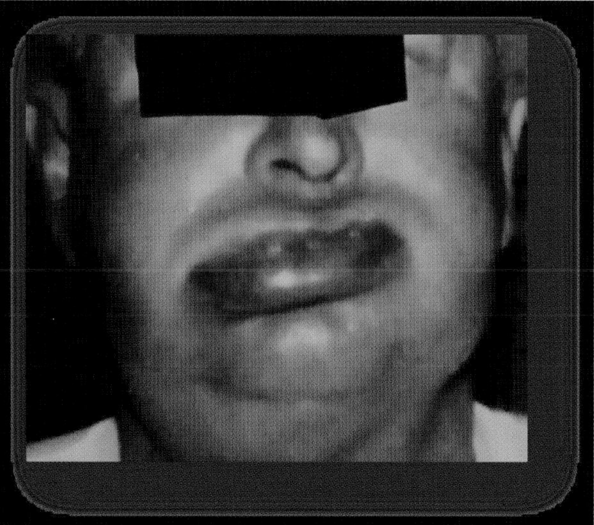

Figure 34.4 Angioedema of the lower lip.

Management

The management of anaphylaxis returns to the concept of safely administering sedation and anesthesia. This includes full monitoring of the patient, with a continuous IV infusion and readily available emergency medications and airway adjuncts, with a

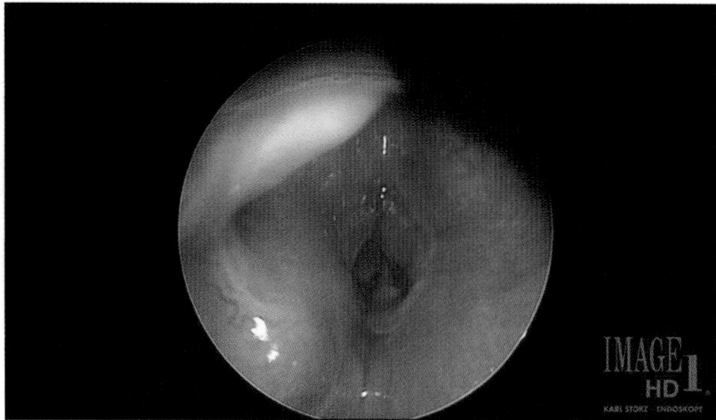

Figure 34.5 Endoscopic view of laryngeal edema. Notice distortion of normal anatomy, which may result in laryngeal obstruction. Airway noise and voice changes in patients capable of speech would be expected. Image courtesy of John D. McAllister, MD.

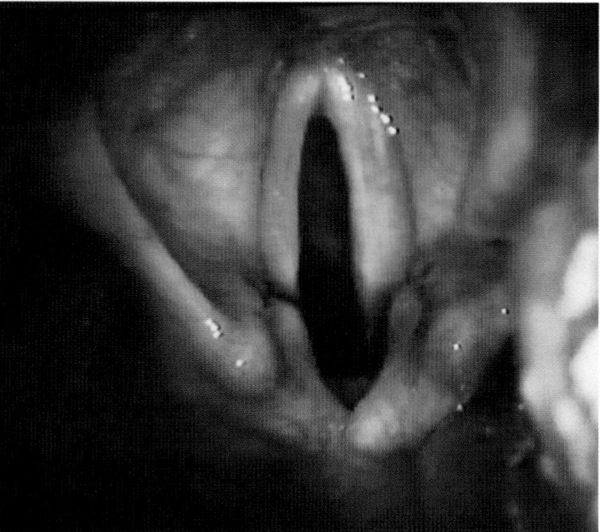

Figure 34.6 Normal larynx, courtesy of H. William Gottschalk, DDS.

prepared and knowledgeable team, each being aware of their responsibility during an emergency. As with any adverse patient response, priority is given to airway, breathing, circulation, and oxygenation. Early activation of EMS is prudent in all situations.

Recognition of symptoms is paramount when selecting appropriate stepwise treatment for an allergic reaction. Anaphylaxis can be mild and resolve spontaneously with the secretion of endogenous epinephrine or angiotensin II, or can be severe and rapidly progress to cardiovascular collapse and death, usually due to respiratory problems (Simons, 2010). Isolated urticaria will often resolve with diphenhydramine, 25–50 mg, by any route, every 6 to 8 hours until resolution.

It is good practice to overestimate the severity of anaphylaxis and favor definitive treatment if unsure of the severity or possible progression of disease. Danger signs (anaphylaxis is unpredictable) include rapid progression, respiratory signs (wheezing), abdominal pain, dysrhythmia, and hypotension. Laryngeal edema may lead to death by asphyxia; early intubation or surgical neck entry may be required.

Epinephrine administration is the most important and effective treatment in a suspected anaphylactic episode (Soar et al., 2008). Epinephrine underutilization and a delay in administration of more than 30 minutes have been associated with poor outcomes (Bock, 2013). Traditionally, the subcutaneous route was the preferred route of administration, but due to the cutaneous vasoconstriction and its absorption pharmacokinetics, the intramuscular route is preferred. Intramuscular administration of 0.3–0.5 mg (0.01 mg/kg; 1:1000 dilution) in the middle lateral thigh demonstrated superior plasma concentrations over a subcutaneous route of administration (Simons et al., 2001). There is little clinical difference between IM and SQ when injected in the deltoid muscle, which may be more accessible in the dental office. It may be necessary to repeat the injection at 5–15 minute intervals, due to inadequate response secondary to underdosing, hypovolemia, or other than supine posturing. Epinephrine increases peripheral vascular resistance, decreases mucosal edema and interferes with mediator release from mast cells and basophils (Vadas and Perelman, 2012). Epinephrine also increases cardiac output and relaxes bronchiolar smooth muscle. Side effects include tremor, palpitations, and headache. Epinephrine can lose therapeutic efficacy in patients taking β blockers. Glucagon (1–5 mg IV slowly, to avoid vomiting and possible aspiration) has both chronotropic and inotropic effects not mediated through β receptors (Thomas and Crawford, 2005). Early administration of inhaled albuterol tends to improve its deeper penetration into the bronchiolar tree, prior to small airway occlusion.

Second-line agents for the treatment of anaphylaxis include antihistamines, of which, diphenhydramine is the most studied. Diphenhydramine is a H1 receptor blocker. It does not relieve airway obstruction, has no effect on mucosal edema, and does not inhibit mediator release. Onset is slow, and may aggravate hypotension, especially when given intravenously. Unlike epinephrine, which can correct the existing situation, histamine only limits its progression. Glucocorticoids have a delayed onset of action and may attenuate prolonged reactions or biphasic reactions. Biphasic reactions consist of recurrent signs and symptoms following apparent resolution without additional exposure to triggers, between 8–12 hours after initial presentation (Sharma et al., 2010). This possibility mandates a period of observation after successful management.

Summary – Management of anaphylaxis Algorithm **(Dewachter et al., 2009):**

1. Stop administration of all drugs, and eliminate spread of antigen (tourniquet?).
2. Call for help.
3. AIRWAY – deliver 100% O_2, prepare to deliver positive pressure ventilation, and use airway adjuncts as required. Intubation and surgical neck entry may be necessary.
4. Establish or maintain wide open IV access. Administer isotonic crystalloids; patient may sequester up to 7 liters of fluid. Place patient in a supine position, and elevate the legs.
5. Administer IM epinephrine (0.3–0.5 mg; 1:1000) into middle lateral thigh or deltoid, with an 1.5" needle to assure IM delivery. Repeat as necessary.
6. Administer albuterol or other rapid-acting inhaled β2 agonist.
7. Administer second-line medication–diphenhydramine, 50 mg IV and dexamethasone 10 mg IV or equivalent.
8. Prepare for EMS transfer.

References

Bock S. Fatal anaphylaxis. In: UpToDate, Simons, F. E. and Feldweg, A. M. (Ed), UpToDate, Waltham, MA. (Accessed on November 25, 2013.)

Dewachter, P., et al. Anaphylaxis and Anesthesia: Controversies and New Insights. *Anesthesiol* **111**: 1141–1150, 2009.

Gruchalla, R. S. Drug allergy. *J Allergy Clin Immunol* **111**: S548–S559, 2002.

Gottesman, B. Anaphylaxis. *Emergency Medicine Reports* **32**: 9–19, 2011.

Kemp, S. Pathophyiology of anaphylaxis. In: UpToDate, Simons, R. E. and Feldweg, A. M. (Ed), UpToDate, Waltham, MA. (Accessed on November 25, 2013.)

Ledford, D.K., et al. perioperative anaphylaxis: clinical manifestations, etiology and diagnosis. In: UpToDate, Adkinson, N. F. and Feldweg, A. M. (Ed), UpToDate, Waltham, MA. (Accessed on November 25, 2013.)

Levy, J. H., et al. Prospective evaluation of risk of protamine reactions in NPH Insulin-dependent diabetics. *Anesth Analg* **65**:739–42, 1986.

Mertes, P. M., et al. Anaphylactic and anaphylactoid reactions occurring during anesthesia in France 1999–2000. *Anesthesiol* **99** : 536–545, 2003.

Mertes, P.M., et al. Anaphylaxis during anesthesia in France : an 8-year national survey. *J Allergy Clin Immunol* **128** : 366–373, 2011.

Ring, J.and Messmer, K. Incidence and Severity of anaphylactoid reactions to colloid volume substitutes. *Lancet* **1**: 466–469, 1977.

Sampson, H. A., et al. Second Symposium on the definition and management of anaphylaxis: Summary report. Second National Institute of allergy and infectious disease/food allergy and anaphylaxis network symposium. *J Allergy Clin Immunol* **17**: 391–397, 2006.

Sharma, R., et al. Management Protocol for Anaphylaxis. *J Oral Maxillofac Surg* **68**: 855–862, 2010.

Soar, J., et al. Emergency treatment of anaphylactic reactions–guidelines for healthcare providers. *Resuscitation*, 77: 157–169, 2008.

Simons, F. E., et al. Epinephrine absorption in adults: Intramuscular versus subcutaneous injection. *J Allergy Clin Immunol* **108**: 871–873, 2001.

Simons, F. E. Anaphylaxis. *J Allergy Clin Immunol* **125**: S161–S81, 2010.

Thomas, M. and Crawford, I. Best evidence topic report. Glucagon infusion in refractory anaphylactic shock in patients on beta-blockers. *Emerg Med J* **22**: 272–273, 2005.

Vadas, R. and Perelman, B. Effect of epinephrine on platelet-activating factor-stimulated human vascular smooth muscle cells. *J Allergy Clin Immunol* **129**: 1329–1333, 2012.

Veien, M., et al. Mechanisms of nonimmunological histamine and tryptase release from human cutaneous mast cells. *Anesthesiol* **92**: 1074–1081, 2000.

35 Anesthetic adversity–neurologic problems

Michael Trofa[1] **and Robert C. Bosack**[2]

[1]University of Connecticut, Department of Oral and Maxillofacial Surgery, Farmington, CT, USA

[2]University of Illinois, College of Dentistry, Chicago, IL, USA

Seizure

A seizure is a paroxysmal, episodic (intermittent and self-limited) abnormal, excessive and synchronous neuronal discharge resulting in an alteration of consciousness and/or motor, sensory, or autonomic changes, accompanied by diagnostic changes in the electroencephalogram (EEG). Seizures are thought to result from an imbalance between inhibitory and excitatory neurons. Seizure classifications are numerous, examples of which are included in Table 35.1, which exposes the variety of possible etiologies. Epilepsy is the propensity to have recurrent, unprovoked seizures (Perks, 2012), while status epilepticus is seizure activity that lasts more than 5 minutes (Lowenstein, 1999). Treatment goals include minimization of both seizure frequency and side effects of anti-seizure medication.

Alterations in seizure thresholds remain attractive etiologies for new onset seizures either during anesthesia or during recovery. Transient metabolic disturbances, such as sleep deprivation, hypoxia, hypoglycemia, hyperventilation, hypovolemia, or fever can lower seizure thresholds. Syncope can be accompanied by a brief salvo of clonic muscular activity. Drug therapy, especially new onset medication or recent changes in dose, notably with tricyclic antidepressants and antipsychotics, can trigger seizure activity, as can illicit drug ingestion, whose content is never known. Local anesthetic toxicity can also manifest in seizure activity. Subtherapeutic levels of anti-seizure medication are also a possibility, secondary to concomitant ingestion of CYP inducers (may take up to 2 weeks to see effect), increased protein binding, or in situations when doses were missed. Many patients may be unable to afford anti-seizure medication and become medically noncompliant especially when seizure activity is infrequent, and drug therapy is viewed as unnecessary. Other patients may become unaccepting and intolerant of adverse side effects of these medications.

Most anesthetic agents possess both proconvulsant and anticonvulsant properties. In general, lower doses tend to be proconvulsant, with the notable exception of opioids (Modica, 1990; Kofke, 2010). Meperidine and its metabolite, normeperidine, can trigger both tonic and clonic activity. Fentanyl, even in low doses, has been reported to cause a generalized seizure (Saboory, 2007). Sevofluane can support seizure activity, especially in children, at high concentrations and during periods of hypocarbia (Constant et al., 2005, Mohanram, 2007). Isoflurane and desflurane have anticonvulsant properties, while N_2O is thought to have a mild suppressant effect. Both methohexital and propofol have been used to treat refractory status epilepticus, yet they can also produce excitatory activity, especially methohexital, which can trigger myoclonic movement. All benzodiazepines are anticonvulsant. Ketamine may facilitate seizures at low doses, but it is thought to be anticonvulsant at anesthetic doses (Myslobodsky, 1981).

Preanesthetic evaluation

Niesen (2010) conducted a 6-year retrospective study of 641 patients with a documented seizure disorder; only 3.4% experienced a perioperative seizure, mostly dependent on the number of antiepileptic medications taken. He concluded that a majority of perioperative seizures in patients with a preexisting seizure disorder are likely related to the patients underlying condition and not the type of surgery or method of anesthesia. These results emphasize the importance of a thorough history (Table 35.2).

Diagnosis

"Everything that shakes is not a seizure" (Shah, 2001). Common movement disorders in the dental office include tremors after injection of local anesthetics with epinephrine or injection of ephedrine. Myoclonic activity (involuntary twitching of a muscle or muscle group) can occur with the use of methohexital and occasionally opioids. Hypocarbic tetany can occur during hyperventilation. Anticholinergic toxicity and inadequately titrated antipsychotic agents can also trigger random movement disorders.

Seizure activity can encompass a full range of clinical expression, but none is more frightful than the generalized tonic–clonic (grand mal) seizure. This seizure classically begins with an epileptic cry, followed by a tonic phase where the extremities stiffen for a period of time. This subsequently gives way to the clonic phase, characterized by rapid and repetitive alternating flexion and extension. During this "ictal" phase, patients can become incontinent of bladder more often than bowel and may appear cyanotic. Tongue biting can occur, which can cause significant hemorrhage. The post-ictal phase presents an exhausted and amnesic patient, often confused and complaining of muscle fatigue and headache.

Anesthesia Complications in the Dental Office, First Edition. Edited by Robert C. Bosack and Stuart Lieblich.

Table 35.1 Seizure classification.

Classification based on etiology	Symptomatic	Stroke
		Lesion
		Infection or trauma
	Idiopathic	No identifiable underlying abnormality
	Altered seizure threshold	Genetics
		Transient metabolic disturbance
		Drugs (prescribed or illicit)
		Subtherapeutic level of anti-seizure medication
Classification to decide therapy	Generalized	EEG abnormality in both hemispheres
	"Localization-related"	Partial – abnormal EEG in part of cortex
		Focal – from a pathologic lesion
	Complex	Loss of consciousness at onset
	Simple	No loss of consciousness at onset

Table 35.2 Salient features of a preanesthetic history for patients with seizure disorders.

- Describe the habitual seizure – triggers, what happens, duration, recovery
- List medications and degree of compliance
- Identify level of control - Ability to drive a car (usually requires a 6 month seizure free period)
- Identify seizure frequency and date of last seizure
- Identify positive or negative trends in seizure frequency or character

Management

Intervention is necessary for all convulsive seizures that have continued 2 minutes longer than the patient's habitual seizures (Perks, 2012) (see Table 35.3). There is little that can be effectively done to a patient who is actively seizing, other than remove harmful or sharp objects from the area. Attempting to restrain the patient is fruitless and can lead to personal harm. Blindly forcing objects into the mouth to keep it open during the seizure often cause more harm than good. Benzodiazepines are first line therapy, with evidence pointing to the fact that the longer the seizure continues, the less effective benzodiazepine therapy becomes (Kapur and Macdonald, 1997). Benzodiazepines should be administered as soon as it is apparent that the seizure is not self-limiting, and depending on the training, experience, and comfort level of the practitioner. EMS triage becomes necessary for prolonged or abnormal seizure activity.

Stroke

Stroke is the acute neurological impairment that follows an interruption in blood supply to the brain, caused by an occlusive clot (ischemic) or rupture of a blood vessel (hemorrhagic) (AHA, 2008). 87% of all strokes are ischemic, which can be due to a thrombotic event (ruptured plaque) in a diseased vessel or an embolic event, when a portion of a peripheral clot in the arterial system separates from its source and travels cephalad until it lodges in a normal vessel, narrower than clot diameter. Therapy is different for these separate events. Tissue plasminogen activator (reperfusion therapy) is indicated for ischemic stroke, but is an absolute contraindication in hemorrhagic stroke. A transient ischemic attack (TIA) is a focal neurologic deficit that resolves completely and spontaneously within 1 hour.

Stroke is the third leading cause of death in the United States (AHA, 2008). Risk factors include hypertension, diabetes, cigarette smoking, hypercoagulable state, atrial fibrillation, recent TIA, carotid stenosis, and polycythemia, among others.

Table 35.3 Early management of seizures in the dental office.

- Protect patient from injury
- Protect patient airway
- Assess ABCs, 100% oxygen if possible
- Check blood glucose (if available)
  - If hypoglycemic
    - Administer 50 ml D50 – intravenously
    - Alternative is glucagon – 1 mg IM (if no IV)
- If seizures >2–3 minutes, 2.5mg IV midazolam or IM
  - Pediatric dose 0.1mg/kg IV or 0.15mg/kg IM
- EMS entry

Table 35.4 Signs of symptoms of stroke.

- Sudden weakness or numbness of the face, arm or leg, especially on one side of the body
- Sudden onset of confusion (difficult to assess if patient is sedated)
- Trouble speaking or understanding
- Sudden trouble in seeing in one or both eyes
- Sudden trouble walking, dizziness, loss of balance or coordination
- Sudden, severe headache with no known cause

Diagnosis

Early recognition of signs and symptoms will facilitate prompt entry into EMS. Most important is the time of symptom onset. If the patient was sedated, the time of symptom onset is defined as the last time the patient was observed to be normal. Signs and symptoms of stroke are listed in Table 35.4.

Further assessment is necessary to rule out stroke mimics, notably seizure and hypoglycemia that can occur in otherwise normal patients presenting for dental care.

The Cincinnati Prehospital Stroke Scale (CPSS) (Table 35.5) is based on physical examination only. The presence of a single abnormality has a sensitivity of 59% and a specificity of 89% (Kothari, 1999). However, if any one of the three signs is abnormal the probability of a stroke is 72%. The Los Angeles Prehospital Stroke Screen (LAPSS) has a sensitivity of 93% and a specificity of 97% (Kidwell, 2000). The examiner rules out other causes of altered levels of consciousness (e.g., history of seizures, severe hyperglycemia or hypoglycemia), then asymmetry is identified in any of the following three examination categories: facial smile or grimace, grip, and arm strength.

Table 35.5 Cincinnati Prehospital Stroke Scale.

- Facial droop (have patient show teeth or smile) (Figure 35.1)
  - Normal – both sides move equally
  - Abnormal – one side does not move as well as the other side
- Arm drift (patient closes eyes and hold both arms straight out for 10 seconds) (Figure 35.2)
  - Normal – both arms move the same or do not move at all
  - Abnormal – one arm does not move or one arm drifts down when compared with the other
- Abnormal speech (have the patient say "you can't teach an old dog new tricks")
  - Normal – patient uses correct words with no slurring
  - Abnormal – patient slurs words, uses the wrong words, or is unable to speak

Management

The overall goal of stroke care is to minimize acute brain injury and maximize patient recovery (Jauch et al., 2010) by appreciating the time-sensitive nature of stroke care. When indicated, IV fibrinolysis should be administered to eligible patients who can be treated in the time period of 3–4.5 hours after symptom onset (del Zoppo, 2009). Patients with acute stroke may be at risk for respiratory compromise from aspiration, upper airway obstruction, and/or hypoventilation. As such, "ABCs" should be closely evaluated and supported, with supplemental oxygen as required, wasting no time to EMS entry and transport. Unless the patient is hypotensive (systolic BP <90 mmHg,) prehospital intervention for blood pressure abnormalities is not recommended (Jauch et al., 2010).

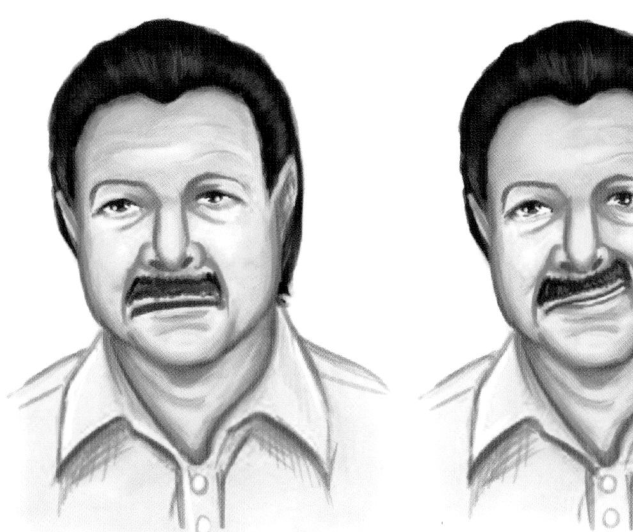

Figure 35.1 Facial droop.

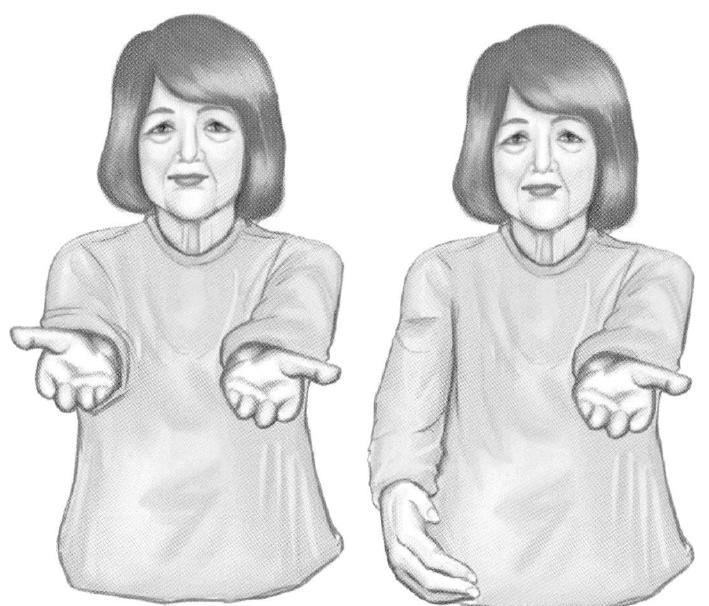

Figure 35.2 Arm drift.

References

American Heart Association. *Heart Disease and Stroke Statistics-2008 Update*. Dallas: American Heart Association, 2008.

Constant, I., et al. Sevoflurance and epileptiform EEG changes. *Paediatr Anaesth* **15**: 266–274, 2005.

Del Zoppo, G. J. Expansion of the time window for treatment of acute ischemic stroke with intravenous tissue plasminogen activator: a science advisory from the American Heart Association/American Stroke Association. *Stroke* **40**: 2945–2948, 2009.

Jauch, E. C., et al. 2010 American Heart Association guidelines for cardiopulmonary resuscitation and emergency cardiovascular care. Part 11: stroke. *Circulation* **122**: s818-s828, 2010.

Kapur, J, and Macdonald, R. L. Rapid seizure-induced reduction of benzodiazepine and Zn^{2+} sensitivity of hippocampal dentate granule cell $GABA_A$ receptors. *J Neurosci* **17**: 7532–40, 1997.

Kidwell, C. S., et al. Identifying stroke in the field. Prospective validation of the Los Angeles prehospital stroke screen (LAPSS). *Stroke* **31**: 71–76, 2000.

Kofke, W. A. Anesthetic management of the patient with epilepsy or prior seizures. *Curr Opin Anaesthesiol* **23**: 391–399, 2010.

Kothari, R. U., et al. Cincinnati prehospital stroke scale: reproducibility and validity. *Ann Emerg Med* **33**: 373–378, 1999.

Lowenstein, D. H., et al. It's time to revise the definition of status epilepticus. *Epilepsia* **40**: 120–22, 1999.

Modica, P., et al. Pro- and anticonvulsant effects of anesthetics [part 1]. *Anesth Analg* **70**: 303–315, 1990.

Mohanram, A., et al. Repetitive generalized seizure activity during emergence form sevoflurane anesthesia. *Can J Anaesth* **54**: 657–61, 2007.

Myslobodsky, M.S., et al. Ketamine: convulsant or anti-convulsant? *Pharmacol Biochem Behav* **14**: 27–33, 1981.

Niesen, A. D., et al. perioperative seizures in patients with a history of a seizure disorder. *Anesth Analg* **1111**: 729–735, 2010.

Perks, A., et al. Anaesthesia and epilepsy. *Br J Anaesthesia* **108**: 562–571, 2012.

Saboory, E., et al. Mechanisms of morphine enhancement of spontaneous seizure activity. *Anesth Analg* **105**: 1729–1735, 2007.

Shah, S. M. Everything that shakes is not a seizure: a primer of movement disorders for emergency physicians. *Emerg Med Reports* **22**: 43–56, 2001.

36 Acute, adverse cognitive, behavioral, and neuromuscular changes

Edward Adlesic[1], Douglas Anderson[2], Robert Bosack[3], Daniel L. Orr[4], and Steven Ganzberg[5]

[1]University of Pittsburgh School of Dental Medicine, Department of Oral and Maxillofacial Surgery, Pittsburgh, PA, USA

[2]Oregon Health Sciences University, Department of Anesthesiology and Peri Operative Medicine, Portland, OR, USA

[3]University of Illinois, College of Dentistry, Chicago, IL, USA

[4]UNLV School of Dental Medicine and University of Nevada School of Medicine, Las Vegas, NV, USA

[5]UCLA School of Dentistry, Century City Outpatient Surgery Center, Los Angeles, CA, USA

Enteral and parenteral sedative/anesthetic agents are administered by dental professionals for at least three reasons: to facilitate and expedite painful or threatening procedures, to humanely mitigate physical and emotional reaction to painful stimuli, and to improve patient satisfaction. These techniques are successful in a vast majority of circumstances, where patients react predictably and sufficiently to the administered medication, followed by uneventful recovery. Unfortunately, there are instances where these techniques are insufficient and unsatisfactory (failed sedation) because of adverse changes in airway, breathing, circulation, or adverse patient response.

Patients do not always respond predictably to sedative/anesthetic medications administered in the dental office. While families and patients are often amused by postanesthetic euphoria, they become dismayed and unsatisfied with negative experiences of agitation or emergence delirium. A wide, variable and sometimes progressive range of adverse patient responses is possible. These include delirium, disinhibition, agitation, violence, movement disorders and fever. Possible etiologies for this diverse clinical spectrum include hypoxia, hypoglycemia, hypovolemia (hypotension), expression of an underlying illness, administered drug effect (adverse, overdose, paradoxical, underdose), illicit drug effect (overdose or withdrawal state), and limited impulse control, among others.

The acute onset of adverse perianesthetic cognitive, behavioral, and/or neuromuscular changes is challenging for the sedation provider and disruptive to daily office flow. The variability of the clinical presentations confounds prevention, recognition, diagnosis, and management of these situations. Many providers may be unwilling or unable (training, licensure) to advance sedation to full general anesthesia to eliminate or postpone adversity. In addition, many offices will not have immediate availability of glucometers, or drugs such as haloperidol or physostigmine. Licensure and consent issues further cloud the acute management of these potentially difficult situations.

Regardless of the etiology, the *initial* approach to these situations includes maintenance of airway, breathing, circulation, and oxygenation, while ensuring the safety of patient, staff, and self. Mild changes can be carefully monitored until stable resolution in a safe, non-stimulating environment. Early entry into EMS is advisable, as definitive diagnosis and treatment often require medical intervention, including diagnostic and supportive/definitive therapy not available in dental offices. The use of reversal agents (naloxone and flumazenil) remains an attractive option, given the premise that the adverse situation developed in an "unaffected" patient *after* drug administration. Unfortunately, reversal may not be an option (lost IV access in an uncooperative patient) and may not be effective, as underlying pathophysiology, once exposed, can persist beyond the triggering event (hysterical conversion reaction, Orr and Glassman, 1985).

This chapter addresses adverse situations and manifestations of toxicity that can present during the administration of office-based sedation/anesthesia. These include serotonin syndrome, anticholinergic syndrome, benzodiazepine disinhibition, agitation, violence, and malignant hyperthermia (MH). The term syndrome implies a variable spectrum of toxicity-related signs and symptoms. Several of these syndromes share clinical features, which emphasizes the importance of a thorough medical history and total situational awareness when evaluating and managing these situations.

Definitions

Adverse cognitive and behavioral fluctuations populate a spectrum ranging from hyperactive to hypoactive (see Table 36.1).

Perception is awareness of the environment via physical sensation (vision, hearing, proprioception).

Cognition is the capacity to process perceptions, applying knowledge and changing preferences. It involves reasoning, memory,

Anesthesia Complications in the Dental Office, First Edition. Edited by Robert C. Bosack and Stuart Lieblich.

Table 36.1 The continuum of adverse cognitive and behavioral changes.

Hypoactive			Hyperactive		
Delirium	Disinhibition	Confusion	Agitation	Aggression	Violence

Table 36.2 Risk factors and precipitating factors for delirium in the dental office.

Delirium	
Predisposing risk factors	**Precipitating factors**
• Age • Male gender • History of psychiatric illness • Dehydration • Polypharmacy • Psychotropic medication • drugs with anticholinergic activity • recent change in medication • substance abuse / withdrawal • Comorbid diseases • Metabolic derangement (hypoxia, hypoglycemia)	• Anesthetic drugs, especially meperidine and drugs with anticholinergic properties (TCAs, atropine, anti-histamines and antipsychotics (Marcantonio et al., 1994) • Hypoxia • Pain • Emotional stress • Metabolic derangement

solving, planning, and execution (executive functioning, Silverstein, 2009).

Confusion is a variable degree of lack of understanding, an inability to correctly perceive or process information.

Delirium is an acute, unpleasant alteration of mood, characterized by a variable and fluctuating disturbance in the level of consciousness, often accompanied by a disturbance of attention and cognitive impairment (disorganized thinking) that cannot be accounted for by preexisting disease (DSM-TR-IV, 2000; Skrobik, 2011). Disturbances in the level of consciousness include a diminished awareness of the environment, altering the ability to focus, sustain, or shift attention. Orientation, thought process, perception, memory, mood, and behavior are among the domains that can be affected.

Postoperative delirium is frequently described in elderly patients after major inpatient surgery. Onset often occurs after 24 hours and up to 7 days after the procedure (Sieber, 2009). Although the pathogenesis is poorly understood and most likely multifactorial, delirium is thought to occur with or result from a combination of increased dopaminergic activity and decreased cholinergic and GABA activity (Boyer and Shannon, 2005; Trzepacz and van der Mast, 2002). Dopaminergic drugs (levodopa and buporprion) can precipitate delirium, while dopamine antagonists (antipsychotics) are often used to manage symptoms. Inflammatory cytokines, the neuroendocrine stress response, and alterations in serotonergic transmission have also been postulated. Delirium can also be a typical or atypical presentation of comorbid disease.

Tune (2001), Inouye (2006), and Steiner (2011a) indicate that vulnerability to delirium depends on both predisposing and precipitating factors, with a predisposed patient more likely to be susceptible to weak triggers and vice versa (see Table 36.2).

Table 36.3 The richmond agitation sedation scale (Sessler et al., 2002).

Score	Term	Description
+4	Combative	Combative, violent, immediate danger to state
+3	Very agitated	Aggressive, pulls or removes tubes or catheters
+2	Agitated	Frequent nonpurposeful movement
+1	Restless	Anxious, but movements not aggressive or vigorous
0	Alert and calm	
−1	Drowsy	Sustained awakening (>10sec) with eye contact to voice
−2	Light sedation	Briefly awakens (<10 sec) with eye contact to voice
−3	Moderate sedation	Movement or eye opening to voice, but no eye contact
−4	Deep sedation	No response to voice, responds to physical stimulation
−5	Unarousable	No response to voice or physical stimulation

Perianesthetic delirious behavior (Silverstein, 2009) describes the emergence agitation (delirium or excitement) often seen in children emerging from anesthesia with volatile agents, in patients after the administration of ketamine or benzodiazepines. This includes disinhibited behavior, where patients are often unresponsive to commands. Physical movement may be difficult to control and occur with strength out of proportion to what is expected from the patient, based on size and muscularity. This behavior is typically self-limiting. Postanesthetic emergence agitation does not appear to be related to postoperative delirium (Steiner, 2011b).

Anxiety is an unpleasant alteration of mood or emotion that is not accompanied by cognitive dysfunction (Hurford, 2012). There appears to be no relationship between anxiety and the occurrence of postoperative delirium in the elderly patient.

Agitation is nonspecific excessive, nonproductive and repetitious motor activity, which can result from pain or anxiety (Hurford, 2012). The Richmond Agitation Sedation Scale has been used to quantify levels of agitation and sedation (Sessler et al., 2002) (see Table 36.3). Agitation introduces the risk of escalation to aggression or violence.

Aggression is forceful, hostile behavior, or attitudes toward another, often with a readiness and intent to confront, attack, and cause harm.

Violence is irrational, physical, compulsive use of brute force to harm self or others. It is associated with vigorous visceral and sympathetic responses. It is usually, but not necessarily, associated with psychiatric illness (personality disorder, bipolar disorder, substance abuse) or drug withdrawal. Oftentimes, violent patients will have committed acts of violence in the past (Fazel et al., 2009; Pulay et al., 2008; Downes, 2009).

Serotonin syndrome

Serotonin (5-HT or 5-hydroxytryptamine) is a neurotransmitter that modulates pain, sleep, appetite, anxiety, depression, migraine and emesis, among others (Dunkley et al., 2003). Serotonin is synthesized from tryptophan and metabolized by monoamine oxidase (MAO).

Table 36.4 A partial list of medications that can increase serotonergic activity (Birmes et al., 2003).

Amphetamines	Ecstasy
	Methamphetamine
	Sibutramine
Analgesics	Fentanyl
	Meperidine
	Tramadol
	Pentazocine
Psychotropic agents	Buspirone
	Lithium
	MAOI
	SSRI
	St. John's wort
	TCA
Antiemetics	Metoclopramide
	Ondansetron
Miscellaneous	Valproic acid
	Cocaine
	Dextromethorphan
	L-tryptophan, 5-hydroxytryptophan

Serotonin syndrome is a predictable spectrum of consequences resulting from overstimulation of serotonin receptors in the central and peripheral nervous systems, which range from barely perceptible to life threatening. Signs and symptoms occur within hours of increased stimulation. Mechanisms include overdose of a serotonergic drug, exposure to a combination of drugs with serotonergic activity, increased serotonin synthesis or release, or reduced serotonin uptake (SSRIs) or metabolism (MAO) (see Table 36.4). Notably, the combination of MAOIs and SSRIs has been documented to be particularly lethal. It has been classically described as a triad of mental status changes, autonomic instability, and neuromuscular hyperactivity (Ables and Nagubilli, 2010); however, this information may not be helpful for accurate clinical diagnosis. Concentration-dependent toxicity results in a symptom spectrum shown in Table 36.5.

Rules for specific and sensitive prediction of serotonin toxicity are included in the Hunter Serotonin Toxicity Criteria (Dunkley et al., 2003), which assesses the following parameters: spontaneous clonus (involuntary, rhythmic muscular contractions and relaxations), inducible clonus, ocular clonus, agitation, diaphoresis, tremor, and hyperreflexia. See Table 36.6.

There are other signs and symptoms of serotonin toxicity that can also occur with other syndromes; lack of specificity limits their values as diagnostic indicators. Mydriasis, tachycardia, and hypertension can occur with serotonin toxicity, anticholinergic excess, and sympathomimetic toxicity. The skin is wet with serotonin toxicity, but dry with anticholinergic toxicity. Neuromuscular tone is increased with serotonin toxicity, but normal in anticholinergic toxicity (see Table 36.7). There are no specific laboratory tests to diagnose serotonin toxicity.

Table 36.5 Symptom spectrum associated with serotonergic toxicity (Boyer and Shannon, 2005).

Severity of reaction	Mental status changes	Autonomic instability	Neuromuscular activity
Mild	Restlessness (akathisia) Anxiety	Tachycardia Mydriasis Shivering Sweating (diaphoresis)	Intermittent tremor Hyperreflexia
Moderate	Agitation	Hypertension	Inducible clonus, legs
	Easily startled	Fever < 104°F	Horizontal ocular myoclonus Sustained clonus
Severe	Confusion Delirium Coma	Fever > 104°F	Leg rigidity

Table 36.6 Hunter serotonin toxicity criteria: decision rules (Dunkley et al., 2003).

In the presence of a serotonergic agent, any of the following predict serotonin toxicity:

1 Spontaneous clonus
2 Inducible clonus and either agitation or diaphoresis
3 Ocular clonus and agitation or diaphoresis
4 Tremor and hyperreflexia
5 Muscle rigidity and temperature > 100.4°F, and either ocular clonus or inducible clonus

Occurrence of serotonin toxicity in the dental office would most likely be serendipitous, following recent alteration in drugs or doses with serotonergic potential (Szakaly and Strauss, 2008). Narcotics, notably meperidine (but also fentanyl), have been known to precipitate toxicity in susceptible patients.

Stepwise treatment is guided by severity. Serotonergic medication should be immediately discontinued. Supportive care and entry into EMS are indicated in all but most mild cases. Cyproheptadine (a serotonin 2A antagonist) is the most widely used antidote (Gillman, 1999), at an initial dose of 12mg PO, followed by 2mg q2h until symptom resolution. Fever and rigidity are medically controlled.

Table 36.7 Distinguishing features of three syndromes that share common features.

	Medical history	Onset	Vital signs	Skin	Muscle tone
Serotonin toxicity	Serotonergic drug	1/2–24 hours	Tachycardia, hypertension, moderate fever	Wet	Increased
Anticholinergic toxicity	Anticholinergic drug	< 12 hours	Tachycardia, hypertension, mild fever	Dry, hot, red	Normal
Malignant hyperthermia	Volatile gas +/or succinylcholine	$^1/_2$ to 24 hours	Tachycardia, hypertension, severe fever, hypercarbia	Wet, mottled	Rigid

Table 36.8 Central and peripheral effects of ach.

D – diarrhea
U – urination
M – miosis, accommodation for near vision
B – bronchoconstriction, bradycardia
E – excitation in the CNS and skeletal muscle (tremor, anxiety, seizures)
L – lacrimation
S – salivation and sweating

Anticholinergic syndrome

Acetylcholine (ACh) is a cholinergic neurotransmitter in both the central and the peripheral nervous systems. Cholinergic synapses are further classified nicotinic (neuromuscular junction, ganglia, and CNS) or muscarinic (salivary and sweat glands, heart and smooth muscle, and CNS). In the CNS, ACh regulates many functions, including the sleep–awake cycle, memory, alertness, orientation, and analgesia (Brown et al., 2004). Muscarinic stimulation by ACh causes effects seen in Table 36.8.

Drugs with anticholinergic properties (see Table 36.10) competitively inhibit binding of ACh to central receptors and peripheral postganglionic cholinergic (muscarinic) receptors supplying smooth muscle (intestine, heart and bronchi), salivary and sweat glands, and the ciliary body of the eye.

A decrease in cholinergic activity can result in a wide variety of both central and peripheral, dose-related signs and symptoms (Schneck and Rupreht, 1989). In the absence of peripheral signs and symptoms, which are uncommon after anesthesia, but easier to diagnose (dry skin and mucous membranes, tachycardia, tremors, blurred vision, and dilated pupils), isolated central symptoms can be difficult to diagnose, and can be confused with prolonged recovery. As ACh receptors are widely distributed within the brain, blockade can lead to a variety of signs including fluctuations between excitation and depression. Central excitatory symptoms include confusion, agitation, delirium, seizures, fever, and ataxia; central depressive symptoms include prolonged somnolence, sedation, and mental impairment. In addition to tachycardia and constipation, cholinergic blockade can lead to signs and symptoms summarized in Table 36.9.

The possibility of anticholinergic toxicity should be entertained in any patient presenting with altered mental status after sedation/anesthesia. In addition to atropine and scopolamine (rarely used), which are tertiary antimuscarinic agents, capable of crossing the blood–brain barrier, there are numerous other medications that can contribute to an anticholinergic burden resulting in toxicity (Table 36.10). Elderly patients are particularly prone to toxicity because of an age-related decrease in cholinergic transmission. Diagnosis of anticholinergic toxicity is imprecise, and often one of exclusion, based on signs and symptoms in addition to recent exposure to medications with anticholinergic properties. The differential diagnoses of anticholinergic toxicity include hypoxia, hypercarbia, malingering, endocrinopathy (hypoglycemia or thyrotoxicosis), or electrolyte disorders.

Treatment of suspected anticholinergic toxicity in patients who have had recent exposure to medications with anticholinergic effects is supportive, including close monitoring of vital signs, protecting the patient from injury, and IV fluids. Physostigmine can be administered when there is a strong suspicion of anticholinergic toxicity. Physostigmine is a tertiary amine (therefore, capable of crossing the blood brain barrier). As an anticholinesterase inhibitor, it competitively inhibits the action of acetylcholinesterase, thereby preventing the degradation of ACh. The resultant increase in ACh competitively displaces muscarinic antagonists from ACh receptors. An intravenous dose of 1–3 mg (0.01–0.04 mg. kg) should be administered slowly to avoid minimize bradycardia and bronchoconstriction, especially in patients with heart block and asthma. Onset is within 5–10 min and duration is 1–2 hours. Seizures, excess salivation, nausea, ocular pain, and blurred vision can occur after administration of physostigmine; these peripheral

Table 36.9 Classic features of anticholinergic toxicity*.

Red as a beet	Cutaneous vasodilation to dissipate heat to compensate for loss of sweating
Dry as a bone	Xerostomia and anhydrosis – dry skin, due to decreased sweating
Hot as hell	Anhydrotic hyperthermia – due to decreased sweating
Blind as a bat	Pupils are dilated (mydriasis) and accommodation is inhibited
Mad as a hatter†	Blockade of CNS muscarinic receptors lead to anxiety, agitation, confusion, delirium, coma and seizures
Full as a flask	Reduced detrusor muscle tone of the bladder decreases urge to urinate and prevents normal opening of urethral sphincter

*Tachycardia and bronchiolar smooth muscle relaxation are also anticholinergic responses not included in the table.
†Mad hatter syndrome refers to an early industrial occupational disease secondary to mercury poisoning. Mercury was used in the manufacture of felt hats. Workers chronically exposed to this cumulative poison developed physical symptoms of "mad hatter syndrome," including trembling (hatter's shakes), loss of coordination, and slurred speech. Mental changes included irritability, memory loss, depression, and other personality changes.

Table 36.10 Select Medications with anticholinergic side effects (Tune et al., 1992; Lieberman, 2004; Brown et al., 2004).

- Antimuscarinics
  - Centrally acting tertiary amines
    - atropine
    - scopolamine
  - peripherally acting quartenary amines
    - glycopyrrolate
- Antihistamines
  - Diphenhydramine
  - Hydroxyzine
- Cardiovascular
  - ACE inhibitors
  - Warfarin
  - Digoxin
- CNS drugs
  - Antipsychotics
  - MAOI
  - SSRI
  - TCA
  - Benzodiazepines
  - Narcotics, including meperidine
- Glucocorticoids
- Anti-parkinson agents
- Antibiotics
- Illicit drugs

signs can be safely reversed with glycopyrrolate, a quartenary amine that will not cross the blood–brain barrier.

Benzodiazepine disinhibition

Benzodiazepines are commonly administered to achieve anxiolysis, amnesia, and sedation to facilitate dental procedures. Although this practice is considered safe and predictable, there are rare instances (< 1%, Dietch and Jennings, 1988) where a paradoxical and unexpected increase in emotional release can occur after the administration of a benzodiazepine. Reported episodes vary in intensity and include confusion, agitation, aggression, violent motor behavior, hostility, rage, dislodging intravenous catheters, screaming, and crying (Mancuso et al., 2004). These reactions are further characterized by four factors: they occur in response to provocation, they are recognized by others but not the patient, and they usually occur with high doses and with drugs of higher potency (Bond, 1998). Parenteral administration of drugs having shorter half-lives can also increase risk.

The exact mechanism for paradoxical benzodiazepine disinhibition is unknown. It can occur with all benzodiazepines administered either parenterally or enterally. Loss of cortical restraint that governs normal social behavior coupled with a reduced ability to perceive social cues to guide normal behavior remains an attractive explanation (Paton, 2002). Although disinhibition is unpredictable, patients who may be more susceptible include those at age extremes, patients with a history of aggression, antisocial personality, alcoholism, or poor impulse control.

Initial treatment is supportive, with maintenance of airway and intravenous access, while protecting the patient from injury. Treatment choices involve changing the depth of sedation by reversing the benzodiazepine with flumazenil or increasing anesthetic depth with additional benzodiazepines, ketamine, hypnotic agents, or volatile agents. Increasing the dose of benzodiazepines can have unpredictable results and may aggravate the situation. Once a deeper level of anesthesia is achieved, emergence can still be accompanied by disinhibitory reactions. Flumazenil is a competitive benzodiazepine antagonist with a 1–2 minute onset after IV administration and a duration of 1 hour. Successful adult doses range from 0.3 to 0.5 mg, which often retain sufficient sedation and amnesia, which allow case completion (McKenzie and Rosenberg, 2010). Pediatric doses of 0.01 mg/kg can be adequate. Redosing may be required as most benzodiazepines have longer half-lives than flumazenil.

Agitation and violence

Agitation, aggression, and violence, although infrequent, can occur in the dental office either before or after sedative/anesthetic drugs are administered. Etiology and treatment approaches are different for each. It should be stated that there is no protocol for prevention or treatment that is 100% successful and that safety for self and others is the top priority. The call for help (EMS and/or police) should not be delayed.

Patients can present to the dental office in an agitated state for many reasons, which can escalate with even the slightest trigger: prolonged waiting time, pain, financial issues, etc. In addition to the disruptive behavior, anyone in close proximity can be at immediate risk for harm. Differential diagnosis includes hypoglycemia, hypoxia, illicit drug exposure (intoxication or withdrawal state), psychiatric disturbance, or a recent change in dose or type of psychiatric medication, among others (Vilke and Wilson, 2009). Factors predisposing to violence are seen in Table 36.11 (Villari et al., 2007). Psychiatric illness, coupled with substance abuse and a prior history of violence, increases the likelihood of violence (Elbogen and Johnson, 2009).

Table 36.11 Predisposing factors for violence.

- Young age
- Male gender
- Lack of education

Lower socioeconomic status

- Unemployed
- Psychiatric illness
  - Personality disorder
  - Poor impulse control
  - Explosive or unpredictable anger/rage
  - Post-traumatic stress disorder
- Intimidating behavior
- Physical agitation

Physical or verbal abuse to others

- Impulsivity

History of violent behavior

- Substance abuse

Although unpredictable, there are three phases of violence (Coburn and Mycyk, 2009). *Anxiety and anger* are often accompanied by loud pressured speech, bodily movements whose only purpose seems to be the expenditure of energy (tense posturing, frequent position changes, pacing, clenching fists), and aggressive acts including hitting self or inanimate objects. *Defensiveness* develops when patients feel that they are losing control and become verbally abusive, irrational, and profane. *Physical aggression* is the third phase.

Prior to the onset of physical aggression, verbal de-escalation can be attempted (Moore and Pfaff, 2014). The call for help should not be delayed. Show concern in a calm and unhurried manner with non-aggressive posturing (sitting position, out of arm's reach, allowing the patient an unobstructed exit path). The patient should not be touched and eye to eye contact should be limited. Voices should not be raised. Take all threats seriously, treat the patient with respect, and address his/her concerns. Verbally agree with requests with limitations (e.g., "Yes, as soon as...." Or "but first we need to ... "). A dominant presence should be maintained, without hint of weakness or vulnerability. If de-escalation is successful, the patient should leave the office immediately and issues postponed for another time.

A different approach is necessary when violent or aggressive acts occur after the administration of sedative, analgesic, or hypnotic drugs in subanesthetic doses (drugs that alter cognition and decision-making). Adequate patient screening and conservative case selection may avert anticipated trouble. Prior anesthetic history, psychiatric and drug (prescribed and illicit) history, and "heightened suspicion" can be used as a basis for case refusal or shift of treatment venue to a non-office location.

When patient control is lost, and the practitioner is unwilling or unable to increase depth of anesthesia (training, licensure), robust and rapid drug reversal can be attempted. Benzodiazepines can be administered in cases of ketamine emergence, with appropriate monitoring of airway and vital signs. Ketamine darts, succinylcholine, or antipsychotics such as haloperidol are unpredictable and/or may worsen the situation. Physical restraint may be necessary to prevent injury to patient, self, and staff. EMS and/or police should be contacted without delay.

Restraint

Several entities in this chapter may be precursors for clinical presentations that can progress to one in which physical restraint is necessary for the protection of the patient and others. Technically, a mouth prop or arm board for catheter stabilization is considered restraint.

Occasionally, more significant restraint measures may be needed. For instance, patients may offer histories of previous untoward physical reactions to anesthesia, thus warning of the possible need for restraint. Prophylactic arm and leg restraint may be suggested to these patients prior to the administration of anesthesia.

More commonly, however, uncontrolled uninhibited physical reactions are not expected and can occur in any patient population. For this reason, practitioners may want to strongly consider obtaining informed consent for emergency restraint. It is also important that responsible third parties, such as parents of children, understand that restraint may be necessary and are not confused in situations that may otherwise be surprising.

Importantly, treatment areas including operatories and recovery rooms should be proactively secured from non-office personnel until the patient is deemed ready for interaction with his lay caregivers. Finally, as mentioned previously, in situations that cannot be adequately controlled, consideration can be given to calling security staff, law enforcement, and/or emergency responders.

Malignant hyperthermia

MH is a rare pharmacogenetic disorder that results in a hypermetabolic crisis of skeletal muscle when exposed to potent volatile inhalation anesthetic agents and/or succinylcholine. With the use of dantrolene the mortality rates in the United States have dropped to 11.7% (Rosero et al., 2009). There are 400 to 1000 suspected cases of MH reported to the MH Association of the United States (MHAUS) each year, and of these cases, approximately 500 are truly MH. Cases are more common in children and adolescents (1:15,000 cases with a peak age of 18.3 years). In adults, the incidence is 1:50,000; males have a greater incidence, while females have a higher mortality rate. The risk of pediatric MH has decreased over the past few years, but this may be related to the decreased use of succinylcholine in these patients (Larach et al., 2008a).

Pathophysiology of MH

Calcium mediates skeletal muscle contractions. In the resting state, calcium is stored in the sarcoplasmic reticulum (SR) and not in the muscle cytoplasm. When ACh binds to the muscle receptors, depolarization occurs, which releases the calcium from the SR. The calcium enters the muscle cytoplasm from the SR by way of the ryanodine (RyR1) receptor channels. Cytoplasmic calcium then binds to troponin, which allows actin to bind to myosin to shorten the muscle fibers and this causes the muscle to contract. This will continue to occur unless there is mechanism to stop the reaction. ATP in the cytoplasm stops the actin–myosin reaction and also pumps the excess calcium back into the SR (Noble 2007) (see Figure 36.1).

During an MH crisis, the RyR1 channel remains open, allowing calcium to flow excessively into the muscle cytoplasm resulting in a hypermetabolic crisis. Aerobic metabolism drives the reaction until oxygen supplies are depleted. Oxygen consumption is increased up

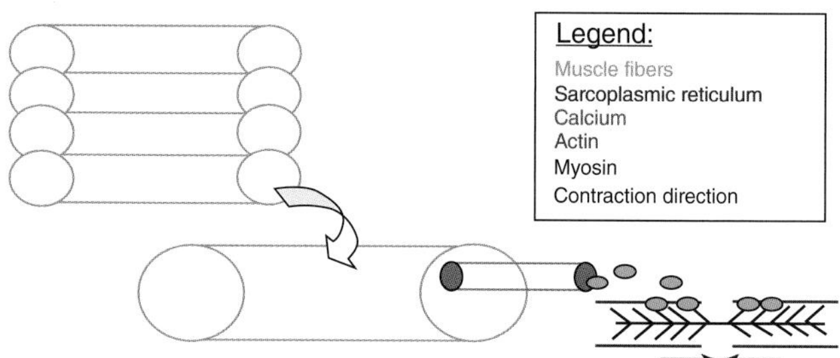

Figure 36.1 In a muscle fiber, Ca^{++} is stored in the sarcoplasmic reticulum (SR). The arrival of an electrical impulse releases the Ca^{++} → Ca^{++} binds to troponin → actin and myosin interact → the muscle fiber shortens. The stored energy in ATP is used in two ways. First, it is used to release the myosin from the actin, leading to muscle relaxation; second, it is used to actively pump Ca^{++} back into the SR. J Perianesth Nurs 22: 341–345, 2007. Used with permission.

to three times normal and the supply of ATP is depleted, trying to pump calcium back into the SR to stop the actin–myosin contractions. Anaerobic metabolism then becomes prominent, leading to metabolic acidosis.

During the period of anaerobic metabolism, the destructive effects of MH are seen. As acidosis develops, cell death occurs, releasing potassium into the circulation, which can be initially detected on the ECG monitor as tall, peaked T waves and small P waves. Muscle necrosis releases myoglobin into the circulation, which increases blood viscosity and capillary obstruction resulting in renal damage in the absence of early treatment. Coagulopathies may be observed.

The untreated hypermetabolic state leads to systemic hypoxia and untreated metabolic acidosis exacerbates renal dysfunction. When persistent hyperkalemia occurs, dysrhythmias may follow leading to cardiac arrest. Disseminated intravascular coagulation frequently develops once temperatures rise above 41.5 C or 106.7 F, which usually culminates in fatality.

MH can occur with the patient's first exposure to a triggering agent, but in at least 30% of cases it can take at least 3 exposures to trigger a crisis, and there is one report where it took up to 10 anesthetic exposures before MH occurred. It is rare to see succinylcholine as a sole triggering agent. In reviewing the current MHAUS registry, in one series, only 6 cases of 500 + documented MH reactions had succinylcholine as the only trigger, and in all of those cases, the dose was > 0.5 mg/kg. The most intense reactions occur when a patient is exposed to a volatile anesthetic gas plus succinylcholine (Rosenberg et al., 2007). Larach (2010) reported that 45% of MH cases occurred after exposure to volatile gases only, 54% occurred after exposure to volatile gases plus succinylcholine, and 0.7% of MH cases occurred after exposure to succinylcholine without volatile gas.

MH reactions are a response to exposure to "triggering agents," which include the potent volatile anesthetic gases and succinylcholine. Patients exposed to both succinylcholine and volatile agents tend to have faster onset MH crisis and more intense reactions.

MH-like syndromes can be triggered by physical stress, overheating, infections, or neuroleptic malignant syndrome. While these reactions are very uncommon, there is evidence to believe that they may be related to MHS, but these reactions are not necessarily life threatening and it is not clear that dantrolene therapy is effective.

Clinical presentation of malignant hyperthermia

The defining clinical sign of MH is a persistently elevated (>55mmHg) $EtCO_2$, despite aggressive positive pressure ventilation. Although tachycardia usually precedes hypercapnia, CO_2 accumulation is the most sensitive sign of MH.

The earliest descriptions of MH included all patients having generalized muscle rigidity along with hyperthermia, acidosis, and high mortality rates. Current data indicates that muscle rigidity may not always be present and hyperthermia is often a late clinical finding. In addition to increases in $EtCO_2$, most patients will show early signs of tachycardia, hypertension, and possibly a drop in SpO_2. Cardiac dysrhythmias secondary to hyperkalemia may be seen as the process progresses. The initial temperature elevation is usually 1° to 2°C every 5 minutes but there may be a delay in onset of temperature elevation. High temperatures of 41.5°C or more lead to coagulopathies with fatal outcomes.

Excessive muscle metabolism and breakdown results in hyperkalemia, hypercalcemia, acidosis, and myoglobinuria (cola colored urine). There is usually an increase in creatine kinase ≥ 20,000 units during the first 24 hours, but this is not always a consistent finding. If detected, this helps confirm the MH diagnosis (Rosero et al., 2009).

Increased muscle mass elevates the risk of death by 14 times and the risk of cardiac arrest by 19 times. The longer it takes for the $EtCO_2$ to peak, the greater the risk of arrest and death. Patients who develop DIC have a 50 times increased arrest rate and 89 times increased death rate.

Postoperative MH

The incidence of postoperative MH is low, only accounting for 1.9% of all cases found in the MHAUS registry. The maximum latency period is unknown, but most cases occur within 0–40 minutes post-op. Unlike classic MH, hyperthermia is not a typical presenting sign. Most of these cases are in fact atypical, and the only abnormality may just be an episode of rhabdomolysis when cola colored urine is noted. These patients should be sent for follow-up muscle biopsy and/or genetic testing to confirm MH susceptibility (Litman et al., 2008).

Recrudescence of MH

An acceptable definition of this reaction is recurrence of a successfully treated MH crisis ≥ 2 hours after the initial event. The incidence is about 20% of MH cases with 50% of these cases occurring in the first 9 hours and 80% occurring within 16 hours. The greater the intensity of the initial reaction, the more likely it is that recurrence will be seen, but there is no correlation to the dose of dantrolene needed to stop the initial MH crisis and the risk of a recurrent reaction.

The odds of recrudescence double in patients with increased muscle mass. The longer it takes for the initial reaction to develop, the more likely you are to see recrudescence. Hyperthermia may be the only classical sign of MH in patients who develop this condition. There are no reports of MH recrudescence with the use of desflurane as the sole anesthetic, so potency and blood:gas solubility may be factors (Burkman et al., 2007). Duration of exposure to a trigger appears to be a risk factor (Hopkins 2007).

Core Temperatures

Temperature monitoring, preferably core monitoring, should be employed for all general anesthetics utilizing triggering agents. Core temperature monitoring is more accurate than peripheral temperature monitoring and includes the use of distal esophagus, rectum, nasopharynx, and tympanic temperatures. In an office, nasopharyngeal and tympanic monitors can be used and accepted by the patient. Peripheral temperatures in the office include mouth, axillae, and forehead temperature strips. While these are not as accurate as core readings, they are acceptable for office-based temperature monitoring. The capnometer remains as the critical monitor since temperature elevation is generally a late sign of MH (Rosenberg et al., 2007; Karlet 1998).

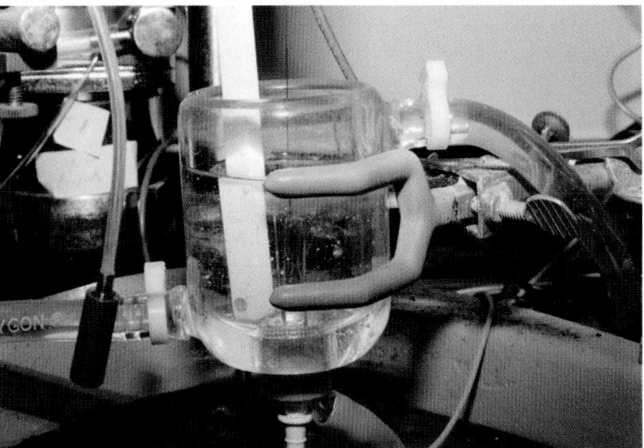

Figure 36.2 Caffeine halothane contracture test, courtesy of Dr. Silas Glisson.

Muscle biopsy: caffeine halothane contracture test (CHCT) (see Figure 36.2)

Introduced in the mid-1970s, muscle testing (see Caffeine halothane contracture test) is still the MHAUS gold standard for the diagnosis of MHS. A strip of muscle (usually vastus lateralis) is harvested and exposed to halothane and caffeine within 5 hours. Muscle contraction is measured against normal values, which provides risk stratification information. Abnormal contraction after exposure to both halothane and caffeine render the patient MH susceptible (MHS). Abnormal contraction after exposure to either halothane or caffeine renders the patient MH equivocal (MHE). No contraction to either agent renders the patient MH normal (MHN). Most US testing centers have guidelines for who can be tested: ASA I and II patients more than 10 years old and 40 kg weight. The sensitivity is reported as 100% (Patients who are MH prone are identified as such) and the specificity is 80–93% (approximately10–20% of patients who are not MH prone are identified as being such) (Hernandez et al., 2009).

Genetic testing & MH

MH is inherited as an autosomal dominant trait. To date, at least two genes have been implicated in MH inheritance. The RyR1 gene (MHS 1) is located on chromosome 19q13.1–13.2 and consists of 106 exons that are all capable of multiple mutations. It accounts for 50–80% of all MH mutations, which lead to a hypersensitive RyR1 channel (Litman et al., 2008; Ibarra, 2006). The second gene is CACNA1 (MHS 5) and accounts for 1% of MH genetic mutations.

One of the problems with genetic testing is that the expression of gene mutations can vary from country to country, local regions in one country, and even in a single family versus the general population (Sumitani et al., 2010). Genetic testing can be partial (Tier 1 testing) where three hot zones on the RyR1 gene are examined for known mutations, or complete (Tier 2 testing) where the entire RyR1 gene is scanned. The hot zones consist of 17 exons and if the scan is limited to just this area, the sensitivity of the test is ~23%. However, if you scan the entire gene, the sensitivity is ~70–80%. Another problem encountered with gene testing is discordance, which can occur in 10% of MH cases. In these cases, patient may be MHS positive by biopsy but there are no genetic mutations found. As a result, genetic testing is not at a stage where it can replace muscle biopsy in all patients.

If a family demonstrates one of the known 29 mutations, a suspect proband can undergo genetic testing first, and if they are positive for the mutation, they are MHS and muscle biopsy can be avoided (Brandom and Rosenberg, 2009).

MH is a heterogenetic disease where more than one gene may have mutations. Patients with two or more mutations are compound heterozygous and will have a greater incidence of MH. In some families that incidence can be 1 in 2000 to 1 in 8500 (Anderson et al., 2008).

Patients should be referred for genetic testing to centers where both testing and genetic counseling can be provided. Results can affect insurance policies, job opportunities, and willingness to have children. While most MHS patients have parents who are also MHS, there can be de novo mutations in a particular patient, which complicates making a correct diagnosis. Typically, a child of any MH-susceptible parent has about a 50% chance of being MHS (Rosenberg, 2010).

Management of MH crisis in the office setting

As the earliest signs of MH are tachycardia and an increase in $EtCO_2$, a capnograph must be used in addition to standard sedation monitors (ECG, NIBP, SpO_2) for patients who have been administered MH triggering agents. If an anesthesia machine with CO_2 absorber is being used with a circle system, the absorber will be hot secondary to an exothermic reaction from increased CO_2 uptake. If succinylcholine is available for emergency use only (such as for emergent treatment of persistent laryngospasm), and not as part of the planned anesthetic where other triggering agents are not used, the availability of advanced monitoring and even emergency medications such as dantrolene continues to be a debate within the dental community. The depth of management will depend on the knowledge and experience of the anesthesia provider and the distance to an emergency facility that can manage MH.

The diagnosis of MH may not be immediately obvious. Tachycardia may be attributed to inadequate anesthesia levels, and there is a wide differential diagnosis for elevated CO_2 levels, especially in open airway cases. In a review of 284 cases, it took an average time of 30 mins to initiate dantrolene once symptoms of MH were recognized by the doctor (Larach et al., 2010). The longer it takes to initiate dantrolene therapy, the greater the likelihood of serious complications (Larach et al., 2008b). Once the diagnosis of MH has been established, however, multiple tasks must be initiated simultaneously.

Emergency Medical Services must be activated immediately. Inform the dispatcher that the emergency is an MH crisis and that dantrolene and an anesthesiologist will be needed in the ED to prevent any delay in further therapy. If potent inhalation anesthetics are being used with a standard anesthesia machine, these agents must be discontinued and preferably, a new source of fresh gas and new breathing circuit used. Oxygen at 100% should be administered. In the dental office, a dental nitrous oxide/oxygen delivery device can be used to deliver 100% oxygen without a residual triggering agent being present, if needed via a Jackson-Rees or other single limb circuit with capnography capability. If this is not available and another "clean" anesthesia machine is not available,

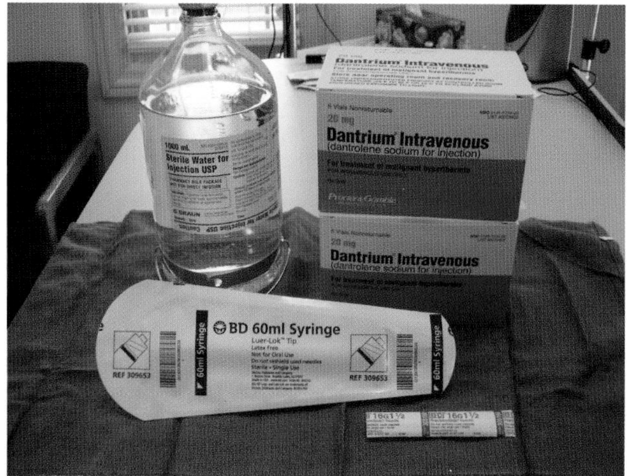

Figure 36.3 Supplies for reconstituting dantrolene.

the breathing circuit should still be changed and 100% oxygen delivered at 10L/min or more. If there is adequate available help, consider changing the CO_2 absorbent canisters. Hyperventilation should be continued to manage hypercarbia. Anesthesia may be maintained with intravenous propofol with or without opioids and ideally the patient should be paralyzed with a non-depolarizing muscle relaxant to facilitate positive pressure ventilation.

Dantrolene should be reconstituted and administered as soon as possible (Figure 36.3). A larger bore IV should be started if possible. Newer formulations of dantrolene can be reconstituted within 30 seconds but sterile water MUST still be used as a diluent. Each vial of dantrolene contains 20 mg of dantrolene plus 3 gms of mannitol and is diluted with 60 ml of sterile water. Mannitol is an osmotic diuretic that aids in flushing the kidneys of myoglobin. Reconstituted dantrolene must be used within 6 hours. The initial dose is 2.5 mg/kg. The event may terminate with just one dose of agent but some cases have required up to 10 mg/kg to stop the reaction. In practice, patient transfer will likely take place well before full dosing of dantrolene has occurred. As an example, a 70-kg patient will require 175 mg of dantrolene or 9 vials. A 20-kg child would require 50 mg or 2.5 vials. Adverse effects of dantrolene include muscle weakness (25% incidence), but cardiac muscle function is preserved. There is a 9 to 11% incidence of phlebitis because of the basic pH of 9.5 (Brandom, 2011).

Fluids should be aggressively administered. Intravenous normal saline, preferably refrigerated, will be the fluid of choice; lactated Ringers (LRs) solution has potassium and calcium added, which should be avoided. Additional IV access should be obtained with larger bore catheters. Low-dose furosemide may be considered in the office setting for increased diuresis prior to insertion of a urinary catheter on admission to the emergency department.

Metabolic acidosis should be treated with 1–2 mEq/kg of sodium bicarbonate if blood gas values are not available, as in the office setting.

Secondary efforts include the placement of ice packs around the axilla, groin, and legs. An orogastric tube can be used for cold saline flushes. The cooling process will need to continue as long as the patient is hyperthermic. Upon arrival in the ED, further cooling measures will be considered as needed. Cooling measures are stopped when the temperature reaches 38°C.

The ECG should be closely monitored for signs of hyperkalemia or other cardiac dysrhythmia. A reduction in the size of the P wave and peaked T waves are initially seen. Widening of the QRS complex implies severe hyperkalemia. Standard emergency and ACLS drugs should already be available. Hyperkalemia results from muscle breakdown, and potassium levels of > 6.0 mE/L are not uncommon. The initial management is hyperventilation and the administration of insulin and dextrose, which shifts potassium ions intracellularly:

1 10 units of insulin + 50 ml of 50% dextrose for adults
2 0.1 units of insulin + 1 ml/kg of 50% dextrose for children
3 Monitoring blood glucose levels within 30 minutes.

Albuterol can also be administered. Additional intravenous sodium bicarbonate may be considered, but this would be ideally administered following laboratory studies that are usually not available in the office setting. It should be noted that calcium channel blockers should not be used with dantrolene because they may further increase the release of potassium from the muscle, leading to serious cardiac dysrhythmias.

On admission to the hospital, arterial blood gases, electrolytes, creatinine, creatine kinase, coagulation studies, etc. will be obtained. The patient will likely be admitted to the ICU even if there is prompt resolution of the event. Oral dantrolene may be considered once the patient has stabilized.

Masseter muscle rigidity (MMR)

There are literature reports of masseter muscle rigidity/spasm following the use of succinylcholine. The mouth is then difficult to open to facilitate endotracheal intubation. This phenomenon is associated with MH and has an incidence of 1:12,000 general anesthetics in children and adults. Limiting studies to only children and adolescents, the incidence increases to 1:100–1:500 general anesthetics involving volatile agents and succinylcholine (Succinylcholine is now contraindicated in children except for emergency treatment of laryngospasm). Patients that are referred for follow-up muscle biopsy show a 50% risk of MH. Most reported cases involve succinylcholine + a volatile gas; however, there are rare reports of intravenous anesthesia + succinylcholine causing MMR.

If a spasm of the muscle does occur, repeat dosing with succinylcholine will not reverse the rigidity. In 30% of cases, MH occurs immediately after the MMR, but the majority of MH cases will take about 20 minutes to develop if it occurs. In these cases, surgery and anesthesia should be stopped, and the patient allowed to awaken, while maintaining ventilation and oxygenation. MH testing can be considered and creatine kinase levels monitored (Brandom and Rosenberg, 2009).

Mimics of malignant hyperthermia

Myodystrophies, particularly Duchenne muscular dystrophy and Becker dystrophy, were thought to be associated with increased risk of MH. In these diseases, patients lack a dystrophin protein that usually stabilizes the muscle cell membrane. If these patients are given succinylcholine or a volatile anesthetic agent, cardiac arrest develops secondary to potassium release from the myocytes. They do not need dantrolene, but need emergency treatment for hyperkalemia. They are not susceptible to MH (Brandom and Rosenberg, 2009). Central core disease and King Denborough Syndrome are two rare muscle disorders with increased MH susceptibility. Hypokalemic and hyperkalemic periodic paralysis may also be associated with MH.

Summary

1 MH many not manifest on first exposure to triggers.
2 MH may be more common than previously thought.
3 Dantrolene should be present when volatile gases or succinylcholine is part of an anesthetic plan. Temperature monitor should be provided, in addition to routine ECG, blood pressure, pulse oximetry, and end-tidal capnography.
4 Intravenous agents, *other than succinylcholine*, are not triggering agents and are safe to use in the office setting provided that an alternative treatment for laryngospasm is available for patients with increased susceptibility to MH.
5 Local anesthesia alone can be used without any special equipment or precautions taken.

References

Ables, A. Z. and Nagubilli, R. Prevention, Diagnosis and Management of Serotonin Syndrome. *Am Fam Phys* **81**: 1139–1142, 2010.

Anderson, A., et al. Identification and biochemical characteristics of novel RyR1 mutation. *Anesthesiol* **108**: 208–215, 2008.

Birmes, P., et al. Serotonin syndrome: a brief review. *CMAJ* **168**: 1439–1442, 2003.

Bond, A. Drug-induced behavioural disinhibition. *CNS Drugs* **9**: 41–57, 1998.

Boyer, E. W. and Shannon, M. The serotonin syndrome. *N Engl J Med* **354**: 1112–1120, 2005.

Brandom, B. and Rosenberg, H. *Clinical Anesthesia*, 6th edn. Philadelphia: Wolters Kluwer, 2009, pp 598–622.

Brandom, B. W., et al. Complications associated with the administration of dantrolene 1987 to 2006: a report from the North American Malignant Hyperthermia Registry of the Malignant Hyperthermia Association of the United States, Anesth Analg **112**: 1115–23, 2011.

Brown, D. V., et al. Anticholinergic syndrome after anesthesia: a case report and review. *Am J Ther* **11**:144–153, 2004.

Burkman, J., et al. Analysis of variables associated with recrudescence. *Anesthesiol* **106**: 902–906, 2007.

Coburn, V. A. and Mycyk, M. B. Physical and chemical restraints. *Emerg Med Clin N Am* **27**: 655–667, 2009.

American Psychiatric Association, *Diagnostic and Statistical Manual of Mental Disorders*, 4th ed. Washington: American Psychiatric Association, 2000.

Dietch, J. T. and Jennings, R. K. Aggressive dyscontrol in patients trated with benzodiazepines. *J Clin Psychiatr* **49**: 184–187, 1988.

Dunkley, E. J. C., et al. The hunter serotonin toxicity crietera: simple and accurate diagnostic decision rules for serotonin toxicity. *Q J Med* **96**: 635–642, 2003.

Downes, M. A. Structured team approach to the agitated patient in the emergency department. *Emerg Med Australasia* **21**: 196–202, 2009.

Elbogen, E. B. and Johnson, S. C. The intricate link between violence and metnal disorder. *Arch Gen Psychiatry* **66**: 152–161, 2009.

Ely, E. W., et al. *Evaluation of delirium in critically ill patients: validation of the confusion assessment method for the intensive care unit (CAM-ICU) Crit Care Med* **29**: 1370–1379, 2001.

Fazel S., et al. Schizophrenia, substance abuse and violent crime. *JAMA* **301**: 2016–2023, 2009.

Gillman, P.K. The serotonin syndrome and its treatment. *J Psychopharmacol* **13**: 100–109, 1999.

Hernandez, J., et al. Scientific advances in genetic understanding and diagnosis of MH. *J Perianesth Nurs* **24**: 19–34, 2009.

Hopkins, P. Recrudescence of malignant hyperthermia. *Anesthesiol* **106**(5), 893–894, 2007.

Hurford, W. E. Delirium and cognitive dysfunction in the perioperative period. ASA Refresher Courses, 2012.

Ibarra, M. C. MH in Japan: mutation screening of entire RyR1 gene. *Anesthesiol* **104**: 1146–1154, 2006.

Inouye, S. K. Delirium in older persons. *N Engl J Med* **354**: 1157–65, 2006.

Karlet, M. MH considerations for ambulatory surgery. *J Perianesth Nurs* **13**: 304–312, 1998.

Larach, M.G., et al. Serious complications associated with malignant hyperthermia events. a NAMH Registry of MHAUS study (abstract A371) In: Proceedings of the American Society of Anesthesiologists Annual Meeting, 2008a.

Larach, M.G., et al. Cardiac arrests and deaths with MH in North America 1987–2006. *Anesthesiol* **108**: 603–611, 2008b.

Larach, M. G., et al. Clinical presentation, treatment, and complications of MH in North America from 1987 to 2006. *Anesth Analg* **110**: 498–507, 2010.

Lieberman, J. A. Managing anticholinergic side effects. Prim care companion. *J Clin Psychiatry* **6**: 20–23, 2004.

Litman, R., et al. Post operative MH analysis of North American registry. *Anesthesiol* **109**: 825–829, 2008.

Malignant Hyperthermia Association of the United States (2010). Clinical practice protocol. www.mhaus.org

Mancuso, C. E., et al. Paradoxical reactions to benzodiazepines: literature review and treatment options. *Pharmacother* **24**: 1177–1185, 2004.

Marcantonio, E. R., et al. The relationship of postoperative delirium with psychoactive medications. *JAMA* **272**: 1518–1522, 1994.

McKenzie, W. S. and Rosenberg, M. Paradoxical reaction following administration of a benzodiazepine. *J Oral Maxillofac Surg* **68**: 3034–3036, 2010.

Moore, G. and Pfaff, J. A. *Assessment and management of the acutely agitated or violent adult*. In: UpToDate, Waltham, MA. Accessed on December 23, 2014.

Noble, K. Malignant hyperthermia: hot stuff. *J Perianesth Nurs* **22**: 341–345, 2007.

Orr, D and Glassman A, Conversion phenomenon following general anesthesia, *J Oral Maxillofac Surg*, **43**:817–819, 1985.

Paton, C. Benzodiazepine and disinhibition: a review. *Psychiatr Bull* **26**: 460–462, 2002.

Pulay, A. J. et al. Violent behavior and DSM-IV psychiatric disorders : results from the national epidemiologic survey on alcohol and related conditions. *J Clin Psychiatry* **69**: 12–22, 2008.

Rosenberg, H., et al. Review of malignant hyperthermia. *Orphanet J Rare Dis* **2**: 21, 2007. www.OJRD.com/content/2/1/21

Rosenberg H. Malignant hyperthermia susceptibility. Gene reviews - NCBI Bookshelf, 2010. www.ncbi.nlm.nih.gov/books/NBK1146 (Accessed May 2011).

Rosero, E., et al. Trends and outcomes of MH in United States 2000–2005. *Anesthesiol* **110**: 89–94, 2009.

Schneck, H. J. and Rupreht, J. Central anticholinergic syndrome (CAS) in anesthesia and intensive care. *Acta Anaesthesiol Belg* **40**: 219–228, 1989.

Sieber, F. E. Postoperative delirium in the elderly surgical patient. *Anesthesiol Clin* **27**: 451–464, 2009.

Silverstein, J. H. Cognition and delirium. ASA Referesher Courses, 2009.

Sessler, C.N., et al. The richmond agitation-sedation scale: validity and reliability in adult intensive care unit patients. *Am J Respir Crit Care Med* **166**: 1338–1344, 2002.

Skrobik, Y. Delirium prevention and treatment. *Anesthesiol Clin* **29**: 721–727, 2011.

Steiner, L.A. Postoperative delirium. Part 1: pathophysiology and risk factors. *Eur J Anaesthesiol* **28**: 628–636, 2011a.

Steiner, L. A. Postoperative delirium, Part 2: detection, prevention and treatment. *Eur J Anaesthesiol* **28**: 723–732, 2011b.

Sumitani, M., et al. Prevalence of MH in Japan. *Anesthesiol* **114**: 84–90, 2010.

Szakaly, B. and Strauss, R. Serotonin syndrome in the oral and maxillofacial surgery office: a review of the literature and report of a case. *J Oral Maxillofac Surg* **66**: 1949–1952, 2008.

Tune, L. E. Anticholinergic effects of medication in elderly patients. *J Clin Psychiatry* **62**: 11–14, 2001.

Tune, L., et al. Anticholinergic effects of drugs commonly prescribed for the elderly: potential means for assessing risk of delirium. *Am J Psychiatry* **149**: 1393–1394, 1992.

Trzepacz, P. and van der Mast, R. The neuropathophysiology of delirium, In Lindesay, J., et al., eds. *Delirium in old age*. Oxford: Oxford University Press, 2002.

Villari, V., et al. Emergency psychiatry. *Minerva Med* **98**: 525–541, 2007.

Vilke, G. M. and Wilson, M. P. Agitation: what every emergency physician should know. *Emerg Med Reports* **30**: 233–243, 2009.

37 Anesthetic problems involving vasculature

Stuart Lieblich
University of Connecticut, Department of Oral and Maxillofacial Surgery, Avon, CT, USA

The provision of ambulatory dental anesthesia is most often administered through the intravenous route. Once intravenous access is obtained, small test doses of the planned medications can be administered so that with close patient observation, the development of allergic or other unusual responses can be readily detected. Importantly, having continuous IV access permits titration of medications along with the access for giving reversal or emergency drugs should the situation arise. Lastly, additional fluids can be given throughout the perioperative period. This "catch up" of fluids for the patient that has been NPO for an interval has been shown to be beneficial in reduction in the perioperative heart rate and reduction in postoperative nausea (Bennett et al., 1999).

Continuous intravenous access is ideally obtained with a catheter over needle system. An 18–20 gauge catheter is sufficient for a 70-kg adult, as there is no indication for a wider bore system in the office setting. Larger bore catheters (14–16) are used for very rapid fluid administration along with blood products. Some practices still elect to use a steel needle (butterfly) system because of decreased cost. However, displacement (infiltration) of the butterfly device during an anesthetic is frequent during patient movement and is problematic, as the procedure must be paused to reestablish intravenous access. Risk factors for displacement of intravenous access are shown in Table 37.1.

Table 37.1 Risk factors for displacement of intravenous access (Infusion Nurses Society, 2006).

- Small, fragile veins
- Placement in areas of movement
- Unstable catheter position in patients with difficult access (obese, pigmented skin)
- Inadequate stabilization
- Patient movement
- Multiple punctures in same vein
- Use of needles vs. catheters
- Rapid cycling of blood pressure cuffs on the arm with IV access

Infiltration and extravasation

The most common complications of intravenous access are infiltration and extravasation. Infiltration and extravasation occur when the tip of the catheter or needle is no longer completely within the vein. This can occur when the needle or catheter erodes or punctures the other side of the vein. In dental anesthesia, patient movement can cause displacement of the needle or catheter either through the wall of the vein (in further advancement) or out of the vein (with retraction). Either process allows the administered fluid to leak into the surrounding tissues.

Infiltration refers to the inadvertent leakage of non-vesicant solution (IV fluids) into the surrounding tissues. The term "vesicant" refers to a fluid that will cause direct tissue damage. Extravasation refers to the inadvertent leakage of a vesicant fluid (antibiotics, diazepam and others) that can cause local sloughing and potential loss of function due to direct nerve damage. As outcome studies are sparse, retrospective, and without clinical trials (unethical), and mild situations often resolve without consequence, there can be an underestimation of the degree of risk and subsequent tissue damage that can occur (Hastings-Tolsma and Yucha, 1994).

Signs of loss of IV access are usually the stoppage or sudden decrease in the rate of the fluid infusion (see Table 37.2). Therefore, a change in rate of a continuous infusion becomes helpful in assuring continuous patency of the catheter-vessel system. The questionable practice of a needle syringe combination without continuously running IV fluids to ensure patency can predispose to infiltration or extravasation. Verifying the continuity of the

Table 37.2 Causes of slow or stopped IV fluid flow.

- Partial catheter obstruction – kink or proximal clot
- Catheter against the wall of a vein or venous valve (positional obstruction)
- Proximal kinking of cannulated vessel
- Failure to release tourniquet, tight clothing proximal to IV site

Anesthesia Complications in the Dental Office, First Edition. Edited by Robert C. Bosack and Stuart Lieblich.

infusion system by lowering the IV bag below the level of the vein and checking for the free return of blood can be done more predictably with a catheter system.

If infiltration occurs and is readily detected, little damage would be expected to occur. A new site of IV access should be established, which causes a delay in the surgical/anesthetic care. If a large quantity of fluids has infiltrated, aspiration prior to removing the failed catheter can be attempted (Camp-Sorrell, 1998). Once the catheter is removed, the arm should be elevated, pressure to the site placed, and at the completion of the procedure, cold compresses to the site. Cold compresses should be continued for 24 hours at home. Inspection of the region, especially distal to the site to ascertain there is no weakness or significant tissue blanching will rule out most episodes of significant tissue damage. Patients should be contacted 24 hours later to ensure that resolution is continuing.

If extravasation (with vesicant) occurs, an antidote (if available) can be administered into the displaced catheter. There are few specific antidotes for agents used in dental anesthesia; fortunately, most are unlikely to cause significant tissue damage. Promethazine has been associated with serious outcomes if extravasation occurs and for that reason many hospitals have removed it from their formulary as an intravenous agent. Since pain is often a heralding sign of extravasation of this drug, the sedated patient may not respond fully to alert the anesthesia team. Consideration of sympathetic blockade and heparin administration is reported, but no successful outcomes are documented (ISMP, 2013). If extravasation of vasopressor agents (epinephrine, phenylephrine) occurs, then reversal with phentolamine can be considered.

Inadvertent intra-arterial injection

One of the most disconcerting complications of intravenous access is the inadvertent intra-arterial injection of agents. Tissue necrosis and distal gangrene have been reported to follow this iatrogenic complication (Lieblich and Topazian, 1988). The clinician needs to verify that the access is indeed intravenous and to carefully observe for any signs of intra-arterial injection, especially with initial doses of medications prior to the patient becoming less responsive. Ghouri (2002) notes the following to be signs of possible intra-arterial injection:

1 Bright red backflow into the tubing after "venipuncture"
2 Pulsatile movement of the fluid in the tubing
3 Backflow even if the bag is higher than the puncture site[1]
4 Pain radiating down the arm, distal to the puncture site.

The use of preoperative sedative medication may blunt the pain response to intra-arterial injection. Propofol is well known to create pain on injection and many patients are not specific as to its location. Fortunately intra-arterial injection of propofol has not been shown to create specific injury (Holley and Cuthrell, 1990). Therefore, consideration of not giving propofol as the initial drug in a newly established vascular access may be more diagnostic for the anesthetist.

There are no specific case-controlled studies comparing the management of inadvertent intra-arterial injection of potentially noxious drugs. Consensus of sparse literature supports leaving the catheter in place. This allows the potential administration of additional therapeutic agents directly into the vessel along with providing access for specific angiography in an advanced setting to determine the extent of the injury. If heparin is not available, then

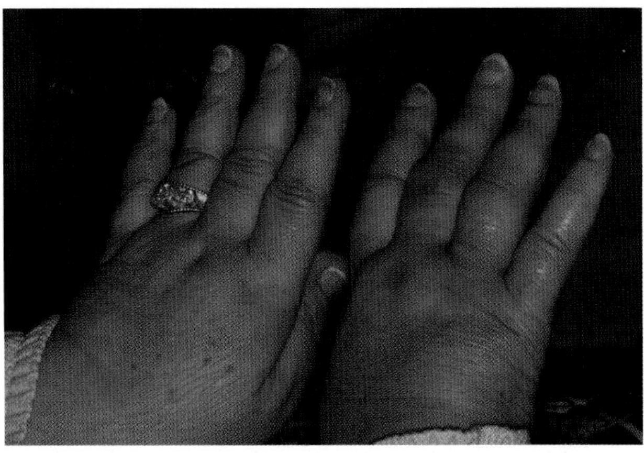

Figure 37.1 This patient complained of pain and swelling in her right hand following administration of diazepam into a small dorsal vein. Urgent removal of all circumferential jewelry, moist heat, and aspirin are indicated, courtesy of Dr. Stuart Lieblich.

0.9% NS should be administered with supplemental pressure to overcome the higher intra-arterial pressures. The use of injections of procaine or lidocaine has been described to reduce vasospasm and improve distal blood flow. Intuitively, it seems beneficial, but animal studies have shown vasodilation for only 10 minutes following injection, and after thiopental injection in a rabbit ear model there were no differences in the procaine vs. placebo group as far as amount of tissue loss was concerned (Kinmonth and Shepherd, 1959).

Besides recognition, avoidance of the arterial puncture is the best strategy. An index of suspicion is necessary following all venipunctures, but especially in individuals with deep or difficult veins to locate. Higher incidences in obese patients, and those with dense or dark-colored skin are reported. Close patient observation with validation of all complaints regarding pain, particularly distally, is necessary.

Thrombophlebitis

Thrombophlebitis is a rare complication in dental anesthesia due to the short duration of the indwelling catheter in contrast to hospitalized patients. Nonetheless, cases have been reported and postoperative complaints of pain, redness, or a palpable cord at the site of the intravenous access should be evaluated by the anesthesia team. Certain agents were notorious for causing these symptoms, particularly diazepam. Diazepam is typically compounded with propylene glycol as a carrier. The incidence of post anesthesia thrombophlebitis has been reported at 7.9% with this agent (Litchfield, 1983), making the substitution of midazolam as the benzodiazepine of choice even more compelling.

If thrombophlebitis occurs the patient may often present with distal edema. As noted in Figure 37.1 if distal edema occurs the patient should be immediately instructed to remove all rings to prevent necrosis. Warm soaks, aspirin, and pain medication may be needed for resolution. Should symptoms persist or a cord in the vein progresses, referral to a vascular specialist and consideration for anticoagulation are indicated.

References

Bennett, J., et al. Perioperative rehydration in ambulatory anesthesia for dentoalveolar surgery. *Oral Surg Oral Med Oral Path* **88**: 279–284, 1999.

[1] Verify that the tourniquet has been removed.

Camp-Sorrell D. Developing extravastation protocols and monitoring outcomes. *J Intravenous Nursing* **21**: 232–239, 1998.

Ghouri, A. F. Accidental intraarterial drug injections via intravascular catheters placed on the dorsum of the hand. *Anesth Analg* **95**: 487–491, 2002.

Hastings-Tolsma, M. and Yucha, C. B. IV infiltration: no clear signs, no clear treatment? *RN* **57**: 34–38, 1994.

Holley, H. S. and Cuthrell, L. Intraarterial injection of propofol. *Anesthesiol* **73**: 183–184, 1990.

Infusion Nurses Society. Infusion nursing standards of practice. *J Infus Nurs* **29**: S1–S92, 2006.

ISMP (Institute for Safe Medical Practices), https://www.ismp.org/newsletters/acute care/articles/20060810.asp (Accessed February 10, 2013).

Kinmonth, J. B. and Shepherd, R. C. Accidental injection of thiopentone into arteries: studies of pathology and treatmen. *Brit Med J* **2**: 914–918, 1959.

Lieblich, S. and Topazian, R. Accidental intra-arterial injection – an update. *J Oral Maxillofac Surg* **42**: 297–302, 1988.

Litchfield NB: Venous complications of intravenous diazepam. *J Oral Maxillofac Surg* **41**: 701–705; 1983.

SECTION 8

Post-anesthetic adversity

38 Nausea and vomiting

Edward Adlesic
University of Pittsburgh, School of Dental Medicine, Department of Oral and Maxillofacial Surgery, Pittsburgh, PA, USA

Introduction

During the "ether era" of anesthesia, postoperative nausea and vomiting (PONV) was expected to occur; it was normal. Rates of 60 to 80% were common. Fortunately, over the past 20 years, the rates of PONV have decreased. Anesthetic agents, especially propofol, used in a total intravenous anesthetic technique (TIVA) have reduced the incidence of early PONV. There are also better antiemetic agents available to prevent and rescue patients with nausea and vomiting. The 5-hydroxytryptamine type 3 (5-HT-3 RA) receptor antagonists are the mainstay of antiemetic therapy. These short-acting agents have been found to be effective postoperatively for the first 24 hours, and there are newer, longer acting 5-HT-3 receptor antagonists that can maintain emesis-free periods for up to 72 hours. Multimodal therapy has also reduced the rates of PONV, especially in patients with multiple risk factors (Le and Gan, 2010).

Definition

Nausea is an unpleasant sensation in the epigastrium and throat associated with the urge to vomit. Symptoms may include pallor, sweating, bloating, and increased salivation. There is a decrease in gastric motility, and the patient may experience mild discomfort up to severe distress. Severe episodes of nausea are more common and can be as disruptive as vomiting, especially in the presence of postoperative pain.

Retching, also called the "dry heaves," is an unproductive effort to vomit. The small intestines contract to prevent gastric emptying, while the gastric contents are stirred by the rhythmic contraction of the diaphragmatic, abdominal, and intercostal muscles.

Vomiting is the forceful expulsion of gastric contents into the oropharynx and nasopharynx. The esophageal sphincter relaxes and gastric contents are expelled by the coordinated contraction of the abdominal, intercostal, and diaphragmatic muscles.

These processes typically will involve unwelcome swings in both the sympathetic and parasympathetic nervous system; pallor, sweating, bloating, salivation and changes in blood pressure and heart rate, which can compromise "unhealthy" patients. Postoperative nausea and vomiting delay discharge, reduce patient satisfaction, may mechanically or chemically interfere with oral wound integrity, aggravating hemorrhage, and in protracted cases, result in fluid and electrolyte abnormalities (hypokalemia and metabolic alkalosis.).

Pathophysiology

The central "coordinating" site for nausea and vomiting is the vomiting center (VC). The VC has also been called the central pattern generator (CPG) because when activated, it stimulates the neurons in the medulla to cause vomiting (Le and Gan, 2010). It receives both sympathetic and parasympathetic input, as well as afferents from the cerebellum, the vestibular apparatus, the "chemo-receptor trigger zone" and higher cortical centers (see Figure 38.1). Multiple emetogenic receptors are found in the CTZ (within the CNS, but not protected by the blood–brain barrier): serotonergic, dopaminergic, histaminic, cholinergic, mu-opioid, and the neurokinergic NK-1. When stimulated, the CTZ can subsequently and directly stimulate the VC or stimulate the adjacent nucleus tractus solitaries, which, in turn, stimulates the VC. The nucleus tractus solitarius also receives peripheral stimulation by way of the sympathetic nervous system and parasympathetic nervous system (glossopharyngeal and vagus nerves) to stimulate the VC. It also receives inputs from the higher cortical centers of the brain in response to sensory stimuli of pain, sight, and smell, as well as psychogenic stimuli of memory and fear.

PONV has been called the "big little problem." Patients are not going to die from this event, and while the morbidity is usually transient and without long-term clinical significance, these episodes can be quite distressing for the patient.

Complications can include pulmonary aspiration of gastric contents, esophageal tears, fractures, wound dehiscence, electrolyte imbalance, and dehydration. Subcutaneous emphysema and airway compromise can occur when air is forced through the intraoral suture lines. There are also reports of intraocular hemorrhage and vision loss from the forces generated in severe PONV (Kovac, 2000; Gan et al., 2007).

Incidence and risk factors

Third molar surgery under general anesthesia with no antiemetic prophylaxis had PONV rates of 20–40% (Fujii et al., 2002, 2008).

The inherent limitations plaguing studies evaluating the efficacy of various therapies are that the etiology of PONV is multifactorial, patients cannot and will not serve as their own control, and no two cases or patients are identical. Nausea and vomiting can be due to ingestion of endogenous material (blood) or exogenous toxins or medicines that irritate gastric mucosa, may indicate a

Anesthesia Complications in the Dental Office, First Edition. Edited by Robert C. Bosack and Stuart Lieblich.

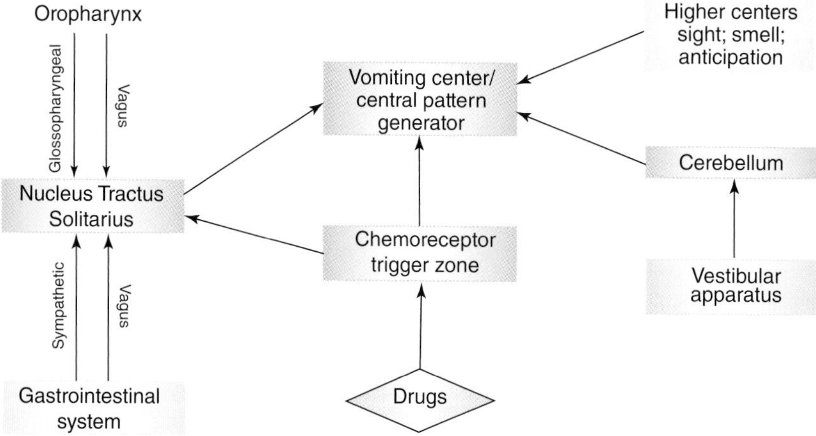

Figure 38.1 Mechanisms of nausea and vomiting, Le and Gan, 2010, with permission.

disease process in the gastrointestinal tract or adjacent organs (viral or bacterial infection, tumor, endocrinopathy), or may be due to CNS influence (hypotension, unpleasant taste or smell, tumor, anesthetic drugs). Overall incidence of PONV approaches 30% of all anesthetics within the first 24 post-surgical/anesthetic hours; this number may be less, but still significant for outpatient dentoalveolar surgery with sedation/anesthesia. PONV can occur as an isolated intraoperative or postoperative event in otherwise healthy patients, or it can occur because of undetected and preexisting diseases or situations, e.g., gastroparesis or lower esophageal sphincter dysfunction. It is important to appreciate that nausea and vomiting in the postoperative period may be due to factors not related to the anesthesia or surgery.

The risk factors for PONV are shown in Table 38.1 (Apfel, 1999). The presence and number of risk factors predicts the presence and duration of PONV (White, 2008).

Some facilities force early PO intake prior to discharge or the patient starts on oral solid foods too soon. It is better to have a patient in the office either rinse the mouth if dry or take a few ice chips. Fluids in the office and a rough ride home again can lead to motion sickness. Upon arrival at home, liquids for 2–4 hours is preferable to solids. Once the liquids are tolerated, solids can be introduced.

Modification of anesthetic risks

The risk of nausea and vomiting can be reduced by modifying the anesthetic technique used. TIVA anesthesia including the use of propofol can reduce the risk by approximately 19%. If nitrous oxide is avoided, the reduction increases to 25%. The use of propofol for maintenance of deep sedation/general anesthesia has the greatest impact of all drug strategies in reducing early PONV. This effect will cover the first few hours postoperatively, but other antiemetics may still be required for long-term protection.

Anxiety will increase nausea and vomiting, so using midazolam to work on the higher cortical centers to decrease noxious stimuli is helpful.

There are multiple reports showing that IV hydration decreases the risk of nausea and vomiting. Maharaj et al. (2005) used IV replacement therapy based upon 2 ml/kg/hr of fasting and found that the incidence of PONV was reduced over a 72-hour period. The frequency of moderate to severe nausea was also reduced, and there was a decrease in postoperative pain and opioid requirements. Holte and Kehlet (2006) in a study on elective fast-tracking surgery found that in minor to moderate non-cardiac surgery, the use of fluids >1 liter improved recovery. Based on the above, it is reasonable to give healthy patients a minimum of 500 ml of an isotonic saline solution of NSS or LR for office surgery, especially in the presence of risk factors for PONV.

Medical management of PONV

Serotonin (5-hydroxytryptamine) receptor antagonists

Serotonin can stimulate the peripheral vagal afferent neurons along the GI tract and the central serotonin receptors in the chemoreceptor trigger zone (CTZ) to stimulate the VC. The 5-hydroxytryptamine type 3 (5-HT3) serotonin receptor antagonists have become the most frequently used agents for both prophylaxis and rescue of PONV. The first-generation 5-HT3 RA are effective for both prevention and rescue. Drugs in this class include ondansetron (Zofran), granisetron (Kytril), and dolasetron (Anzemet). Side effects include headache, dizziness, and flushing at the IV site. Ondansetron is the most widely used drug, at a dose of 4mg IV. As expected, 5-HT3 antagonists lose efficacy in the presence of SSRI medication. With therapeutic failure, an antiemetic drug from another class should be used (Candiotti et al., 2007).

Ondansetron is also supplied as an 8 mg freeze-dried oral disintegrating tablet (ODT). It dissolves on the tongue so there is no need to swallow a pill with water. It is absorbed by the GI tract and not the oral mucosa.

Dexamethasone

Dexamethasone is a potent steroid medication often used in dental surgery to decrease postoperative swelling and inflammation. At a dose of 4mg IV, it is a potent antiemetic agent, whose efficacy is similar to that of 4 mg of ondansetron (Gan et al., 2007). Side effects include GI irritation, anxiety, hyperglycemia, and perineal itch (especially if the drug is injected as a rapid, IV bolus). Dexamethosone will cause a transient increase in blood glucose levels.

Table 38.1 Risk factors for nausea and vomiting.

PREOPERATIVE	Age	Children and adolescents are more likely to have PONV
	Gender	Females are 3x more likely to experience PONV, and episodes are often more severe
	Positive past history	Past history of motion sickness or PONV
	Smoking	Smoking decreases PONV by 1/2
	Endogenous catecholamines	Associated with hypotension/ anxiety
	Gastroesophageal dysfunction	Increased tendency for reflux with obesity and/or GERD
PERIOPERATIVE	Anesthetic drugs	• Nitrous oxide, especially in higher concentrations • Opioids • All volatile gases • Etomidate and ketamine (esp PO) • Risk of PONV with general anesthesia is 9x more than local anesthesia
	Duration of surgery	Surgery longer than 30 min can increase PONV × 59% (Cameron and Gan, 2003)
	Hypoxemia	
	Oropharyngeal irritation	
	Anesthetic course	"Stormy" anesthetics predispose to PONV
POSTOPERATIVE	Premature ambulation	Trigger both dizziness and hypotension
	Pain	
	Orthostatic hypotension	
	Opioid usage	
	Hypoxemia	
	Premature oral intake	Especially swallowed blood (emetogenic). Mandatory PO intake prior to discharge can aggravate PONV
	Tactile stimulation of oropharynx	
	Elimination of previously administered antiemetic	
	Hypoglycemia	
	Agitation	

Dopamine (D2) receptor antagonists

These agents act on the D2 receptors found in the CTZ and area postrema. The drugs in this category include the phenothiazines and benzamides. Butyrophenone (droperidol) is also a dopamine receptor antagonist, which has an FDA black box warning due to a questionable risk of lethal cardiac dysrhythmias (Nuttal et al., 2013).

Prochlorperazine (Compazine™) is the most frequently used phenothiazine for prophylaxis or rescue from PONV. The dose is 5-10 mg IV or IM given at the end of the surgery. The side effects of phenothiazines are one of the reasons their use for PONV has decreased. Patients can experience restlessness, diarrhea, and agitation. The elderly and children can have prolonged sedation and hypotension especially with intravenous doses. Extrapyramidal reactions including torticollis, tongue protrusion, and lip smacking have occurred as well as supraventricular tachycardia. 25mg suppositories are available for adults. This dose is decreased to 0.1mg/kg PR for children.

Promethazine (Phenergan™) is classified as both phenothiazine and antihistamine. Most of its antiemetic effect is not on the D2 receptor but on the histamine-1 receptor. It is both a prophylactic and a rescue agent. The prophylactic dose is 12.5mg IV or IM at induction. Reports of extensive tissue injury and necrosis along with amputations from inadvertent arterial injections and intravenous extravasations have been documented by multiple sources. Sheth (2005) reported that the incident rate ratio for promethazine was higher than that for all other antiemetics combined. The complications were highest in patients older than 65. Injectable promethazine contains phenol, a tissue irritant, and has a pH of 4.0 – 5.5, which makes the drug corrosive to soft tissue. The intima of the blood vessels are damaged, which causes extravasation of the drug into the soft tissue leading to inflammation and then necrosis. Nerves in the field have also been damaged. The worst damage is with inadvertent intra-arterial injections. Patients will complain of severe burning in the extremity, followed by pain, erythema, swelling, vessel spasm, and phlebitis. As the injury persists, nerves are directly damaged by the phenol, sometimes leading to arm paralysis. The tissues become necrotic and gangrene develops. Surgical interventions include fasciotomy, skin grafts, and at times amputation of digits or hand.

If a choice is made to administer the drug IV, a maximum dose of 12.5 mg should be diluted with 20 ml saline and delivered slowly over 10 minutes from the distal-most port in the tubing of a continuously running IV solution in the largest caliber vein available.

Metaclopramide (Reglan™) is a benzamide D2 RA at the peripheral GI tract receptors and the CTZ receptors. The drug also has prokinetic activity to increase gastric emptying, which is useful in the obese and GERD patient. It can be used for prophylaxis and rescue at a dose of 10 mg IV Q 4 – 6 h. The 2007 SAMBA guidelines did not recommend the use of 10 mg of metaclopromide because studies only showed a 50% decrease in PONV at that dose. Recent data has shown that at doses of 25 – 50 mgs IV metaclopramide did decrease PONV for up to 24 hours. However, there are concerns about developing tardive dyskinesia with this agent; multiple law suits have been filed. It is highly unlikely to see tardive dyskinesia with short-term use of the drug; this effect, while very rare, is most likely to occur with chronic use (Gan et al., 2007; Apfel, 2008).

Trimethobenzamide (Tigan™) is another benzamide agent that acts as both a D2 receptor antagonist and a H-1 receptor antagonist. Years ago, it was a popular antiemetic agent and can still be found in some of the commercial emergency kits sold to dentists. However, the FDA claims that trimethobenzamide suppositories are ineffective for both adults and children. There are more effective agents available, so this drug is not a first-line agent.

Antihistamines

The drugs in this category include diphenhydramine (Benadryl™), dimenhydrinate (Dramamine™, an aminophylline salt of diphenhydramine), cyclizine (Marezine™), and promethazine (Phenergan™). These agents are histamine −1 receptor antagonists with activity in the CTZ, VC, and the vestibular system. The parenteral dose of diphenhydramine is 25–50 mg in the adult. The side effects of these two agents include sedation, prolonged recovery, dry mouth, blurred vision, confusion, and possible urinary retention due to anticholinergic properties. They are usually not first line drugs of choice for PONV, but they do play a role in middle ear surgery. Low dose of diphenhydramine at the start of surgery may decrease motion sickness in susceptible patients living long distances from the office (Scuderi, 2003).

Anticholinergics

Scopolamine has been used as a transdermal patch with an onset of 2–4 hours, which is not typically used in the office. Its parenteral use is limited by its ability to cross the blood–brain barrier causing disorientation. Intravenous atropine can be used as an adjunctive agent, but there are no references found that consider this use as a primary management tool for PONV.

Propofol

Propofol has antiemetic properties but the mechanism is unknown. It is effective for early PONV (0–6 hours), but its action diminishes rapidly after that. Other agents will be necessary for coverage beyond the first few hours, especially for patients with multiple risk factors (Fujii et al., 2002, 2008).

Multimodal therapy

Studies have shown that different classes of antiemetics act independently of each other, so risk reductions with multiple agents were additive. Each agent was found to decrease the risk by ~10% (Gan, 2009). This reduction in PONV will level off at ~10% no matter how many agents are used, and the best results for multimodal therapy will occur when agents from multiple categories are used. Multimodal therapy should be used in patients with moderate risk factors (two risk factors) and high risk factors (three or more risk factors) (White et al., 2008).

Suggested office protocols

PONV prophylaxis is not a universal requirement for all surgical procedures; however, prevention is more successful than risk. Surgeons need to evaluate the patient's risk factors and the anesthetic techniques that will be used. The overall incidence of PONV in surgery without prophylaxis is 20–30%; in third molar surgery the range is 20 to 40%. Most patients do not experience nausea and vomiting in the office. It is usually after discharge, occurring during the first 3 days postoperatively in 50–78% of the cases.

High risk patients (3 or more risk factors) have less PDNV if three or more antiemetics are used instead of monotherapy. While low dose intraoperative opioids have little effect on nausea and vomiting, postoperative opioids do, so this risk must be included in your assessment for PONV and PDNV. In ambulatory surgery, a more liberal use of antiemetics can be considers as discharged patients have less access to the surgeon, and the surgeon has limited treatment options for rescue at home. In surgical cases where nausea and vomiting will adversely affect wound healing and surgical outcomes or in patients with moderate to severe risk factors, matching the number of antiemetics to the number of risks is an acceptable approach (Kolodzie and Apfel, 2009).

In low risk patients, their approach uses either no antiemetic or dexamethasone 4 mg IV at induction. If the patient has two risk factors, dexamethasone 4 mg IV at induction is augmented with TIVA anesthesia. In high risk patients (three to four risk factors), they make two separate recommendations.

A patient with three risk factors will receive dexamethasone and TIVA anesthesia, and the 5-HT-3 RA (Kolodzie and Apfel, 2009).

Post discharge nausea and vomiting

Post discharge nausea and vomiting can be more difficult to treat than nausea and vomiting in the office. The patient has been discharged so there is no immediate access to the patient; there is no IV in place to provide fluids, analgesics, or rescue agents.

Oral agents are of little benefit, as the pill will often be regurgitated prior to absorption. The only other route available is by suppository, which many patients find objectionable. Tigan as a suppository has been found to be ineffective in children and adults. The other two agents left are prochlorperazine and promethazine.

The PR (per rectum) dose of prochlorperazine in the adult is 25 mg BID, and 12.5 mg BID in the elderly; the PR dose of promethazine in the adult are 12.5–25 mg Q 4 to 6 h prn and 12.5 mg Q 4 to 6 h in the elderly. In the elderly, these agents can cause dysphoria and sedation. In children, they can cause significant sedation; the FDA has issued a black box warning for these drugs when used in children under the age of 2 years because of risk of fatal respiratory depression. If these agents are to be used in children, it is wise to discuss dosing with a pharmacist.

Ondansetron 8mg ODT BID for 1 to 3 days can be used to control PDNV successfully, although its use for this indication is off-label. Davis et al. (2008) used 8 mg ondansetron ODT tablets to prevent PDNV in children undergoing outpatient tonsillectomy and adenoidectomy in ASA 1 and 2 patients weighing at least 25 kg. The prophylactic dose was 8mg upon arrival at home, followed by 8 mg BID dosing for 1–2 days. A 4 mg ODT is also available.

Protracted, severe nausea and vomiting that is unresponsive to these at home therapies can be referred to the emergency room for rehydration and the administration of one or more rescue agents that may not be available in the office.

References

Apfel, C. Simplified Risk Score for Predicting PONV. *Anesthesiol* **91**: 693–700, 1999.

Cameron, D. and Gan, T. J. Management of postoperative nausea and vomiting in ambulatory surgery. *Anesthesiol Clin N Amer* **21**: 347–365, 2003.

Fujii, Y., et al. Small doses of propofol prevents PONV after third molar surgery. *J Oral Maxillofac Surg* **60**: 1246–1249, 2002.

Candiotti, K., et al. Granisetron versus Ondansetron for breakthrough PONV after Prophylaxis. *Anesth Analg* **104**: 1370–1373, 2007.

Davis, P., et al. Effects of ondansetron ODT for prevention of at-home emesis after ENT surgery. *Anesth Analg* **106**: 1117–1121, 2008.

Fujii, Y., et al. Propofol alone and combined with dexamethasone for PONV in adult third molar surgery. *Br J Oral Maxillofac Surg* **46**: 207–210, 2008.

Gan, T., et al. Society for ambulatory anesthesia guidelines for management of PONV. *Anesth Analg* **105**: 1615–1678, 2007.

Gan, T. Management of PONV. *ASA Refresher Course in Anesthesiology* **37**: 69–80, 2009.

Holte, K. and Kehlet, H. Fluid therapy in elective fast track surgery. *J Am Coll Surg* **209**: 971–989, 2006.

Kolodzie, K. and Apfel, C. Nausea and vomiting after office based anesthesia. *Curr Opin Anesthesiol* **22**: 532–538, 2009.

Kovac, A. Prevention and treatment of PONV. *Durgs* **59**: 213–243, 2000.

Le, T. and Gan, T. 2010 update on management of PONV and PDNV in ambulatory surgery. *Anesthesiol Clin* **28**: 225–249, 2010.

Maharaj, C. H., et al. Pre-operative intravenous fluid therapy decreases nausea and vomiting. *Anesth Analg* **100**: 675–682, 2005.

Nuttal, G. A., et al. Does low-dose properidol increase the risk of polymorphic ventiruclar tachycardia or death in the surgical patient? *Anesthesiol* **118**: 382–386, 2013.
Scuderi, P.E. Pharmacology of antiemetics. *Int Anesthesiol Clin* **41**: 41–66, 2003.
Sheth, H. S. Promethasine package insert. *Ann Pharmcother* **39**: 255–261, 2005.
White, P. Relationship between risk factors and early vs. late emetic symptoms. *Anesth Analg* **107**: 459–463, 2008.
White, P., et al. Impact on current antiemetic practices on patient outcomes. *Anesth Analg* **107**: 452–458, 2008.

39 Post-anesthetic recall of intraoperative awareness

Robert C. Bosack
University of Illinois, College of Dentistry, Chicago, IL, USA

Patients who wish to be sedated or "asleep" during their office-based dental procedure typically have the expectation that they will feel or remember nothing. "Wake-up issues" trigger anxiety, as patients are fearful of both "waking up in the middle" as well as "not waking up" at the end of the procedure. Unfortunately, this expectation of amnesia and depth of anesthesia may be difficult or impossible to meet, depending on the health of the patient, the nature of the procedure and anesthesia and/or the training and expertise of the anesthetist. The dental literature is silent regarding the incidence of breakthrough memories of "anesthetic awareness," possibly because it is rarely guaranteed; however, cases alleging unexpected awareness with recall are beginning to appear in medico-legal circles, especially when professional fees are tendered reflecting the administration of general anesthesia. Awareness includes hearing drills or conversation, pain, helplessness, panic and inability to speak, among others. An understanding of etiology, risk factors, prevention and management of awareness with recall requires knowledge of the process of memory formation.

Definition

Much has been studied and written about consciousness, learning and memory; yet little is fully understood. Memory is a thing in a place in the brain (Martinez and Kesner, 1998), a retrieval and playback of thought stored in a pattern of neural connections. It is a constructive, dynamic process designed to fine tune behavioral responses and NOT to faithfully record experiences. The very usefulness of memory depends on the ability to extract and generalize from past experience, adaptive responses and rules to improve survival and maximize pleasure.

Memory begins with an awareness of sensory input – seeing, hearing, thinking, smelling, tasting or touching (Atkinson and Shiffrin, 1968) (Figure 39.1). This input is immediately transferred to working memory (short term memory) for immediate use, where thought and reasoning are added. Short-term memory is limited in capacity and, without rehearsal, becomes transient, fleeting and easily overwhelmed by new incoming information. Subsequently, short term memory either vanishes or proceeds to the process of consolidation and creation of long term memory, with the expectation that it can be located and retrieved for future use. Consolidation is a time-dependent process that unfolds in the subsequent minutes to hours (and even years, Reasor and Poe, 2008), a process that is fragile and vulnerable in its earlier stages to disruption by interference. Consolidation (in the hippocampus, with rich expression of $GABA_A$ receptors) involves the formation of a permanent memory trace, which is then stored back in the cortex where the stimulus was first discovered. This trace requires neurochemical, neuroanatomic and electrophysiologic synaptic changes – in accord with the Hebbian tenant of "use-dependent neural plasticity" (Hebb, 1949). When retrieved, the engram is brought back into working memory, where it once again becomes labile, re-edited and reconsolidated. Fortunately, long-term memory is subject to decay (forgotten), otherwise, accumulation of insignificant details would needlessly clog the mind. As might be expected, emotionally charged events (accompanied by increased sympathetic discharge) are easier to consolidate, thus more difficult to forget (Cahill and Alkire, 2003). The amygdala is a key player in emotional modulation. From the foregoing, it becomes apparent that multiple loci (cortex, hippocampus, amygdala) participate in memory formation with robust and complex communication between these regions.

Memory is either explicit (conscious) or implicit (unconscious) (Tulving, 1972). Explicit memory (declarative) requires awareness – an intentional or conscious recollection of prior experience or learned fact. Explicit memory is further categorized as episodic ("I remember visiting the Eiffel Tower last summer with my family") or semantic ("Paris is the capital of France") – impersonal, generic factual information. Implicit memory involves a change in subsequent performance produced by prior experience without conscious recollection or awareness of that experience. In this context, the adolescent patient who can give no reason for hysterical crying in recovery might be reacting to subconscious awareness during a light and stormy anesthetic.

Amnesia is the loss of long term, explicit, episodic memory as reflected in the inability to recall. Anterograde amnesia is the inability to retain information for some period of time after the triggering event – trauma, surgery or drug administration. Retrograde amnesia is the inability to retain information for some period of time prior to the triggering event. Brain trauma and electroconvulsive therapy (ECT) can induce varying amounts of occasionally permanent retrograde amnesia, typically involving events immediately prior to the insult, adding credence to a time-dependent consolidation hypothesis.

Anesthesia Complications in the Dental Office, First Edition. Edited by Robert C. Bosack and Stuart Lieblich.

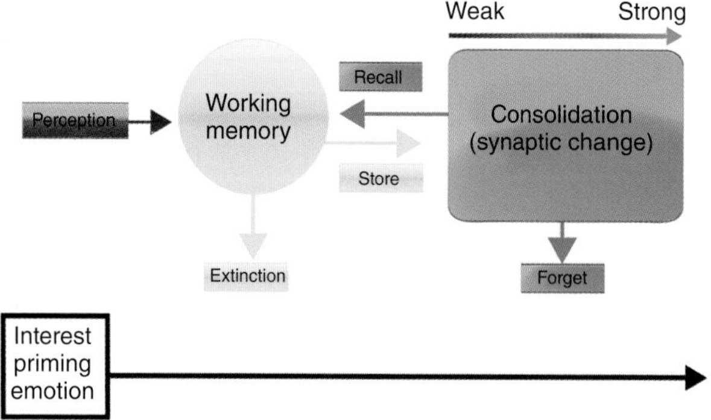

Figure 39.1 Memory Formation.

It is impossible to create memory during deeper stages of anesthesia because patients are unconscious and unaware of their surroundings. Propofol, benzodiazepines, ketamine, nitrous oxide and volatile agents, among others, are known to cause to anterograde amnesia, even in concentrations less than that required to eliminate attention. This is thought to occur by interference with either consolidation (Ghoneim, 2004) or forgetting (Veselis and Pryor, 2010) via enhancement of the $GABA_A$ receptor (propofol, benzodiazepines) or blockade of the NMDA receptor (ketamine, nitrous oxide) (Newcomer et al., 2000; Krystal et al., 1994). Specifically, these drugs are thought to impair long-term potentiation by interference with the production of memory related proteins (Nagashima et al., 2005; Alkire and Guzowski, 2008). These drugs do not affect short term memory, as evidenced when patients effectively communicate and follow commands during sedation, but have no recall during recovery. This common phenomenon provides repeated proof that perianesthetic conscious awareness is not always sufficient to produce post-anesthetic recall. It is interesting to note that anesthetic drugs affect only recent or fragile memory, without interference with remote, long standing memory, providing additional credence to the temporal principle of memory formation. Increasing the concentration of these drugs however, progressively impairs the ability to attend to stimuli, which eventually eliminates attention to input and any possibility of short or long term memory.

Etiology

Intraoperative awareness is due to insufficient anesthesia because of inadequate drug delivery or patient factors. Patient risk factors include a history of prior awareness, $GABA_A$ receptor mutation leading to resistance, accelerated drug metabolism [chronic drug or alcohol abuse, female sex, young age, concomitant exposure to known CYP 430 inducers (carbamazepine, glucocorticoids, phenytoin, barbiturates, St. John's Wort, smoking), red hair (Liem et al., 2004)] and obesity (difficult airways, increased volume of distribution). Factors relating to the insufficient delivery of anesthesia include unintentional underdosing (dosing error, lack of vigilance, pump or vaporizer malfunction), intentional underdosing (early termination of drug administration to facilitate discharge, conservative drug administration in unhealthy patients or patients with difficult airways) or inherent difficulty with total intravenous anesthesia (TIVA) mandating an open airway with spontaneous ventilation.

Incidence

The incidence of post-anesthetic recall of perioperative events for hospital based general anesthetics is estimated at 0.1–0.2% (Ghoneim, 2007). The incidence is much higher in dental offices providing light, moderate or deep sedation to maintain patent airways, spontaneous ventilation and time-efficient discharge to home, and in accord with training, licensure and practitioner comfort. Estimates of awareness are confounded by several factors including the timing and nature of the patient interview. Early questioning can augment or imprint a memory which otherwise might have been forgotten, while the nature of the probing questions might invite associations of questionable recall with awareness. Patients may not become aware of recall until weeks after the procedure or may be unwilling to report awareness spontaneously for fears of retaliation or appearing ungrateful. Finally, emotionally charged recall may be repressed, only to result in symptoms of post-traumatic stress disorder (PTSD), as may occur when patients retain implicit (unconscious) rather than explicit memory (Andrade and Deeprose, 2007). Practitioners should be aware that some patients might falsely claim awareness.

Prevention

There are many opportunities to prevent awareness during anesthesia, includeing sufficient understanding and vigilant dosing of anesthetic and amnestic medication and management of patient expectations regarding limitations of intended depth of anesthesia and its consequences. Avoidance of painful stimulation by efficacious use of local anesthesia and systemic analgesics eliminates awakening stimuli. Vigilant monitoring with a rapid correction of signs of autonomic hyperactivity, including patient movement, tearing, sighing, tachycardia, hypertension and tachypnea will also minimize awareness. It is paramount to realize that a failure to respond to commands or a lack of sympathetic discharge or patient movement is not a guarantee of unconsciousness or lack of awareness. Auditory processing is often maintained during general anesthesia (Schwender et al., 1998), therefore, operatory conversation should be kept to a minimum, including the avoidance of any inciting remarks about surgery or patient appearance. Similarly, reassuring comments can be beneficial. Bispectral (BIS) analysis is helpful to assess the level of consciousness, but is unable to monitor the ability to form and retrieve memory (Avidan et al., 2011). BIS is insensitive to nitrous oxide and ketamine (Dahaba, 2005).

Consequences and treatment

The consequences of awareness with recall range from nothing to fulminant PTSD (Leslie et al., 2010; Bruchas et al., 2011). Table 39.1 reveals key features of PTSD, which, by definition linger for more than 1 month, and cause significant stress and disruption of social or occupational functioning. Complaints of intraoperative awareness should immediately be met with acceptance, empathy, validation and, if possible, explanation. Early dismissal or denial can exacerbate PTSD. Table 39.2 includes a series of questions (Liu et al., 1991), which will aid in determining the extent of recall. Notice the absence of inflammatory or suggestive questions such as "can you remember when my drill broke in your jaw". Treatment includes cognitive behavioral therapy and drug therapy by appropriate health care professionals (Lennmarken and Sydsjo, 2007).

Table 39.1 Features of post-traumatic stress disorder.

- Re-experiencing – Continual (spontaneous or cued) reliving the traumatic memory – intrusive memory – flashbacks, nightmares
- Avoidance – Avoidance of stimuli associated with the event
- Emotional dysfunction – numbing, forgetting, social detachment, diminished range of affect
- Hyperarousal – nightmares, sleep disturbance, difficulty concentrating

Table 39.2 Questions to determine the extent of recall of intraoperative awareness.

What was the last thing you remember before you went to sleep?
What was the first think you remember after you woke up?
Can you remember anything in-between these periods?
Did you dream during your operation?

Management

Knowledge of the neurophysiology of memory provides key management strategies of unexpected intra-operative awareness with the threat of recall.

1 Avoid conversation to minimize retrieval. If necessary – overwrite the engram during vulnerability, alter its significance, misdirect, trivialize to avoid emotional modulation – "we're just getting started"
2 Overload working memory at the time of the awakening
3 Prevent retrieval, rehearsal and consolidation in the early post op period – redirect conversation
4 Interfere with consolidation by immediate redosing to stage III or deep stage II anesthesia
5 Do not interfere with working memory extinction

References

Alkire, M. T. and Guzowski, J. F. Hypothesis: suppression of memory protein formation underlies anesthetic-induced amnesia. *Anesthesiol* **109**: 768–770, 2008.

Andrade, J. and Deeprose, C. Unconsicous memory formation during anesthesia. *Best Prac Res Clin Anaesthesiol.* **21**: 385–401, 2007.

Atkinson, R. C. and Shiffrin, R. M. Human memory: a proposed system and its control processes. In: Spence, K. W. and Spence, J. T. *The Psychology of Learning and Motivation*, Vol. **2**. New York: Academic Press, 1968.

Avidan, M. S., et al. Prevention of intraoperative awareness in a high-risk surgical population. *N Engl J Med* **365**: 591–600, 2011.

Bruchas, R. R., et al. Anesthesia awareness: narrative review of psychological sequelae, treatment and incidence. *J Clin Psychol Med Settings* **18**: 257–267, 2011.

Cahill, L. and Alkire, M. T. Epinephrine enhancement of human memory consolidation: Interaction with arousal at encoding. *Neurobio Learn Mem* **79**: 194–198, 2003.

Dahaba, A. A. Different conditions that could result in the bispectral index indicating an incorrect hypnotic state. *Anesth Analg* **101**: 765–773, 2005.

Ghoneim, M. M. Incidence of and risk factors for awareness during anaesthesia. *Best Prac Res Clin Anaesthesiol* **21**: 327–343, 2007.

Ghoneim, M. M. Drugs and human memory (Part 2). *Anesthesiol* **100**: 1277–1297, 2004.

Hebb, D. O. *Organization of Behavior*. New York: Wiley, 1949.

Krystal, J. H., et al. Subanesthetic effects of the noncompetitive NMDA antagonist, ketamine, in humans. *Arch Gen Psych* **51**: 199–214, 1994.

Lennmarken, C. and Sydsjo, G. Psychological consequences of awareness and their treatment. *Best Prac Res Clin Anaesthesiol* **21**: 357–367, 2007.

Leslie, K., et al. Posttraumatic stress disorder in aware patients from the B-aware trial. *Anesth Analg* **110**: 823–828, 2010.

Liem, E.B., et al. Anesthetic requirements is increased in redheads. *Anesthesiol* **101**: 279083, 2004.

Liu, W., et al. Incidence of awareness with recall during general anesthesia. *Anaesthesia* **46**: 435–437, 1991.

Martinez, J. and Kesner, R. *Neurobiology of learning and memory*. Orlando: Academic Press, 1998.

Nagashima, K, et al. Propofol inhibits long term potentiation but not long term depression in rat hippocampal slices. *Anesthesiol* **103**: 318–326, 2005.

Newcomer, J. W., et al. NMDA receptor function, memory, and brain aging. *Dialogues Clin Neurosci* **2**: 219–232, 2000.

Reasor, J. D. and Poe, G. R. Learning and memory during sleep and anesthesia. *Int Anesthesiol Clin* **46**: 105–129, 2008.

Schwender, D., et al. Colnscious awareness during generral anaesthesia: Patients' perceptions, emotions, cognition and reactions. *Br J Anaesth* **80**: 133–139, 1998.

Tulving, E. Episodic and semantic memory. In: Tulving, E. and Donaldson, W., eds. *Organization of Memory*. New York: Academic Press, 1972.

Veselis, R. A. and Pryor, K. O. Propofol amnesia – What is going on in the brain? In: Hudetz A. and Pearce, R. *Suppressing the Mind: Anesthetic Modulation of Memory and Consciousness*. New York: Humana Press, 2010.

40 Delayed awakening from anesthesia

Stuart E. Lieblich
University of Connecticut, Department of Oral and Maxillofacial Surgery, Avon, CT, USA

Following the completion of the surgical procedure and anesthesia, the goal is to have the patient return to a full level of consciousness to facilitate safe discharge under the watch of a responsible adult. Drugs that redistribute rapidly (propofol) or are inactivated rapidly (remifentanil,) facilitate a rapid return to a conscious state. However, there are occasional circumstances where a patient does not recover as rapidly. Although prolonged recovery is often dismissed as normal pharmacologic variability, it is important to be mindful of possible non-pharmacologic causes, which if left untreated, may result in adverse outcomes. The signs (and symptoms) of metabolic disorders often present in differently in sedated patients versus patients who are not sedated. In general, causes of delayed awakening can be separated into drug effects, pathophysiologic effects and surgical causes. These will be reviewed individually (see Table 40.1).

Table 40.1 Select causes of delayed awakening in the dental office.

Pharmacologic	Drug overdose
	Synergistic drug reaction
	Adverse drug reaction
Metabolic	Hypoxia
	Hypoglycemia
	Hypovolemia
	Hypercarbia - acidosis
	Hypothermia
Neurologic	Stroke, seizure

Surgical effects

Following the completion of the surgery, there is less stimulation to the patient. As the medications may now have a more profound effect without painful stimulation, a persistent state of unconsciousness or lack of response may occur. Monitoring of the airway and vital signs while waiting for termination of drug effect is preferred over repeated physical stimulation to achieve an awake state, which does nothing to hasten drug action or recovery time. Notwithstanding the foregoing, physical stimulation may be necessary to encourage ventilation or sufficiently awaken the patient to enhance airway tone and avoid obstruction.

Drug effects

The persistence of an anesthetic drug effect is the most likely cause of delayed awakening in the dental anesthesia setting. This can occur with patients who are pharmacologically prone to a greater than expected drug response or prolonged drug action, or in cases of drug overdose. The combination of benzodiazepines and opioids has synergistic effects that enhance the sedative aspects of each (Vittanen et al., 1999). If the patient is over "narcotized," they may present with pinpoint pupils; however, excessive benzodiazepines will not present with a specific clinical sign. Reversal of drug effect with naloxone or flumazenil can be considered, however, this will prolong monitored recovery in the office as the clinical duration of the reversal agent is shorter than the duration of the drug being reversed, inviting resedation. Given the modest doses commonly used in dental anesthesia, along with the usual lack of a neuromuscular blocking agent, a rapid awakening would be expected.

The possibility of dosing error by any member of the anesthesia team should also be considered. Certain agents, midazolam in particular, are formulated with different concentrations (5 mg/mL and 1 mg/mL). If the team is expecting one concentration and an inadvertent substitution occurs, a 5 fold increase in medication can be mistakenly delivered. In addition, it is possible that the patient may have self-medicated, with either prescribed or illicit drugs prior to anesthesia. (see Figure 40.1). In these cases, reversal as noted above should rapidly awaken the patient and be diagnostic as well.

For continuously infused drugs such as propofol, which are primarily dependent on redistribution for awakening, it is valuable to review the context sensitive half-life of the drug. In general an 80% reduction in effect site concentration is required for recovery to occur. With longer infusions, the context sensitive curves are not linear. A 2 hour infusion will take 36 minutes for recovery but if the dose is doubled it will take 105 minutes. Halving the dose leads to a 10 minute recovery (Hughes et al., 1992). There is no reversal agent for propofol.

Adverse drug combinations, although rare in the dental office may also prolong recovery. An example is exposure to a combination of drugs with anticholinergic properties that can lead to prolonged somnolence. This topic is covered in Chapter 36.

Anesthesia Complications in the Dental Office, First Edition. Edited by Robert C. Bosack and Stuart Lieblich.

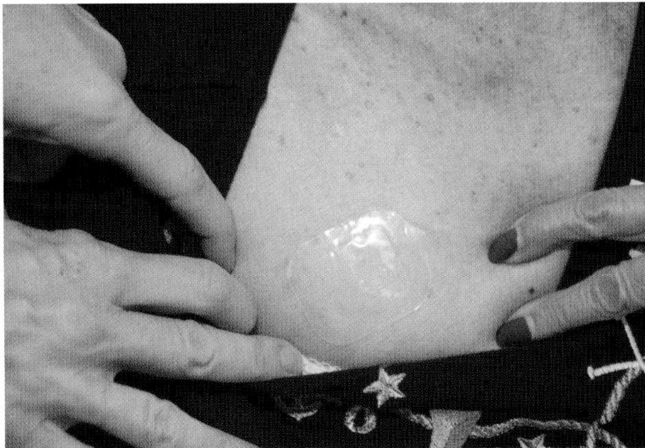

Figure 40.1 Apnea and delayed recovery occurred with this patient, who later revealed the use of a fentanyl patch for arthritic pain.

Patient genetic factors can alter drug effects. The classic example of an enzyme deficiency of plasma cholinesterase is known to cause extremely prolonged recovery from the administration of succinylcholine. Although succinylcholine is not commonly used, the possibility remains that certain patients will react more profoundly to different medications. Since many patients have never had anesthesia before, there is no history to help predict responses to various medication used for dental anesthesia.

Recovery after inhaling anesthetic vapors is dependent on both pulmonary ventilation and pulmonary perfusion. After the anesthetic is turned off the partial pressure of the gas in the alveoli will determine the level of consciousness. In general once the partial pressures reach 30% MAC, the patient will awaken. The rate at which that occurs is dependent on the tidal volume, the perfusion of the lungs and the duration of exposure to the anesthetic vapor. Typically, the use agents with low solubility hasten both time of onset and offset. Once the patient reaches the 30% level and awakens, the potential for resedation from the anesthetic gas does not occur.

Pathophysiologic changes

In all cases of delayed awakening, the adequacy of respiration should be immediately assessed. Retention of carbon dioxide despite adequate oxygen saturation can lead to CO_2 narcosis and delay recovery. Although the CO_2 levels necessary cause narcosis are high, this scenario is possible with a COPD patient, who is hypoventilating during the administration of supplemental O_2.The use of end tidal CO_2 monitoring is especially beneficial in this circumstance. Since many anesthetic drugs are highly protein bound, retained CO_2 leads to acidosis and an increase in the amounts of free circulating drugs due to displacement from the plasma proteins.

During anesthesia, muscle relaxation can compromise respiratory function. The diaphragm relaxes, causing cephalad shifting of abdominal contents. The reduction in vital capacity, notably in patients with obesity, can lead to CO_2 retention. CO_2 retention is also likely in patients with obstructive sleep apnea, who require diligent monitoring of ventilation, especially in the early post-anesthetic period, following the cessation of the surgical stimulus.

Table 40.2 Management of delayed awakening from anesthesia (adapted from Sinclair and Faleiro, 2006).

1 ABC – verify ventilation, oxygenation, check blood pressure and ECG
   (a) Administer 100% O_2
   (b) Positive pressure ventilation, airway adjuncts as necessary
2 Consider drug reversal
   (a) Flumazenil for benzodiazepine
   (b) Naloxone for opioids
   (c) Physostigmine for anticholinergic toxicity
3 Check blood glucose (fingerstick)
   (a) Correct hypoglycemia with 50% dextrose
   (b) EMS triage for patients with hyperglycemia
4 Check body temperature
5 Check neurologic status
   (a) Painful stimuli to elicit focal neurologic deficits
   (b) Evaluate symmetry of movement and strength if patient awake
   (c) Evaluation sensation and speech
6 EMS triage without improvement

Management

Prolonged somnolence after the administration of reversal agents should trigger concern of pathophysiologic (metabolic) alteration. Following verification of adequate oxygenation and blood pressure (i.e., basic ABC's) other potentially reversible causes should be immediately entertained (see Table 40.2). Presumed hypovolemia is easily corrected with Trendelenberg positioning and an isotonic fluid challenge.

Blood glucose levels from a fingerstick blood sample should be determined in all patients, including diabetic patients. Patients with depleted nutritional stores (anorexia or drug abuse) are prone to hypoglycemia. High or low blood glucose levels can delay the emergence from anesthesia. Hypoglycemia will create lethargy, confusion and focal neurologic deficits especially in the elderly. Hypoglycemia is corrected with the slow intravenous administration of 25 – 100 ml of a 50% dextrose solution. Hyperglycemia can cause persistence of unconsciousness due to the formation of a hyperosmolar state with diuresis. The fluid deficit is associated with drowsiness and may cause reduction in the rate of the redistribution of the anesthetic drugs. In extreme hyperglycemia with ketoacidosis cerebral edema may occur and with confounding signs and symptoms of a CVA. This scenario is unlikely in the dental office.

Electrolyte abnormalities and hypothermia have been associated with delayed recovery in the hospitalized patient. Clinically significant electrolyte abnormalities are uncommon in the typically healthier patient receiving anesthesia in a dental office. Futhermore, dental offices are not equipped to measure plasma electrolyte concentrations. Hypothermia is a known cause of delayed awakening, but is unlikely in the dental setting. Lowered core temperatures reduce cardiac output thereby delaying the redistribution of drugs. Neurologic changes including confusion, apnea and unconsciousness is noted with severely lowered temperatures. Body temperature can be easily measured to rule out hypothermia.

Other unexpected events such as a cerebrovascular accident (CVA) may have occurred during the sedation/anesthetic aspect of the procedure. Lateralizing or decorticate/decerebrate posturing with painful stimulation mandates immediate transport to an advanced care facility. Suspicion of a CVA may be raised if the patient becomes acutely hypertensive. Fundoscopic examination for the presence of papilledema may also be diagnostic for hypertensive stroke. If suspected, careful lowering of blood pressure can be considered, but the risk of exacerbating the neurologic injury by creating relative hypotension needs to be weighed against the concern of the hypertension.

References

Hughes, M. A., et al. Context-sensitive half-time in multi-compartment pharmacokinetic models for intravenous anesthetic drugs. *Anesthesiol* **76**: 334–341, 1992.

Sinclair, R. C. F. and Faleiro, R. Delayed recovery of consciousness after anaesthesia. *Cont Ed Anaesth Crit Care Pain* **6**: 114–118, 2006.

Vittanen, H. H., et al. Premedication with midazolam delays recovery after ambulatory sevoflurane anesthesia in children. *Anesth Analg* **89**: 72–79, 1999.

41 Safe discharge after office-based anesthesia

Stuart Lieblich[1] and Peter M. Tan[2]

[1] University of Connecticut, Department of Oral and Maxillofacial Surgery, Avon, CT, USA
[2] Private Practice, P.A. Frederick, MD, USA

Recovery from sedation or anesthesia to the pre-anesthetic physiologic state is a variable continuum, affected by patient parameters (concomitant disease states, level of hydration, plasma protein concentration, receptor number and sensitivity, propensity to nausea and vomiting, etc.) as well as administered drugs (types, routes, duration and total dose). Criteria for choosing an appropriate time for "safe" discharge from office to home under the care of a vested escort (who has been instructed on the importance of continual observation to prevent patient injury) are continually scrutinized and subject to debate. There are many different criteria to assess adequate recovery, which attests to the complexity of this subject, and indicate that an "ideal" set of parameters has yet to be devised. Protocols and guidelines are important aids to determine evidence-based parameters necessary for consistent and safe discharge, which anticipates and prevents late complications. Inappropriate (premature) discharge invites airway obstruction, orthostatic intolerance and falls, nausea and vomiting, among others.

Early recovery occurs when anesthetic or sedative drugs are no longer administered. Patients should be observed in appropriately staffed and equipped areas until they are near their baseline level of consciousness, when the risk of cardiorespiratory depression and hypoxia is eliminated. Early recovery can be prolonged when sedation becomes more profound because surgical stimulation or pain is eliminated. Intermediate recovery ends when the patient is discharge ready. Intermediate recovery can be prolonged by delayed drug absorption following non-intravenous administration. Slow drug elimination, which becomes necessary for termination of effect of some long-acting orally administered drugs can also prolong sedation and intermediate recovery. As an example, exposure to clarithromycin or anti-viral agents which inhibit CYP enzymes needed to metabolize benzodiazepines can delay elimination. Late recovery marks the return to the pre-anesthetic physiologic state (McGrath and Chung, 2003).

Discharge criteria should be relevant, practical and germane to the level of anesthesia practiced. For example, knowing that a patient can move all four extremities after single drug benzodiazepine sedation seems irrelevant. However, ensuring the ability to safely and steadily ambulate without assistance implies the ability to move four extremities and predicts safety at home when using stairs or bathrooms.

Using a standardized system for discharge has the benefits of verifying that all the aspects have been evaluated by the team prior to discharge. This permits documentation of objective criteria that the patient was ready for discharge in care of a responsible, but non-medically trained escort. The most common standardized criteria is the Modified Aldrete Score, with a score ≥9/10 indicating discharge readiness (Aldrete, 1995) (see Table 41.1). Although valuable to document that the patient's vital signs are returned to normal, it does not take into account issues such as the *presence of pain, nausea or vomiting, the ability to ambulate or the presence of bleeding from the surgical site.* These latter issues are pertinent for dental anesthesia cases where the patient's vital signs are not expected to have been significantly affected by the anesthetic. These other factors are recorded in the post-anesthetic discharge scoring

Table 41.1 "Modified aldrete score" (Aldrete, 1995).

- *Activity*: able to move voluntarily or on command
  - 4 extremities – 2
  - 2 extremities – 1
  - Zero extremities – 0
- *Respiration*
  - Able to deep breath and cough freely – 2
  - Dyspnea, shallow or limited breathing – 1
  - Apneic – 0
- *Circulation* – hemodynamic stability
  - BP ±20 mmHg of preanesthetic level – 2
  - BP ±20–50 mmHg of preanesthesia level – 1
  - BP ±50 mmHg of preanesthesia level – 0
- *Consciousness*
  - Fully awake – 2
  - Arousable on calling – 1
  - Not responding – 0
- *O_2 saturation*
  - Able to maintain SpO_2 >92% on room air – 2
  - Needs supplemental O_2 to maintain SpO_2 >90% – 1
  - SpO_2 <90% with supplemental O_2 – 0

Anesthesia Complications in the Dental Office, First Edition. Edited by Robert C. Bosack and Stuart Lieblich.

Table 41.2 The post-anesthesia discharge scoring system (PADSS) (Marschall and Chung, 1997).

- *Vital signs* – must be stable and consistent with age and pre-operative baseline
  - BP and pulse within 20% of preoperative baseline – 2
  - BP and pulse within 20–40% of preop baseline – 1
  - BP and pulse >40% of preoperative baseline – 0
- *Activity level* – patient must be able to ambulate at pre-op level
  - Steady gait, no dizziness, or meets preop level – 2
  - Requires assistance – 1
  - Unable to ambulate – 0
- *Nausea and vomiting* – patient should have minimal nausea and vomiting before discharge
  - Minimal – successfully treated with oral medication – 2
  - Moderate-successfully treated with IM medication – 1
  - Severe – continues after repeated treatment – 0
- *Pain* – patient should have minimal to no pain before discharge, level of pain should be acceptable to the patient. Pain should be controlled by oral analgesics. The location, type and intensity of pain should be consistent with anticipated post-op discomfort.
  - Pain acceptable – 2
  - Pain not acceptable – 1
- *Surgical bleeding* – post-op bleeding should be consistent with expected blood loss for the procedure
  - Minimal – does not require dressing change – 2
  - Moderate – up to 2 dressing changes – 1
  - Severe – more than 3 dressing changes required – 0

system (PADSS) (Marschall and Chung, 1997) (Table 41.2) and may be a useful tool. Like the Modified Aldrete Score, the PADSS also evaluates five key parameters with a score ≥9/10 considered fit for home discharge. Parameters missing from PADSS include *SpO_2, respiratory status and level of consciousness.* It is important to note that these scoring systems were devised for hospitalized patients and assessed readiness for discharge from PACUs or to "fast track" patient from operating rooms to "step-down" units, bypassing the PACU. Neither was devised to assess "home readiness." White and Song (1999) combined features of the Modified Aldrete and PADSS.

Discharge criteria for office-based anesthesia

Requiring patients to void or tolerate oral fluids is no longer supported and has been shown to lead to unnecessary patient delays (Ead, 2006; Awad and Chung, 2006). In fact, premature PO intake can be emetogenic. It may be difficult to determine "normal vital signs" when measured in an anxious patient immediately prior to a dental procedure or venipuncture. Younger patients are prone to greater swings in heart rate and are usually able to tolerate them. After the administration of anesthetic or sedative medications in the dental office, the following criteria can be used to assess home readiness. Patients who meet these criteria are assumed to have the ability to move all four extremities and be fully awake.

1. *Vital signs* – blood pressure and pulse rate should be within 20% of pre-operative values.
2. *Respiration* – should be able to take a deep breath and cough forcefully
3. *Activity* – should be able to ambulate with minimal assistance and without dizziness
4. *SpO_2* – should be able to maintain SpO_2 at or above 94% on room air, or pre-anesthetic level, whichever is greater
5. *PONV* – patients should have minimal nausea or vomiting before discharge
6. *Surgical site* – pain should be that as expected and tolerable by the patient, bleeding must be controlled
7. *Escort* – upon discharge, the patient should be left in the care of a vested, informed escort, who will transport the patient to home. The level or duration of home monitoring by the vested escort is difficult to standardize.
8. *Written and verbal instructions* should be provided, along with 24 hour phone access.

Situations that would warrant a longer period of observation would include cases where reversal agents such as flumazenil or naloxone were administered. As noted in the previous chapters these agents have a shorter duration in reversal activity than the original sedative drug. Consideration for at least a full 60–90 minutes of monitored observation is indicated. Should patients start to desaturate or exhibit signs of re-sedation, the time interval should be extended. Patients at risk of airway compromise, such as those with obesity and/or obstructive sleep apnea may require a longer observational interval, especially if narcotic analgesics have been prescribed.

It is important to clearly communicate postoperative instructions to the escort both verbally and in writing. If a narcotic analgesic is prescribed cautions as to the sedative and possible loss of balance needs to be reinforced to the caregiver at home. A trained professional should be available to answer post-anesthetic questions that may arise to determine if the reactions are significant and if advanced care is needed.

References

Aldrete, J. A. The post anaesthesia recovery score revisited [letter]. *J Clin Anesth* **7**: 89–91, 1995.

Awad, I. T. and Chung, F. Factors affecting recovery and discharge following ambulatory surgery. *Can J Anesth* **53**: 858–872, 2006.

Ead, H. From aldrete to PADSS: reviewing discharge criteria after ambulatory surgery. *J PeriAnesthesia Nursing* **21**: 259–267, 2006.

Marschall, S. and Chung, F. Assessment of "home readiness": discharge criteria and post-discharge complications. *Curr Opin Anaesthesiol* **10**: 445–450, 1997.

McGrath, B. and Chung, R. Postoperative recovery and discharge. *Anesthesiol Clin N Am* **21**: 367–386, 2003.

White, P. F. and Song, D. S. New criteria for fast-tracking after outpatient anesthesia: a comparison with the modified aldrete's scoring system. *Anesth Analg* **88**: 1069–1072, 1999.

SECTION 9

When bad things happen

42 Morbidity and mortality

Lewis Estabrooks
OMSNIC, Rosemont, IL, USA

Analysis of allegations of office-based anesthesia mortality

Anesthetic complications

A wide variety of complications can occur with any medical intervention.

In 22 years of reviewing anesthesia claims and incidents of Oral and Maxillofacial Surgeons' (OMS) anesthesia morbidity and mortality at OMS National Insurance Company (OMSNIC) RRG, what stands out is the superlative safety record of office-based anesthesia provided by the anesthesia teams to their patients. OMSNIC currently insures over 80% of the OMS who are eligible to be insured. Over those two decades about 60 million office-based procedures with anesthesia were provided with a mortality frequency of less than 1/365,500 per encounter. It is clear that due to a lack of fully understanding the risks involved in delivery of care, the public assumes that if a patient enters a dental office they should leave alive. This perception leads to immediate and negative media coverage when a death occurs. All dental professionals should strive to eliminate preventable complications, and manage unpreventable adversity to the standard expected of the profession.

There are several reported cases each year where a patient, sitting in the waiting room before being called in for a consult or surgery, loses consciousness before any treatment is provided. On many occasions, the rapid resuscitative response to maintain and/or establish an airway and assess the cardiac status with appropriate monitors, which is an integral part of oral surgery training, assists patients' survival of an acute myocardial infarction. Unfortunately, there is little recognition for this life-saving treatment. Yet, if this had occurred minutes later in the dental chair after receiving local anesthesia, sedation, or any treatment, the office team would have been put on the defensive.

There are many other times that a thorough history reflects changes or symptoms that precipitate a referral or request for a consult, which results in a diagnosis benefitting a patient. Some signs recognized by oral surgeons have been such changes in behavior that demonstrate early strokes, diabetes, congestive heart failure, and pulmonary diseases, including pulmonary edema, pulmonary emboli, pneumonia, and asthma. Certainly the use of monitors and the taking of vital signs have led to referrals for evaluation of hypertension and cardiac arrhythmias. One such case finding actually led to the diagnosis of a pheochromocytoma.

The profession deserves accolades for these early recognitions. However, similarly to most events in life, what is remembered is the occurrence of the adverse event. Thus, OMSNIC and the profession spend a lot more time reviewing and analyzing the troubling events. There is an innate desire to do the best for our patients and to do what we do to the best of our abilities. Through continuing education – repeated simulation training, risk management, and anesthesia morbidity and mortality conferences – the anesthesia team is able to recognize opportunities for their own improvement in delivering better patient care.

From the review of OMSNIC's anesthesia cases, the most frequent allegations against the anesthesia team were identified. The actions that contributed to either the cause of an adverse anesthesia event or the failure in resuscitation were the focus of further review. Certainly, once a cardiorespiratory event occurs, not all patients will survive even with an excellently executed resuscitation. In some cases, not all the records could be retrieved for analysis. On occasion, treating doctors have sent the patient's original chart of the resuscitation treatment and all the anesthesia monitor documentation along with the EMTs to the hospital. This decision is often made in the judgment of the best patient care. However, when the records get misplaced or lost during the chaos of transport or at the hospital, allegations and assumptions can be made that are not easily refuted without a contemporaneously documented record.

The anesthesia team's documentation has historically relied on having a printout from the BP, pulse oximeter, and ECG monitors. The anesthesia team would print this out at the end of a case and attach it to the anesthesia record. Often when EMTs arrive they disconnect and replace all office equipment with their own monitors. A number of the OMS monitors did not have memory and instantaneously lost all the data once they were disconnected. Because most state dental boards have a requirement to report the emergency transport of a patient or the death of a patient within a specific limited time frame, the doctor then is recreating the lost material. Many doctors displayed a tendency to report what should have been done rather than what was actually done and recall timing of monitor readings that support a sequence of actions. Eventually, the original record may be recovered within the hospital chart, and discrepancies or inconsistencies between the two charts, even if minor, can be used by plaintiffs' attorneys to discredit the integrity of the anesthesia team's treatment.

To best protect oneself, have contemporaneously recorded monitor results in the chart that are printed. Make sure monitors allow the office to retrieve patient data for some period of time after the monitors are disconnected. Office charts including H&P, X-rays, consents, anesthesia records, and resuscitation records should always remain in the office. Copies can be made for the EMTs and hospital.

Anesthesia Complications in the Dental Office, First Edition. Edited by Robert C. Bosack and Stuart Lieblich.

Review of office anesthesia mortality

To best ascertain areas of risk associated with office anesthesia mortality, all of the allegations made were quantified. Most cases had multiple allegations. Not all allegations are based in fact but every allegation requires additional defense effort. Case reviews also focused on any weakness found in the treatment choice or the record keeping of treatment rendered.

1 The most frequent allegation was the loss of adequate oxygenation, which was alleged in almost all cases. The first symptoms were usually a declining SpO_2 or a difficulty with air exchange. On induction, there could be apnea that did not resolve and then progressed to hypoxia oftentimes associated with a mechanical (anatomic) airway obstruction. During the maintenance phase of the anesthetic, agitation probably due to hypercarbia or hypoxia was the earliest recognized sign. In addition, while under anesthesia, vomiting, aspiration laryngospasm, bronchospasm, wheezing, and changes in blood color were all signs associated with a declining SpO_2. After emergence from sedation/anesthesia, symptoms of shortness of breath, chest pain, and diaphoresis were associated with pending myocardial infarctions, pulmonary emboli, and congestive heart failure.

   Anatomic challenges to airway maintenance were most frequently associated with obese patients with short thick necks. Many charts did not preoperatively record the height, weight, or BMI, but this information was acquired from autopsy data. Unfortunately, more than half of the charts did not document a Mallampati classification. This documentation at least demonstrates that the airway was assessed. Many times a plaintiff's expert will assume that an obese patient has sleep apnea. A recorded positive history of a diagnosis of sleep apnea with the need for CPAP requires supporting documentation as to the thought process for the selected sedation/anesthesia and recovery. A variety of physical findings, such as trismus from TMJ disorders, infection, adhesions, and scar tissue from radiation and surgery were found to contribute to interference with the maintenance or reestablishment of an adequate airway. Congenital findings of retrognathia and pathologic findings of tongue and laryngeal carcinoma along with significant infection have also compromised the airway.

2 The second most frequent allegation was delay in recognition of the onset of the fatal event. The assumption was if only the doctor had recognized the symptoms earlier, then he could have intervened to prevent the fatal outcome. The plaintiff's expert usually sites such things as inadequate monitoring because the doctor did not document or did not use SpO_2, CO_2, ECG, or BP monitors. Failure to document auscultation after intubation to confirm tube placement was a common allegation. Moreover, failure to palpate and document a pulse when there were ventricular arrhythmias and possible electrical mechanical dissociation delayed in diagnosing a cardiac problem. Far too often, the doctor would first assume that abnormal monitor findings were due to equipment malfunction and waste precious time setting up new monitors that confirmed the original findings. There were even cases where the anesthesia team had turned the monitor alarms down or off because they were annoying. This becomes extremely difficult to defend.

3 The third most frequent allegation was very similar to the second but states that there was a delay in instituting the proper rescue. In addition to all of the allegations of failure to recognize, further allegations included the doctor failed to initiate the proper resuscitation protocols in a timely manner. The doctor might have thought the symptoms would reverse on their own and done nothing until the case had spiraled down. Even going through a proper differential analysis of why something is occurring, it is always easier for a plaintiff's expert to be a Monday morning quarterback and testify that the final causative diagnosis should have been considered sooner. An example is when the doctor observes the SpO_2 declining and is unable to ventilate with positive pressure O_2 even after placing an oral airway. Then, a muscle relaxant is given and the patient successfully intubated only to determine that the chest wall is rigid and still cannot be ventilated. Now, considering a bronchospasm, the doctor treats the situation as such, but the case has deteriorated beyond salvage. Unfortunately, there are cases when the anesthesia team did not make sure that all their equipment was in working order, fit together properly, and was readily accessible.

4 The fourth most frequent allegation was failure to appropriately resuscitate. This is alleged whenever one is unable to reestablish an adequate airway. Most frequently, the doctor fails at conventional intubation attempts and does not have an LMA. Then, they fail at a surgical airway or create additional complications. Sometimes, when the doctor is successful with intubation, there is no confirmation with a CO_2 monitor or with documented auscultation of the breath sounds. Far too often the doctors have successfully intubated a patient and state that the SpO_2 has returned to normal; however, when the patient arrives in the emergency room the ER doctor documents that the SpO_2 is low and the tube is in the esophagus. Certainly during transport from the dental chair to the EMTs' gurney and transport to the hospital a tube can become displaced. Thus, it is imperative there are recorded printouts and documentation to support the success of the resuscitation before transport.

   This allegation is often accompanied with a wrong diagnosis allegation. An example is when the team notices the SpO_2 is declining. They suction, do a chin thrust, and ventilate with oxygen. The doctor can ventilate and observes the chest rise and even auscultates and hears breath sounds but the SpO_2 continues to drop. Because there is no oxygenation of the blood, the doctor now feels he has to attempt to intubate because incorrectly he still considers this an airway problem. We see this more frequently in light sedation cases where the doctor does not use an ECG monitor and so has no idea of the cardiac status. Moreover, there may be failure to palpate for a pulse. If there is no circulation of blood then the blood will not get oxygenated. Thus, precious time has been wasted trying to intubate when the doctor was confident in ventilating the patient. If one can ventilate there is no immediate reason to intubate.

   An additional allegation under inappropriate resuscitation is that the team gave the wrong drug for the symptoms or gave the wrong dosage. One such case was a middle-aged woman who, after receiving 2 milligrams of midazolam, developed wheezing and shortness of breath. The SpO_2 was in the 70s. The doctor correctly diagnosed an acute allergic reaction and decided to give IV epinephrine. Because he had recently attended an ACLS course, and they had given 3 mg of epinephrine for resuscitation, he gave the same dose. His actions produced a severe tachycardia and hypertension that resulted in an acute MI and death.

   Instituting the wrong algorithm interferes with a timely and proper rescue. Plaintiffs' experts frequently point to the failure to immediately give reversal agents when a problem develops. In addition, some treating doctors feel that reversal agents are their safety net. It usually takes several minutes for that agent to work and if there is a compromised cardiac circulation it may take much longer. Of course, one has to make the correct diagnosis to follow the correct ACLS, AAOMS's Office Anesthesia Manual protocols, or the state's office anesthesia permit recommendations. Since oral surgeons do not deal with emergency situations daily, many have found it helpful to have preprinted algorithms for various emergencies with proper medication dosages for adults and children readily available in each operatory.

5 The fifth most frequent allegation was an inadequate preanesthetic history. This is easily pled when the patient checks off on the history form some type of medical problem and there is no documented follow-up evaluation by the reviewing team member. Something as simple as "are you seeing a doctor?" is checked "yes" but the treater never documents why. There have been several cases where the patient did not have a diagnosis or needed laboratory data back. Yet, the doctor in her deposition admits that had she only known what those results were, she would not have done the case. Thus, it is imperative to document your exploration of all positive responses on the patient's health history. If your best judgment is that further clarification or consultation from the treating doctor is needed – do so – and chart it. Sometimes, it is the anesthesia team that first recognizes a pending medical problem and makes the initial referral for evaluation and treatment.

All clinicians rely on patient honesty in order to make correct treatment decisions. Unfortunately, patients do not always provide complete or accurate information. This may occur because they have forgotten or they do not understand the relevancy to a dental and anesthetic procedure. Sometimes patients just lie. As an example, substance abusing patients may be less than forthright in conveying an accurate history for fear that they will not get the requested treatment. If there is any suspicion of an untruthful history, it is incumbent on the clinician to continually and persistently pursue information gathering (leading questions, search for needle marks, etc.) until such suspicions are either confirmed or put to rest.

There also are patients with severe medical problems that have had outpatient anesthesia services denied because of their medical condition. One such case was a patient scheduled for replacement of a failing prosthetic mitral valve. She developed acute dental pain and an abscess and had been refused surgery at several offices that day due to her medical status. She had appropriately been given antibiotics and pain medication but she wanted the tooth out that day. The ER referred her to the OMS on call and he saw her as an emergency in his office. She did not check off any health history findings. She was NPO so the OMS put her to sleep for a single extraction. She arrested in the office and was unable to be resuscitated. There is certainly contributory negligence on behalf of the patient in such a case. However, the doctor was criticized because he did not auscultate the heart and lungs before administration of an anesthetic. He admitted if he had auscultated the heart he definitely would have heard the prosthetic heart valve and seen the scar on her chest and at such time he would have explored her history in more depth and probably not treated her.

6 The sixth most frequent allegation was questioning the judgment of the doctor to perform the anesthetic in an office setting. This is included in almost every office-based anesthetic mortality. It is easy for the plaintiff's side to find hospital-based anesthesiologists and nurse anesthetists to testify that the only safe place for anesthesia is in the hospital setting administered by someone other than the operator. They do not understand the office anesthesia team concept and have a hard time showing any safety statistics better than the OMSNIC data of a mortality rate of less than 1 in every 365,500 office anesthesia administered cases. The difficulty for defense sometimes lies in the lack of documentation when the chart is compared to the hospital anesthesia record. We also see both oral surgeons and anesthesiologists challenge an OMS' decision to treat a certain medical risk patient in the office. The real question should be, "Was the administration and resuscitation done at the same standard as if the patient had been in the hospital?" Just because one OMS's comfort level handling a medically compromised patient in the office is different than that of another OMS, such a choice is not necessarily negligence.

7 The seventh most frequent allegation was challenging the judgment on which anesthetic drugs the doctor selected to administer. There are multiple acceptable anesthetic techniques with variations on sequence and dosing. It becomes easy to find someone who will state they use a different technique that would have been better. All patients need to be considered as individuals with drug selection and administration personalized for each case. There is no place for "cook book" anesthesia where every patient regardless of age and health is treated the same.

8 The eight most frequent allegation was the decision to even use sedation or a general anesthetic. OMSNIC's OMS reported two-thirds of their twenty-nine million office anesthetic cases in the last 11 years were deep sedation/general anesthetics, while one-third were considered conscious sedation cases. Nearly one half of the mortalities were in this later group. Only conjecture can explain this finding. It may be that the anesthetic team did not feel it was necessary to use an ECG monitor since only sedation was being administered. So they did not recognize a cardiac event until unexpectedly the patient lost consciousness. It could also be that some patients progressed to a deeper plane of anesthesia than expected and the team did not recognize the problems. It could be that this group of patients had more recognized comorbidity so they were administered sedation rather than general anesthesia. Again, the choice of an anesthetic technique is determined by the anesthetist's best judgment and experience with that type of patient. Documentation of one's thought process while considering the various options along with a patient's informed consent can help support the decision.

9 The ninth most frequent allegation was failure to regain consciousness. There have been several cases where all the vital signs have remained stable throughout the case and during the anticipated recovery. Reversal drugs have been given and the patients eventually transported to the hospital because they failed to respond. Several cases have been diagnosed as acute strokes – both ischemic and hemorrhagic. There are several incidents of young healthy people who failed to properly emerge from anesthesia. After being transported and worked up with head CTs they acutely awakened as if nothing ever happened. There are about a half dozen such case histories where no one has been able to pinpoint why there was such a delay.

10 The tenth most frequent allegation was inadequate assistance, which always brings into question the training of the entire anesthetic team. It is ironic that the anesthesiologist and nurse anesthetist who provide anesthesia in OMS offices (about

3%) essentially use the existing OMS personnel and do not bring other assistants with them. Yet these groups are the most vocal plaintiffs' experts. There have also been office anesthetic mortalities when anesthesia was administered by a physician anesthesiologist, dental anesthesiologist, or nurse anesthetists. Whenever and wherever an emergency develops everyone is immediately activated and the entire team needs to respond appropriately. The anesthesia team needs to have practiced simulated emergencies on a regular basis to ensure competency. Thus, it is always helpful when the office can produce their clinical training schedules and records of the types of simulated cases. The best test of competency is when you feel comfortable that in an unanticipated emergency your trained team could resuscitate you. The office needs to have current ACLS and BLS cards as well as a current office inspection with any active required state anesthesia permit.

Emergency Medical Services (EMS) responds to 911 calls and should be activated earlier rather than later. They deal with acute emergencies and as a rule, do an excellent job. It is desirable to invite local EMS professionals into the office to familiarize them with the nature of anesthesia care being rendered, the resuscitative equipment available and instructions on how they should enter the surgical area when called. Allow them to explain how they function, what guidance they receive for emergencies, and what they would like from you if they are summoned. Their documentation of the time of contact and arrival and their initial assessment of the situation upon arrival goes a long way in supporting your team. It always helps when the office monitor times are accurate and correspond to the documented time that the EMS has recorded. Some EMS units will allow you to ride with them during transport while others will not. Having this clear before they ever arrive for an emergency eliminates a conflict. When there is a mutual respect for each other's capabilities there will be less confusion and better coordinated treatment during any rescue.

The dental profession needs to continually demonstrate competency and safety of the office-based anesthesia team model. This can be done via frequent simulation training with the entire team, improved documentation of thought processes involved in the selection of the patient, the anesthetic and the location of care; and the use of the most advanced and complete monitoring available for each patient. Checklists are key reminders of appropriate steps to ensure proper evaluation, management, recovery and rescue (if needed) to the standards that the dental profession demands.

43 Death in the chair: a dentist's nightmare

Glen Crick
Chicago, IL, USA

Introduction

Very few people die during or as a result of undergoing a dental procedure, but the unfortunate fact is that patient deaths do occur.

Very little information is available about the frequency of death or serious injury as a result of undergoing a dental procedure in the United States. There are no national mandatory reporting requirements to capture information about such incidents and many state dental licensing or certification boards do not require dentists to report when a death or serious injury occurs. Even in states that mandate reporting, statistics may not be available regarding patient death or serious injury if the incident does not result in sanctions against a dentist. Nonetheless, experts agree that patient mortality and morbidity are influenced more by the use of anesthesia than any other element of dental practice.

The point of this chapter is not to tell dentists how to avoid a death in their practice. That is the role of dental educators and experts in dentistry, anesthesiology, and related fields. The author of this chapter is an attorney who has represented a number of dentists during the course of investigations and prosecutions following cases in which a patient death occurred. The focus of this chapter is on the investigation that will follow the serious injury or death of a patient as a result of a dental procedure, the questions that will be asked, and the aspects of a dentist's practice that will be examined in detail. Suggestions regarding how a dental practice may prepare for an emergency also will be made.

While it is hoped that the information presented here will be of value in helping avoid such an incident, its intent is to help a dentist prepare for and withstand the investigation that will follow a dental death or the serious injury of a patient.

The assumption

When a dental death occurs, there is an assumption on the part of the public and even among other dentists that the treating dentist did something wrong. Therefore, following the death or serious injury of a patient, there will be an investigation by any number of entities, including

- the state dental licensing board and/or other entity that regulates the practice of dentistry
- the local state's attorney and/or the police
- the Federal Drug Enforcement Agency (DEA)
- any entity that licenses the facility
- attorneys on behalf of the patient's family or estate
- the news media.

Questions that will be asked

During the course of an investigation, questions will be asked about:

- the dentist
- the patient
- the anesthesia used
- the office equipment
- the dental assistants
- how the dentist and staff reacted to the emergency
- drugs administered as a result of the emergency
- records of the procedure and the emergency

About the Dentist

- Was the dentist properly licensed?

A dentist must hold a valid, active license in the jurisdiction where he or she practices. A dentist who treats patients before he or she has been issued a license in the jurisdiction of practice, or whose license has expired, has committed a criminal offense. It is important for a dentist to be issued a license before beginning to practice in a particular jurisdiction and to renew all licenses in a timely manner.

- Was the dentist trained and qualified to perform the procedure?

It is not enough for a dentist to hold a license to practice dentistry. Generally, and in particular, when a patient death or injury occurs, a dentist will be asked to prove that he or she was adequately trained and qualified to perform the procedure the patient underwent.

- Was the dentist authorized and trained to administer anesthesia?

Most states require special licensure for a dentist to be authorized to administer anesthesia.

- Was the dentist authorized to sedate the patient to the level reached?

Levels of sedation are defined either by statute or rule within a particular jurisdiction, or by reference to an existing standard. Levels of sedation may range from "light conscious" to "general." The issue is whether the patient was taken to an unintended level of sedation.

- Was the dentist adequately trained and certified to deal with an emergency?

The laws within the jurisdiction of a dental practice may require training and certification in Basic Life Support or Advanced Cardiac Life Support as a qualification for a dentist to sedate a patient to a particular level. It is important that all such required certifications be current. An expired certification may indicate that the dentist's knowledge in life-saving practices is not current.

- Was the dentist present throughout the procedure?

Some jurisdictions require the treating dentist to be chair-side the entire time a patient is sedated. These requirements may vary,

Anesthesia Complications in the Dental Office, First Edition. Edited by Robert C. Bosack and Stuart Lieblich.

depending on the level of intended sedation. Even in jurisdictions that do not specifically require a treating dentist or a dentist administering anesthesia to be present throughout sedation, a dentist is well advised to remain in the room with the patient any time a patient is under anesthesia.

About the patient

- Was the patient a proper subject for the procedure?

A dentist should carefully screen every patient who will be sedated while undergoing dental treatment. Having a patient fill out a routine personal history form might not be enough. The patient also should be interviewed about known and suspected medical conditions, preferably by the treating dentist. Any time a patient reports that he or she is under the care of a physician for a condition that could render the patient a poor candidate for a procedure or for sedation, the physician should be contacted to request medical clearance. Specific concerns are heart condition, uncontrolled diabetes, asthma, and morbid obesity. In cases where the decision has been made to sedate a medically compromised patient, it is wise to consider administering the procedure at a hospital or an ambulatory surgical treatment center where equipment and assistance are immediately available if something goes wrong.

- Was the patient adequately advised of the risks involved?

In addition to having a patient sign a standard "Informed Consent" form, the treating dentist or another responsible individual in the practice should discuss the specific risks of the procedure and the sedation that will be involved. It is a good idea to have the patient initial and date certain paragraphs of the patient medical history form and to note in the patient's treatment record that a discussion regarding known risks took place.

- Was the patient sedated to or beyond the desired level?

Patients react differently to anesthesia. Some will reach a deeper level of sedation with much less anesthesia. When a deeper level of sedation than intended is reached, the questions will become whether the amount of anesthesia administered to the patient was based on some logical basis and whether the anesthesia was titrated.

- Was the patient constantly monitored while being sedated?

Even in jurisdictions where there is no specific requirement that the dentist administering anesthesia be present the entire time a patient is under it, someone must actively monitor the patient while he or she is under sedation. Further, the person who monitors the patient should not be "multi-tasking" while doing so.

About the anesthesia

- Was the anesthesia appropriate for the patient and for the procedure?

Not all types of anesthesia are appropriate for all patients. A dentist is wise to review the drug manufacturer's instructions and warnings about contraindications for use, especially when dealing with patients who are medically compromised or taking medication.

- Was the anesthesia calculated based on the patient's age, weight, or by some other method?

A dentist must be able to explain why a particular amount of anesthesia was used. The great danger is falling into a routine. When something goes wrong, it never is a good idea to explain, "That's the way we always do it." A dentist should consider all circumstances surrounding a patient's case (medical history, dental procedure being conducted, drug allergies, etc.) and decide how much anesthesia to administer on a case-by-case basis.

- Was the anesthesia selected and prepared by the treating dentist?

The overall responsibility for the anesthesia used on a patient rests with the treating dentist. At the same time, a particular medical practitioner such as a medical doctor trained in anesthesiology may have more expertise in such matters. An anesthesia "cocktail" to be administered to a patient should be mixed only by the treating dentist or by a certified, registered nurse anesthesiologist who will administer the anesthesia. Mixing the anesthesia is too important a task to leave to an assistant, however well qualified.

- Was the anesthesia properly titrated?

Anesthesia should be administered slowly, until the desired level of sedation is achieved. It is dangerous to assume that, based on "experience," a certain amount of anesthesia will always result in the same level of sedation for patients of a particular age and weight. Anesthesia affects different people differently, and the dosage always should be titrated.

About the assistants

- Were the assistants trained according to individual state requirements?

State law where a dental practice is located should be reviewed to determine the number of chair-side assistants required when a patient is sedated to a certain level, and the training required for those assistants. In states where the law is silent on this matter, a dentist is held to the local "standard of care." Standard of care may be explained as what a reasonable and prudent dentist would do under similar circumstances. In states where there appears to be no legal guidance on this matter, it is suggested that a dentist follow other established standards for assistants, such as those found in the "American Academy of Pediatric Dentistry's 2010–11 Definitions, Oral Health Policies, and Clinical Guidelines," found on the American Academy of Pediatric Dentistry's website: http://www.aapd.org/media/policies.asp.

- Were the assistants certified in basic life support for healthcare professionals?

Not only should chair-side assistants be trained in Basic Life Support, their certifications also must remain current.

- Were the assistants trained to respond to an emergency?

It is in the best interest of a dentist and the dental practice to train all assistants in emergency preparedness and response. Drills are an effective method for reinforcing emergency training. It is also helpful to maintain a training log showing the employees' training and their participation in practice drills.

About the equipment

- Was the required equipment present and in good working order?

To learn the minimum equipment requirement for sedating patients to certain levels, research the laws governing dental practice in the state where the practice is located. As previously noted, in states where the law is silent, the "standard of care" will prevail, so it is recommended that a dentist adhere to other published standards, such as those of the American Academy of Pediatric Dentistry, published online at http://www.aapd.org/media/policies.asp. Not only must the required equipment be present it also must be in good working order. Routinely inspect equipment to ensure that it is fully functional.

About Dentist and staff reaction to the emergency

- How well did the dentist and staff react to the emergency?

Things do go wrong. How well the dentist and staff reacted to the emergency is the big question. Obviously, the better prepared for an emergency the practice is, the better, and the keys to preparedness are training and practice drills.

About drugs used during the procedure and the emergency

- Were all of the drugs and medicines used for the procedure and in the emergency supplies current?

In the event of a dental death, investigators will pay particular attention to drugs and medicines administered to the patient. There should be no expired drugs used in a procedure and none in the emergency supplies.

About the record of the procedure and the emergency

- Were adequate records of the procedure and the reaction to the emergency maintained?

The dentist's treatment record for the patient will be examined. The dentist's notes should be comprehensive and legible. All notes should be entered into the treatment record as soon as practical after the incident. Details that come to the attention of the dentist after his or her initial entry in the record may be included as addenda. *Once the original record has been created, it should never be altered.*

About whether the incident was properly reported

- Did the dentist report the incident, per all state law requirements?

A dentist should check the laws of their jurisdiction to determine whether and to whom he or she is required to report if a patient dies as a result of a dental procedure. Be sure to check your state's reporting requirements, including the timeline for doing so. It is imperative that such report, if required, be filed in a timely manner. It should also be noted that *statements made in the report will be considered admissions*, and may be admitted into evidence in any formal evidentiary hearing or trial that could result from the occurrence.

The investigation

An investigation into the serious injury or death of a patient most often will include an inspection of

- the facility
- the equipment used
- emergency supplies or kits.

The investigation also will consist of

- interviews of dentist, staff, and others
- a review of records kept
- verification of licensure and training of all involved dentists and staff.

The facility

When a dental patient dies or has been seriously injured, an investigation by any one of the entities referred to in the beginning of this chapter will ensue, and it is expected that investigators will inspect the practice location. During the initial inspection of the facility, investigators will examine whether emergency lighting and emergency oxygen delivery systems are present, and where controlled substances are stored. Investigators will also observe the cleanliness and organization of the facility.

The equipment used

Equipment, particularly the one that was used for monitoring and for the emergency, will be inspected. The investigators also may ask the dentist or a member of his or her staff to demonstrate how the equipment works and may ask when it was last inspected.

Emergency supplies or kits

The location where emergency drugs are stored (such as a cabinet or emergency cart) will be inspected, any controlled substances present will be inventoried, and any empty drug containers or expired drugs will be noted.

Dentist's interview

It is to be expected that an investigator will want to interview the dentist or dentists involved in the treatment. It is important for a dentist being investigated to remember that he or she

- is *not* required to submit to an interview
- may consult with legal counsel and insist that counsel be present during an interview.

The interview of a dentist following an adverse incident focuses on answering the question, "What did the dentist do wrong?"

Note: For additional information about how a dentist can protect his or her rights during the course of an investigation, refer to the article, "What to Do When Investigated," found at www.cricklaw.com.

Staff interviews

Investigators likely will want to interview staff members, particularly those who were present prior to and during the emergency. Like dentists, staff are not required to be interviewed and should not be encouraged or discouraged to do so. All staff should be told it is their decision whether to be interviewed. It is a good idea to make staff aware that investigators might attempt to contact them at home during non-business hours, and attempt to intimidate them into being interviewed. Investigators look for inconsistencies between what the dentist says happened and what the staff says happened.

Verification of training and continuing medical education

During the course of the investigation, the dentist will be asked to provide proof of life support training and certification and completion of the required continuing medical education. A dentist also may be asked to provide proof of specialized training, anesthesia training, and training regarding the specific procedure undertaken.

Records

A dentist may also expect that *all* records will be reviewed, including

- the patient treatment record
- the anesthesia record
- controlled substances records.

Patient treatment record and anesthesia log

Investigators will request a copy of the complete record of treatment of the patient. An outside expert most likely will review all records, particularly the anesthesia record. A dentist also may expect to be asked to discuss and explain the record.

At minimum, any time a patient is sedated, the dentist should keep the following records:

- medical history of the patient
- record of the patient evaluation prior to the procedure
- patient's "informed consent" for the procedure to be performed and administration of anesthesia
- preoperative, intraoperative, and pre-discharge blood pressure, pulse, respiration, and oxygen saturation measurements
- record of EKG or other monitoring during the procedure

- drug names and dosage amounts of all drugs used during the procedure
- identification of the individual who administered the drugs and times of their administration over the course of the procedure
- documentation of the anesthetic encounter, consistent with currently accepted standards of anesthetic practice.

Anesthesia record

An anesthesia record is a time-based record containing the name, route, site, times, dosage, and patient effects of administered drugs. Such a record is examined for
- who administered the drugs
- whether the patient's vital signs were taken before, during, and after the procedure and emergency.

Controlled substances records

During the course of the investigation, particularly if DEA investigators are involved, it is expected that an inventory of all controlled substances on hand will be taken. Tablets will be counted and liquid amounts estimated. The controlled substances records that will be reviewed are
- initial, annual, and biennial controlled substances inventories
- DEA 222 Forms
- invoices and other records reflecting purchase and receipt of Schedules III, IV, and V controlled substances (totals will be recorded)
- any "Patient Controlled Substances Record" required by the laws of the jurisdiction
- logs of controlled substances wasted, returned, and destroyed.

Note: For a thorough discussion about controlled substance record keeping requirements under Illinois and federal law and how an audit is conducted, see the article, "Controlled Substances Record Keeping Requirements for Illinois Healthcare Practitioners," found at www.cricklaw.com.

Finding fault

In a number of cases where an adverse incident occurred during or as a result of a dental procedure, dentists are commonly criticized for one or more of the reasons listed below.
- The patient was medically compromised and patient screening did not reveal the medical condition.
- A medical condition was known, but the dentist proceeded without obtaining medical clearance from the patient's primary-care physician.
- More anesthesia than necessary was administered to the patient, based on his or her age and weight.
- The anesthesia administered was not titrated and the patient reached a deeper level of sedation than intended.
- The facility where the procedure took place did not have the required equipment or the required equipment did not function properly.
- The patient was not adequately monitored.
- Staff were not properly trained and supervised.
- There was a perceived failure to adequately and properly respond to the emergency.

Although they cannot be said to cause or contribute to an adverse incident, there are two other "reasons" that dentists are criticized following such an incident, as listed below.
- Failure to adequately document the procedure.
- Failure to properly report the adverse incident within the required time frame.

Suggestions for protecting your practice

Establish written protocols

While not required, written protocols for preparing patients, preparing and administering anesthesia, and undertaking different dental procedures will establish consistency in the standard of care provided at a dental office. Following are recommended protocols that may help a dentist involved in a dental death to better withstand each phase of the ensuing investigation.

Screen patients and obtain "informed consent"

To give "informed consent" for receipt of a dental procedure and to undergo sedation, an individual patient must have adequate reasoning faculties and be in possession of all relevant facts when giving such consent. Factors such as age, mental retardation, mental illness, or intoxication may render a patient unable to give consent. In addition, a dentist must make a patient aware of all pertinent information, such as known risks and possible consequences, for his or her consent to be considered valid.

Thorough patient screening is essential. The key element of a successful screening is to take a detailed medical history to determine any preexisting medical conditions or any drug allergies. If a medical condition is revealed during a patient screening that might make the procedure and/or administration of anesthesia ill advised, the patient's primary-care physician should be contacted to obtain medical clearance for the dental procedure. Such approval should be documented.

A dentist may require patients to initial and date important health history questions and to sign and date the "Informed Consent Form."

If there is any doubt about whether a patient is appropriate for sedation, a dentist should obtain medical clearance from the patient's primary care physician or treating specialist.

Recommendations about sedation equipment

Laws in various states prescribe the equipment that must be present. Most jurisdictions require that, at minimum, a facility be equipped with
1 a sphygmomanometer and a stethoscope
2 an oxygen delivery system with full face masks and connectors capable of delivering oxygen to the patient under positive pressure, and a backup system
3 emergency drugs and equipment appropriate to the medications administered
4 suction equipment
5 an emergency back-up lighting system that will permit the completion of any operation underway
6 a pulse oximeter.

In addition, a facility where deep sedation or general anesthesia is administered should be equipped with
1 a laryngoscope, complete with selection of blades and spare batteries and bulbs in sizes appropriate to the patient population being served
2 endotracheal tubes and connectors and face masks in sizes appropriate for the patient population being served, and a device capable of delivering positive pressure ventilation
3 tonsillar or pharyngeal suction tips adaptable to all office outlets
4 nasal and oral airways in sizes appropriate to the patient population being served
5 a device for monitoring temperature (such as temperature strips or a thermometer)
6 electrocardioscope and defibrillator

7 equipment for establishing an intravenous infusion
8 an operating table or operating chair that permits appropriate access to the patient and provides a firm platform for managing cardiopulmonary resuscitation
9 a recovery area with available oxygen, lighting, suction, and electrical outlets.

Note: A patient should remain in the recovery area until the individual retains the ability to independently and consciously maintain an airway and respond appropriately to physical stimulation and verbal command. The recovery area may be the operatory.

General recommendations concerning anesthesia

Selection and administration

Select anesthesia that is appropriate for the patient and for the procedure. The patient's age, weight, general health, and any known medical conditions must be taken into account when deciding upon which anesthesia to be administered. IN addition, sedation agents should be titrated until the desired level of sedation is achieved.

Preparation

If anesthesia is drawn, mixed, or otherwise prepared by anyone other than the dentist administering the sedation, it is important to put in place a detailed, written protocol. It is also advised to label syringes and cross-check preparations.

Taking and recording vital signs

Vital signs must be taken preoperatively, intraoperatively, and postoperatively. It is a good practice to take and record respiration, regardless of whether the dentist believes it to be necessary. Recording respiration is required by law in certain jurisdictions.

Monitoring

It is essential to adequately monitor a patient who is under any kind of sedation. In addition to preventing the patient's head from dropping and thereby cutting off oxygen, consistent monitoring will immediately reveal difficulty in breathing and other signs of distress. A patient must be monitored from the time sedation is administered until he or she is thoroughly recovered and ready to leave the facility.

Record keeping recommendations

Patient treatment records

Always include in a patient's treatment record

- patient's medical history
- treatment plan
- informed consent for the procedure and the anesthesia
- treatment provided
- drugs administered (a copy of the anesthesia record is sufficient)
- description of any emergency.

Patient controlled substances records

- Record each controlled substance administered separately in a "Patient Controlled Substance Record."
- Use a separate page or pages for each dosage form of a controlled substance administered or dispensed (for example, "Hydrocodone, 10 mg tablet").
- Make a separate entry on the particular controlled substance dosage form page showing
- patient's name
- date the substance was administered or dispensed
- amount of the substance administered or dispensed

Recommendations about emergency supplies and lighting

Maintain a separate emergency kit with emergency drugs and equipment appropriate to the medications administered in each operatory. To guarantee the equipment is up to date and functioning properly and that drugs and medications have not expired, conduct regularly scheduled inspections of required equipment and emergency kits. Emergency lighting should be more than just a flashlight.

Recommended procedures for handling a patient in distress

A written emergency plan usually is not required by law. However, it is strongly suggested to have an emergency plan in place that describes assigned roles and duties in the event of an emergency, and that provides for drills and cross-training.

Remember the Dentist is in charge

The dentist performing the procedure must immediately take charge and provide direction to others who assist in the emergency. The less preparation, training, and drills that have occurred before the incident, the more important it is for the dentist to provide direction. In theory, the dentist remains in charge of the emergency situation until the patient is stabilized or until the dentist is relieved by a medical doctor at the hospital emergency room.

Call 911

A staff member should be designated to call 911 immediately and instructed to stay on the line with the operator until first responders have arrived.

Lie patient on firm surface

Unless the dental chair can achieve *a fully supine position*, remove a patient who is not breathing from the chair and lay the individual on the floor.

Clear airway

Be sure that any gauze, dams, blocks, or debris are removed from the patient's mouth before beginning CPR.

Begin CPR

Use of an Ambubag with positive pressure oxygen is the preferred method for CPR, but mouth-to-mouth resuscitation may be administered if circumstances dictate. Be prepared to have the patient intubated, if necessary, and to have someone properly trained to perform this procedure.

Appoint a timekeeper

If there are an adequate number of well-trained staff on hand, one staff member should be appointed as or assume the role of timekeeper, and keep a log of

- what occurs, including the time drugs and reversing agents are administered and the amounts administered
- who administers CPR

- who enters and leaves the room
- other notable occurrences.

Administer appropriate reversing agents

When circumstances allow, record the amount of each reversing agent administered and the time it was given.

Notify all staff

Staff members not directly involved in the emergency should calmly be made aware that an emergency exists. When possible, assign someone to meet the "first responders." Clear the path for the first responders to easily and quickly reach the emergency. Note that in urban areas there may be more than one team of first responders.

Inform the patient's companions

Notify anyone who accompanied the patient of the incident. Take care, though, to keep him or her from interfering with life-saving efforts.

Dismiss other patients

When possible, it is best to dismiss other patients without attempting to reschedule their appointments. Rescheduling can take place at a later time.

Recommended procedures for handling first responders

Although the dentist is still in charge, common sense should be used and conflict avoided.

Allow first responders to take over

Even though the dentist is in charge, it may be necessary to allow the first responders to take over CPR.

Provide essential information

Describe the "what," "when," and "who." Explain to first responders how long the patient has been in distress, the drugs administered, the reversing agents and stimulants administered, the patient's known health history, the procedure performed, and provide any other pertinent information.

Recommended procedures for removing the patient to a hospital

Whenever possible, the dentist should accompany the patient in the ambulance to the hospital. *Do not simply go on to treat the next patient!*

At the hospital, a dentist should identify himself or herself to emergency room staff and provide all relevant information. The dentist also should meet with friends and family of the patient and, without making admissions, answer their questions.

It is important for a dentist meeting with friends and family to listen and really hear what the patient's friends and family are saying. It is not only the polite and civilized thing to do, it is also a way for the dentist to gain information about the patient, such as a preexisting medical condition undisclosed on the patient's medical history form or during the consultation. If the patient is admitted to the hospital, the dentist should frequently call to obtain updates about his or her condition.

What to do immediately after an incident

Cancel appointments

Direct staff to cancel all remaining patient appointments.

Identify all employees and others present during the incident

Safeguard the appointment book and/or patient sign-in sheet, and identify who was present in the operatory and in the clinic during the incident.

Complete patient treatment record

Complete the patient treatment record in as much detail as possible. Note that this report should be factual and procedural, not speculative. Secure the print-outs of any monitors that were used.

Notify malpractice insurance carrier

As soon as possible, a dentist should notify his or her malpractice insurance carriers to seek instructions.

Do not ask staff to prepare written reports

As soon as possible, arrange to have staff "debriefed" by an attorney. The results will become "attorney work product," rather than discoverable notes or reports.

Seal or safeguard operatory

Do not immediately clean the operatory. It is important to identify and record the equipment used during the procedure and during the emergency.

Safeguard drugs and syringes

Identify and secure the drugs administered to the patient, including the vials from which drugs were drawn and, depending on the circumstances, drugs from the same lot. Save and secure any syringes used.

Safeguard equipment

Identify, inventory, and (when practical) secure all equipment used during the procedure. Determine if the equipment works properly.

Inspect required equipment

Following an incident and prior to resuming practice, to ensure that all of the required equipment is on hand and functioning properly, a dentist should review the list of equipment required for administering conscious sedation, deep sedation, or general anesthesia.

Inventory all drugs on hand

It is advisable to replace and replenish supplies of drugs used, particularly reversing agents and stimulants from an emergency kit. Remove and segregate any expired drugs.

Debrief staff

During the debriefing period, do not discourage staff from talking about what happened. Arrange to have staff debriefed by an attorney. After they speak with the attorney, a dentist should consider holding an in-house "debriefing" session to discuss and review with staff which protocols were properly followed, and which ones were not.

Provide counseling

Life-threatening emergencies and deaths that occur in a dental setting can be very traumatic, particularly for younger, less experienced staff who never dealt with such circumstances in the past. A dentist may wish to arrange for staff to see a counselor. It also is not a bad idea for the dentist to talk with a counselor following a traumatic event.

Retain and consult with legal counsel

A dentist who experiences a dental death or the serious injury of a patient is wise to seek legal counsel as soon as possible. A question that may arise is whether separate counsel is necessary because of licensure issues. Separate counsel is advisable if a dentist's malpractice insurance policy does not provide coverage during licensure and regulatory investigations, or if legal counsel recommended or provided by the insurance carrier is not experienced in representing dentists involved in dental death investigations and prosecutions.

Report the incident

If required within the jurisdiction where the practice is located, be sure to report the incident.

Post-emergency don'ts

He following is a list of what *not* to do in the case of a dental emergency.

- *Do not* just go on to the next patient.
- *Do not* alter or recreate a record.
- *Do not* ask staff to write a narrative report.
- *Do not* talk to the press.
- *Do not* submit to an investigative interview without counsel present.

Conclusion

Life-threatening dental emergencies are rare, but they do occur. It is far better to plan for, train for, and practice responding to an emergency before one actually occurs.

44 Legal issues of anesthesia complications: risks or malpractice

Arthur W. Curley
Bradley, Curley, Asiano, Barrabee, Abel & Kowalski, PC Larkspur, CA, USA

Oral and intravenous sedation have become essential to the delivery of many forms of modern dental care. Even with the use of profound local anesthesia, many procedures, such as periodontal surgery, placement of dental implants, or removal of impacted teeth, would not be accepted by many patients without sedation. Pediatric sedation allows for the delivery of significant care without the attendant fear and resistance associated with physical restraints and controls. Indeed, some procedures, such as orthognathic surgery, nerve repair, and placement of zygomatic implants, realistically could not be provided without conscious sedation or general anesthesia. The application of sedation has become routine for many practitioners. However, despite improved monitoring and the use of more predictable anesthetic agents, there remains the risk of significant complications every time a patient is sedated. Irrespective of whether complications are an unavoidable risk or the result of substandard care, they involve issues of law as well as issues of medicine. This chapter reviews the legal principles, cases, and offers recommendations for compliance with the legal standard of care.

The law of anesthesia

There are three basic elements required for a patient to prevail in a claim for malpractice: (1) *negligence*; (2) *causation*; and (3) *injury*. All three must be present before a patient is entitled to payment for any damages suffered. *Negligence* (aka malpractice) can be defined as failure to meet the standard of care, engaging in unprofessional conduct, or violation of a statute.[1]

Standards of care, generally

The *standard of care* is the most common measure of dental negligence. It is defined as what a reasonable and prudent practitioner would do, or should have done, or should have avoided doing, in the same or similar circumstances, in the same or similar locality, and during the same period of time. The source of any particular standard of care, with some exceptions, is generally not found in any legal treaty, statute, or text. Rather, it is determined by the opinions of expert witnesses as to the standards in the dental community. Upon the review of records and testimony in a case, experts render opinions as to whether there was a violation of the standard of care. A typical malpractice claim is heard by the *finder of fact*, a jury, or a judge sitting in place of a jury, determining which side's experts are to be believed.[2] Until recently, standard of care evolved slowly because of the legal qualifier of *the same* or similar locality during the same time period, sometimes called the *local standard of care qualifier*. In the modern era of communications via e-journals, video continuing education (CE) programs, and other technological advances, the legal trend is to recognize a national standard of care. Therefore, the prudent practitioner must remain aware of the evolving, as well as the current, standards of care.

Written standards of care

Expert witnesses may bolster their opinions by citing authoritative or well-recognized texts, peer-reviewed journals, or treatises.[3] However, whether a text is considered authoritative or well-recognized is determined by a judge, who considers expert witness testimony as to the qualifications of the text or journal on an issue, before it can be read to a jury. Written guidelines by healthcare organizations can be used as a standard of care if they were so intended by the author(s). Guidelines, such as those of the American Heart Association, are documents that also may be considered evidence of the standard of care.[4] The guidelines of the American Society of Anesthesiologists (ASA) were intended to set standards of care to reduce morbidity and mortality.[5] Accordingly, these guidelines are part of the typical oral and maxillofacial residency program and may be admitted in most courts as evidence of standards of care for anesthesia. Therefore, surgeons providing anesthesia must consider those guidelines. For example, experts have testified that failure to rate a patient as ASA 1 to 4 may be evidence of substandard care in the event of an anesthesia complication. On the other hand, the Parameters of Care of the American Society of Oral & Maxillofacial Surgeons are specifically meant not to be standards of care. However, some courts have allowed their admission as evidence.[6] Surgical technologies, such as ECG monitors, come with manufacturer's guidelines. Although not specifically stated or intended as setting standards of care, courts have allowed experts to testify that a defendant's failure to adhere to the manufacturer's guidelines, such as routine calibration, is a violation of the standard of care.

Violation of a statute or code

An exception to the traditional expert witness-defined legal standards of care is a violation of statute or code not necessarily included

Anesthesia Complications in the Dental Office, First Edition. Edited by Robert C. Bosack and Stuart Lieblich.

in licensing regulations. Such statutes typically are found in state penal and/or civil codes and, in some cases, Federal statutes. Violation of a statute intended to provide protection or safety to the public is presumed to be evidence of negligence. Examples of this would be statutes regarding the recordkeeping for medications. If a patient had a problem that could have been caused by the dose of a medication and the doctor's recordkeeping was not in compliance, such treatment would be presumed to have violated that standard of care if the harm that occurred was in the realm of what the statute was intended to prevent.[7] It is important for the prudent practitioner to maintain basic knowledge of the laws regarding anesthesia and recordkeeping for all patients. Specifics as to those laws often can be obtained from the web pages of dental licensing agencies.[8]

Licensing agencies

Regulations set forth by a state's licensing agency, a violation of which is commonly referred to as *unprofessional conduct,* are also exceptions to the traditional expert witness-defined legal standards of care. Such regulations typically include the scope of practice (i.e., what any healthcare provider is allowed to do as determined by his/her license). While generally similar from state to state, regulations can be very specific. For example, in California, there are specific regulations regarding the administration of oral and conscious sedation as well as general anesthesia. They include permit requirements,[9] in office evaluation,[10] recordkeeping,[11] emergency medications and dosing,[12] informed consent,[13] use of auxiliaries,[14] monitoring, and morbidity and mortality reporting.[15] Violation of such regulations may be considered unprofessional conduct and a form of negligence. In such cases, expert testimony may not be required to prove substandard care.[16]

Requisite proof

The amount of evidence required to prevail, called the *burden of proof* in a malpractice case, is a *preponderance,* or a simple majority (more than 50%), of the evidence, and not evidence beyond a *reasonable doubt* (more than 90% of the evidence), as in criminal cases.[17] Records are the most common source of evidence of the quality of care provided. This author has cross-examined many expert witnesses who have testified that, "If it isn't written or noted, it didn't happen." Therefore, the detail and quality of dental records are essential in reducing the risks of being subject to a malpractice claim in the event of a complication of anesthesia.

Causation

In order to win a malpractice suit, a patient also must prove *causation,* which is evidence that substandard care probably resulted in some injury.[18] As with the standard of care, most of the proof of causation comes by way of expert testimony after evaluation of the evidence, most often the anesthesia and resuscitation records. Therefore, it is important to record the absence of any significant problems during and after the application of anesthesia in order to avoid blame for complications caused by other factors beyond the control of the healthcare provider.

Conduct of others

Under the law, for a patient to recover damages malpractice need not be the sole cause of the injury but merely a substantial factor, even if there are other causes. Those other causes can be the negligence of other persons or entities. An example would be when a doctor is administering anesthesia, the patient stops breathing, 9-1-1 is called, and the EMT fails to properly intubate the patient who suffers toxic hypoxia. Two principles are applicable in this example. First, basic tort law holds that a negligent person is liable for all the consequences of that negligence, including exposure to the negligence of others.[19] In such cases, the patient need only bring a suit against the first healthcare provider. Second, the law in most states provides for apportionment of fault between negligent persons, even those that are not named defendants in a suit.[20]

Evidence and the nature of litigation

A lawsuit alleging anesthesia malpractice or substandard care primarily involves issues of fact, the plaintiff versus the defendant and staff recollections, interactions with other healthcare providers, and competing expert opinions. Litigation outcomes are most often determined by the credibility of witnesses. One measure of credibility is the presence or absence of supporting or contrary documentation and physical evidence. As a defense attorney, my recommendations for resolution of an anesthesia suit often are based upon the quality of the documentation, in addition to the conduct and testimony of the parties. In the final analysis, when there is polar testimony, the witness or the party with the best supporting documentation most often prevails in the test of credibility before a jury or judge.

Complications: risk or substandard care

A complication can be a risk of the application of anesthesia or the result of substandard care. It is generally accepted that when a patient experiences an unavoidable and unintended harm or injury during or after an application of anesthesia, whether it be short-term and moderate or catastrophic and permanent, he/she has experienced a complication. While there is no statute or code specifically stating when a complication is evidence of a risk versus evidence of substandard care, the following guidelines will offer a working model based upon this author's litigation experience.

A risk is a complication that can happen despite the application of reasonable skill, care, and technology. Skill is the operator's physical interactions with the patient, such as protecting the airway during the extraction of an impacted third molar. Care is the evaluation and management of the patient before, during, and after treatment. Technology is the instrumentation that provides for greater skill and care, such as a PO_2 monitor, or a precordial stethoscope. Thus, by contrast, if injury to a patient could have been avoided with the application of appropriate skill, care, or technology, then experts may opine that the occurrence of such a complication is evidence of substandard care. The contrary is that, if the complication could still have occurred despite the application of appropriate skill, care, and/or technology, its occurrence is not evidence of substandard care.

Classifications of complications

In the experience of this author, legal issues associated with complications of the application of anesthesia fall into four classifications:

1 Patient candidacy, selection, and preparation
2 Anesthesia selection, delivery, dose, and duration

3 Monitoring and evaluation before, during, and after application of anesthesia or
4 Resuscitation and staff/team response.

The majority of significant anesthesia claims involve either the need for or failure of resuscitation. The first three elements lead up or contribute to the need for resuscitation.

Patient candidacy, selection, and preparation

From a legal perspective, documentation of the process of evaluating a patient's candidacy for conscious sedation or general anesthesia is as important as the process itself. Cases involving candidacy issues have involved lack of documentation to support the ASA rating, inadequate health history documentation, failure to obtain medical clearance, or NPO status.

Merely checking an ASA rating box in the records without supporting documentation of the basis for such a determination can create issues of fact in the event of a complication. Issues of fact are determined by juries. The records should reflect knowledge of and specifics as to the elements that lead to the ASA rating. The health history form and consultation notes should detail and reflect an interactive process. The form should be signed and dated by the patient and/or guardian and then the doctor to confirm the interactive process. No exceptions should be allowed, not even for close friends and family members. In one case defended by this author, an oral surgeon performed orthognathic surgery on his wife. Because he "knew her," the ASA work-up and history documentation was scant at best. Following the surgery, for unrelated reasons, the surgeon and his wife separated, and then she filed for divorce, and malpractice. Allegations of lack of informed consent and inadequate evaluation were included in the malpractice claim. The testimonies of the parties were polar opposites. The wife claimed that they "never talked." The defendant surgeon chose to settle the malpractice claim due in part to the lack of documentation. Similar malpractice claims have been brought by family members of a referring general dentist, employees of the surgeon, or the spouse of a long-time friend of the defendant. The lesson is to have consistent documentation protocols for all patients, without exception. Also, it is recommended that the questions on health history forms provided to prospective patients be evaluated annually to be sure that they are up to date. When health history forms completed by patients are evaluated, notations should be made to reflect that the process occurred. Positive responses to questions should be circled or highlighted and any discussions about a positive response should be charted. For example, if a patient responds positively to a question about asthma, and upon further evaluation it is recommended that the patient use his/her inhaler just before induction of anesthesia, that advice and the patient's compliance or lack thereof should be noted. Failure to note that an evaluation took place because "evaluation would be our routine" creates an issue of fact in the event of a complication such as a laryngospasm. Because of anesthesia, a patient may not recall using the inhaler, and testify that he/she was not told to do so.

In some cases, depending on the information learned during the health history evaluation, obtaining medical clearance may be appropriate. Documenting medical clearance has become essential in this era of complex treatments for chronic and systemic diseases. In the event of a significant anesthesia complication such as hypoxia or death, the patient or his/her heirs can bring suit against all the healthcare providers involved in the case. The allegations can involve claims of lack of medical clearance on the part of the surgeon and, in some cases, inappropriate issuance of medical clearance on behalf of the patient's physician. The law allows alternative and contrasting theories to be alleged at the same time.[21] Such a tactic is designed to pit the defendants against each other. In a recent case, a 21-year old patient with a history of an immune disorder that can cause facial swelling in response to trauma was seen for removal of third molars by an oral surgeon. The surgeon knew of the condition and recalled that he was given clearance by the referring doctor, but he had no documented proof. Surgery was performed using IV anesthesia without immediate evidence of a complication. However, the patient experienced significant postoperative swelling and died 12 days later. The oral surgeon and referring doctor were sued. At trial, the defendant had no physical evidence to support the claim of having obtained medical clearance, and the referring doctor, also a defendant, denied giving any approval. The jury found against the surgeon, dismissed the referring doctor, and awarded over $11 million in damages to the patient's heirs. The claim could have been avoided had the surgeon insisted upon written medical clearance. That can be accomplished by either having the medical healthcare provider sign and return a letter approving the use of sedation/general anesthesia for the specific patient or, in the case of oral approval, sending a confirming letter by fax. In most states, if the doctor receiving a fax does not object to or contradict the confirming fax within two business days, the statements therein can be used as an admission of accuracy of the statements in the fax.[22] Appendix A is a sample form for a confirming fax. After a verbal discussion approving the use of anesthesia, a confirmation form should be filled out and sent by fax. Then, what is typically called a fax "activity report" should be printed to accompany it.[23] This report is generated by an automated feature on most modern fax machines. The activity report and the original letter should be put together in the chart where they serve as the proof that approval and clearance for ambulatory anesthesia was obtained.

Anesthesia selection, delivery, dose, and duration

The choice of anesthesia, methods of delivery, dose, and duration are typically not sources of claims unto themselves. However, following the occurrence of a significant complication, the anesthesia records may be examined carefully by attorneys or investigators of a licensing agency. Comparisons will be made between the ASA rating, body weight, vitals, surgery goals, and the nature of the anesthesia provided. The records should reflect that the type and dose of anesthesia was matched to the patient rather than delivered in a "one-size-fits-all" method. Also, if there are appropriate options for the level of anesthesia for the planned surgery, there should be documentation of discussing those options with the patient, the patient's selection, and his/her reasons. Further, because such discussions are considered part of the informed consent process, they should be acknowledged by the patient and documented. Otherwise, there is the risk that the patient will deny having been given options of different levels of anesthesia and being able to choose one with less potential for the type of complication the patient experienced. This is particularly true when the patient is either not fully compliant with pre-surgical instructions or a borderline candidate. For example, in one case defended by this author, a patient advised the surgeon that he was not fully NPO, because he had a meal about 4 hours before surgery. The doctor advised the patient of the risks. But, the patient said it was a very small meal, and he insisted it was ok to go ahead with IV anesthesia, rather than just local anesthesia, because he had set aside the time, had taken time off work, and had his wife there to give him a ride. Those discussions were poorly documented and not signed by the patient. During surgery and anesthesia, the patient vomited and aspirated. Significant airway spasms occurred, the patient could not be intubated easily, became hypoxic, and then acidic. The surgeon never recovered the airway, and the patient died. The doctor and the EMTs observed that the vomit appeared consistent with a large meal and one ingested much less than 4 hours before surgery. However, due to the lack of documentation as to the decision to proceed with surgery, the subsequent wrongful death suit brought by the heirs had to be settled with a significant payment.

Monitoring and evaluation before, during, and after application of anesthesia

ASA standards apply not only to patient selection but also to the monitoring of a patient during and after the application of anesthesia until discharge. Allegations of substandard care involving anesthesia monitoring typically have come from three areas: (1) maintenance and calibration of monitoring equipment; (2) staff/anesthesia team protocols and training; and (3) documentation of monitoring and evaluation.

Use of monitoring equipment that is not maintained and calibrated can be worse than not using it at all because of the potential for false readings. In one case, a minor patient on IV sedation experienced what appeared to be a drop in PO_2 and an ECG flatline. Movement of the leads showed some spikes in the ECG. The machine had a history of such problems. Therefore, the surgeon called for switching the ECG machine with one in another room. Upon starting up the other machine, the ECG was again flat. At that time, resuscitation was initiated and an EMT was called. The patient had moments of ECG activity during resuscitation, but was found by the Emergency Department (ED) team to be hypoxic and acidotic. Resuscitation was ultimately unsuccessful, and the patient died. During subsequent litigation for wrongful death brought by the child's parents, it was determined that the ECG equipment used was not subject to regular maintenance. Also, a precordial stethoscope had not been employed. The allegations were that with maintained and calibrated equipment, resuscitation would have begun sooner and would have had a greater chance of success.

In another case, there was no office procedure for recording the results of monitoring during resuscitation. Once the patient's status became an issue, all documentation stopped due to lack of protocols for recordkeeping during an emergency. Those notes had to be created well after the event. Because the doctor and one staff person went to the ED with the patient, some entries made the next day were guesses. The result was that chart notes with inconsistencies were compared to those created by the EMT and the ED. A wrongful death suit was filed and subsequently had to be settled for the maximum allowed under the laws of that state.

Resuscitation and staff/team response

It has been the experience of this author, and the report of colleagues that resuscitation and staff/team responses to complications of anesthesia are more determinative as to whether a complication results in litigation than any other aspect of anesthesia care. Generally, successful resuscitation and staff/team response to complications of anesthesia are seldom followed by litigation. The reasons are the same as the basic elements of malpractice litigation; i.e., negligent care must cause an injury before there can be an award of damages. While there may be some perception of injury because a patient experienced a successful resuscitation, most injuries are generally not serious enough to merit the time and expense of litigation.

Legal issues with resuscitation and staff/team response begin with early recognition of the onset of the complication and a timely response within the standard of care. Despite effective monitoring and evaluation of a patient during anesthesia, the surgeon and staff still must respond in an effective and timely manner. That requires training and experience. Experience comes from practice drills, and, perhaps most importantly, preparation for complications, even those that are uncommon or rare, but still known to occur.

In one case defended by this author, a 78-year-old male was seen for removal of impacted third molars under IV anesthesia. About halfway through surgery, his vitals began to drop and a laryngospasm was noted. Efforts were made at intubation. After three failed attempts, another doctor was called in to try another approach. Only then was 9-1-1 called. After the fifth try at intubation, some success was achieved. However, by that point, the patient was hypoxic and acidotic, as determined by the ED staff. Because of lack of meaningful ECG activity after 72 hours, life support was discontinued. A malpractice suit was filed by the surviving spouse. In litigation, it was learned that the surgeon did not have any formal written protocols for resuscitation and did not consider or attempt a cricothyroidotomy but, instead, made multiple attempts at intubation. Experts for the plaintiff stated that the surgeon stayed with the attempts at intubation too long, probably because of concerns about scarring and long-term effects of a cricothyroidotomy. The doctor did not make the decision to elevate the resuscitation efforts in the face of persistent low PO_2 readings.

Reactions to anesthesia drugs are not the only reason for complications. Airway blockage can create significant problems during surgery with conscious sedation and general anesthesia. In two recent pediatric cases, patients inhaled objects during treatment while under sedation. One case involved a 2x2-inch gauze, and the other a cotton roll. In both cases, the airway was completely blocked. Resuscitation efforts involved the use of cotton pliers or fingers to try to clear the blockages. In both cases, the attempts resulted in swelling and bleeding that frustrated subsequent resuscitation attempts. Both patients died. Suits were filed by the surviving parents and investigations opened by the respective licensing boards. Note that some states require dentists to report in writing any death or significant hospitalization associated with the application of conscious sedation or general anesthesia.[24] Experts for the plaintiffs in both cases opined that the doctor was not prepared for such a complication and did not have the appropriate equipment, such as McGill forceps, to retrieve the foreign objects, in addition to not having adequate protection of the airway in place. When the defense in each case attempted to attribute the complication to unexpected and inappropriate behavior by the patients who were children, the opposing experts stated that when patients are under the effects of sedation or general anesthesia, particularly children, the standard of care requires preparation for unexpected but known potential complications. Indeed, in response to such events, some states recently have mandated that dentists providing anesthesia must have training in airway blockage resuscitation and the use of McGill forceps.[25]

Even with training and preparation, staff protocols for documentation are essential, regardless of the resuscitation techniques employed. One case defended by this author is particularly illustrative of all of the foregoing. A five-year-old patient was seen for IV anesthesia in order to allow for significant dental treatment. During surgery, the airway closed down. 9-1-1 was called, and unsuccessful attempts were made at resuscitation. The patient died in the ED. Suit was filed by the surviving parents against the general dentist and the oral surgeon who provided the anesthesia. During the course of litigation, it was discovered that the surgeon did not have trained staff at the surgery, and, instead, utilized the staff of the general dentist. This is common in cases of itinerant surgeons providing surgery and/or anesthesia in the offices of general dentists. In this case, when the emergency was declared, the staff did not have any emergency/resuscitation forms or documentation protocols and, therefore, wrote notes of the event on the paper tray cover. Also, the surgeon had not completed the notes of the patient's preanesthesia evaluation, intending to do so right after surgery. After the EMT took the patient, the doctor and the chairside staff person went to the hospital. A remaining staff person cleaned up the operatory, discarding the written notes on the paper tray cover, which he/she assumed was trash. The next day when the doctor returned to the office to complete the notes, they had to be done from memory, including such information as the ASA rating, health history evaluation, doses, monitoring, and resuscitation response. Those notes were subsequently provided in the course of litigation and the licensing board investigation. However, unknown to the defendant doctor, when the EMT arrived, they requested a copy of the chart to take with them, much of which was incomplete. Therefore, there were two sets of records. The surgeon had guessed at the times and other aspects of the event, and the ones that were selected were in conflict with some of the times and observations recorded by 9-1-1 phone services and the EMT. Finally, a recorded transcript of an untrained staff person's 9-1-1 call, which was obtained in litigation, disclosed that when she was asked if the doctor had performed CPR on the patient, the staff person replied, "No." She did not know what CPR meant. The case was settled for the maximum allowed by the laws of that state.

Preparation for complications

Training for delivery of conscious sedation or general anesthesia typically includes recognition and response to emergent complications. Delay in recognition and resuscitation can result in claims of substandard care. Plan for and be ready for the unexpected. Then react promptly. It is better to have to explain the application of resuscitation that may not have been necessary than to have to explain a death or brain damage from an untimely or ineffective resuscitation.

Maintain and calibrate all monitoring and resuscitation equipment and keep logs of the completion of those tasks. See that staff is trained for resuscitation, including regular drills. Maintain up-to-date (reviewed annually) "crash cart" equipment, including medications (Discard and replace any that have expired.). Make the use of resuscitation equipment and drugs part of the drills (Use the expired medications for practice.). In one case evaluated by this author, during a resuscitation emergency, the doctor called for the start of D50W, which was stored on a shelf. An untrained staff person grabbed a bag off the shelf and started the drip. In the same area where the D50W bags were stored, other similar-looking bags were stored. The staff member grabbed the wrong bag and started the IV, and the surgeon did not verify the selection. The resuscitation was unsuccessful, and the patient died.

Have staff trained and drilled in recordkeeping during and after resuscitation. Also, do not hesitate to call 9-1-1. It is better to send an EMT home without a patient due to a successful resuscitation than to have the patient taken to the ED with a serious complication and unsuccessful resuscitation.

Conclusions

While complications from anesthesia may not always be preventable, experts have opined that the standard of care includes that the surgeon and staff to be trained for all known potential complications of anesthesia, be prepared for complications, respond in a timely manner, and apply appropriate resuscitation. Proving that the occurrence of a complication was the manifestation of a risk and not substandard care comes by way of well-planned and well-executed documentation before, during, and after the application of anesthesia, including resuscitation, where indicated. Having the knowledge and training to deal with complications is not adequate if the application is ineffective. To be effective, the doctor and staff/anesthesia team routinely should practice and video record (for team review and learning) mock emergencies and resuscitation. Finally, do not hesitate to react. This author has not seen a claim for unnecessary or successful resuscitation but has seen many suits for delayed, ineffective, and/or poorly documented cases that have resulted in profound or fatal complications.

Endnotes

1 Available at: http://www.medicalmalpractice.com/dental-malpractice.cfm Accessed April 8, 2011
2 Available at: http://www.dentalbeacon.org/para3.htm Accessed April 8, 2011
3 California Evidence Code Section 721
4 Available at: http://www.americanheart.org/presenter.jhtml?identifier53047051. Accessed April 8, 2011.
5 Available at: http://www.asahq.org/For-Healthcare-Professionals/Standards-Guidelines-and-Statements.aspx Accessed April 8, 2011
6 Available at: http://www.aaomsstore.com/p-65-aaomsparameters-of-care-clinical-practice-guidelines.aspx. Accessed April 8, 2011.
7 Available at: http://www.courts.michigan.gov/mcji/negligence-Ch10-19/negligence-ch12.htm Accessed April 8, 2011
8 Available at: http://www.dbc.ca.gov/lawsregs/index.shtml Accessed April 8, 2011
9 California Business and Professions Code, Sections 1646 – 1646.9 (2011)
10 California Code of Regulations, Section 1043.3(a) (2011)
11 California Code of Regulations, Section 1043.3(b) (2011)
12 California Code of Regulations, Section 1043.3(c) (2011)
13 California Business and Professions Code, Section 1682(e) (2011)
14 California Business and Professions Code, Section 1750.4-5 (2011)
15 California Business and Professions Code, Section 1680(z) (2011)
16 California Evidence Code Section 669 (2011)
17 Weiner v. Fleischman (1991) 54 Cal. 3d 476, 483 [286 Cal. Rptr. 40, 816 P.2d 892]
18 Viner v. Sweet (2003) 30 Cal. 4th 1232, 1239 – 1240 [135 Cal. Rptr. 2d, 629, 70 P.3d 1046]
19 Espinosa v. Little Company of Mary Hospital (1995) 31 Cal. App. 4th 1304 [37 Cal. Rptr. 2d 541]
20 Alaska Stat. Section 09.17.080 (2011)
21 Federal Rules of Civil Procedure, Section 8(d)(2)
22 California Evidence Code Section 250

23 Available at: http://www.tcnj.edu/˜helpdesk/documents/Canon%20eManuals/Canon%20Color%20eManual/iRADV_C5051_Manual_us/contents/adfunc_005cdk/func.html Accessed June 1, 2011

24 California Business and Professions Code Section 1680(z)

25 California Business and Professions Code Section 1016 (a)(C)(ii)(1–3)

Appendix A

[*Doctor's letterhead with telephone number*]

Date: __________________ **Fax No.** __________________

Dear Dr.____________________,

This fax will confirm our conversation of today wherein we discussed your patient and his/her

condition(s) of

and our proposed treatment of

[ ] with local anesthesia [ ] with epinephrine [ ] with [ ] without IV Sedation
scheduled for______________**. In response, you recommended the following:**

Thank you for your advice in this matter. Please immediately advise us before the next business day if this letter is not accurate or if the patient's condition should change significantly before our scheduled treatment/operation as noted above. Otherwise, we will proceed as noted and will assume the foregoing is a correct statement of your advice.

[Doctor's printed name and signature]

THE DOCUMENT BEING FAXED IS INTENDED ONLYFOR THE USE OF THE INDIVIDUAL OR ENTITY TO WHICH IT IS ADDRESSED, AND IT MAY CONTAIN INFORMATION THAT IS PRIVILEGED, CONFIDENTIAL, AND EXEMPT FROM DISCLOSURE UNDER APPLICABLE LAW.
IF THE READER OF THIS MESSAGE IS NOT THE INTENDED RECIPIENT, YOU ARE HEREBYNOTIFIED THAT ANY DISSEMINATION, DISTRIBUTION, OR COPYING OF THIS COMMUNICATION IS STRICTLY PROHIBITED. IF YOU HAVE RECEIVED THIS COMMUNICATION IN ERROR, PLEASE NOTIFY US IMMEDIATELY BY TELEPHONE, AND RETURN THE ORIGINAL MESSAGE AT THE ABOVE ADDRESS VIA THE UNITED STATES POSTAL SERVICE.

SECTION 10

When should you say no

45 When should you say no?

Andrew Herlich[1,2] and Robert C. Bosack[3]

[1] University of Pittsburgh School of Medicine, Department of Anesthesiology, Pittsburgh, PA, USA
[2] UPMC Mercy, Pittsburgh, PA, USA
[3] University of Illinois, College of Dentistry, Chicago, IL, USA

The goal of this final chapter is to identify and implement a decision-making process that ends in safe, patient-focused care in the dental office, where medical resources may be limited. The anatomical systems and disease processes that are likely to impact planning by the dental anesthesia provider are reviewed with clinical emphasis. Training, experience, and ability of both doctor and staff to perform as a team are also extremely relevant to the decision-making process. Cautionary steps are identified in terms of preparation of the patient, the practitioner, the staff, and the equipment to improve safety and patient comfort. The synthesis of these processes results in the delivery of appropriate anesthesia to the appropriate patient in the appropriate location.

Refusing to provide treatment (anesthesia) is a difficult decision-making process. The obvious cases for refusal are easy to identify: morbid obesity with obstructive sleep apnea (OSA) and decompensated heart failure. The not-so-easy cases to identify and refuse might be a combination of mild obesity and limitation of mouth opening, with a blood pressure of 175/105 mmHg and a PVC burden of 12 per minute. Decisions should not be made solely on patient factors, but should also include planned depth of anesthesia and back-up emergency plans, particularly as they relate to airway management. Indeed, the "cannot ventilate, cannot intubate" predicament can be largely dependent on the skill of the practitioner. Arbitrary depth of anesthesia limit setting may not mitigate airway risk.

When you should say no

The frequency of anesthesia refusal or case refusal is rare. However, these instances are firm and obvious.

1. No informed consent with *written confirmation of the process.* Informed consent is the process of informing the patient of the reasonable risks and benefits of the procedure; the paperwork is the written confirmation of the process.
2. No regulatory authority or licensure. An example of such is a situation in which the practitioner does not have a permit to administer sedation or general anesthesia in the office. Another example of this situation is the lack of transfer of care agreement with the closest hospital if an untoward event requires such a transfer.
3. A complex patient disease or problem of which the practitioner has no knowledge or understanding of the possible consequences of treatment. An example is a patient with a incompletely repaired congenital heart defect, where the practitioner has not received a thorough consultation from the cardiologist regarding the ability of the patient to withstand the possible stressors of planned surgery or anesthesia. Even a free-standing surgicenter may not be sufficiently prepared to handle these complex patients.
4. A patient with a medical comorbidity that is not optimally managed from an acute or chronic care perspective. Examples of such comorbidities are uncompensated congestive heart failure, poorly treated hypertension, a stroke or MI in the past 30 days, or untreated OSA. Patients with end-stage diseases of the liver, neurological, cardiovascular, or pulmonary systems are not appropriate candidates for office-based procedures.
5. A practitioner or the staff does not have any experience in treating the disease process or the equipment to manage the procedure.

Ahmad (2010) outlined several other clinical situations that were considered to significantly increase risk when a procedure was performed in the office-based environment. These situations include severe neuromuscular disorders such as athetoid disease, myopathic diseases (muscular dystrophy, MD), uncontrolled hypertension, unstable angina, the presence of an AICD, coagulopathic diseases, severe OSA, morbid obesity, recent stroke, or severe hepatobiliary disease.

The safety of office-based anesthesia

Office-based anesthesia has a relatively high level of safety. However, the data supporting this statement may not be completely accurate. Information may be based on voluntary reporting, which often reflects less morbidity than would mandatory reporting. Furthermore, data may reflect treatment completed at locations other than the office, that is, hospitals or free-standing surgery centers. If the data is derived from mandatory reporting data banks, the data is likely to be unbiased; if the data is interpreted by the authors, bias can occur.

Bhanaker et al. (2006), Robbertze (2006), and Metzner et al. (2009) have summarized closed claim reports (litigated and settled). Adverse events that may have been reported to state regulatory agencies but did not result in a malpractice and closed claim were not available. The data and conclusions from these reports are similar; "monitored anesthesia care" in locations outside of the operating room typically involved older and sicker patients. The most frequent adverse event was inadequate ventilation and oxygenation, because of an absolute or relative overdose of anesthetic medication, coupled with suboptimal monitoring and vigilance.

Anesthesia Complications in the Dental Office, First Edition. Edited by Robert C. Bosack and Stuart Lieblich.

Airway risk becomes the most significant anesthetic complication in the dental office. It is discussed in detail in Chapters 2 and 33.

Vila et al. (2003) reviewed data reported to the Florida Board of Medicine during a 2-year period. A 10-fold increased risk of adverse events was noted when procedures were performed in an office setting, as compared to ambulatory surgery facilities. In most instances, an anesthesiologist was not present and a significant number of facilities were not accredited. A high proportion of the adverse outcomes involved cosmetic surgery. These outcomes may not be comparable to the oral and maxillofacial surgery office, where practitioners have received significant anesthesiology training, as compared with non-anesthesiologist physicians. Reports by Perrott et al. (2003) and D'Eramo et al. (2008) included voluntary reporting or reporting with satisfaction data that alters the precision of the data. Although patient satisfaction is an important measure, it is not necessarily a factor in patient safety.

Although reports of pediatric morbidity and mortality are sparse, rare adverse events in the office-based setting are often catastrophic and quickly become fodder for the lay press. Cote (2000a,b) and van der Griend (2011) have published meaningful data.

Current reports suggest that 1/3 of all contributing factors to successful malpractice claims could have been prevented by a surgical checklist (de Vries et al., 2011). Other adverse events included preventable medication errors. The use of a surgical safety checklist such as the WHO checklist that identifies issues of correct organ (tooth) and laterality (left vs. right) among other important issues PRIOR to proceeding with sedation, analgesia, and surgery would drastically reduce these adverse events (de Vries, 2010). The checklist has not been studied in the office-based environment; there are few doubts that it would save a wrong tooth or wrong side surgery (de Vries et al., 2008).

Preparation of the anesthesia team

Medical error is ubiquitous and inevitable. High fidelity simulation and team training must be supplemented with in situ simulation, mental practice, and hybrid simulation to promote shared mental models of teamwork and task accomplishment (Petrosoniak and Hicks, 2013; Ostergaard et al., 2011). Crisis resource management is the ability to translate knowing what to do into effective task performance during an emergency. CRM intends to optimize and utilize all available resources. It becomes an effective process to mitigate the inherent risk of dental anesthesia.

Key points of crisis resource management

- Before the emergency
  - Anticipate and plan.
  - Frequent rehearsal.
  - Establish role clarity – pre-assigned role assignments.
  - Know the environment – equipment location, monitors, drugs, etc.
  - Create cognitive aids.
- During the emergency
  - Call for help early.
  - Mobilize all resources.
  - Use all available information.
  - Set priorities dynamically – "assess – diagnose – treat" looping.
  - Use cognitive aids.
  - Communicate effectively – closed loop.
  - Distribute the workload.
  - Exercise leadership, allocate attention wisely.
  - Identify and compensate for human flaws.

Preoperative preparation and testing

Preoperative preparation in the medically complex patient should consist of a direct communication between the primary care physician and the dental professional. It is preferable to obtain a statement in writing, declaring that the patient is in the *best possible condition* considering the patient's baseline disease. If the patient is not optimal, then every attempt should be made to optimize the patient prior to performing elective oral and maxillofacial surgery.

Chung et al. (2009) reported no difference in the frequency of adverse events for ASA I/II based on the presence or lack of preoperative testing. Any laboratory testing or physiological testing should be performed based upon surgical need only. This would include fasting blood sugar for diabetic patients (especially if NPO), INR, and platelets and WBC count for patients receiving treatment affecting these values and counts. For instance, routine hemoglobin and hematocrit in a large study of outpatient procedures found that 75 of 9584 ASA I/II patients had a measurable hemoglobin of less than 9 grams. Only four of those needed to be transfused prior to the elective procedure. None of the 75 patients had an adverse outcome. The anemia evaluation safely took place after the elective surgical procedure (Olson et al., 2005). Patients with hemoglobin >6 g/dl should be able to tolerate a well-conducted anesthetic in the absence of other comorbidity (Practice guidelines, 2006).

Organ systems and anesthesia risk

Eating disorders

Eating disorders are prevalent worldwide with clinical presentations ranging from morbid obesity to emaciation. Although BMI (kg/m^2) values are often dismissed as inaccurate and not completely indicative of the health of the patient, they do serve as a reference guideline to aid in patient evaluation.

Important risk factors associated with obesity that are most relevant in office-based anesthesia include drug accumulation in ubiquitous fat stores, increased risk of airway obstruction, and decrease in the functional residual capacity ("oxygen gas tank") because of upward pressure on the thoracic cage by the enlarged abdomen, aggravated by supine posturing. Given the fact that adipose tissue is metabolically active, these changes decrease the time from apnea to oxygen desaturation. Stated another way, obese patients have a smaller oxygen "gas tank," which is more difficult to fill and quicker to empty." Other common comorbidities include cardiovascular disease and diabetes, among others. In addition, patients with obesity tend to always be on some type of diet, with or without prescribed or over-the-counter medication. Special positioning may be necessary to maintain an open airway during sedation (see Figure 45.1). Intravenous access may be difficult and is often abandoned after three unsuccessful attempts. A technique to promote visual prominence of veins includes the temporary occlusion of the upper arm with a blood pressure cuff pumped and maintained below systolic pressure and above diastolic pressure during repeated grasping of a tennis ball to provide resistance to otherwise effortless hand pumping (Figure 45.2). It is safer to titrate all sedative drugs based on lean body weight (with the exception of succinylcholine, which is dosed on total body weight) (Ingrande and Lemmens, 2010). Local anesthesia should be a mainstay of the anesthetic regimen for patients with obesity: if necessary, supplemental sedation should be a secondary process and used judiciously. Intravenous acetaminophen can be useful in patients where the respiratory depression of opiates is not tolerated,

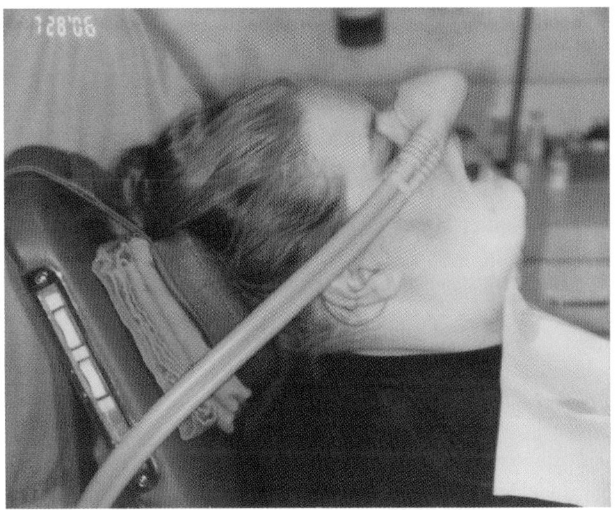

Figure 45.1 Special positioning to maintain the airway in patients with obesity.

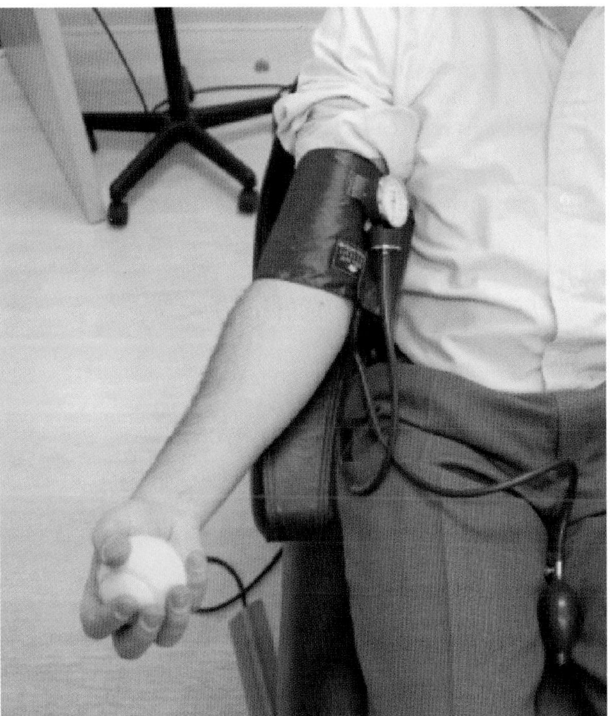

Figure 45.2 A method to improve venous prominence prior to venipuncture.

ketorolac is contraindicated, or opiates result in severe nausea and vomiting (Jahr and Lee, 2010).

Any history of anorexia or bulimia, whether in the recent or distant past, should trigger a heightened awareness of their propensity for anesthetic adversity, as permanent cures remain elusive. Denial is near universal, as these "failures of will" are associated with shame and embarrassment. Mere suspicion is often sufficient for diagnosis. Thorough preoperative evaluation should address anesthetic concerns of blunted autonomic responses (bradycardia and hypotension), exaggerated drug response (hypovolemia, decreased plasma proteins and fat and muscle compartments), and electrolyte disturbances, which are often severe and may cause cardiac dysrhythmias that may be life threatening (Suri et al., 1999).

Psychiatric illness

Psychiatric illness is among the most common of all human afflictions. Anesthesia risk for office-based procedures includes the level of management of the disease and complications of psychotropic medical therapy, including overdose, withdrawal, or adverse drug interaction. Drug toxicity may not be evident until the patient becomes hemodynamically challenged during the neuroendocrine stress response and/or administration of sedative/hypnotic drugs. Poorly controlled psychiatric illness may pose a significant challenge to patient cooperation during or after anesthesia. Hypotension, tachydysrhythmias, and excessive sedation are distinct possibilities during anesthesia for patients taking psychotropic agents. Special caution is required for patients taking monoamine oxidase inhibitors, with adverse drug interaction possible with meperidine or indirect-acting amines, such as ephedrine. All psychotropic agents should be continued in the perioperative period.

Substance abuse has become common place and denial is near universal. Again, suspicion clinches diagnosis, and refusal to treat must occasionally be based on "gut feelings." There is no way to determine what drugs are actually being ingested.

Cardiovascular diseases

Cardiac disease should be optimized whenever possible prior to elective dental procedures with or without office sedation. Evaluation and risk modification is best guided by the latest recommendations from the American College of Cardiology/American Heart Association Task Force on Practice Guidelines (Fleisher et al., 2007). Patients who should undergo evaluation prior to dental treatment include those with unstable coronary syndromes, decompensated heart failure with symptoms at rest, severe valvular diseases, or hemodynamically significant dysrhythmias.

Recent angioplasty with stent placement requires dual antiplatelet therapy (aspirin and clopidogrel (Paxil®)) for 6 weeks after insertion of bare metal stents and 12 months after insertion of drug-eluting stents in order to avoid life-threatening re-thrombosis. Elective surgery should be delayed until patients have completed the recommended course of treatment. Abrupt discontinuation of these agents has been associated with a rebound prothrombotic state (Newsome et al., 2008). The perioperative management of patients that take long-term continuous antiplatelet therapy is based on the relative risks of bleeding and thrombosis. Literature is silent regarding the thrombotic risk of routine tooth extraction in patients where antiplatelet therapy is continued; consultation is advisable (van Kuijk et al., 2009). If the surgery is emergent, then halting the clopidogrel should be chosen and aspirin continued. Clopidogrel should be reinstituted immediately after surgery or as soon as possible from a safe surgical perspective. When the risks of perioperative hemorrhage exceed the benefits of thrombosis prevention, consideration to discontinue or alter anticoagulation therapy, or modify therapy can be entertained in consultation with the appropriate physician (Hall and Maxer, 2011).

Special precautions should be taken if electrocautery is necessary for patients with a pacemaker or AICD. In these instances, consultation is mandatory regarding possible device reprogramming or the use of a magnet to "blind" the device to external interference. During the period of AICD suspension, an external pacer must be applied to the patient. Consequently, these patients are not suitable candidates for office-based surgery because the required resources are not readily available. One may proceed with caution with the caveats of judicious local anesthesia/sedation and limited surgery (ASA 2011).

A patient with an unstable TIA or recent stroke should be treated in a similar manner as a patient with instable angina or one with a recent MI. Patients with uncontrolled atrial fibrillation, renal disease, or recent stroke are at risk for an acute perioperative stroke. These patients should not be treated in the office or any other facility for that matter until their neurovascular status has been stabilized (Mashour et al., 2011).

Endocrine diseases

Several endocrinopathies require special attention. The patient with uncontrolled hyperthyroidism should never be anesthetized until thyroid function is controlled. Most anesthesiologists agree that unless the surgery is life saving and outweighs the risks of perioperative thyroid storm, surgery must be postponed. Obviously, these patients are unsuitable candidates for office-based or ambulatory surgery center procedures (Kohl and Schwartz, 2010).

Diabetic patients, whose diseases are optimized and stable are often safely managed in the office setting. Fasting blood sugars should be measured prior to anesthesia in patients who have been NPO, with a desirable range between 80 and 200 mg/dl. Levels greater than 200 mg/dl lead to urinary glucose spilling, with possible dehydration and acidosis. Levels less than 60 mg/dl invite autonomic instability. Oral agents and non-insulin injectable medications can be omitted on the day of surgery for most patients. Consultation regarding the management of insulin therapy improves patient management (Joshi et al., 2010). Hemoglobin A1c values often predict the presence and severity of comorbid cardiovascular disease.

The use of exogenous steroids is the subject of much scrutiny. The most common usage by oral and maxillofacial surgeons is for the reduction of postoperative nausea and vomiting as well as surgical edema. RARELY, is it required for adrenal insufficiency. A patient who has adrenal insufficiency is not a candidate for office-based surgical procedures at any time unless the patient is stabilized.

Respiratory considerations

The evaluation of pulmonary risk for office sedation considers the likelihood of airway irritation, laryngospasm, and exacerbation of bronchospastic diseases. Recent upper respiratory tract infections, especially in pediatric and asthmatic patients, can be problematic. The use of opioids blunts the ventilatory response to hypercarbia, causing hypoxemia.

Cigarette smoking is not a contraindication to office-based surgery; however, the benefits of smoking cessation are numerous, including reduction in carbon monoxide levels (which falsely elevate SpO_2), reduction of nicotine-induced sympathetic stimulation, and reduction of direct airway irritation by smoke pollutants (Kuri et al., 2005).

Control of asthma is a requisite for elective procedures, especially if airway manipulation is planned. The definition of controlled asthma is less than two rescue albuterol nebulizers per week, no emergency room visits, and no more than one systemic steroid course on an annualized basis as well as no daytime or nighttime attacks (National Heart, Lung, Blood Institute, 2007).

If general anesthesia is required at any point in the patient treatment plan, inhaled and/or intravenous preoperative steroids and bronchodilators reduce the rate of postoperative pulmonary problems (Tirumalasetty and Grammer, 2006). Parenteral anesthetic agents that are less likely to produce bronchospasm are propofol, ketamine, fentanyl, and midazolam. Histaminergic agents include morphine, methohexital, and succinylcholine, which should be avoided in asthmatic patients. If feasible, airway manipulation should be avoided in patients with asthma. If airway manipulation is necessary, it should be done under deep anesthesia. As mentioned previously, optimal control of asthma should be achieved prior to elective anesthesia or surgery.

Patients with diagnosed or suspected obstructive sleep present with multiple risk factors, including a host of comorbid diseases (dysrhythmias, cardiovascular disease, obesity, and gastroesophageal reflux disease, among others). As OSA is underdiagnosed, suspicion should clinch diagnosis, and airway compromise, either during or after office-based anesthesia, is both possible and frequent, especially when opioids are used.

Neurologic diseases

Patients with debilitating neurological conditions may not be suitable candidates for office-based anesthetics and procedures. End-stage multiple sclerosis (MS), MD, difficult-to-control epilepsy, advanced Parkinson's disease or patients with any dystonia are examples of such poor candidates. Parkinsonian and end-stage MS patients frequently have problems with positioning, spasticity, ability to control secretions, and expressive cognitive function. They may be more prone to hypotension from parenteral anesthetic agents. Antispasticity medication, such as baclofen, must be continued through the perioperative period to avoid seizures, hyperthermia, and hypertension, which can result from abrupt withdrawal. The patient with Duchenne's and Becker's MD have sensitivity to succinylcholine and inhaled volatile anesthetics that mimic malignant hyperthermia reactions. These patients are NOT MH positive but their reaction to triggering agents mimics MH (Gurnaney et al., 2009).

Pediatric patients

Preoperative evaluation of the pediatric patient should include chronic illnesses, current and frequent URI, asthma, significant heart murmur, activity restrictions, NPO status, and consent issues. Adolescent females who are or have been pregnant are generally considered emancipated minors. Consequently, in most jurisdictions, they may give their own consent. However, the prudent clinician will check with each state's laws to determine the validity of the emancipated minor. All institutionalized patients must have clear direction of health guardianship prior to proceeding. Under no circumstances should one proceed until consent is obtained.

A child with the "runny nose" presents the dilemma to the clinician of when is it safe to proceed. Irrespective of systemic implications of the "runny nose," it is clear that these children are at an increased risk for airway problems irrespective of the process being acute, chronic, or environmental. A recent comprehensive study characterized when there is increased risk for pediatric patients. Included in the increased risk were the following issues: inhalation induction, intravenous maintenance, uncuffed endotracheal tube, and airway management performed by a non-pediatric anesthesiologist (von Ungem-Stemberg et al., 2010). The temptation for the "snatch and grab" in the child with a URI with "just a little nitrous" has the potential risk of perioperative pulmonary complications including laryngospasm and bronchospasm.

Children with untreated or unresolved OSA are not suitable candidates for office-based procedures. Children with airway

Box 45.1 Take home points

1 Sedation/anesthesia in the dental office is elective. There is no reason to be aggressive with patient selection or technique.
2 Choice of location is important.
3 The decision to defer "sick" patients is easy. Risk assessment for borderline "judgment" cases may not be as easy.
4 There are patients that are unsuitable for office-based anesthesia.
5 Getting away with aggressive choices does not infer safety or suitability.
6 Training, simulation, and frequent rehearsal will improve patient care.

anomalies, and complex cardiac anomalies with OR without surgical correction are also unsuitable candidates for office-based procedures that require sedation. Despite surgical correction of the cardiac lesion, the pathophysiology may persist.

Children with heart murmurs should be characterized prior to any sedation. Innocent murmurs are generally asymptomatic, soft, early systolic, and disappear with positioning. However, despite these generalities, pediatricians frequently refer these murmurs for echocardiographic confirmation (Danford et al., 2002).

Geriatric patients

The elderly patient is not necessarily at risk by age alone although there may be hidden problems that create uncertainty. The elderly are more at risk by disease processes and comorbidities than the younger patient (Pasternak, 2007). Judicious dosing is mandatory because of increased drug sensitivity, pronounced hemodynamic effects, reduced clearance, and increased volume of distribution, especially in patients older than 70 years (Lortat-Jacob and Servin, 2007).

Postoperative delirium and cognitive dysfunction increases with age. Use of drugs that may increase the possibility of delirium and dysfunction such as midazolam should be carefully considered prior to administration. It is clear that postoperative delirium and cognitive dysfunction increase the early risk for postoperative morbidity and mortality (Monk et al. 2008). Consideration should be made to minimizing long treatment times in favor of shorter, less stressful, times. Less sedation and anesthesia may lessen the frequency and severity of postoperative delirium and cognitive dysfunction.

In summary, careful planning and preparation of staff, equipment, and most importantly the patient will reduce unfavorable outcomes. Understanding each patient's limit of tolerance will help the clinician decide if the "not ever" is just "not today." Not ever is a wise decision when the risks of proceeding outweigh the benefits of waiting (Box 45.1).

References

Ahmad, S. Office-based anesthesia: is my anesthetic care any different? assessment and management. *Anesthesiol Clin* **28**: 369–384, 2010.

American Society of Anesthesiologists. Practice advisory for the perioperative management of patients with cardiac implantable electronic devices: pacemakers and implantable cardioverter-defibrillators. an update report by the American Society of Anesthesiologists Task Force on perioperative management of patients with cardiac implantable electronic devices. *Anesthesiol* **114**: 247–261, 2011.

Bhanaker, S. M., et al. Injury and liability associated with monitored anesthesia care: a closed claims analysis. *Anesthesiol* **104**: 228–234, 2006.

Chung, F., et al. Elimination of preoperative testing in ambulatory surgery. *Anesth Analg* **108**: 467–475, 2009.

Cote, C., et al. Adverse sedation events in pediatrics: a critical incident analysis of contributing factors. *Pediatr* **105**: 805–814, 2000a.

Cote, C., et al. Adverse sedation events in pediatrics: analysis of medications used for sedation. *Pediatr* **106**: 633–644, 2000b.

Danford, D. A., et al. Echocardiographic yield in children when innocent murmur seems likely but doubts linger. *Pediatr Cardiol* **23**: 410–414, 2002.

D'Eramo, E. M., et al. Anesthesia morbidity and mortality experience among massachusetts oral and maxillofacial surgeons. *J Oral Maxillofac Surg* **66**: 2421–2433, 2008.

de Vries, E. N., et al. WHO's checklist for surgery: don't confine it to the operating room. Letter to the editor. *Lancet* **372**: 1148–1149, 2008.

de Vries, E. N. Effect of a comprehensive surgical safety system on patient outcomes. *N Engl J Med* **363**: 1928–1937, 2010.

de Vries, E. N., et al. Prevention of surgical malpractice by use of a surgical safety checklist. *Ann Surg* **253**: 624–628, 2011.

Fleisher, L. A., et al. ACC/AHA 2007 Guidelines on perioperative cardiovascular evaluation and care for noncardiac surgery: executive summary: a report on the American College of Cardiology/American Heart Association Task Force on practice guidelines (Writing Committee to revise the 2002 guidelines on perioperative cardiovascular evaluation for noncardiac surgery) *Circ* **116**: 1971–1996, 2007.

Gurnaney, H., et al. Malignant hyperthermia and muscular dystrophies. *Anesth Analg* **109**: 1043–1048, 2009.

Hall, R. and Maxer, C. D. Antiplatelet drugs: a review of their pharmacology and management in the perioperative period. *Anesth Analg* **112**: 292–318, 2011.

Ingrande, J. and Lemmens, H. J. M. Dose adjustment of anaesthetics in the morbidly obese. *Brit J Anaesthesia* **105**: i16–i23, 2010.

Jahr, J. S. and Lee, V. K. Intravenous acetaminophen. *Anesthesiol Clin* **28**: 619–645, 2010.

Joshi, G. P., et al. Society for ambulatory anesthesia consensus statement on perioperative blood glucose management in diabetic patients undergoing ambulatory surgery. *Anesth Analg* **111**: 1378–1387, 2010.

Kohl, B. A. and Schwartz, S. How to manage perioperative insufficiency. *Anesthesiol Clin* **28**: 139–155, 2010.

Kuri, M., et al. Determination of the duration of preoperative smoking cessation to improve wound healing after head and neck surgery. *Anesthesiol* **102**: 892–896, 2005).

Lortat-Jacob, B. and Servin, F. Pharmacology of intravenous drugs in the elderly. In: Sieber, F., ed. *Geriatric Anesthesia*, New York: McGraw-Hill, 2007, pp 91–103.

Mashour, G. A., et al. Perioperative stroke and associated mortality after noncardiac surgery. *Anesthesiol* **114**: 1289–1296, 2011.

Metzner, J., et al. The risk and safety of anesthesia at remote locations: the US closed claim experience. *Curr Opin Anesthesiol* **22**: 502–508, 2009.

Monk, T. G., et al. Predictors of cognitive dysfunction after major noncardiac surgery. *Anesthesiol* **108**: 18–30, 2008.

National Heart, Lung, Blood Institute, National Asthma Education and Prevention Program, Expert Panel 3: guidelines for the diagnosis and management of Asthma, (2007) http://www.nhlbi.nih.gov/guidelines/asthma/asth.gdln.pdf (Accessed August 18, 2011).

Newsome, L., et al. Coronary Artery Stents: II. Perioperative Considerations and Management. *Anesth Analg* **107**: 570–590. 2008.

Olson, R. P., et al. The prevalence and significance of low hemoglobin in ASA 1 or 2 outpatient surgery candidates. *Anesth Analg* **101**: 1337–1340, 2005.

Ostergaard, D., et al. Simulation and CRM. *Best Prac Res Clin Anesthesiol* **25**: 239–249, 2011.

Pasternak, L. R. Preoperative screening for outpatient surgery in geriatric patients. In: Sieber, F., ed. *Geriatric Anesthesia*. New York: McGraw-Hill, 2007, pp. 173–179.

Perrott, D. H., et al. Office-based ambulatory anesthesia: outcomes of clinical practice of oral and maxillofacial surgeons. *J Oral Maxillofac Surg* **61**: 983–995, 2003.

Petrosoniak, A. and Hicks, C. M. Beyond crisis resource management: New frontiers in human factors training for acute care medicine. *Curr Opin Anesthesiol* **26**: 699–706, 2013.

Practice Guidelines. Perioperative blood transfusion and adjuvant therapies. an updated report by the American Society of Anesthesiologists Task Force on perioperative blood transfusion and adjuvant therapies. *Anesthesiol* **105**: 198–208, 2006.

Robbertze, R. Closed claims review of anesthesia for procedures outside the operating room. *Curr Opin Anesthesiol* **19**: 436–442, 2006.

Suri, P., et al. Unrecognized bulimia nervosa: a potential cause of perioperative cardiac dysrhythmias. *Can J Anaesth* **46**: 1048–1052, 1999.

Tirumalasetty, J. and Grammer, L. C. Asthma, surgery, and general anesthesia: a review. *J. Asth* **43**: 251–254, 2006.
van der Griend, B. F., et al. Postoperative mortality in children after 101,885 anesthetics at a tertiary pediatric hospital. *Anesth Analg* **112**: 1440–1447, 2011.
Vila, H., et al. Comparative outcomes analysis of procedures performed in physicians offices and ambulatory surgery centers. *Arch Surg* **138**: 991–995, 2003.
van Kuijk, J., et al. Timing of noncardiac surgery after coronary artery stenting with bare metal or drug-eluting stents. *Am J Cardiol* **104**: 1229–1234, 2009.
von Ungem-Stemberg, B. S., et al. Risk assessment for respiratory complications in paediatric anaesthesia: a prospective cohort study. *Lancet* **376**: 773–783, 2010.

SECTION 11

Appendices

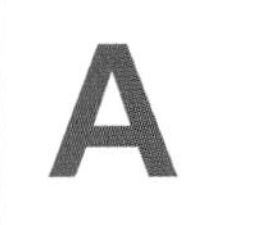

A pilot's perspective on crisis resource management

David Yock
Southwest Airlines Dallas, TX, USA

Although flying an airplane and administering anesthesia seem to be on different ends of the spectrum, I want to assure you they are much closer, or should be much closer, than you think. A long history of increasing technology and advancement along with unnecessary death and destruction have shaped the airline industry. As aircraft speeds increased, the air traffic system became more and more advanced, and the amount of aircraft in the skies increased. While this was good economically, the stresses and struggles of an airline pilot increased substantially, which paved the way to increased accidents. In addition to these issues, pilots were idolized because they were considered to have a very prestigious job of adventure, excitement, and respect. With this prestige came a public perception of infallibility as well. This perception helped feed the ego of an airline pilot. This added to what could have been the demise of the airline industry.

Airline cockpits usually had three pilots: a captain, a first officer, and a second officer. Each pilot had his/her specific duties but the captain was the boss. Many airline pilots were military trained and with that training came regimented and unwavering response to hierarchy. Prestige, respect, unquestioned command, and irreproachability unfortunately enhanced already inflated egos, engendering a "Sky God" mentality, which lead to many problems in the cockpit. Aircraft accidents increased as did cockpit errors. Aircraft were crashing not because they pilots did not know how to fly the aircraft, but simply because they did not know how to work together as a team. Most pilots did not want to question the captain because doing so could have been met with career-ending consequences.

By 1979, the airline community wanted to change the way pilots were operating. NASA put together a workshop with the hope of improving aviation safety. They collected information by using flight recorders and voice recorders. We call these the "black boxes," which are installed in airliners and are used to record flight inputs to the aircraft controls, noise, and voices during a flight. With the information collected, they immediately determined two things. First, that 70% of accidents had little to do with actually flying the aircraft and second, that crews were having problems *responding appropriately to each other*. They also determined that there was *uneven workload* among the pilots that caused *high stress* and *loss of situational awareness*. Cockpit Resource Management was created, where interpersonal skills were developed and taught in classrooms and simulator environments.

NASA sponsored a second workshop in 1986. They knew aviation was getting better but also knew they could improve substantially by expanding on a few things. They realized that the initial workshop focused on issues in the cockpit but found they could better solve problems in the cockpit by actually using all available resources outside the cockpit as well. Safety and efficiency was promoted and the CRM became Crew Resource Management. This form of CRM is what is in use today.

CRM, whether it be in aviation or medicine, seeks to minimize unpredictable and inevitable human error and its consequences. Rapidly changing, high stakes situations invite stress and foster time urgency, with deleterious effects on judgment and performance. CRM helps reduce errors by detecting the errors early in the error chain to allow corrective action to improve outcomes.

Teamwork is primary to good CRM. The airline team consists of the captain, first officer, and flight attendants in the aircraft and maintenance crew, ground crew, dispatch, and air traffic control outside the aircraft. Each team member or crew member has a part to play and is cross-trained and usable should a bad situation arise. It is imperative that each member be respected by all crewmembers and each member understands his/her role before deleterious situations arise. The captain remains the leader of the crew but, unlike the cockpits of the past, encourages open communication among crew members.

Standardization, risk management, decision making, and situational awareness are all major parts of CRM. Correlating these parts is essential to gaining a greater understanding of what CRM is and how to put it to use. Standardization is essentially having all team members on the same page. Each member is clearly aware of the standard operating procedure (SOP) or the method of accomplishing a task and his/her part in accomplishing that task. SOPs create predictability because procedures are done the same way every time. SOPs require regular training and understanding that if one team member chooses to deviate from them, mention should be made to another team member immediately. Standardization, as you can now see, opens the lines of communication and keeps every team member on the same page. A great benefit to good SOPs is the fact that team members can be changed with no effect on the operation. For example, when pilots are switched in the cockpit, it makes no difference if these pilots have flown together before or if they have never met before. These pilots will operate their aircraft the same way as the next pilot because they are "standardized." They know their jobs the same way as any other pilot with the same position using the same SOPs.

Anesthesia Complications in the Dental Office, First Edition. Edited by Robert C. Bosack and Stuart Lieblich.

Table A.1 Aviation acronyms.

"IMSAFE"
*I*llness
*M*edication
*S*tress
*A*lcohol
*F*atigue
*E*xperience
"DECIDE"
*D*etect that a decision needs to be made
*E*valuate all options
*C*hoose best option
*I*mplement your choice
*D*etect that your choice has a result
*E*valuate the result

Understanding risk factors is also a great way to help improve CRM. It is important to realize that every human action involves risk. Risk is cumulative and may create a "snowball effect" if the risk is not kept under control. Because of this, a team member needs to create personal limits and be aware of what those limits are at all times. To help mitigate risk, proper equipment must be used for a task and a proper team must be used. In aviation, the acronym IMSAFE (see Table A.1) is a personal guideline to optimize human performance to reduce risk by reducing the possibility of error. Very simply put, do not try to work while you are sick. Illness, stress, fatigue, and alcohol lead to performance decrement. Medication (prescribed or illicit) can impair judgment. Proper rest prior to a procedure is essential to keeping one's mind alert and being able to make good decisions. Finally, experience is necessary to keep risk down. Continuing education and forethought can keep a bad situation from ever arising. By linking risk factors and becoming the risk manager, you only continue to increase safety in your operation. We must remember to not sacrifice safety for selfish goals. These goals include anything that rushes a procedure or takes a short cut to rush instead of focusing on the task at hand and giving 100% each and every time.

Differing personalities and attitudes also affect the dynamic decision-making process. The acronym "decide" (Table A.1) is very important to recognize in regard to CRM. This acronym identifies proper decision-making skills.

Hazardous attitudes can adversely affect productive team functioning. Identifying a team member with one or more of these attitudes may be cause for elimination from that team due to the negative potentials that may be imposed. An anti-authority attitude is one that refuses to listen to anyone, the "don't tell me" attitude. An impulsive attitude is one where the team member refuses to consider options, procedures, or policies. They want to "do it now." The invulnerability attitude is one where the team member feels invincible, the "it won't happen to me" attitude. The macho attitude is one where the team member thinks "I can do it anything." The possibilities pique with the resignation or "why bother" attitude.

The final main part of CRM is the ability to maintain situational awareness – awareness of self, of other team members, and of the aircraft. SA is fundamental to proper decision-making by understanding what you perceive. Without SA, task performance is blind. We need to have an open mind, be able to take criticism, and be well aware of our surroundings. Situational awareness can be hampered in many ways. At all times, members need to keep their heads in the game and be aware that other team members are also in the game.

Situations that interfere with situational awareness

- Departure from standard operating procedures
- Nobody functions as team leader
- Communication breakdown
- Ambiguity among team members
- Unresolved discrepancies
- Preoccupation or distraction
- "Bad feelings"

An important resource for good CRM is a checklist. Airline pilots use checklists regularly and continue to improve on them as well. Checklists help create standardization. They also help maintain good situational awareness by keeping an orderly flow to the process. This streamlined flow reduces the stress of a situation and essentially becomes a member of the team. Checklists are typically short, concise, and easy to read. These lists not only make sure certain items are accomplished for a procedure but also prompt members of the team to stay engaged and alert throughout the procedure. In an airline cockpit, there are typically several types of checklists for different types of situations including normal, abnormal, and emergency. These checklists are used in normal flying events and training events to make sure they are being used properly and understood completely. Checklists simply become another member of your team.

CRM incorporates all available resources. Focus is maintained on behaviors and how they affect safety because safety is the number one priority. CRM is a continuous process where active participation in training is encouraged. Once CRM is developed and used, the results become self-evident. CRM cannot be accomplished overnight with a one-time training event. It cannot be forced upon any individual. All participants must understand CRM and be willing to participate in operational settings as well as training events. It only makes sense that training events are not individually oriented but team oriented. Through training, emergency procedures must be discussed and practiced and industry issues must be discussed with education in mind that process, procedure, and errors are all taken into account. Mistakes must not be in vain; those who ignore them are destined to repeat them. CRM may be awkward at first, but once it becomes routine, structure, increased situational awareness, and team building concepts will fall into place.

For today's airline pilot, preparation begins the day prior to flight using the IMSAFE acronym. There are a series of checklists run before, during, and after the flight. Crew briefings, continuous monitoring, and planning are second nature because of the structure of a typical flight operation. Should a problem arise, checklists, discussion, and problem-solving skills become key. These are all taught and practiced regularly. Crisis resource management has become deeply ingrained in the specialty of anesthesiology. In my opinion, the routine anesthetic is no different than the routine of an airline flight.

B Medical emergency manual for the general practitioner

Robert C. Bosack
University of Illinois, School of Dentistry, Chicago, IL, USA

Busy clinicians require information that can be rapidly accessed and put to immediate use, especially when the need is urgent. With this in mind, the fifth edition of *Medical Emergencies in the Office* provides a fresh approach to aid the dentist in the medicolegal responsibility of anticipation, prevention, diagnosis, and management of acute medical problems that can present during the day-to-day practice of dentistry. Because these events are infrequent, training and experience are limited. Recall, decision-making, and performance are diminished in times of stress and time urgency. The ONLY way to effectively manage these situations is to have well-rehearsed SYSTEMS in place to help guide you and your staff in the management of emergent situations.

Repeated exposure to this information via continuing education, journal articles, and frequent, documented physical rehearsal of written emergency policies is mandatory, including clear role assignment for office staff, whose help during emergent times is invaluable and can be life saving. The following key duties, listed in no specific order, should be reviewed and assigned so that on any given day, and with any given staff, each member will have a clear understanding of their expected behavior in the event of an emergency:

- Assist with airway, CPR, and drug preparation/administration.
- Bring drugs, oxygen, airway devices, etc. to site of emergency.
- Document all interventions with timetable.
- Provide information to accompanying parties.
- Vacate or reschedule other patients, as necessary.
- Call 911, escort paramedics to the site of emergency.
- Provide written records to paramedics.
- Notify local hospital ER by telephone.

Awareness, diligence, anticipation, and flawless, repeated task performance – patient histories, vital signs, injection technique – are just a part of the overall relentless attention to detail that is necessary to achieve excellence in the clinical practice of dentistry.

The intent of this document is to provide a sound basis for clinical judgment, followed by a summary of rational, practical, and *easily referred to* guidelines for the diagnosis and treatment of medical emergencies (symptoms) in the dental office. A basic kit is suggested. Knowledge and competence in drug/device usage should guide your selection. Drugs should be checked for expiration at least two times per year, and equipment should be kept in working order. All members of the staff should be currently certified in CPR.

Dental practitioners should recognize that each case is different and that this guide is meant as an overview, rather than a strict protocol for treatment of all cases. The patient's history, always the most important step, should give the clinician an advantage in determining the cause of the problem. If an anticipated problem occurs, then the emergent situation can be managed in an orderly manner. It is not an expressed goal to make an accurate diagnosis; rather, the focus is on symptom recognition and emergent treatment of those symptoms as necessary to save a life, until further help arrives.

History and focused physical examination

The primary goal in the management of medical emergencies is prevention, ideally achieved with a thorough, directed *history*, updated at each visit, and a focused *physical examination*. Although emergencies, such as syncope or first-time chest pain can occur in otherwise ostensibly healthy patients, urgent situations are more likely to involve patients with concurrent medical problems, such as asthma, cardiovascular disease, seizure disorders, allergy, or diabetes. Therefore, when the respiratory, cardiovascular, neurologic, immunologic, or endocrine systems are involved, thorough questioning is necessary – specifically related to triggers, onset, signs, symptoms, and relieving or palliative factors. For example, a patient relates that he/she gets chest pain with one flight of stairs that is always relieved by rest and occasionally by one nitroglycerin tablet. If chest pain occurs in the office, the dentist will stop the procedure, check vital signs, provide oxygen, and administer a nitroglycerin tablet, as the patient predicted might happen. IF this is unsuccessful, EMS should be contacted immediately, while administering a second nitroglycerin tablet. Note that this event was "outside" the patient's normal response—a possible indication that something more serious is occurring and that additional measures will be necessary. Similarly, if a patient has an asthmatic attack that does not resolve with one puff of his rescue inhaler (that he/she previously stated always worked in the past), this also would be an indication to contact EMS and encourage preparation for further treatment options.

Many patients are poor historians; they may not remember or may not understand the nature of their diseases. Current medications relate to the nature of the disease. If a complete history or medication list is unavailable, invasive treatment should be deferred until this information is obtained.

Many patients do not regularly visit their physician, yet they can still have undiagnosed disease. Here, the identification of the following risk factors may be the only clue that trouble might occur.

Anesthesia Complications in the Dental Office, First Edition. Edited by Robert C. Bosack and Stuart Lieblich.

These risk factors include obesity, smoking, sedentary lifestyle, poor dietary choices, regular alcohol consumption, and a positive family history of cardiovascular disease or diabetes.

The following questions should be included in your preoperative evaluation and documented history, as they relate to the likelihood of medical problems occurring in your office. Your history form should have areas for checking yes *or no*, as it is equally important to document negative findings (medicolegal). The answers to these questions provide a framework for further investigation into your patient's medical conditions that may affect the care that you render.

1 Are you currently under a physician's care? For what?
2 Have you been in the hospital during the past 2 years? For what?
3 List all current medications.
4 List all allergies, with specific reference to antibiotics, codeine, aspirin, and latex.
5 Are you subject to fainting, dizziness, or seizures?
6 Do you have asthma or any shortness of breath with normal activity?
7 Are you or could you be pregnant?
8 Have you had any of the following?
   (a) chest pain, heart attack, bypass, angioplasty, or pacemaker
   (b) any trouble with heart valves
   (c) high blood pressure
   (d) stroke
   (e) diabetes
9 Are you able to take care of yourself and perform usual household tasks, including the ability to climb 1 – 2 flights of stairs?

Coupling a history with a focused physical examination, to include general observation of the patient, blood pressure, pulse rate and rhythm, and auscultation of the lungs (in asthmatic patients to check for wheezing) will usually, but not always, enhance predictability of trouble during a dental appointment. Blood pressures greater than 180/110mmHg, resting pulse rates that are excessively fast (>170bpm), excessively slow (<50bpm), or irregular should invite suspicion and the possible need for additional medical intervention to optimize the patient's health prior to elective or semielective dental work.

To review, a history and physical examination involves the identification of systems problems and their current level of control or severity to assess the likelihood that signs or symptoms of decompensating disease might occur during dental treatment. Rapid screening of all systems, noting all current medications and compliance, guides the astute clinician to further focused questioning.

Identifying the "at risk" patient

After an accurate medical history is obtained, a decision must be made regarding the ability of the patient to tolerate the planned treatments. Dentistry involves a wide variety of procedures, occasionally uncomfortable, that can lead to emotional and/or physical distress due to or in spite of the use of local anesthesia. The three procedures most likely to cause this stress are local anesthetic injection, dental extraction, and endodontic manipulation. In the past, the identification of patients who can "safely" tolerate these procedures has been difficult, nonspecific, and subjective.

Risk of a cardiac event during dental treatment

In 2007, the American College of Cardiology and American Heart Association updated recommendations to identify patients who may be unable to safely tolerate non-cardiac surgical procedures. Specifically, *the document focuses on the estimation of risk* of a cardiac event during non-cardiac surgery, in an operating room, under general anesthesia. These concepts do apply to dental manipulation, which is considered *minor, low risk surgery*, having an arbitrary upper limit of prolonged, single visit multiquadrant extractions or reconstruction.

Patients with the following active cardiac conditions may be unable to tolerate invasive dental procedures. Medical consultation / referral is advised prior to treatment.

1 *Unstable coronary syndromes*
   (a) recent myocardial infarction (within 1 month)
   (b) unstable angina (non-provoked chest pain)
2 *Decompensated heart failure*
   (a) patients with congestive heart failure who have excessive swelling around the ankles, who easily become short of breath, or who cannot sleep supine (among many other findings)
   (b) any shortness of breath not associated with physical exertion
3 *Severe cardiac valvular disease or arrhythmias*
   (a) always provoking symptoms of dizziness or light-headedness
4 *Recent pacemaker or implanted cardiac defibrillator*
5 *Orthostatic intolerance – inability to stand without getting dizzy.*

Risk of a non-cardiac event during dental treatment

The document above does not address risk for non-cardiac issues such as syncope, asthma attack, stroke, seizure, hypoglycemia, or allergy, among others. These issues will be covered in the following sections.

General concepts regarding common "emergencies"

"Fight or flight"

Some patients may not be "mentally prepared" or able to tolerate needle penetration, extraction, or other perceived threats. Exaggerated anticipation or mild discomfort can trigger various somatic responses. Usually, these reactions will be revealed as an increase in sympathetic tone leading to what is classically described as the "fight or flight" response. As expected, signs and symptoms include a rapid heartbeat, rapid breathing (hyperventilation), agitation, "feelings of panic or loss of control," elevated blood pressure, and inappropriate sweating (in the absence of exercise or ambient heat).

It is important to realize that other challenges to the patient will also, at least initially, result in this hyper-adrenergic response. Allergy, local anesthetic toxicity, heightened response to exogenous vasoconstrictors (also seen with frank overdose or intravascular injection), breathing difficulty, hypoglycemia, and early syncope can all demonstrate the same initial presentation. Because of these similarities, an accurate and thorough medical history becomes paramount in aiding treatment decisions.

Chest pain can also, at least initially, be a trigger of the fight or flight response. A complaint of new onset chest pain should never be taken lightly.

Psychogenic reactions

Psychogenic reactions are, by far, the most common cause of patient difficulty in the dental office. Apprehension and fear are among the most potent mental stressors that a patient may endure. These situations herald a variety of responses, including inappropriate and unrestrained behavior, hyperventilation, syncope, or near-syncope, all with attendant changes in heart rate, respiratory rate, and blood pressure. Nausea and vomiting are also possible. Occasionally, patients may demonstrate a red "blush" over the lower face, anterior neck, and upper chest when challenged by a stressful situation. This is in direct contradistinction to the raised, pruritic (itching) hive that may be seen with cutaneous allergy, after antigenic challenge. These events can be minimized in severity and frequency by practitioner empathy, limit-setting, and by taking the necessary time to establish rapport with each patient prior to treatment. Fortunately, most isolated psychogenic reactions are short-lived and often resolve with appropriate practitioner intervention.

Recognizing the emergent situation

Medical emergencies vary in presentation, duration, and severity depending on a host of factors. In general, any deviation from "normal," whether that refers to physical status or appropriate interaction with one's environment, should be considered a harbinger of trouble. It is common for the practitioner to "deny" that bad things are happening. Unfortunately, this often leads to a delay in appropriate treatment that can have devastating consequences.

Emergencies will present as:

- Loss of consciousness
- Respiratory distress
- Altered patient status
  - "Feeling sick"
  - Increased anxiety
  - Pain
  - Pallor
  - Inappropriate sweating
  - Tremors
  - Rash
  - Headache
  - Confusion

General treatment protocol for medical emergencies

1 Maintain the airway! – chin lift, jaw thrust
2 Terminate the procedure - remove any hardware or loose objects from the mouth
3 Reposition the patient – supine on a firm, flat surface
   - With cardiac or respiratory distress in a conscious patient, semirecumbent positioning may be preferred.
4 If the patient is in the late stages of pregnancy and is conscious, semirecumbent positioning with knees flexed is preferred. If pregnant and unconscious, supine with right hip elevation is necessary.
5 Activate the emergency medical system (EMS) at any time when you do not "feel comfortable" with a circumstance AND with any patient who is unconscious or is losing consciousness (except in cases of uncomplicated vasovagal syncope).
6 Assess and monitor airway and breathing.
7 Assess circulation, and take vital signs.
8 Administer oxygen.

Activating emergency medical systems

The "call for help"

When you take the time to think about this, the 911 call is a frightful and stressful experience. When the office is unprepared, it becomes chaotic - your patient is not doing well, and you are coming to the realization that you are unable to improve the situation and will need help right away. Concern about blame and guilt can surface, usually inappropriately.

There are many reasons why the call for help is necessary. As an example, assume a 55-year-old male has started to complain about chest pain, and then becomes pulseless. His wife and two other patients are in the waiting room, one hygiene chair is filled, and another patient is waiting for local anesthesia to take effect. Who will call 911? Who will help you with CPR? Who will bring oxygen to the room? Do you have an AED? Is there a face mask readily available, or will you do unprotected mouth-to-mouth rescue breathing? Who will document the event? Who will direct the paramedics to the appropriate area? How will his wife react when she sees paramedics entering your office? Should you say something to her in advance, and if so, what should be said and who will say it? Will you follow the patient to the hospital? How will you handle the other patients in the midst of treatment? The answers to these questions should be determined in advance. The specific roles and assigned duties will depend on the nature of the practice, layout of the office, and number of staff members present on any given day. A partial list of tasks that should be pre-assigned includes the following:

- Team leader tasks
  - establish the diagnosis, and direct the call for 911
  - maintain the airway
  - CPR as necessary
  - administer necessary drugs
- Assistant tasks
  - bring drugs and equipment to the patient
  - assist with CPR
  - draw up drugs

Drug	Name	Indication	How supplied	Dose/route
Sympathomimetic amine	Epinephrine (Adrenalin™)	Allergy Asthma	1:1000 Ampoule, pre-filled syringe	.1 - .3cc subQ or IM injection
β_2 agonist	Albuterol inhaler (Ventolin™, Proventil™)	Allergy Asthma	Inhaler	Metered puff
Antihistamine	Diphenhydramine (Benadryl™)	Allergy	Elixir	25 – 50mg orally
Vasodilator	Nitroglycerin	Chest pain	Tablet / sublingual spray	.4mg subL, dissolve in mouth
Sugar	Glutose™, Orange juice, etc	Hypoglycemia	Tube	Oral
Oxygen		All	Tank	Mouth / nose
Aspirin		Chest pain	325mg tablet	Chew, dissolve in mouth

- administer medication as needed, under the supervision of the team leader
- record events
- call to 911
- manage other patients in the office
- manage family or accompanying parties to the patient

Each office is unique and may have a rotating staff, such that some members will change from day to day. Writing out "task cards" and distributing them each day will guide the coordinated performance of duties. The most important caveat is to avoid panic and remain as calm as possible to promote clarity of thought and optimal performance of intended actions.

Office emergency kit (minimum)

1 Oxygen source and delivery mask
2 Sugar source (glucose paste, orange juice, Glutose™)
3 Diphenhydramine elixir (Benadryl™)
4 Epinephrine 1:1000, 1mg/cc (Epipen™, TwinJect™, syringe and ampoule) – more than one dose should be available
5 Albuterol inhaler (Proventil™, Ventolin™)
6 Nitroglycerin (.4mg tablets or sublingual spray)
7 Aspirin tablet

Syncope

Disease

Syncope is a transient, abrupt loss of consciousness and postural tone secondary to inadequate cerebral blood perfusion. Vasovagal syncope is the most frequent cause of unconsciousness in the dental office, and is usually triggered by anxiety, pain, sight of blood, etc. The term vasovagal describes two pathophysiologic parameters that often occur simultaneously. "Vaso" refers to vasodepressor – causing a decrease in vascular tone and blood pressure; "vagal" refers to a heightened cardioinhibitory vagal response causing a decrease in heart rate.

Classic vasovagal syncope occurs in susceptible patients in the following manner. A perceived threat – sight of blood, needle, anticipation of discomfort, etc. triggers a fight or flight sympathetic response where the heart rate is increased and blood is diverted to the larger muscle groups (legs) in anticipation of activity. The patient, however, sits still in the chair, which diminishes venous return to the heart, because of the lack of lower extremity muscular activity pumping blood back to central circulation. The result is a rapidly beating heart with no blood to pump. Cardiac output falls, leading to diminished blood flow to the brain. In susceptible patients, a heightened vagal response causes the heart to slow down excessively, further decreasing cardiac output. If the brain is deprived of enough oxygen, the patient will lose consciousness and control of the airway. In some cases, resolution is spontaneous, while others may proceed to a short salvo of seizure activity. This muscular activity augments venous return sufficiently to restore cerebral perfusion and consciousness.

When "passing out" is more serious than "vasovagal syncope"

Deviation from any of the following "classic" features of vasovagal syncope should invite suspicion of more serious etiology:

Classic syncope

- quick onset, temporary, limited duration, quick recovery
- brief prodromal warning symptoms – sweating, anxiety, feeling of warmth
- usually young, otherwise healthy, fearful patients
- patients look "pale," not blue
- incontinence is rare
- seizure activity; if it occurs, is brief in duration
- *chest pain* before passing out

Warning signs

- gradual loss of consciousness – deterioration over several minutes
- very sudden drops or falls (no prodrome or warning), frequently causing injury; may be assumed to be a sign of significant cardiac or neurologic trouble until proven otherwise
- incontinence of bladder, but especially bowel
- prolonged seizure activity and/or prolonged recovery
- geriatric patients who "pass out"
- any loss of consciousness with cyanosis (blue coloration)

History

Question the patient concerning prior history of syncope, nature of provoking factors, occurrence of seizure activity, prior medical work-up, etc. The more frequent the episodes, the more likely the problem may present.

Diagnosis

Clinical syncope (or near syncope, where the patient feels bad, but never quite loses consciousness) occurs as follows. A prodromal feeling of warmth, sweating, and (skin turns pale, esp. face, lips and oral mucosa) and patient awareness of a rapid heartbeat (palpitations) will manifest. As the event progresses, the patient becomes cold and clammy. In some cases and occasionally regardless of appropriate treatment, loss of consciousness, with loss of airway and spontaneous respirations can occur, oftentimes followed by two to three myoclonic (jerking) movements. In other cases, a full progression to unconsciousness will not occur; the patient will instead feel bad for 10 or more minutes.

When syncope leads to seizure activity, one must entertain a diagnosis of neurologic seizures. The seizure activity associated with syncope is of short duration, rarely involves injury, usually is not accompanied by incontinence, and ends with a quick return to normalcy. The seizure of neurologic origin usually occurs without warning, is of longer duration, can involve injury and incontinence, and is followed by significant postictal depression.

The patient experiencing syncope will turn pale, but not cyanotic (blue), which might be an indication of serious cardiac or pulmonary trouble.

Treatment

1 Maintain airway; supplemental oxygen.
2 Terminate procedure; remove loose objects from mouth.
3 Trendelenburg positioning – patient supine with legs higher than the heart. If semiconscious, encourage repetitive leg movement to augment venous return.
4 Prevent injury if the patient is convulsant.

If there is no improvement with this protocol, activate EMS and consider other possible etiologies, such as primary seizure disorder, stroke, allergy, hypoglycemia, or myocardial infarction.

Chest pain – myocardial infarction

Disease

Chest pain

Angina pectoris is typically a transient, substernal, squeezing or pressure type of pain that can spread across the chest and may radiate to any area above the diaphragm. It is important to realize that myocardial embarrassment without chest pain is possible and that patients may present with "anginal variants" such as nausea, vomiting, dizziness, palpitations, or shortness of breath. Angina is due to an imbalance between myocardial oxygen demand and oxygen supply. Events that increase oxygen demand, such as exertion, stress, or anxiety can precipitate angina, while rest, oxygen, or vasodilators relieve angina by improving oxygen supply. The most frequent cause of stable angina is narrowing of the coronary vessels by atherosclerotic plaques. Unstable angina occurs without warning or worsens rapidly (crescendo) and may not respond to vasodilator therapy. Unstable angina is presumed to be caused by a blood clot lodging in and obstructing a coronary vessel. This scenario requires immediate medical attention.

Myocardial infarction

Heart attack is usually, but not always, preceded by angina and is indicative of death of those heart muscle cells supplied by the obstructed coronary vessel. A small or minor heart attack may go unnoticed by the patient and may not cause significant pump or conductive tissue problems, while a major heart attack can be heralded by severe chest pain, electrical instability (rhythm abnormalities), and even death, as the heart fails to be an effective pump. For purposes of this monograph, the usual symptom of a heart attack is chest pain that persists for longer than 2 minutes in a patient with a negative cardiac history, or chest pain that is refractory to three challenges of sublingual NTG over a 15-minute period, in a person who normally depends on NTG to relieve chest pain.

History

A thorough cardiac history is necessary. Consultation with the patient's physician should be obtained prior to treating any patient with a history of an attack within the last 6 months. In patients with ongoing anginal problems, document frequency of attacks, precipitating events, and response to NTG. This will be your "road map" to manage chest pain, should it occur during dental treatment.

Diagnosis

Substernal pressure, pain, squeezing, fullness, tightness, and heaviness with or without radiation are typical "hard" symptoms of myocardial ischemia. "Soft" anginal variants include nausea, vomiting, sweating, shortness of breath, dizziness, disorientation, and lethargy. Loss of consciousness, loss of pulse, and death are the ultimate sequelae.

Treatment

1 Terminate the procedure, and remove any loose dental hardware.
2 Reposition the patient
   (a) if conscious, semirecumbent or as the patient prefers
   (b) if unconscious, supine on a flat, firm surface, ready to perform external cardiac compressions if pulselessness occurs
3 Administer 100% O_2.
4 Obtain and continuously monitor airway and vital signs
5 If conscious, administer one aspirin (160-325mg) to be chewed and absorbed in the mouth (not swallowed). Quick release aspirin crystals are now available for this purpose.
6 For NTG-dependent patients with a prior anginal history, *and* if *the systolic BP is >90mmHg,* give one NTG (.4mg) tablet and allow to dissolve sublingually. If chest pain persists, administer a second and third tablet, if necessary, at 5 minute intervals. If chest pain still persists after three doses of NTG over a 15 minute period, assume MI, activate EMS, and monitor pulse and respiration, being prepared to commence CPR if necessary, in a pulseless, breathless patient.
7 For patients without a cardiac history, when chest pain persists longer than 2 minutes, assume MI, activate EMS, and monitor vital signs.
8 Any change in location, severity, or duration of chest pain constitutes unstable or "preinfarction" angina; EMS should be summoned immediately.

Breathing disorders—asthma

Disease

Asthma is recurrent, reversible hyperresponsiveness of the tracheobronchial smooth muscle to various stimuli, with overlying acute and chronic inflammation of the airway mucosa. It is considered an obstructive disease because air flow is hindered when the diameter of the conducting bronchi and bronchioles is reduced by smooth muscle spasm, edematous mucosa, and excessive secretions/mucus plugging. As would be expected, the obstruction to air movement occurs primarily with active expiration when lungs AND airways are squeezed and narrowed by the diaphragm and intercostal muscles. Inspiration, on the other hand, tends to dilate the airways as the chest volume is increased and connective tissues tug on the airways, increasing their diameter. It is easy to appreciate that an asthma attack is characterized by a dynamic hyperinflation of the lungs – each breath becomes more difficult to take as the lungs expand further and air is trapped. The patient panics as he/she feels the need for more air, but cannot breathe it in! This results in the inability to move oxygen from the atmosphere to the alveolar capillary membrane, resulting in suffocation and tissue hypoxia as its most severe expression.

The prevalence of asthma is increasing, with a predilection for patients <18 years; however, all people of ages are affected. Usual triggers include environmental irritants (tobacco smoke), strong odors, emotional upset, cold air, and exercise, to name a few.

History

The disease is classified according to the frequency and severity of symptoms. Mild intermittent disease can often be controlled with a "rescue" β_2 agonist inhaler (albuterol) that relaxes bronchiolar smooth muscle and dilates the airways. If this fails to control the disease, classification is advanced to mild or severe *persistent,* now requiring other medications, including inhaled or systemic steroids and leukotriene inhibitors (e.g., montelukast – Singulair™.) Airway hyperreactivity tends to last for several weeks after a recent attack, increasing its likelihood for recurrence during this period. The following are considered risk factors that can increase the likelihood of an asthmatic attack occurring in your office. Be vigilant – "out of the blue" attacks are also possible.

Warning signs

1 Recent attack
2 Need for two or more different medications
3 Noncompliance with medications
4 Poorly controlled and/or longstanding disease
5 Active wheezing
6 Upper respiratory infection in asthmatic patients
7 Prior history of sudden, severe exacerbations
8 More than two hospitalizations or three ER visits within the last year for asthma

Diagnosis

- Patient in distress – leaning forward
- Chest tightness
- Wheezing
- Cough
- Shortness of breath – gasping for air

Treatment

1 Terminate the procedure.
2 Administer one or two puffs of a β_2 agonist (albuterol) – EARLY.
3 Administer supplemental oxygen.
4 Activate EMS if situation fails to improve.
5 With deteriorating condition, failure of multiple puffs of inhaler, and help not being immediately available, administer .3cc (.3mg) of 1:1000 epinephrine subcutaneously or intramuscularly and be prepared to re-administer a second dose in 5 minutes should this be necessary. This dose can be reduced to .1cc in small patients. Refer the section titled "The epinephrine injection."

Breathing disorders—hyperventilation

Disease

Hyperventilation is respiration in excess of the current metabolic demand. It is usually psychogenic in origin, secondary to anxiety or fear. Hyperventilation expresses as an increase in tidal volume and/or increase in respiratory rate. Too much oxygen is not a clinical problem; rather, it is the overelimination of CO_2 that leads to difficulties. Hypocarbia is associated with respiratory alkalosis, which causes a decrease in serum ionized Ca^{++} levels. Hypocalcemia lowers threshold potentials, leading to neuromuscular irritability and tetany as its most severe expression.

History

Hyperventilation usually appears in apprehensive patients who initially attempt to hide their fear. It can be associated with "panic attacks." Many patients may not be willing to volunteer this information, even with direct questioning.

Diagnosis

Diagnosis is relatively straightforward; the increase in rate or volume of ventilation is easily noticed and heard. If allowed to persist, hypocarbia and alkalosis will result, causing a constriction of cerebral blood vessels leading to lightheadedness and impairment of consciousness. Neuromuscular irritability leads to complaints of numbness or tingling of the extremities, muscle pain, cramps, spasms, trismus, and generalized stiffness.

Treatment

1 Terminate the procedure.
2 Verbally calm the patient – may have to be firm.
3 Have the patient breathe into a paper bag in order to rebreathe and accumulate CO_2 to bring these levels back to normal.

Breathing disorders—emphysema

Disease

Emphysema is a pulmonary response to chronic exposure to noxious stimuli, characterized by abnormal permanent enlargement (coalescence) of distal air spaces and loss of elasticity in the lung parenchyma. This causes premature airway collapse prior to alveolar emptying on necessarily active expiration, resulting in air trapping and an inability to exhale. The end result is an inability to move air with subsequent decreased oxygenation of tissues.

History

Usually, the patient is aware of this diagnosis. It occurs in susceptible patients secondary to chronic exposure to noxious stimuli.

Diagnosis

The emphysematous patient is usually thin, barrel-chested, and prefers to exhale through "pursed lips" – necessary to keep the airways open. Typically, these patients prefer to lean forward to help with their breathing. When severe, the patient quietly gasps for air, speaks in short phrases, and is intolerant to any but the mildest physical activity when the disease is severe. Often times, supplemental oxygen is necessary, usually administered through nasal prongs. It is possible for these patients to decompensate and become very short of breath during dental appointments.

Treatment

1 Recognize the signs and symptoms.
2 Allow the patient to breathe as he/she requires – he/she may not be able to tolerate prolonged periods with a wide open mouth.
3 Supplemental oxygen – 2-3 liters per minute.
4 β_2 agonist inhaler (albuterol) as necessary.

Hypoglycemia

Disease

HYPOGLYCEMIA can readily present as an emergent situation in the dental office. It can occur in diabetic patients who have taken hypoglycemic agents (oral pills or insulin) and have not been supplied sufficient calories. In this instance, basal levels of blood

Insulins

Duration	Insulin preparation	Onset	Peak	Duration
Rapid acting	**Lispro (Humalog™) Aspart (Novolog™)**	**5–15 min**	**30–90 min**	**4 - 6 hours**
Short acting	**Insulin (Regular)**	**30–60 min**	**2–4 hours**	**5–10 hours**
Intermediate acting	Isophane (NPH, Humulin N, Novolin N)	2–4 hours	4–10 hours	10–18 hours
	Insulin Zinc (Lente, Humulin L, Novolin L)	2–4 hours	4–12 hours	12–20 hours
Long acting	Extended Insulin Zinc Ultralente	6–10 hours	10–16 hours	18–24 hours
	Glargine (Lantus)	2–4 hours	Continuous	24 hours
Premixed insulins				
Humulin 70/30	70% NPH +30% regular	30–60 min	Dual	10–16 hours
Humulin 50/50	50% NPH +50% regular	30–60 min	Dual	10–16 hours
Humalog 75/25	**75% NPL* +25% lispro**	**5–15 min**	**Dual**	**10–16 hours**
Novalog 70/30	**70% NPL* +30% aspart**	**5–15 min**	**Dual**	**10–16 hours**

*NPL = neutral protamine lispro, functionally identical to NPH (neutral protamine hagedorn).

glucose are excessively decreased, leading to signs and symptoms of low blood sugar. It is important to note that there are some patients who are not diabetic who can experience episodic hypoglycemia (e.g., after eating). Treatment considerations are the same, however. The brain has a continual need for glucose and, in the acute situation, is unable to utilize any other metabolic substrate. When glucose levels fall, signs and symptoms relating to a compromised nervous system will appear.

Diabetes mellitus is a progressive disease of glucose dysregulation and carbohydrate intolerance. In this disease, insulin is either lacking or ineffective in escorting blood glucose intracellularly, where it is broken down to create energy for cellular metabolism. The resultant excess blood sugar (chronic HYPERGLYCEMIA) is toxic to all cells and promotes osmotic diuresis. Type I diabetics have an absolute insulin deficiency and always require exogenous insulin. Type II diabetics have impaired "insulin functioning" – not enough, ineffective, or insulin receptor resistance – and may require insulin in addition to oral medication to keep blood sugar levels in an appropriate range.

History

Currently, many patients have undiagnosed diabetes – this will lead to hyperglycemia, which rarely presents as an office emergency. Diabetic patients who may be prone to hypoglycemia will have already been diagnosed, and will be currently taking insulin or oral agents to control their blood sugar. SPECIFICALLY,

- They took insulin, but did not eat or eat enough.
- They took insulin, but are in a hypermetabolic state (fever, exercise, stress).

Drugs capable of lowering blood sugar

Oral hypoglycemic agents

- Diabinese™ (chlorpropamide)
- Micronase™, Diabeta™ (glyburide)
- Glucotrol™ (glipizide)
- Glucophage™ (metformin)
- Glucovance™ (metformin + glyburide)

Diagnosis

Hypoglycemia affects both the autonomic nervous system and the central nervous system.

Signs and symptoms of ANS dysfunction can appear with mild hypoglycemia (50–70mg/dl) and can include the following:

- Weakness
- Hunger
- Anxiety
- Hypotension
- ↑ sympathetic discharge (fight or flight)
  - Inappropriate sweating
  - Tachycardia – palpitations (being aware of one's heartbeat)
  - Trembling
  - Peripheral vasoconstriction (cold, clammy hands)
  - Nausea and vomiting
  - Piloerection

Signs and symptoms of CNS dysfunction usually appear with moderate to severe hypoglycemia (20 – 50mg/dl) and can include the following:

- Decreased spontaneity
- Mood alteration
  - Inability to concentrate
  - Mood alteration
  - Belligerence
- Dizziness, confusion, lethargy
- Headache
- Slurred speech
- Loss of consciousness
- Seizures

The loss of consciousness that is seen with severe hypoglycemia is usually slow in onset, heralded by a gradual decline in cerebral functioning. In contrast, the loss of consciousness that is seen with vasovagal syncope is usually sudden, although patients experiencing vasovagal syncope may experience some warning – sweating, palpitations, etc.

Treatment

1. Any diabetic patient demonstrating slow, bizarre behavior should be assumed to be hypoglycemic and managed as such until proven otherwise.
2. The treatment of suspected hypoglycemia is to give sugar orally if the patient is conscious – orange juice, candy bar, glucose syrup, etc. Putting food or liquid in the mouth on an unconscious patient can lead to airway embarrassment.
3. If the patient is unconscious, contact EMS, maintain airway, and breathing and circulation. Protect the patient from harm in the event of seizure activity.

Allergy

Disease

Allergy is a hypersensitive immunologic state acquired by exposure to a particular antigen; subsequent re-exposure produces a heightened capacity to react. Allergic reactions have variable clinical manifestations ranging from MILD, DELAYED ONSET to IMMEDIATE, ACUTE ONSET and LIFE THREATENING. The severity and time from exposure to symptom appearance vary with the degree of antigenicity, route of exposure, dose of antigen, as well as host factors. This discussion focuses on TYPE I (immediate hypersensitivity) reactions, where an antigen cross-links preexisting IgE antibodies on mast cells and basophils, stimulating the release of histamine (causing increased capillary permeability and vasodilation) and SRS-A (causing bronchiolar constriction), among a veritable plethora of other mediators, all producing similar effects.

History

Direct questioning concerning allergy to frequently used drugs in the dental office should include reactions to *penicillin, codeine, iodine (surface disinfectants),* and *latex*. These should be noted in the chart. The question of local anesthetic allergy occasionally surfaces. Allergic reactions to amide-type anesthetics are extremely rare, while allergy to esters (such as Hurricaine™ or Cetacaine™) is more common, as these drugs are metabolized to the notoriously allergenic PABA (para-amino benzoic acid). Direct questioning about the occurrence of rash, itching, and rhinitis should all but eliminate the possibility of local anesthetic allergy. If in doubt, it is not wise to challenge your patient with a "test dose," as even minute amounts of allergen can trigger full-blown anaphylaxis in susceptible patients.

Diagnosis

Diagnostic features of allergy can involve any or all of the systems noted in the next section. Milder reactions usually involve only one or two systems, with cutaneous manifestations common as an initial presentation. When multiple systems are involved, with severe and rapid escalation, the patient may report a feeling of "impending doom," and generalized anaphylaxis may be approaching. Any combination of symptoms can occur within 5 – 30 minutes, or several days after exposure to an antigen. True, life-threatening anaphylaxis is quite rare, especially in the dental office; however, case reports occasionally surface involving the administration of penicillin derivatives to penicillin-allergic patients for antibiotic prophylaxis. As stated above, the patient may report a feeling of intense itching, flushing, giant hives, piloerection, cramping, nausea, vomiting, and wheezing.

Signs and symptoms of allergy

- Cutaneous
  - Urticaria (hive)
  - Angioedema (asymmetrical swelling in loose tissues)
  - Pruritis (itching)
  - Erythema (rash)
  - Wheal formation
  - Warm, red skin
  - Periorbital swelling
- Exocrine
  - Watery eyes
  - Running nose
- Respiratory
  - Difficulty in breathing
  - Bronchoconstriction – wheezing, shortness of breath
  - Laryngeal edema (change in tone or pitch of voice)
- Cardiovascular
  - Hypotension
  - Tachycardia - palpitations
  - Generalized *collapse and loss of consciousness*
- Gastrointestinal
  - Cramping
  - Nausea / vomiting
  - Incontinence

Many of these reactions may be confused with other diagnoses, all having several symptoms in common. Bronchoconstriction also occurs in the asthmatic patient – in many instances, asthmatic patients have multiple allergies. Differentiation of the various possible etiologies is secondary and should not delay palliative treatment of signs or symptoms. Tachycardia and palpitations are seen in most reactions – these are classic fight or flight signs. Early syncope can mask as early allergy – however, one would not expect rash formation with syncope, and the skin in syncope or hypoglycemia is moist and cold, while the skin in anaphylaxis is warm and dry.

Visual manifestations of allergy

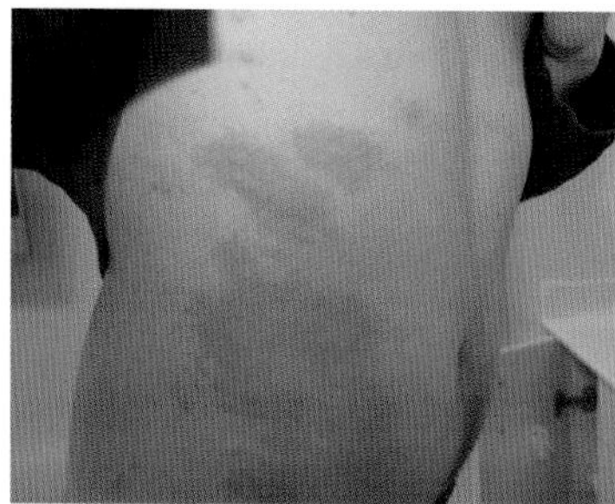

Note raised, itching *hive* on right lateral chest and abdominal wall, representing a reaction to penicillin.

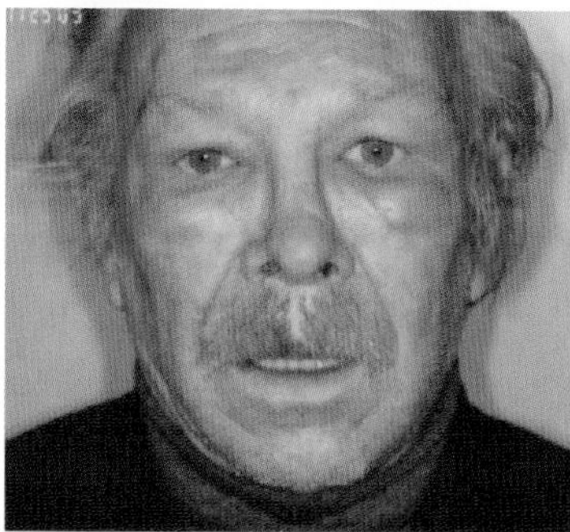

Note *periorbital swelling, watery eyes, rhinitis "runny nose."* This patient "looks bad." This particular case represents a reaction to clindamycin.

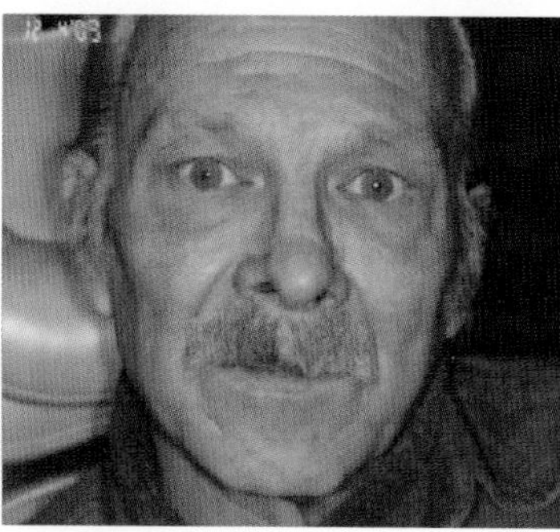

This is the same patient as above, 3 days after the allergic reaction resolved, and now appears *normal.*

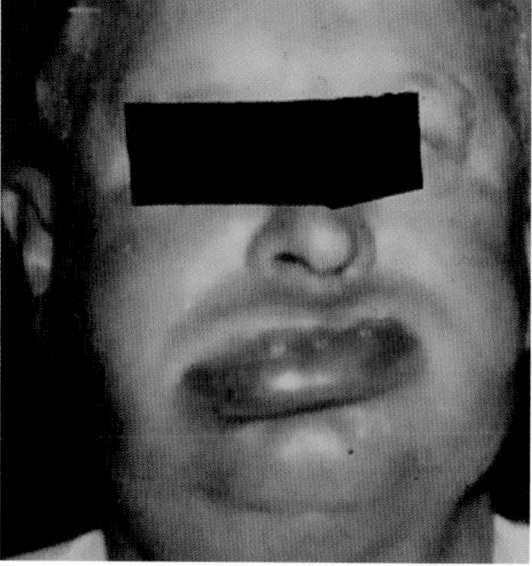

This is a clinical example of *angioedema of the lower lip.* Note asymmetric contortion secondary to fluid accumulation in loose tissue layers. Angioedema can also occur in the soft laryngeal tissues, leading to upper airway obstruction.

Treatment

Mild

Treatment should be tailored to the severity and rapidity of symptom onset. Mild, cutaneous, or exocrine reactions can often be managed by *eliminating the allergen* (if possible) and taking *oral diphenhydramine (Benadryl™) 25-50mg QID* for several days as needed to control signs and symptoms. Consultation with the patient's physician or an emergency room is recommended.

Severe

The appearance of any other signs or symptoms, and especially with rapid onset, including wheezing, change in voice, difficulty in breathing, tachycardia, or hypotension should prompt immediate contact with EMS. While waiting for their arrival, the *airway is maintained, oxygen and β_2 agonist bronchodilators should be administered (inhaled albuterol), and when urgency dictates, .3mg of 1:1000 epinephrine solution should be injected subcutaneously or intramsuclarly, every 5 minutes as necessary until help arrives.* Epinephrine is life saving in anaphylaxis, but its effect is short lived. Refer the section titled "The epinephrine injection."

Seizures

Disease

A seizure is an abnormal, paroxysmal neuronal discharge in the brain, characterized by an attack involving changes in the state of consciousness, motor activity, and/or sensory phenomena. Usually, the attack is *sudden* in onset and brief in duration. Etiology includes genetic predisposition, brain lesions, trauma, infection, or *non-compliance with anti-seizure medication.* There is no identifiable cause in a majority of cases.

Classification is wide and varied with signs and symptoms ranging from simple, episodic short-lived absence seizures (spell); complex seizures involving a loss of consciousness and/or involuntary motor or autonomic discharge; or the frightening display of tonic (sustained muscular contraction) – clonic (twitching) contortions of the trunk and extremities, usually lasting between 2 and 5 minutes, followed by postictal depression that can last for several hours. Some patients may be able to anticipate their seizure activity, while in others the occurrence is without warning.

Common medications include phenytoin (Dilantin™) and barbiturates, among several others.

History

Question the patient concerning the type, frequency, duration, sequelae, warning signs, and instigating factors of the seizure. The patient should be able to describe what may happen, the likelihood that it will happen, and what you should do about it if it happens. Noncompliance with medication and limited effectiveness of current medication are important issues that should increase anticipation of a seizure. Usually, seizure patients who are allowed to drive a car are considered to be adequately controlled.

Diagnosis

Diagnosis is straightforward and requires only visual detection. The patient may demonstrate a blank stare or absence spell, facial muscle twitching, loss of consciousness, nausea, vomiting, possible airway obstruction, and/or incontinence.

Differential diagnosis

Seizure activity can also occur with syncope and severe hypoglycemia. Seizure activity that can occur during syncope is much shorter duration, usually consisting of 1 – 2 clonic jerks with a rapid recovery to normalcy. Seizure activity associated with hypoglycemia occurs with gradual onset in a patient who has already lost consciousness.

Treatment: (grand mal)

1. Terminate the procedure.
2. Remove all dental hardware (clamps, bands, etc.) with the appearance of prodromal signs.
3. Protect the patient from injury – you cannot and should not restrain the patient during a seizure – rather, remove objects that may be in the way of his motion to avoid cuts or punctures.
4. Maintain the airway – this is easy to say and hard to do during the seizure – if the patient loses his airway during the seizure, it may be impossible to extend the neck and protrude the jaw. The use of hard objects to forcefully pry the jaws apart is not recommended. If possible, suction should be nearby in the event of hemorrhage as a result of tongue or cheek biting.
5. Continue to support the airway in the lethargic, post-ictal stage.
6. Contact EMS with prolonged or unusual seizure activity (something different than what patients report as their 'normal seizure).
7. The use of benzodiazepines to control seizure activity in the office by those unfamiliar with their parenteral usage is not recommended and may exacerbate post-ictal depression.

Stroke

Disease

A stroke is a sudden disruption in the flow of blood to a region of the brain. Deprived of oxygen, the affected area of the brain can be either injured or succumb to cell death. There are two types of stroke:

1. Ischemic (80%) – caused by stationary (thrombotic) or moving (embolic) blood clots. This is more common in older patients.
2. Hemorrhagic (20%) – occurs when a blood vessel in the brain leaks or ruptures, secondary to an inherent vascular weakness or severe hypertension. More common in middle-aged patients.

History

Strokes are usually sudden and unexpected in onset; therefore, history may not be helpful, except in cases where the patient has risk factors and has suffered strokes in the past. Risk factors include, but are not limited to, male gender, advanced age, sedentary lifestyle, cigarette smoking, obesity, and hypercholesterolemia.

Diagnosis

1. sudden, severe headache with no known or apparent cause
2. sudden weakness / loss of sensation on one side of the face or unilateral extremity
3. sudden dimness or loss of vision, especially unilateral
4. loss of coherent speech or trouble talking or understanding speech
5. unexplained dizziness, unsteadiness or sudden falls, especially with any of the other signs above.

TIA – Transient ischemic attack is a focal, temporary loss of neurologic function, secondary to ischemia. The TIA is abrupt in onset, LESS than 1 hour in duration, and resolves without residual signs. A TIA is an important warning sign for stroke. Since the initial presentation of a TIA is identical to stroke, it should be managed in a similar emergent manner.

Treatment

If a stroke is due to an occlusive clot (as diagnosed on CT scan) AND these patients are treated with thrombolytic agents within 3-4.5 hours of symptom onset the frequency of irreversible brain injury decreases. As such, signs and symptoms of stroke should be considered an emergent situation, requiring *immediate activation of the EMS.* Your role will be recognitive, supportive, and intermediary. Supplemental oxygen and supine posturing can be considered, but both can worsen a cerebral bleed.

Disorders of blood pressure

Baseline blood pressures should be measured on all dental patients. Otherwise normotensive patients presenting with low blood pressure can be at increased risk of syncope (80/50mmHg), while patients with sustained high blood pressure can be at risk of myocardial ischemia or cerebral hemorrhage (230/120mmHg) as well as damage to the eyes, kidneys, and other organ systems.

Elective treatment is deferred for patients with blood pressures greater than 180/110mmHg, while immediate consultation with the patient's physician or the emergency room is indicated with pressures >220/120mmHg. These numbers are approximate values; each case should be managed on an individual basis, with consideration of other risk factors, such as type and urgency of surgery, general health of the patient, and consultation with the patient's treating physician.

Should a patient develop headache, confusion, or nausea during an appointment CONCOMITANT with a significant rise in blood pressure over baseline, treatment should be stopped, and immediate medical consultation obtained. Reassure your patient and consider oxygen. There is no indication for the parenteral use of antihypertensive agents (or vasopressors) in the general dental office to treat abnormalities of blood pressure by those practitioners unfamiliar with their usage.

Management of foreign bodies displaced beyond the oropharynx

Prevention

The introduction of small objects into the mouth invites the possibility of their displacement beyond the throat. An oropharyngeal drape (rubber dam, 4 × 4 gauze) should be used to reduce the possibility of accidental aspiration or ingestion. If this is not possible (e.g., patients prone to gagging,), instruments should be tethered to suture or floss to aid in their retrieval. A numeric inventory of small parts on the operative tray should be maintained.

Diagnosis

USUALLY, but not always, aspirated objects will produce a coughing reflex, while ingested objects will produce no response or possibly a gag response if the ingested object is large.

Treatment

When an object is lost to the hypopharyngeal region in an already supine patient, do not allow the patient to sit up. Keep the patient supine or Trendelenberg (*head down*), lying on the *right side.* If the patient is upright, reposition as above, unless the patient is in a coughing paroxysm. The best chance for retrieval occurs with the patient in this position. Right-sided Trendelenberg posturing lessens the force of gravity pushing the object in a more caudal direction, and in cases of aspiration this may keep the object to the right mainstem bronchus, where it is most often located and from where spontaneous or endoscopic retrieval is easier. If unsure of the location of a foreign body, radiographs should be obtained – PA and lateral chest films to check for aspiration and/or a flat plate of the abdomen (KUB) to localize an ingested item. All lost objects must be retrieved or followed to elimination with x-rays, if radiographically identifiable.

Ingestion of small, blunt objects – tooth, cotton roll, small implant hardware may be managed by radiographic documentation of passage with the help of high fiber diet. Consultation with a physician may be warranted.

Ingestion of large, blunt objects or any sharp object – endodontic file, bur, scalpel blade, suture needle, or large implant hardware should be immediately referred to a general surgeon, gastroenterologist, or emergency facility.

Aspiration of small, blunt objects will often be accompanied by coughing. Immediately place patient to a right-sided Trendelenberg, encourage a slow inhalation (to minimize deeper aspiration) followed by a forceful cough. One CANNOT assume that an aspirated object has been eliminated simply because a coughing paroxysm has stopped. Referral is necessary in cases of unsuccessful retrieval.

Aspiration of large and/or sharp objects should be immediately referred to an emergency facility for management. Maintain vigilance and anticipate airway compromise. DO NOT encourage coughing if the lost object is sharp. A Heimlich maneuver should be performed with airway obstruction.

The epinephrine injection

Performing an extraoral epinephrine injection, in order to save the patient's life, can be daunting for even the most experienced clinicians. Careful planning and rehearsal are the only two ways to prepare for this procedure. To reiterate, the two indications for parenteral epinephrine in the dental office are asthmatic bronchospasm unresponsive to inhaled β_2 agonists AND severe and worsening allergic reactions.

In the United States, epinephrine is available in three forms: the Epipen™ (Dey Pharmaceuticals), the TwinJect™ (Verus Pharmaceuticals), or in an ampoule. The ampoule will require a simple maneuver (see subsequent text) to fill a syringe; however, it is the most cost effective.

The epinephrine ampoule and tuberculin syringe are available at most local pharmacies. The Epipen™ contains one injection only, and is available in both adult and pediatric doses. The TwinJect™ contains two injections, first as an autoinjector, and a second as a regular pre-filled syringe contained within the apparatus; it is also supplied in both adult and pediatric doses. It is important to note that with true anaphylaxis, one dose of epinephrine may not be sufficient and repeated dosing may be necessary within 5–10 minutes.

Instructions for use of these two devices can be viewed at the following websites:

- TwinJect™ - www.twinject.com
- Epipen™ - www.allergic-reactions.com/howtouse.aspx.

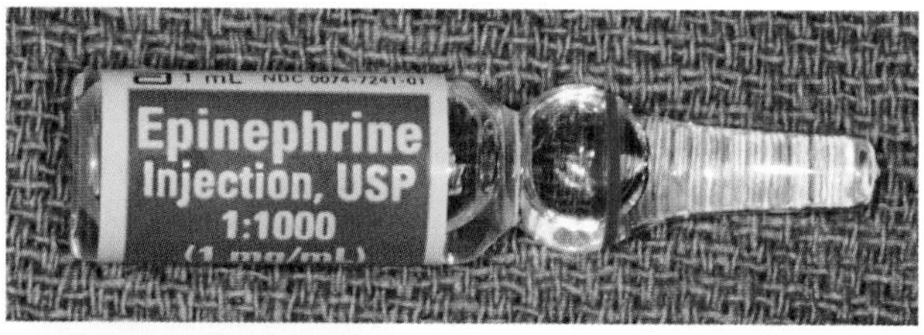

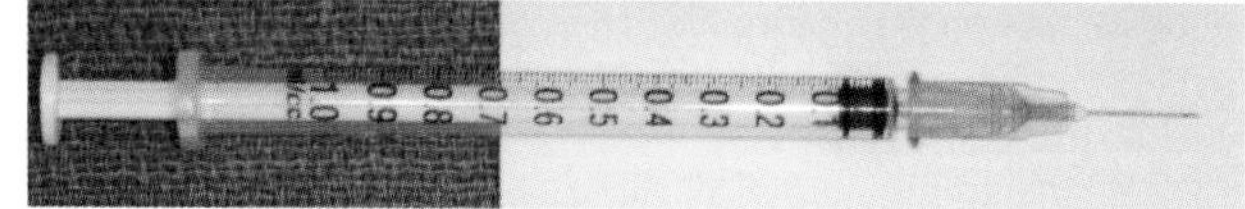

Preparing medication for injection from a glass ampoule

1 READ THE LABEL!
   - Verify that the ampoule contains the drug you wish to administer.
   - Check expiration date.

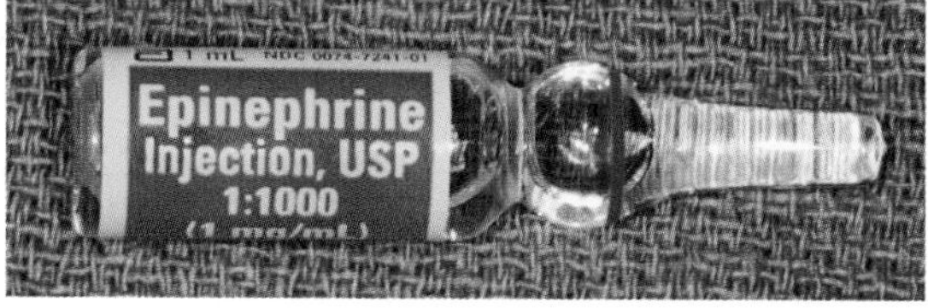

2 Break the ampoule
- Flick the upper stem with your fingernail to bring all liquid down to the main portion of the ampoule.
- Grasp with thumbs and index fingers and briskly snap off the top.

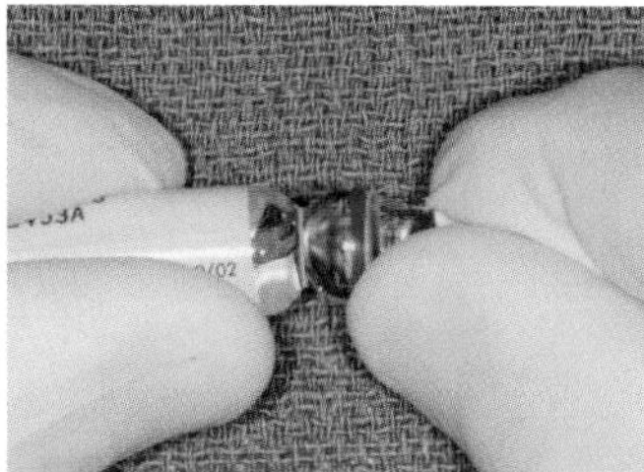

3 Tip the ampoule and withdraw medication into a tuberculin syringe
- Place tip of needle at the bottom *wall* of the ampoule as shown, and withdraw; this minimizes the possibility of aspirating small pieces of broken glass that may have fallen to the bottom of the ampoule.

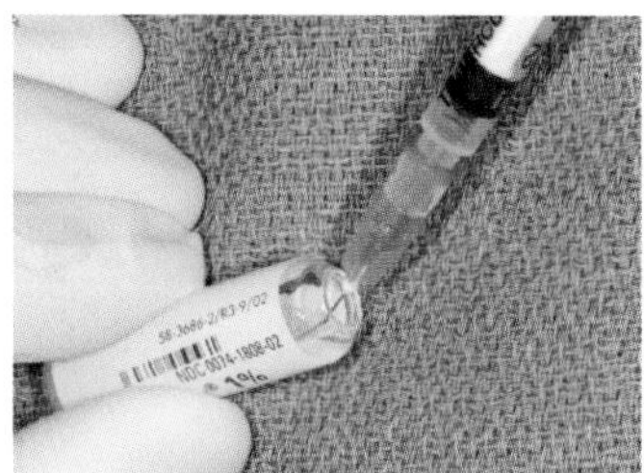

4 Express any air bubbles from the syringe
- Flick the syringe with the needle up to allow air to come to the top and express the bubbles.
- Ready to inject.

Where should the epinephrine injection be given?

Epinephrine is rapidly metabolized once it reaches the blood stream; therefore, the 1:1000 (1mg/cc) concentration should be administered in a location where absorption is slower to promote a reasonably sustained effect. Any location with subcutaneous fat is acceptable. Intramuscular injections (tongue, floor of mouth) can also be administered; however, absorption will be quicker, duration will be shorter, and undesirable side effects (tachycardia, agitation) may be exaggerated. The intramuscular injection is deeper than the subcutaneous route and a longer needle is used in trajectory perpendicular to the skin.

The fat over the back of the upper arm is a readily accessible location when patients are in the dental chair. The needle should be inserted at a 45° angle into the layer of fat that is pinched by the non-dominant hand. Aspiration is not necessary. 0.3cc of a 1:1,000 solution should be administered in an adult, while 0.1cc of a 1:1,000 solution is sufficient in a small child. In many cases, this dose must be repeated every 5 minutes.

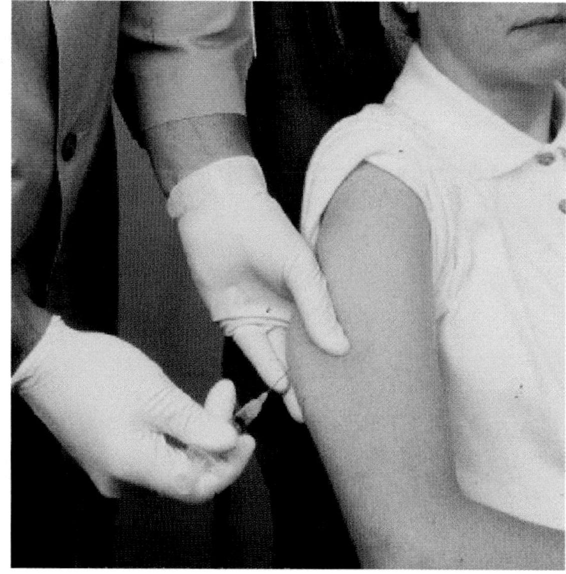

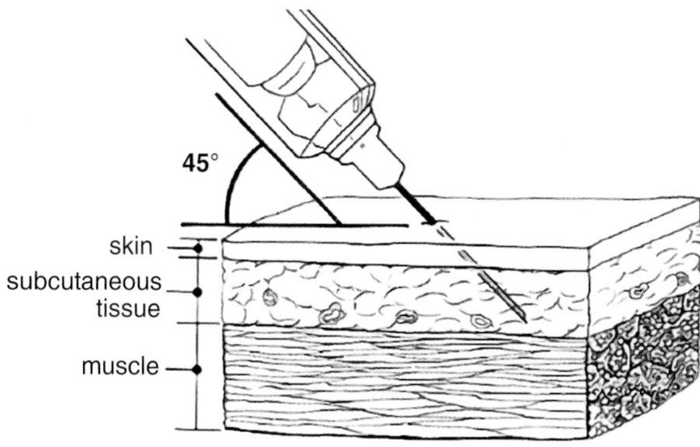

The purpose of this document is to provide information, rather than advice or opinion. It does not attempt to establish a standard of care and should not be construed as doing so. It should not be used to establish liability, error, or duty on the part of the practitioner. It should not be used or referred to in any court or peer review proceeding. Licensed healthcare professionals accessing this presentation agree to assume full responsibility for the use of this information and hold harmless any third party, including Robert C. Bosack, DDS (and any of his affiliated corporate entities) for any claim, loss, injury, or damage arising from the use or dissemination of this information. As each patient is different; this manual, at best, can offer only guidelines in management of medical emergencies. As new research and clinical experience continually broaden our knowledge, changes in treatment and drug therapy naturally follow, which can lead to changes in the recommendations, concepts, and guidelines presented herein. Practitioners are advised to continually seek confirmation of this material with other reputable sources and are advised to keep abreast of all current information as it becomes available.

References

Bennett, J. D. and Rosenberg, M. B. *Medical Emergencies in Dentistry*. Philadelphia: W. B. Saunders, 2002.

Fleisher, L. A., et al. ACC/AHA 2007 guidelines on perioperative cardiovascular evaluation and care for noncardiac surgery: executive summary. *Circulation* **116**: 1971–1996, 2007.

Gaba, D. M., Fish, K. J., et al. *Crisis Management in Anesthesiology*. Philadelphia: Churchill Livingstone, 1994.

Miller, R.D., et al. *Miller's Anesthesia*. 7th edn. Philadelphia: Churchill Livingstone Elsevier, 2010.

Malamed, S. *Medical Emergencies in the Dental Office*. 6th edn. St. Louis: Mosby, 2007.

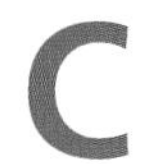

Malignant hyperthermia Q & A

Edward C. Adlesic[1] and Steven I. Ganzberg[2]

[1] University of Pittsburgh School of Dental Medicine, Department of Oral and Maxillofacial Surgery, Pittsburgh, PA, USA

[2] UCLA School of Dentistry, Century City Outpatient Surgery Center, Los Angeles, CA, USA

Are MHS employees at risk for MH in your office?

In reviewing the literature, no reports were found documenting any risk to MHS staff participating in general anesthetics using volatile gases in the office. However, there should be adequate ventilation and scavenging of gases in the operatory. When properly provided for, the vast majority of the exhaled gases are eliminated. A call to the MHAUS consultant line also reflected a similar opinion (personal communication).

Are MHS patients safe to sedate or anesthetize in the office setting?

Nitrous oxide, local anesthetics, intravenous anesthetics, sedatives, and opioid drugs are not triggering agents, so moderate or deep sedation and intravenous general anesthesia can be provided for these patients if certain precautions are taken. Since succinylcholine is a possible trigger, a rapid acting non-depolarizing muscle relaxant will be needed for emergency treatment of persistent laryngospasm unresponsive to positive pressure oxygen and deepening of the anesthetic level. Rocuronium 0.6 – 1 mg/kg, with the dose dependent on the degree of hypoxia, patient age and other patient factors, would appear to be the drug of choice. If used, the clinician should be prepared to ventilate the patient for an extended period of time. The dentist may elect not to treat these particular patients or to use an anesthetic technique that employs reversible agents only (benzodiazepines and opioids) so that laryngospasm can be managed with reversal of sedative level.

Must dantrolene be kept in the office if the only triggering agent present is succinylcholine for emergency use?

There has been concern in the OMFS community regarding the need to stock dantrolene when the only triggering agent present is succinylcholine and its use is very rare and frequently in low doses. Succinylcholine when used alone appears to be a very weak MH trigger. Informal polling at meetings indicates that most providers of deep sedation in a dental office have never used succinylcholine to break a laryngospasm, so they do not stock dantrolene. Others believe that dantrolene should be kept even for this rare event. Rodrigues (2008) indicated that unless all triggering agents can be eliminated from an office, a minimum amount of dantrolene should be stocked. It is recommended that at least 12 vials with enough sterile water for reconstitution should be kept in the office to allow for administration of an initial dose of dantrolene for most adult patients. MHAUS recommends that 36 vials of dantrolene be available if any triggering agents *may* be used at any time. This discussion continues without a consensus opinion.

How long do you keep MHS patients in the office after a procedure, even if only local anesthesia was used?

In the past, a recovery time period of 4 hours has been recommended. Then the recovery period was decreased to 2.5 hours. Brandom and Rosenberg (2009) recommended that patients who have surgery in an ambulatory center should be kept for 2 hours postoperatively if no triggering agents were used. According to Rosenberg in an MHAUS newsletter in 2005, MHS patients do not need a prolonged recovery period, and can be treated similarly to any other patient. In an ambulatory setting that time frame now would be ~1 hour, and during that period of time, the patient should be watched for signs of MH: increases in $EtCO_2$, muscle rigidity, tachycardia, and dysrhythmias. The surgeon may also consider keeping a few urine dip sticks to monitor for blood in the urine; if there is a deep color reaction for blood in the urine, it is safe to assume that myoglobin is present. If there is no blood in the urine after 1 hour, there was no MH reaction (Brandom, 2009).

If you do not use triggering agents of any kind, you have no reason to keep dantrolene in the office. If a suspected MH reaction did occur, one should provide supportive care and call EMS for rapid transport to an ED capable of treating suspected MH.

Local anesthetics are not triggering agents and general dental practitioners and other dental specialists are not able to provide any monitoring except for blood pressure, pulse, respirations, and visual inspection. It would seem that no additional monitors or training is needed for these groups.

Silver Bullets for MH reactions

For MHS patients for whom the OMFS provides TIVA anesthesia care, what drug can be used for persistent laryngospasm requiring drug therapy when succinylcholine is contraindicated? At present, there are no rapid onset, short-acting neuromuscular blockers that approach the pharmacokinetics of succinylcholine. Rocuronium

Anesthesia Complications in the Dental Office, First Edition. Edited by Robert C. Bosack and Stuart Lieblich.

may be used for emergency treatment of laryngospasm since at higher doses of 1 mg/kg; onset of vocal cord paralysis may be 30 – 60 seconds. If rocuronium is used, the surgeon must be comfortable with long-term (30 - 60+ minutes) patient ventilation, generally with advanced airway devices and anesthetic maintenance.

A recent drug of interest is Sugammadex, a selective relaxant binding agent that can reverse the effects of steroidal non-depolarizing agents. An intubating dose of rocuronium was reversed in 2 minutes with an 8 mg/kg dose of Sugammadex. Unfortunately, it was denied approval in the United States because of allergic reactions, but it is used in Europe.

References

Brandom, B, and Rosenberg, H. *Clinical anesthesia*, 6th edn Philadelphia: Wolters Kluwer, 2009, pp 598 – 622.

Brandom B. Ambulatory surgery and malignant hyperthermia. *Curr Opin Anesthesiol* **22**: 744 – 747, 2009.

Rodrigues, J., et al. Successful management of malignant hyperthermia during orthognathic surgery: case report. *J Oral Maxillofac Surg* **66**: 1485 – 1488, 2008.

Index

Page references followed by *f* indicate an illustrated figure; followed by *t* indicate a table and followed by *n* indicate a note.

A

acidic epinephrine-containing solution, reinjection, 212
ACLS. *See* Advanced Cardiac Life Support (ACLS) algorithms
acute intoxication, 86
Addison's disease, 68
adenosine (Adenocard®), 195
adjustable gastric banding, 67
adrenocortical insufficiency (AI)
  adrenal function testing, 69
  ambulatory anesthesia, 68
  anesthetic management, 69
  antifungal agents and, 68
  primary, 68
  secondary, 68
  steroid equivalency chart, 68, 69*t*
Advanced Cardiac Life Support (ACLS) algorithms, 189, 228, 228*f*, 229, 229*f*
advanced heart blocks, 43
adverse drug interactions with vasoconstrictors
  monoamine oxidase inhibitors, 211, 211*t*
  nonselective β blockers, 210, 210*t*
  phenothiazines and α blockers, 210, 210*t*
  physiologic homeostasis, 210
  tricyclic antidepressants, 210, 211*t*
aging
  cardiovascular system, 98
  central nervous system, 97
  physiologic changes, 97, 98*t*
  renal system, 99
  respiratory system, 98–99
agitation and violence
  differential diagnosis, 265
  etiology and treatment, 265
  ketamine emergence, benzodiazepines, 265–266
  restraint, 266
  verbal de-escalation, 265
AI. *See* adrenocortical insufficiency (AI)
airway management
  complete obstruction, 181
  endotracheal tube, 183, 183*f*
  glottic and subglottic obstructions, 181
  Magill forceps, 183, 183*f*
  nasopharyngeal, 182, 182*f*
  oropharyngeal, 182, 182*f*
  partial obstruction, 181
  sedatives, narcotics and hypnotics, 181
  subdiaphragmatic, 181
  supraglottic (*see* supraglottic airway (SGA))
  ventilation with full face mask, patient with morbid obesity, 181, 181*f*
airway obstruction
  bag-valve mask, with oxygen reservoir, 231, 232*f*
  CVCI (*see* cannot ventilate, cannot intubate (CVCI))
  description, 231
  obstructive problems (*see* obstructive airway problems)
  physiologic problems (*see* physiologic airway problems)
  tray (*see* airway tray)
airway tray, 232*f*
  requirements, 231
  respiratory and mechanical problems, 231, 232*t*
alcohol abuse, 76, 85
allergy
  and anaphylaxis (*see* anaphylaxis)
  description, 251
  drugs, 252
  penicillin, 253*f*
  signs and symptoms, 251, 253*t*
alpha-2 agonists and dexmedetomidine
  adverse effects, 139
  organ systems, 139
  pharmacodynamics, 139
  pharmacokinetics, 139
Alzheimer's disease, 83, 84, 101, 215
American Society of Anesthesiologists (ASA), 9, 67, 163, 240, 241, 307
amide local anesthetics, 87, 130*f*, 208
amphetamines, 67, 76, 157
Amsorb, 148
anaphylaxis
  algorithm, 254
  angioedema of lower lip, 251, 253*f*
  antigen-specific IgE antibodies, 251
  classic signs, 251, 252*f*
  clinical features, 251, 253*t*
  diagnosis, 252
  diagnostic criterias, 251–252
  grades, 252
  hive located proximally on dorsal wrist, 251, 252*f*
  laryngeal edema, endoscopic view, 251, 254*f*
  management, 253–254
  non-immunologic reactions, 251
  normal larynx, 251, 254*f*
  penicillin allergy, 251, 253*f*
  prevention, 252–253
  risk factors, 251
  select inflammatory mediators, 251, 252*t*
Anectine®, 192
anesthesia refusal, 315
anesthesia team, 95, 272, 295–298, 316
anesthetic pharmacology
  central opioid receptors, 123
  impulse and $GABA_A$ and NMDA receptors, 123–124
  local, 129–131
  receptor concept, 123
angina/cardiac ischemia/infarct
  myocardial oxygen demand, 227, 227*t*
  sedated patient, 227
  ventricular ischemia, 227
angiotensin-converting enzyme (ACE) inhibitors, 27, 31, 89, 159
antacids, 20, 21, 238
anti-arrhythmic agents
  adenosine, 195
  amiodarone, 195
  calcium channel blockers, 195–196
  lidocaine, 195
anticholinergic (ACh) syndrome
  central and peripheral effects, 264, 264*t*
  central excitatory symptoms, 264
  cholinergic neurotransmitter, 264
  features, 264, 264*t*
  medications, 264, 264*t*
  treatment, 264
anticholinergics, 280
anticoagulation agents, 108–109
anticonvulsants, 196
antihistamines, 197, 279–280
  agents, 152
  autacoids, 151
  distribution, metabolism and elimination, 152
  mechanism and action site, 152
  in office-based anesthesia, 152
  organ systems, 152
antihypertensive agents
  β blockers, 194
  nitroglycerin, 194–195
antimuscarinics
  atropine and glycopyrrolate, 151, 152*t*
  mechanism and site of action, 151
  muscarinic receptor sites, 151, 152*t*
  pharmacodynamics and pharmacokinetics, 151
antiplatelet therapy, 31, 107–108
antithrombotic therapy, 107
anxiety disorders
  PTSD patients, 72
  symptoms, 71, 72*t*
aortic regurgitation, 34
aortic stenosis, 33–34
aspiration/foreign body ingestion
  acidic fluid, 239
  fasting guidelines, 238, 239*t*
  inadequate oropharyngeal drape, 238, 239, 239*f*
  risk factors, 238, 238*t*
  signs and symptoms, 239
  suspected/confirmed treatment, 239
  water absorbent foampad, oropharyngeal partition, 238, 239, 239*f*
aspirin
  acute coronary syndrome, 196
  in asthma, 54
  platelet cyclooxygenase inhibition, 108
  and thienopyridines, 108

Anesthesia Complications in the Dental Office, First Edition. Edited by Robert C. Bosack and Stuart Lieblich.

asthma
  anesthetic management, 54
  aspirin, 54
  bronchodilator response, 52
  lung volumes and capacities, 52*f*, 53
  medications, 53, 54*t*
  respiratory disease patients, 52–54
  risk assessment, 53
  severity and treatment recommendations, 53, 54*t*
  symptoms, 52
  treatment, 52–53
  triggers, 52
atrial fibrillation, 38, 39*f*, 107, 108, 159, 194
atrial kick, 33
atropine
  antimuscarinic anticholinergic drug, 196
  emergency drugs, 196
  and glycopyrrolate, 151, 152*t*
AuraOnce disposable laryngeal mask, 243, 243*f*
autacoids, 151
autism, 83–84

B
barbiturates
  adverse effects, 135–136
  methohexital and thiopental, 135
  organ systems, 135
  pharmacodynamics, 135
  pharmacokinetics, 135
benzodiazepines
  adverse effects, 139
  clinical characteristics, 203, 203*t*
  CNS depressants, 158
  disinhibition, 265
  fetal clefting, 119–120
  glucuronide, 157
  and metabolic inducers, 157
  and metabolic inhibitors, 158
  organ systems, 139
  pharmacodynamics, 138
  pharmacokinetics, 138–139
bispectral (BIS) analysis, 284
bleeding disorders
  anticoagulation agents, 108–109
  hemostasis, 103
  presurgical evaluation, 103
  thrombus formation, 103, 104*f*
  von Willebrand factor (vWBF), 104–105
bleomycin, 114, 145
blood urea nitrogen (BUN) and creatinine, laboratory evaluation, 16
BLS healthcare provider algorithm, 228, 228*f*
body mass index (BMI), 65, 66*t*
bradydysrhythmias
  escape beats, 42
  sinus bradycardia, 41–42
breast milk and infant formula, 19
bronchodilators, 52, 54, 137–138, 197, 318
bronchospasm
  anesthetic drugs, 237
  bronchial airway hyper-responsiveness, 236
  differential diagnosis, during anesthesia, 237, 237*t*
  inhaled SABA during facemask ventilation, 237, 237*f*
  inhaler adapter, 237, 237*f*
  inhaler placed in 60cc syringe, 237, 237*f*
  Luer Lock adapter on 90° connector, 237, 237*f*
  pulmonary history signaling increased risk, 236, 236*t*
  risk factors, 236, 236*t*
  SABAs, 236–237
BURP maneuver, 243, 245*f*

C
CAD. *See* coronary artery disease (CAD)
caffeine halothane contracture test (CHCT), 267, 267*f*
calcium channel blockers, 195–196
cancer
  airway considerations, 115
  cardiac toxicity, 115
  chemotherapy, 113–114
  classification and treatment, 113
  gastrointestinal considerations, 115
  hematologic considerations, 115
  malignancy
    chronic and acute pain, 114
    drug metabolism, 114
    vascular access, 114
  metabolic imbalances, 115
  nervous system considerations, 115
  psychological distress and depression, 114
  pulmonary toxicity, 115
  radiation, 114
  renal and hepatic failure, 115
  surgery, 114
  vascular access, 114
cannot ventilate, cannot intubate (CVCI)
  airway evaluation, 240
  American Society of Anesthesiologists, 240, 241*f*
  description, 240
  difficult airway definitions, 240, 240*t*
  office-based sedation/anesthesia (*see* office-based sedation/anesthesia)
  videolaryngoscopy, 241
capnography
  bronchospasm, 167, 168*f*
  capnogram, 167, 167*f*
  CO_2 sampling, 165, 166*f*
  divided cannula, 165, 166*f*
  $EtCO_2$, 167, 167*f*, 168*f*
  nasal cannula, 165, 166*f*
  respiratory membrane, 165
  ventilatory changes, 167
  waveform loss, 167, 167*f*
cardiac and cardiovascular studies, 17–18
cardiac dysrhythmias, 37–38
cardiac rhythm disorders
  dynamic ECG interpretation, 36*t*
  ECG tracing, 35, 36*f*
  heart, electrical system, 35*f*
  rhythm disorders, 35
  sinus rhythm, 35*f*
cardiac toxicity, 115
cardiopulmonary resuscitation (CPR), 178, 179
cardiovascular disease patients
  blood pressure, 26
  bradydysrhythmias, 41–42
  cardiac dilatation, 25
  cardiac dysrhythmias, 37–38
  cardiac muscle hypertrophy, 25
  cardiac rhythm disorders, 35–36
  cardiovascular implanted electronic devices (CIED), 43–44
  cardiovascular system, 25
  conduction disturbances, 42
  congestive heart failure, 45–47
  coronary artery disease, 29–33
  coronary perfusion, 25
  heart block, 42–43
  hypertension, 26–29
  implantable cardioverter defibrillators, 44–45
  pacemakers, 44
  systemic blood pressure, 25
  tachydysrhythmias, 38–40
  valvular heart disease, 34–35
  ventricular tachydysrhythmias, 40–41
cardiovascular implanted electronic devices (CIED), 43–44
cardiovascular problems
  blood pressure determinants, 219, 220*f*
  clinically significant variances, drugs selection, 221, 221*t*
  emergencies, 220
  mean arterial pressure, 219, 220*f*
  mechanisms, 219
  organ systems and anesthesia risk, 317–318
  patient resilience and reserve, 220, 220*t*
  perianesthetic
    cardiovascular adversity, 219, 220
    hypertension (*see* perianesthetic hypertension)
    hypotension (*see* perianesthetic hypotension)
  PSVT (*see* paroxysmal supraventricular tachycardia (PSVT))
  PVCs (*see* premature ventricular complexes (PVCs))
  sinus tachycardia, 225, 225*f*
  syncope (*see* syncope)
cardiovascular risk assessment
  ASA physical status score, 9, 10*t*
  dental patients evaluation, 9
  examination, 10–11
  extent of risk, elements, 10
  physical symptoms, 9
  preexisting diseases, 9
  resilience, 9–10
  screening questions, 10*t*
  surgery and anesthesia, elements, 10, 11*t*
carpopedal spasm, 232, 232*f*
central pattern generator (CPG), 277
cerebral palsy, 81–82, 82*t*
CHCT. *See* caffeine halothane contracture test (CHCT)
chemotherapy, 107, 113–114, 115, 145
chest wall rigidity, 233
Child-Turcotte-Pugh score, 86, 86*t*
cholinergic crisis, 81
cholinergic deficiency, 99
chronic bronchitis and emphysema, 55
chronic kidney disease (CKD), 89–90, 90*t*. *See also* renal disease
chronic obstructive pulmonary disease (COPD), 55, 56, 144–145, 189, 194
CIED. *See* cardiovascular implanted electronic devices (CIED)
The Cincinnati Prehospital Stroke Scale (CPSS), 258, 259*t*
clear liquids, 19
coagulation studies, 16
cocaine, 76, 210
complete airway obstruction, 181
complete blood count, laboratory evaluation, 16
complications. *See also* localized complications
  anesthesia selection, delivery, dose, and duration, 309–310
  anesthetic, 4, 4*t*
  definition, 3
  monitoring and evaluation, anesthesia, 310
  morbidity and mortality, 295
  patient candidacy, selection, and preparation, 309
  perianesthetic, 4
  perioperative pulmonary, 11*t*
  preparation, 311
  resuscitation and staff/team response, 310–311
  scope, 4
  simulation technique, dental anesthesia, 178
  supplemental oxygen administration, 51–52
  surgical neck entry, 244
  systemic, 208–211
congestive heart failure
  anesthetic concerns, 46–47
  definition, 45
  pathophysiology, 45–46
  risk assessment, 46
  treatment

digoxin, 46
diuretics, 46
continuing education (CE) programs, 307
COPD. *See* chronic obstructive pulmonary disease (COPD)
coronary artery disease (CAD)
active cardiac conditions, 31, 32*t*
anesthetic concerns, 32–33
definition, 29
myocardial oxygen balance, 30*t*
pathophysiology, 29–30
risk assessment, 31–32
risk factors, 29*t*
spectrum, 30*t*
treatment
angiotensin-converting enzyme (ACE) inhibitors, 31
antiplatelet therapy, 31
beta-blockers, 30
lifestyle modification, 30
nitrates, 31
corticosteroids, 53, 68, 69, 81, 197, 253
CPG. *See* central pattern generator (CPG)
CPR. *See* cardiopulmonary resuscitation (CPR)
CPSS. *See* The Cincinnati Prehospital Stroke Scale (CPSS)
cricoid pressure, 21, 239
cricothyrotomy
Shiley low pressure cuffed tracheostomy, 246, 247*f*
shoulder support, neck extension, 246, 247f
surgical tray, 246, 247*f*
Trousseau dilator (Kelly hemostats), 246
crisis resource management (CRM), 4, 316
adverse outcomes, 173
clinicians, 174
communication, 175
computerized full-body simulator, 173
decision-making during, 175
description, 173
elements, 173, 174*t*
errors, 173, 174
hazardous attitudes, 175
latent factors, 174
situational awareness, 173
The Swiss cheese model, 174, 174*f*
training, 175
CRM. *See* crisis resource management (CRM)
crystalloids *vs.* colloids, 187–188
CVCI. *See* cannot ventilate, cannot intubate (CVCI)
cyanosis, 11, 165*t*, 208, 232, 239
cyclooxygenase (COX) enzymes, 159
cytochrome P450 inducers, 158, 158*t*

D
dantrolene (Dantrium®), 192
decision-making process
anesthesia/case refusal, 315
cardiovascular diseases, 317–318
eating disorders, 316–317
endocrine diseases, 318
geriatric patients, 319
neurologic diseases, 318
office-based anesthesia, 315–316
pediatric patients, 318–319
preoperative preparation, 316
preparation, anesthesia team, 316
psychiatric illness, 317
respiratory considerations, 318
deep sedation, limitations, 204
delayed awakening, anesthesia
airway and vital signs, 287
drug effects, 287–288
management, 288–289
pathophysiologic changes, 288
surgical procedure and anesthesia, 287
dental death
after incident, 304–305
anesthesia, recommendations, 303
assumption, 299
emergency supplies and lighting recommendations, 303
fault, 302
first responders, recommended procedures, 304
informed consent, 302
investigations
anesthesia, 300
assistants, 300
dentist, 299–300
drugs, procedure and emergency, 301
emergency, dentist and staff reaction, 300–301
equipment, 300
incident report, 301
patient, 300
record, procedure and emergency, 301
patient identification, 304
patient in distress, recommended procedures, 303–304
post-emergency don'ts, 305
record keeping recommendations, 303
sedation equipment, recommendations, 302–303
written protocols, 302
depolarization, 79
desflurane, 147, 148, 257, 267
dexamethasone, 64, 197, 278
dextrose-containing solutions, 188
diabetes mellitus (DM)
anesthetic management, 63–64
daily glucose control, 61
description, 61
drugs for, 61
hemoglobin A1c values, 63*t*
hypoglycemia, 62–63, 64
insulin pump and transcutaneous glucose sensor, 63*f*
insulin, subcutaneous injection, 61, 62*t*
long-term blood glucose control, 61
non-insulin injectables, 61, 62*t*
oral antihyperglycemic agents, 61, 62*t*
direct laryngoscopy
anteriorly tilted larynx, 243, 245*f*
BURP maneuver, 243, 245*f*
The King Vision videolaryngoscope, 244, 246*f*
McGrath Mac® Videolaryngoscope, 244, 245*f*
oral, pharyngeal and laryngeal axes, 243
proper laryngoscope hand position, 243, 245*f*
videolaryngoscope mitigation, 243
DM. *See* diabetes mellitus (DM)
dopamine (D2) receptor antagonists, 279
Down syndrome, 83
drug interactions
anesthetic agents, 155
antagonism, 155–156
benzodiazepines, 157–158
epinephrine, 157
opioid agonists (*see* opioids)
pharmaceutical, 156–157
pharmacodynamic, 156
pharmacokinetic, 156
potentiation, 156
propofol and ketamine, 155
risk factors, 155
synergistic effects, 156
triazolam, 156
unexpected drug effects, 156
drug tolerance, 76

E
eating disorders
anorexia nervosa, 75
cardiac conduction abnormalities, 75
organ systems and anesthesia risk, 316–317, 317*f*
preexisting hypotension, 75
self-imposed disorders, 75
ECF. *See* extracellular fluid (ECF)
ECT. *See* electroconvulsive therapy (ECT)
ectopic beats
tachydysrhythmias, 38, 39*f*
ventricular tachydysrhythmias, 40–41, 41*f*
electrocardiogram, 17
electrocardiography (ECG)
electrodes, 167
lead II, 167, 168*t*
rhythm, 168
electroconvulsive therapy (ECT), 283
Emergency Department (ED) team, 310
emergency drugs
ACLS, 189
anesthesia and sedation, 189
anti-arrhythmic agents (*see* anti-arrhythmic agents)
anticonvulsants, 196
antihistamines, 197
antihypertensive agents (*see* antihypertensive agents)
aspirin, 196
atropine, 196
bronchodilators, 197
corticosteroids, 197
group drugs, adverse event, 189, 190*t*
management drugs, adverse events, 189, 190*t*
morphine, 196
muscle relaxants (*see* muscle relaxants)
oxygen administration, 189–190
reversal agents (*see* reversal agents)
vasopressors (*see* vasopressors)
EmergencyMedical Services (EMS), 298
EMLA®. *See* Eutectic Mixture of Local Anesthetics (EMLA®)
endocrinopathies patients
adrenocortical insufficiency (AI), 68–69
diabetes mellitus (DM), 62–64
obesity and post-bariatric surgery, 65–68
thyroid disorders, 64–65
endotracheal tubes, 183, 183*f*
Enk oxygen flow modulator®, 245, 246*f*
enteral sedation agents
non-benzodiazepine hypnotics, 133
termination, 134
triazolam, 133
zaleplon, 133
zolpidem, 133
ephedrine, 38, 47, 77, 157, 193, 224, 227
epinephrine
MAOIs, 157
and non-selective β blockers, 157
reversal, 210
TCAs and SNRIs, 157
vasopressors, 192–193
errors
anesthetic, 3, 4*t*
definition, 3
human condition, 3–4
scope, 3
triggering events, 3, 4*t*
escape beats, 42
Eutectic Mixture of Local Anesthetics (EMLA®), 203
extracellular fluid (ECF), 185
eye surgery, 145

F
FDA pregnancy risk categories, 119, 119*t*
fetal hypoxemia
benzodiazepines, 119–120
drug-free blood, 119
FDA pregnancy risk categories, 119, 119*t*
first trimester, 118

fetal hypoxemia (*continued*)
ketamine, 120
local anesthetics, 119
nitrous oxide, 120
opioids, 120
second trimester, 118–119
sedatives and hypnotics, 120
vasoconstrictors, 119
first degree heart block, 42, 42*f*
flumazenil (Romazicon®), 191
foreign body ingestion
Magills forceps, 239
perforation, 240
pulmonary assessment, 239
trachea and mainstem bronchi, 239, 240*f*
The 4–2–1 rule, maintenance fluid requirements, 186–187, 186*t*
fresh frozen plasma (FFP), 109
functional hypovolemia, 85

G
gamma-aminobutyric acid channel ($GABA_A$), 123, 124*f*
gastric prokinetics, 20–21
gateway drug, 76
geriatric patients
age (*see* aging)
anesthetic management, 99, 100*t*
dental professionals, 97
perioperative complications, 100–101
pharmacologic considerations, 99
preanesthetic evaluation, 99
glomerular filtration rate (GFR), 89
glottic and subglottic obstructions, 181
glottic obstruction
laryngeal edema, 236, 236*f*
laryngospasm (*see* laryngospasm)

H
heart block
advanced heart blocks, 43
first degree heart block, 42, 42*f*
second-degree heart block, Mobitz I, 42–43, 43*f*
hemophilia
A and B, 105–106
and inhibitors, 106–107
hemostasis, 85, 86, 103, 104, 110, 159, 188
heparin-inducted thrombocytopenia (HIT), 108
hepatic disease
acute intoxication, 86
amide local anesthetics, 87
Child-Turcotte-Pugh score, 86, 86*t*
chronic liver disease and cirrhosis, 86
hyperdynamic circulation, 86
liver disease, 85–86
parenteral anesthetic agents, 86
pseudocholinesterase concentration, 87
risk assessment, 86
Hunter serotonin toxicity criteria, 263, 263*t*
hypertension
anesthetic concerns, 29
autoregulation, 28, 29*f*
blood pressure classification, 26*t*
definition, 26
hypertensive crises, 26
pathophysiology, 26–27
risk assessment, 28–29
treatment
angiotensin receptor blockers (ARBs), 27
angiotensin-converting enzyme (ACE) inhibitors, 27
beta-adrenergic blockers, 27–28
calcium channel blockers (CCBs), 28
diuretics, 27
hyperthyroid disease, 64–65
hyperventilation
abnormal cortical state, 232
alkalosis, 231
carpopedal spasm, 232, 232*f*
definition, 231
intra-/postanesthetic delirium, 232
postanesthetic delirium, 231
treatment of, 232
hypothyroid disease, 65
hypoventilation
definition, 232
drug reversal, 233
narcotics, time to peak effects, 232, 233*t*
respiratory depression, 232
slow/absent ventilation, 232

I
ICF. *See* intracellular fluid compartments (ICF)
iGel™, supraglottic airways, 182, 183*f*
impaired disorders development
Alzheimer's disease, 84
autism, 83–84
Down syndrome, 83
implantable cardioverter defibrillators, 44–45
inadvertent intra-arterial injection, 272
individual gases
desflurane, 147
isoflurane, 147
sevoflurane, 148
volatile anesthetic agents, 147, 147*t*
infiltration and extravasation
catheter/needle, 271
causes of slow/stopped IV fluid flow, 271, 271*t*
dental anesthesia, 272
non-vesicant solution (IV fluids), 271
informed consent, 300, 302, 308, 309, 315
inhalational anesthetic agents
nitrous oxide (*see* nitrous oxide pharmacology)
pharmacodynamics, 146
pharmacokinetics, 146–147
intracellular fluid compartments (ICF), 185
intramuscular and subcutaneous administration, 204
intraoperative awareness
amnesia, 283
amygdala, 283
description, 283
drugs, 284
ECT and brain trauma, 283
etiology, 284
explicit and implicit memory, 283
incidence, 284
management, 285
memory formation, 283, 284*f*
perianesthetic conscious awareness, 284
prevention, 284
PTSD (*see* post-traumatic stress disorder (PTSD))
intravenous access
catheters, 271
inadvertent intra-arterial injection, 272
infiltration and extravasation, 271–272, 271*t*
reversal/emergency drugs, 271
risk factors for displacement, 271, 271*t*
thrombophlebitis, 272, 272*f*
intravenous administration, sedation failure, 203–204
intravenous fluid (IVF) therapy
4–2–4 rule, maintenance fluid requirements, 186–187, 186*t*
common crystalloid solutions, components, 187, 187*t*
compartments in body, 185, 186*f*
crystalloids *vs.* colloids, 187–188
current ASA NPO guidelines, 185, 186*t*
dextrose-containing solutions, 188
fluid loss, 185
physical examination, 185–186
surgical and anesthetic treatment, 185
tonicity, 188
investigation, dental death
anesthesia record, 302
controlled substances records, 302
dentist's interview, 301
emergency supplies, 301
equipment used, 301
facility, 301
records, 301–302
staff interviews, 301
training and continuing medical education, verification, 301
isoflurane, 147, 148
IVF. *See* intravenous fluid (IVF) therapy

K
ketamine, 120
adverse effects, 138
in office-based anesthesia, 138
organ systems, 138
pharmacodynamics, 137–138
pharmacokinetics, 138
King LT airway, 243, 244*f*
King LT(S)–D™, 182, 183*f*
The King Vision videolaryngoscope, 244, 246*f*

L
laboratory evaluation
basic metabolic panel, 16*f*
BUN and creatinine, 16
potassium, 15–16
serum glucose, 16
sodium, 15
cardiac and cardiovascular studies, 17–18
coagulation studies, 16
complete blood count, 16, 17*t*
liver function tests, 16–17
pre-anesthetic testing rationale, 15*t*
pregnancy tests, 17
radionucleotide angiography, 18
radionucleotide tests and cardiac catheterizations, 18
stress tests, 18
LAPSS. *See* Los Angeles Prehospital Stroke Screen (LAPSS)
laryngeal edema, 236, 236*f*
laryngeal mask airway (LMA), 234
laryngospasm
bronchospasm, 235
intravascular access, 236
negative intrathoracic pressures, 235
risk factors, 235, 235*t*
treatment, 235
videolaryngoscope view, 234, 235*f*
latent errors, 3
law of anesthesia, 307
LBW. *See* lean body weight (LBW)
lean body weight (LBW), 68
legal issues, risks/malpractice
causation, 308
conduct, 308
Doctor's letterhead with telephone number, 312
law of anesthesia, 307
licensing agencies, 308
litigation, evidence and nature, 308
negligence, 307
requisite proof, 308
risk/substandard care, 308
standards of care, 307
violation of statute/code, 307–308
lipophilic drugs, 136*f*
liver function tests, laboratory evaluation, 16–17
LMA. *See* laryngeal mask airway (LMA)
local anesthetic failure

acidic epinephrine-containing solution, reinjection, 212
inability, mandibular block, 211, 211*f*, 212*f*
infiltration into inflamed tissues/near painful regions, 211
nonmyelinated c fibers, 211–212
local anesthetic pharmacology
1.8cc cartridge, 130
dose numbers, 130
drug properties, 129
Ester and Amide local anesthetics, 129, 130*f*
maximum allowable doses, 130, 131
properties, 129, 130*t*
sodium (Na^+) channels, 129
local anesthetic systemic toxicity, 207, 208*f*, 208*t*
local (topical) hemostatic measurement, 109–110
local standard of care qualifier, 307
localized complications
injection pain and transient facial blanching, 212, 212*f*, 213*f*
local anesthetic failure (*see* local anesthetic failure)
needle breakage (*see* needle breakage)
nerve injury, 216–217
opthalmologic complications, 214–215, 215*f*
tissue injury (*see* localized tissue injury)
unintended nerve involvement, 213–214, 214*f*
vascular injury (*see* vascular injury)
localized tissue injury
after mandibular block injection, 215, 215*f*
lip biting, 215, 216*f*
lip sucking, 215, 216*f*
physical and/or chemical injury, 215
post inadvertent tongue biting after mandibular block anesthesia, 215, 216*f*
post-mandibular block trismus, 215, 215*f*
Los Angeles Prehospital Stroke Screen (LAPSS), 258
lost airway algorithm, dental professional, 246–248
Lou Gehrig's disease, 79
low molecular weight heparins (LMWH), 109*t*
Luer Lock adapter on 90° connector, 237, 237*f*

M

Magill forceps, 183, 183*f*
malignant hyperthermia (MH)
CHCT, 267, 267*f*
clinical presentation, 267
core temperatures, 267
crisis management, 268–269, 268*f*
and genetic testing, 267–268
hypermetabolic crisis, 266
MMR, 269
myodystrophies, 269
pathophysiology, 266, 266*f*
postoperative, 267
recrudescence, 267
risk of pediatric, 266
malignant hyperthermia (MH)., 147
Mallampatti classification, 13
marijuana, 76
Masseter muscle rigidity (MMR), 269
McGrath Mac® Videolaryngoscope, 244, 245*f*
mean arterial pressure (MAP), 89
metabolic syndrome, 66, 66*t*
MH. *See* malignant hyperthermia (MH)
minimum alveolar concentration (MAC), 147
mitral regurgitation, 34
mitral stenosis, 34
mitral valve prolapse (MVP), 34
R. *See* Masseter muscle rigidity (MMR)D

monoamine oxidase inhibitor (MAOIs) drugs, 157, 211, 211*t*
mood disorders
antimanic agents, 73
bipolar illness, 73
depression, 72, 72*t*
drugs, 72, 74*t*
lithium, 73
management, 73*t*
monoamine oxidase inhibitors (MAOI), 73
selective serotonin reuptake inhibitors (SSRI), 72
tricyclic antidepressants, 72–73
morbidity and mortality
allegations, anesthetic complications
anesthesia team's documentation, 295
cardiorespiratory event, 295
office charts, 295
office anesthesia mortality, review
airway maintenance, anatomic challenges, 296
challenging the judgment, 297
decision to use sedation or general anesthetic, 297
delay in event recognition, 296
delay in instituting rescue, 296
doctor judgment, 297
failure to regain consciousness, 297
failure to resuscitate, 296
inadequate assistance, 297
inadequate preanesthetic history, 297
loss of adequate oxygenation, 296
morphine, severe pain management, 196
motor neuron disease
amyotrophic lateral sclerosis (ALS), 79–80
spinal muscular atrophy, 79
multimodal therapy, 280
multiple sclerosis, 81
muscarinic receptor sites, 151, 152*t*
muscle relaxants
dantrolene, 192
succinylcholine, 192
muscular dystrophy, 81
MVP. *See* mitral valve prolapse (MVP)
Myasthenia gravis, 80–81

N

naloxone (Narcan®), 191
nasopharyngeal airway, 182, 182*f*
needle breakage
medial pterygoid space, 215, 216*f*
three-dimensional reconstruction, 215, 217*f*
negative pressure pulmonary edema (NPPE), 238
negligence, 307–308
neurologic disease
cerebral palsy, 81–82, 82*t*
impaired disorders development, 82–84
motor neuron disease, 79–80
multiple sclerosis, 81
muscular dystrophy, 81
Myasthenia gravis, 80–81
Parkinson disease, 80
seizure disorders, 82–83, 82*t*
nitrous oxide pharmacology
adverse effects, 144–145
chemical structure, 144*f*
clinical use, 145
concomitant administration, 146
oversedation, 146
pharmacodynamics, 143
pharmacokinetics, 143–144
physical properties, 143
physiologic effects, 144
safety measurement, 145–146
sedation, 146
N-methyl D-aspartate (NMDA) receptor, 123–124, 125*f*
nonmyelinated c fibers, 211–212
non-rebreather mask, 189
nonselective β blockers, 210, 210*t*
nonsteroidal anti-inflammatory analgesics (NSAIDs)
ACE inhibitors, 159
and immunosuppressive drugs, 159–160
lithium and, 160
maintenance, 159
and warfarin (Coumadin), 159
non-surgical weight loss, 66–67
NPO guidelines
ASA guidelines, 19, 20*t*
breast milk and infant formula, 19
clear liquids, 19
critical values, 19
preoperative therapeutics
antacids, 20
cricoid pressure, 21
gastric prokinetics, 20–21
PPIs and H_2 blockers, 21
pulmonary aspiration risk, 19, 20*t*
solid foods and nonhuman milk, 19–20
NPPE. *See* negative pressure pulmonary edema (NPPE)

O

obesity and post-bariatric surgery
adjustable gastric banding, 67
body mass index (BMI), 65, 66*t*
lean body weight (LBW), 68
metabolic syndrome, 66, 66*t*
non-surgical weight loss, 66–67
obese patient, anesthetic management, 67–68
obstructive sleep apnea (OSA), 66
osteoarthritis, 66
problematic tracheal intubation, 66
ventilation–perfusion mismatching, 66
obstructive airway problems
blood soaked, untethered gauze pack hypopharynx, 234, 235*f*
glottic (*see* glottic obstruction)
proper placement, oropharyngeal airway, 234, 234*f*
quadruple airway maneuver, 234, 234*f*
"rocking boat" movement, 233
SGA obstruction, 233, 233*f*
subglottic (*see* subglottic obstruction)
supraglottic devices, 234, 234*f*
tethered throat pack, hypopharynx, 234, 235*f*
triple airway maneuver, 233*f*, 234
obstructive disease, 52
obstructive sleep apnea (OSA), 66
airway dilators, 57
airway patency, 57*f*
anesthetic concerns, 58–59
cardiovascular consequences, 57–58
description, 56–57
pathophysiologic repetitive cycle, 57, 57*f*
predisposing factors, 57
risk assessment, 58
office-based anesthesia
anesthetic monitoring, 163, 164
direct visualization, 163
pretracheal auscultation (*see* pretracheal auscultation)
pulse oximetry (*see* pulse oximetry)
vigilance, 163
office-based sedation/anesthesia
ACh (*see* anticholinergic (ACh) syndrome)
aggression and violence, 262
agitation, 262, 262*t* (*see also* agitation and violence)
anxiety, 262
benzodiazepine disinhibition, 265
cognition, 261–262
confusion, 262
continuum of, 261, 262*t*
delirium, risk factors and precipitating factors, 262, 262*t*
description, 241
licensure and consent issues, 261
likelihood of

office-based sedation/anesthesia (*continued*)
 airway collapse with sedatives, opioids/hypnotics, 242, 242*f*
 direct laryngoscopy (*see* direct laryngoscopy)
 intubation, 244
 mask ventilation, 242, 242*f*, 243*f*, 243*n*
 SGA (*see* supraglottic airway (SGA))
 surgical neck entry (*see* surgical neck entry)
 lost airway algorithm, dental professional, 246–248
 MH (*see* malignant hyperthermia (MH))
 perception, 261
 perianesthetic delirious behavior, 262
 safety, 315–316
 sedative/anesthetic medications, 261
 serotonin (*see* serotonin (5-HT/5-hydroxytryptamine))
open airway general anesthesia, 204
opioids, 120
 abuse, 76
 adverse effects, 140
 agonists
 and benzodiazepines, 158
 meperidine, 158–159
 organ systems, 140
 pharmacodynamics, 139–140
 pharmacokinetics, 140
Oral and Maxillofacial Surgeons' (OMS), 295
oral dabigatran, 109
oral sedation
 agents, 201
 in dental patients, 202
 difficult patients, 203
 empiric dosages, 202–203, 203*t*
 latency period, drug, 202
 oral titration, multiple/stacked dosing, 201
 residual effects, 203
organ systems and anesthesia risk
 cardiovascular diseases, 317–318
 eating disorders, 316–317
 endocrine diseases, 318
 geriatric patients, 319
 neurologic diseases, 318
 pediatric patients, 318–319
 psychiatric illness, 317
 respiratory considerations, 318
oropharyngeal airway, 182, 182*f*, 234*f*
orthostatic hypotension, 222
osteoarthritis, 32, 66

P

PABA. *See* para-amino benzoic acid (PABA)
pacemakers, 35, 38, 43, 44, 317
PADSS. *See* post-anesthesia discharge scoring system (PADSS)
para-amino benzoic acid (PABA), 253
parenteral anesthetic agents, 86
 barbiturates (*see* barbiturates)
 non-barbiturate intravenous anesthetics (*see* propofol)
parenteral moderate sedation, 203
Parkinson disease, 80
paroxysmal supraventricular tachycardia (PSVT), 38–39, 40*f*
 ACLS adult tachycardia (with pulse), 227
 adenosine, 226–227
 bidirectional pathway, 226, 226*f*
 carotid sinus massage, 226, 226*f*
 description, 225, 226*f*
partial airway obstruction, 181
pediatric patients
 airway, 93, 94*f*
 cardiovascular system, 93–94
 pharmacodynamics, 94, 94*t*
 preoperative evaluation, 94–95
 pulmonary system, 93
 sedative/anesthetic techniques, 95–96
percutaneous cannulas, 245–246, 247*f*
percutaneous catheter
 cricothyroid membrane identification, 245
 Enk oxygen flow modulator®, 245, 246*f*
 intravenous catheter, 244, 246*f*
perianesthetic complications, 4
perianesthetic hypertension
 acute increases in blood pressure, office based anesthesia, 224, 224*t*
 afterload and myocardial wall tension, 224
 drugs/treatment thresholds, 224
 hydralazine, peripheral arteriolar dilator, 225
 hypertensive urgencies, 224
 nitroglycerin, venous dilator, 224–225
perianesthetic hypotension
 acute decreases in blood pressure, office based anesthesia, 223, 223*t*
 anesthetic drugs administration, 223
 arterial blood pressure, 223
 ephedrine and phenylephrine, 224
peripherally inserted central catheters (PICC), 114, 114*f*
pharmacokinetic profile
 biotransformation and elimination, 127
 body tissue compartments, 125, 125*t*, 126*f*
 distribution and drug clearance, 124
 drug accumulation, 126, 126*f*
 gastrointestinal enzymes, 125
 graphic depiction, 126, 126*f*
 short-acting drugs, 126
 vessel-rich structures, 126
phenothiazines and α blockers, 210, 210*t*
phenylephrine, 65, 193–194, 224
physiologic airway problems
 chest wall rigidity, 233
 hyperventilation (*see* hyperventilation)
 hypoventilation/apnea (*see* hypoventilation)
physiologic homeostasis, 210
physostigmine drug, 191–192
PONV. *See* postoperative nausea and vomiting (PONV)
post-anesthesia discharge scoring system (PADSS), 291, 292
postoperative cognitive deficit or decline (POCD), 100–101
postoperative nausea and vomiting (PONV)
 anesthetic risks modification, 278
 definition, 277
 5-HT-3 RA receptor antagonists, 277
 incidence and risk factors, 277–278, 279*t*
 medical management
 anticholinergics, 280
 antihistamines, 279–280
 dexamethasone, 278
 dopamine (D2) receptor antagonists, 279
 multimodal therapy, 280
 propofol, 280
 serotonin (5-hydroxytryptamine) receptor antagonists, 278
 office protocols, 280
 pathophysiology, 277, 278*f*
 post discharge, 280
post-traumatic stress disorder (PTSD)
 features, 284, 285*t*
 recall extent, intraoperative awareness, 284, 285*t*
potassium, laboratory evaluation, 15–16
pre-excitation syndromes, 39–40
pregnancy tests, laboratory evaluation, 17
pregnant patients
 anxiety and pain, 117
 cardiovascular system, 118
 central nervous system, 118
 gastrointestinal system, 118
 morbidity, 117
 respiratory system, 117–118
premature ventricular complexes (PVCs)
 β blocker therapy, 227
 during anesthesia, 227
 angina/cardiac ischemia/infarct (*see* angina/cardiac ischemia/infarct)
 ectopic beats, 40–41, 41*f*
 hypoxia/sympathetic stimulation, 227
 sinus bradycardia, 227, 227*t*
preoperative preparation and testing, 316
pretracheal auscultation
 headsets, 163, 165*f*
 weighted bell placement, 163, 166*f*
problematic tracheal intubation, 66
propofol, 280
 adverse effects, 137
 organ systems, 137
 pharmacodynamics, 136
 pharmacokinetics, 136–137
prosthetic heart valves, 35
proton pump inhibitors (PPIs) and H_2 blockers, 21
pseudocholinesterase concentration, 87
PSVT. *See* paroxysmal supraventricular tachycardia (PSVT)
psychiatric illness
 abnormal behavior, 71
 American Psychiatric Association, 71
 anxiety disorders, 71–72
 disorder, 71
 eating disorders, 75–76
 mood disorders, 72–73
 organ systems and anesthesia risk, 317
 patient management, 76–77
 problematic psychogenic issues, 71
 psychiatric disorders, 71, 72*t*
 substance abuse, 76
 thought disorders, 73–75
psychological precursors, 3
PTSD. *See* post-traumatic stress disorder (PTSD)
pulmonary risk assessment
 anesthetic drugs, 11
 examination, 11–12
 oxygenation, 11
 perioperative pulmonary complications, risk factor, 11*t*
 smoking, 11
 symptoms and diseases, 11
 upper airway risk assessment, 12–13, 12*f*–13*f*
pulmonary toxicity, 115
pulse oximetry
 cardiopulmonary monitoring, 165*t*
 depth of sedation, 165*t*
 hemoglobin, 164
 oximeter functions, 164
 oxygen–hemoglobin dissociation curve, 164, 166*f*
PVCs. *See* premature ventricular complexes (PVCs)

Q

"quadruple" airway maneuver, 234, 234*f*
Quelicin®, 192

R

radionucleotide angiography, 18
renal disease
 anatomy, nephron, 90, 90*f*
 CKD (*see* chronic kidney disease (CKD))
 classification, 89
 comorbidities, 90–91
 description, 89
 risk assessment, 91–92
 treatment, 91
reperfusion therapy, 258
requisite proof, legal issues, 308
respiratory disease patients

asthma, 52–54
chronic bronchitis and emphysema, 55
complications, 51–52
lung volumes and capacities, 49
obstructive disease, 52
obstructive sleep apnea (OSA), 56–59
perianesthetic complications, 51–52
respiratory system macroscopic level, 50*f*, 51*f*
restrictive disease, 55–56
smoking, 56
supplemental oxygen administration, 49–52
upper respiratory tract infection, 56
ventilation, 49
reversal agents
agonists, 190
antagonists, 191
blockers, 191
flumazenil, 191
naloxone, 191
physostigmine, 191–192
Revised Cardiac Risk Index, 10
The Richmond agitation sedation scale, 262, 262*t*
risk assessment
ASA physical status, 9
cardiovascular, 9–11
definition, 9
pulmonary, 11–13
risk/substandard care, 308
rivaroxaban, 108–109
Rusch QuickTrach® TELEFLEX MEDICAL, 245–246, 247*f*

S
SABAs. *See* short-acting β–agonists (SABAs)
safe discharge
early recovery, 291
home readiness, 292
intermediate recovery, 291
late recovery, 291
modified aldrete score, 291*t*
office-based anesthesia
60–90 minutes, monitored observation, 292
airway compromise, risk, 292
normal vital signs, 292
postoperative instructions, 292
parameters missing from PADSS, 292
post-anesthesia discharge scoring system (PADSS), 292*t*
standardized system, 291
time for, 291
second-degree heart block, Mobitz I, 42–43, 43*f*
sedation failure
continuum of depth, 201, 202*t*
deep sedation, 204
intramuscular and subcutaneous administration, 204
intravenous administration, 203–204
normal distribution curve, 201, 202*f*
office-based sedation, 201, 201*t*
open airway general anesthesia, 204
oral sedation (*see* oral sedation)
parenteral moderate sedation, 203
patient preparation, 201
underdosing and overdosing, 201
sedative/anesthetic techniques, 95–96
seizure
anesthetic agents, 257
benzodiazepines, 258
classification, 257, 258*t*
description, 257
diagnosis, 257
disorders, 82–83, 82*t*
early management, dental office, 258, 258*t*
preanesthetic evaluation, 257, 258*t*
transient metabolic disturbances, 257
serotonin (5-HT/5-hydroxytryptamine)
features, 263, 263*t*
Hunter serotonin toxicity criteria, 263, 263*t*
MAO synthesis, 262
medications, 263, 263*t*
mydriasis, tachycardia and hypertension, 263
receptor antagonists, 278
stepwise treatment, 263
symptom spectrum, 263, 263*t*
serotonin-norepinephrine reuptake inhibitors (SNRIs), 157
serum glucose, laboratory evaluation, 16
sevoflurane, 148
SGA. *See* supraglottic airway (SGA)
Shiley low pressure cuffed tracheostomy, 246, 247*f*
short-acting β–agonists (SABAs), 236–237
simulation technique, dental anesthesia
advantages, 177
cardiac problems, 178
definition, 177
in designing, 178–179
diabetic patients, complications, 178
drug complications, 178
on emergencies, 178
evaluation, 177
full body computer controlled simulators, 177
occurrences, 178
people training, 177
students and junior resident practitioners, 178
task trainers, 177
teaching and assessment, 177
video recording, 178
virtual reality, 177
sinus bradycardia, 41–42, 227, 227*t*
sinus pause, 42, 42*f*, 222
sinus tachycardia, 225, 225*f*
smoking, 11, 56, 237
sodium, laboratory evaluation, 15
solid foods and nonhuman milk, 19–20
sphygomomanometry
blood pressure measurement, 168
measurement intervals, 168–169
stethoscope, 168
spironolactone, 46
standards of care, 307
status epilepticus, 196
stress tests, 18
stroke
acute neurological impairment, 258
CPSS, 258, 259*t*
LAPSS, 258
management, 259, 259*f*
risk factors, 258
signs of symptoms, 258, 258*t*
tissue plasminogen activator, 258
subdiaphragmatic obstruction, 181
subglottic obstruction
aspiration/foreign body ingestion (*see* aspiration/foreign body ingestion)
bronchospasm (*see* bronchospasm)
foreign body ingestion (*see* foreign body ingestion)
NPPE, 238
substance abuse, 76
succinylcholine (Anectine®), 192
supplemental oxygen administration
nasal cannula, 49, 53*f*
nasal hood with passive fit, 49, 53*f*
nasal mask with tight fit, 49, 53*f*
non-rebreather, 50
non-rebreather mask, 49, 53*f*
perianesthetic complications, 51–52
ventilation, 49–50
supraglottic airway (SGA)
AuraOnce disposable LMA, 182, 182*f*
higher ventilator pressures, 183
iGel™, 182, 183*f*
King LT (S)-D™, 182, 183*f*
obstructive airway problems, 233, 233*f*
placement and ventilation
AuraOnce disposable laryngeal mask, 243, 243*f*
igel, non-inflatable supraglottic airway, 243, 244*f*
King LT airway, 243, 244*f*
potential problems with LMA placement, 243, 244*f*
supraventricular tachydysrhythmias, 38, 39*f*
surgical neck entry
complications, 244
cricothyrotomy (*see* cricothyrotomy)
percutaneous cannulas, 245–246, 247*f*
percutaneous catheter, 244–245, 246*f*
psychological reluctance, 244
The Swiss cheese model, 174, 174*f*
syncope
classic vasovagal, healthy patients, 222, 222*t*
etiology, 221, 221*t*
metabolic derangements, 222
neurologic seizures diagnosis, 223
orthostatic hypotension, 222
patient with pre-syncopal signs, 222, 222*f*
rhythm strip, 222, 223*f*
sinus pause, 222, 222*f*
treatment protocol, 223
vasovagal (neurocardiogenic), 221–222
warning signs, 222, 223*t*
systemic complications
acquired methemoglobinemia, 208, 208*n*
adverse drug interactions with vasoconstrictors, 210–211, 210*t*, 211*t*
allergic reactions, 208–209, 209*t*
local anesthetic systemic toxicity, 207, 208*f*, 208*t*
psychogenic reactions, 207, 207*f*
vasoconstrictor additives, 209–210

T
tachydysrhythmias
atrial fibrillation, 38, 39*f*
ectopic beats, 38, 39*f*
paroxysmal supraventricular tachycardia (PSVT), 38–39, 40*f*
pre-excitation syndromes, 39–40
supraventricular tachydysrhythmias, 38, 39*f*
TBW. *See* total body water (TBW)
thought disorders
adversemetabolic effects, 75
anticholinergic effects, 74
anticholinergic syndrome signs, 75*t*
anti-histaminic effects, 75
antipsychotic medication, 74
α1-blockade, 75
neuroleptics, 74
non-specific D2 blockade, 75
potency, 74
psychosis, 73
QT prolongation, 75*t*
schizophrenia, 73, 74*t*
thrombocytopenia, 86, 87, 103, 107, 115
thrombophlebitis, 272, 272*f*
thyroid disorders, 64–65
TIA. *See* transient ischemic attack (TIA)
tissue plasminogen activator, 258
TIVA. *See* total intravenous anesthesia (TIVA)
total body water (TBW), 185
total intravenous anesthesia (TIVA), 284
trachea and main stem bronchi, 239, 240*f*
transient ischemic attack (TIA), 258
triazolam
dosage, 133
long-acting metabolites, 133
oral administration, 133
plasma concentrations, 134, 134*f*

triazolam (*continued*)
  sublingual incremental dose, 133–134
tricyclic antidepressants (TCAs), 157, 210, 211*t*
triple airway maneuver, 233*f*, 234
type I immediate-onset hypersensitivity reactions, 209, 209*t*

U
unprofessional conduct, licensing agency, 308
upper airway risk assessment, 12–13
  cricothyroid location, 13, 13*f*
  Mallampatti classification, 13
  mask ventilation, 12
  past medical history, 12
  preanesthetic/sedation evaluation, 12
  rapid assessment, 12*f*, 13
  vocal cords visualization, 12*f*, 13
upper respiratory tract infection, 56

V
valvular heart disease
  aortic regurgitation, 34
  aortic stenosis, 33–34
  mitral regurgitation, 34
  mitral stenosis, 34
  mitral valve prolapse (MVP), 34
  prosthetic heart valves, 35
vascular injury
  immediate periorbial hematoma, 213, 214*f*
  infratemporal hematoma, 213, 213*f*
vasoconstrictors, 119
  additives, 209–210
  local anesthetic pharmacology, 129
vasopressors
  ephedrine, 193
  epinephrine, 192–193
  phenylephrine, 193–194
  vasopressin, 193
vasovagal (neurocardiogenic) syncope, 221–222
VC. *See* vomiting center (VC)
ventilation, 49, 164*t*, 233, 246
ventilation–perfusion mismatching, 66
ventricular tachydysrhythmias, 40–41
violation of statute/code, 307–308
volatile anesthetics, 144, 144*t*
vomiting center (VC), 277
von Willebrand factor (vWBF)
  antifibrinolytic agents, 105
  coagulation factor replacement products, 105, 105*t*
  tranexamic acid, 105
  treatment, 104
  type I and III, 104

W
warfarin, 109, 159
white coat syndrome, 32

Z
zaleplon, 133, 191, 201
zolpidem, 133, 191, 201